Pediatric Imaging for the Emergency Provider

Pediatric Imaging
for the Emergency
Provider

Pediatric Imaging for the Emergency Provider

Robert Vezzetti, MD, FAAP, FACEP
Assistant Professor
Pediatric Emergency Medicine/Pediatrics
Associate Program Director, Pediatric Residency Program
University of Texas Dell Medical School/Dell Children's Medical Center
Austin, TX
USA

Jestin Carlson, MD, MS
Director of Resident Research
Emergency Medicine
Saint Vincent Hospital, Allegheny Health Network
Erie, PA
USA

Debra Pennington, MD, FACR
Affiliate Faculty
Department of Diagnostic Medicine
Dell Medical School at the University of Texas
Austin, TX
Adjunct Assistant Professor
Texas A&M Health Science Center College of Medicine
Round Rock, TX
USA

ELSEVIER

Elsevier
1600 John F. Kennedy Blvd.
Ste 1800
Philadelphia, PA 19103-2899

PEDIATRIC IMAGING FOR THE EMERGENCY PROVIDER

ISBN: 978-0-323-70849-4

Library of Congress Control Number: 2020947886

Senior Content Strategist: Kayla Wolfe
Content Development Manager: Meghan B. Andress
Content Development Specialist: Erika Ninsin
Senior Project Manager: Manchu Mohan
Design: Ryan Cook
Illustrator: Muthukumaran Thangaraj
Marketing Manager: Kathleen Patton

Printed in China

Last digit is the print number: 9 8 7 6 5 4 3 2 1

Dedication

To my wife and children, who have tolerated my home and career shenanigans with love and patience in so many ways and made my life absolutely wonderful; to my patients, who have taught me the many joys of Pediatrics and humbled me with their trust; and to all my colleagues, whom I have had the privilege of working with and learning a great deal from.

Robert Vezzetti

I would like to thank my wife and children for all their support, without which much would not be possible. I would also like to thank every patient that has entrusted me with their care during many of the most challenging events of their lives. These encounters have helped me to continue to grow as a healthcare provider and I continue to be touched by the human spirit during these encounters.

Jestin Carlson

To all I have worked with through a rewarding career in pediatric radiology - from mentors, colleagues, trainees, technologists, imaging personnel, and administration to the precious children and families that we serve. I am humbled and feel blessed to have worked with and learned from all of you. Also, to my husband and our girls, with love and thanks for always being there.

Debra Pennington

List of Contributors

Coburn Allen, MD
Associate Professor
Pediatric Emergency Medicine/Pediatrics/Pediatric
   Infectious Disease
Fellowship Director, Pediatric Emergency Medicine
   Fellowship
University of Texas Dell Medical School/Dell Children's
   Medical Center
Austin, TX
USA

Jestin Carlson, MD, MS
Director of Resident Research
Emergency Medicine
Saint Vincent Hospital, Allegheny Health Network
Erie, PA
USA

Tina Chu, MD
Assistant Professor
Pediatric Emergency Medicine/Pediatrics
University of Texas Dell Medical School/Dell Children's
   Medical Center
Austin, TX
USA

Ada Earp, DO, FAAP
Clinical Assistant Professor
Pediatric Emergency Medicine/Pediatrics
University of Texas Dell Medical School/Dell Children's
   Medical Center
Austin, TX
USA

Michael Gorn, MD
Clinical Assistant Professor
Pediatric Emergency Medicine/Pediatrics
University of Texas Dell Medical School/Dell Children's
   Medical Center
Austin, TX
USA

Greg Hand, MD
Resident Physician
Emergency Medicine
Carl R. Darnall Army Medical Center
Uniformed Services University of the Health Sciences
Bethesda, MD
USA

Guyon Hill, MD
Emergency Medicine Faculty
Carl R. Darnall Army Medical Center
Uniformed Services University of the Health Sciences
Bethesda, MD
Attending Physician
Pediatric Emergency Medicine
University of Texas Dell Medical School/Dell Children's
   Medical Center
Austin, TX
USA

Sujit Iyer, MD
Associate Professor
Pediatric Emergency Medicine/Pediatrics
Associate Fellowship Director
Pediatric Emergency Medicine Fellowship
University of Texas Dell Medical School/Dell Children's
   Medical Center
Austin, TX
USA

Malia J. Moore, MD
Associate Program Director
Simulation Director
Emergency Medicine Faculty
Carl R. Darnall Army Medical Center
Assistant Professor of Military/Emergency Medicine
Uniformed Services University of the Health Sciences
Bethesda, MD
USA

Erin Munns, MD
Fellow Physician
Pediatric Emergency Medicine
University of Texas Dell Medical School/Dell Children's
   Medical Center
Austin, TX
USA

Bhairav Patel, MD
Assistant Professor, Department of Diagnostic Medicine,
   Dell Medical School
Associate Chair of Education, Department of Diagnostic
   Medicine, Dell Medical School
Dell Children's Medical Center
Austin, TX
USA

Debra Pennington, MD, FACR
Affiliate Faculty
Department of Diagnostic Medicine
Dell Medical School at the University of Texas
Austin, TX
Adjunct Assistant Professor
Texas A&M Health Science Center College of Medicine
Round Rock, TX
USA

Tim Ruttan, MD
Clinical Assistant Professor
Pediatric Emergency Medicine
University of Texas Dell Medical School/Dell Children's
    Medical Center
Austin, TX
USA

Anna Schlechter, MD
Fellow Physician
Pediatric Emergency Medicine
University of Texas Dell Medical School/Dell Children's
    Medical Center
Austin, TX
USA

Mary Teeler, BS
Candidate for MD/MPH at Louisiana State University
    Health Science Center
New Orleans, LA
USA

Winnie Whitaker, MD, FAAP
Clinical Assistant Professor
Pediatric Emergency Medicine/Pediatrics
University of Texas at Austin Dell Medical School
Austin, TX
USA

Christopher Michael Wright, MD
Resident Physician, Pediatrics
Pediatric Residency Program
University of Texas Dell Medical School/Dell Children's
    Medical Center
Austin, TX
USA

Robert Vezzetti, MD, FAAP, FACEP
Assistant Professor
Pediatric Emergency Medicine/Pediatrics
Associate Program Director, Pediatric Residency Program
University of Texas Dell Medical School/Dell Children's
    Medical Center
Austin, TX
USA

Preface

The practice of medicine requires the thoughtful gathering and consideration of historical and physical examination findings, allowing the clinician to synthesize an appropriate plan of care that best serves the needs of the patient and their family. The variation of presentation of disease and trauma pathology can make this process complex.

In clinical practice, this process may be simplified and a working diagnosis supported or repudiated through the use of ancillary testing as a complement to this process. However, constraints of time, available institutional resources, patient financial concerns, and the innate clinician desire to arrive at a diagnosis, especially a correct one, all factor into the utilization of available testing modalities a clinician may choose from. Radiographic testing is employed quite frequently in the emergent or urgent setting. There are myriad diagnostic imaging modalities available today. This, along with advances in imaging technology and techniques, can present the clinician with a dilemma: which modality to use?

Additionally, particularly in the pediatric patient, there are concerns about ionizing radiation. While the degree of ionizing radiation exposure can be attenuated by pediatric-specific imaging protocols and improved imaging techniques, it remains a significant concern. An effort should be made to employ appropriate imaging technology that minimizes ionizing radiation exposure by adhering to ALARA (As Low As Reasonably Achievable) guidelines. Difficulty potentially arises when a clinician, tasked with managing multiple patients of differing levels of clinical severity, speaking to families, and working with other medical professionals, is burdened by not always having easy access to these accepted and recommended guidelines in a concise and organized resource.

The purpose of this textbook is to assist the busy clinician with choosing an appropriate radiologic imaging modality when such a test is clinically indicated for the pediatric patient. The format is case-based and designed for easy reference of a variety of commonly-employed imaging modalities that are used for the evaluation, diagnosis, and management of pediatric illness and injury that are encountered in the urgent/emergent setting. While the emphasis is on radiographic investigation, each chapter contains a succinct didactic and management discussion. This text is designed to assist the health care provider who cares for children in a general setting where pediatric subspecialty support may not be readily available, those providers who care for children in settings where such support is plentiful, and every environment in between.

Pediatric patients are not, as the old adage goes, just small adults. This holds true for imaging the pediatric patient. On behalf of my fellow editors and authors, it is our sincere hope this textbook will provide a readily accessible and useful resource for any health care professional who has the privilege of caring for children.

Robert Vezzetti, MD, FAAP, FACEP
Jestin Carlson, MD, MS
Debra Pennington, MD, FACR

Acknowledgement

We would like to thank the many physicians whose time and dedication to excellence in patient care made this work possible. We are in your debt.

Contents

Pediatric Imaging for the Emergency Provider

Pediatric Imaging
for the Emergency
Provider

Introduction

1 Imaging Modalities in the Pediatric Patient: How to Choose

DEBRA PENNINGTON, MD, FACR

To Image or Not to Image?

Quality in health care, as defined by the U.S. Agency for Healthcare Research and Quality, is "doing the right thing for the right patient, at the right time, in the right way to achieve the best possible results."[1] When a pediatric patient presents in the emergency setting, the decision of which, if any, imaging test should be performed can be challenging. Factors to consider include patient factors, such as age, developmental stage, and coexisting illness, and facility factors, including available expertise in pediatric imaging, clinical support such as pediatric surgical services, and whether sedation capabilities are available if needed. One must consider whether the imaging test answers the clinical question, as well as myriad other questions: Can the child cooperate for the study? Can intravenous (IV) access be obtained if necessary? Is a test necessary or can the diagnosis be made clinically, either at presentation or after an observation period? Can testing be delayed until other resources are available (e.g., the only pediatric sonographer arrives at 7:00 a.m.)? Do the benefits of the test results outweigh potential risks? One must consider whether an imaging strategy follows the "ALARA" principle: keeping patient exposure to ionizing radiation "as low as reasonably achievable" (see Chapter 2) while ensuring diagnostic quality of the imaging. If considering a test involving ionizing radiation, is there an alternative mode of making the diagnosis with less risk (e.g., rapid magnetic resonance imaging [MRI] for hydrocephalus in a patient with a ventricular shunt)? There may be a role for shared decision making, educating the patient or the parent/guardian, and involving them in the decision. The clinician should also consider whether the patient is best served by imaging at the current facility or whether the patient should be transferred to a more specialized facility for diagnosis and management.

Transition to Evidence-Based Medicine

Traditionally, medical decision making has been based on an individual practitioner's experience and what the practitioner had learned from what has been termed "eminence-based medicine"; however, more recently, there has been a transition to evidence-based medicine, with a major goal of improving outcomes for patients.[2] "Eminence-based medicine" has been described as reliance on learning from experts, especially those encountered through medical training, national publications, and meetings, and this approach relies on years of practice experience. In evidence-based medicine, it is assumed that a single practitioner does not arrive at an unbiased assessment through experience alone. In this paradigm, assessment of appropriate medical care should be based upon evidence-based research. The practitioner does not just accept information from the expert but assimilates and critically assesses the research evidence in literature to guide a clinical decision. In this process, one formulates a clinical question, identifies pertinent medical literature, judges the quality of studies, produces a summary of evidence, and applies evidence to arrive at appropriate clinical action. For an individual clinician, with the volume of medical literature and the pace of imaging innovation, this task can become overwhelming, especially for one practicing in an emergency center environment, caring for patients with a wide variety of illnesses and injuries. A need for evidence-based imaging guidelines and support has developed.

EVIDENCE-BASED IMAGING FOR THE EMERGENCY PATIENT

With increased availability and complexity of imaging technologies, the use of medical imaging can significantly increase without resulting in clinical gains and benefits for patients. A goal for evidence-based imaging is to ensure that patients receive quality care and the benefits of imaging, while minimizing risk. In 2015, the Society for Academic Emergency Medicine convened a multidisciplinary conference "Diagnostic Imaging in the Emergency Department: A Research Agenda to Optimize Utilization."[3,4] Citing the increased use of diagnostic imaging in the emergency setting, the goals of this conference were to establish a priority research agenda for emergency diagnostic imaging, in order to guide the design of future investigations, and to develop evidence-based knowledge to improve quality, safety, and outcomes for patients. One of the priority topics was clinical decision rules (CDRs). CDRs are evidence-based algorithms derived from research and used to provide guidance for clinical decision making. CDRs can potentially reduce the use of diagnostic tests, reduce inappropriate variation in practice, and empower the clinician with risk assessments for a given set of clinical symptoms and signs.

CLINICAL DECISION SUPPORT (CDS)

CDRs are a form of CDS (CDS, or CDSM for clinical decision support mechanism). Appropriate use criteria (AUC, or AC for appropriateness criteria®), such as those established by the American College of Radiology (ACR), are also a component of CDS. CDS, including AUC, such as the Pediatric Emergency Care Applied Research Network (PECARN) head injury rule and the Canadian Assessment of Tomography for Childhood Head Injury (CATCH) rule,[5] enables provider education and provides evidence-based guidance for imaging.

A widely utilized CDR, the PECARN head injury rule, was developed using a large, multicenter prospective cohort to identify children at very low risk of clinically important traumatic brain injury (TBI) who could safely avoid computed tomography (CT). TBI prediction rules assist with decision making by identifying patients at either low risk for TBI, for whom CT scans may be safely avoided, or at high risk for TBI, for whom CT scans may be indicated.[5] PECARN head injury prediction rules have been externally validated, shown to be reliable in clinical practice, with both excellent sensitivity and negative predictive value for clinically important TBI.[3,6] Prediction rules are best applied together with clinical judgment, based on factors including practice setting and clinician experience.[5]

With the increased availability and complexity of advanced diagnostic imaging, it is important to realize that increased utilization of an imaging technology can decrease diagnostic yield and create harm due to unnecessary imaging. CDS can provide evidence-based guidance to diminish this effect. In a recent study, providers were given a choice of whether to use a CDS tool in the decision to order a CT scan for pulmonary embolus (PE). The percentage of positive tests for PE increased (38% higher diagnostic yield) when providers chose to use CDS, as compared to when providers chose not to use the CDS tool.[7]

CDSMs can be integrated into clinical pathways and electronic health information systems, to be readily available to the clinician at the time of order entry. The ACR AC are a helpful resource for imaging evaluation guidance and are available, along with other evidence-based AUC guidelines, in the CareSelect Imaging product (National Decision Support Company, Madison, Wisconsin). The ACR AC are also available for free online at https://www.acr.org/Clinical-Resources/ACR-Appropriateness-Criteria®. In the United States, CDS vendors are required to provide a free online version of their product.

Although CDS tools are of value, individual practitioner experience and judgment remain important,[5] as does the value of the radiologist consultation. As part of a study about how software-based CDSMs may integrate with current imaging CDS, pediatric emergency department physicians were interviewed. The emergency physicians emphasized that although they were optimistic that the newly provided CDSM may improve workflow, they stated that CDSMs are not a "fix-all": radiologist consultation remained a valuable component of imaging CDS, and they sought out guidance through discussion with the radiologist, especially when a clinical scenario did not fit well within existing clinical pathways. The clinicians asserted that consultation with a radiologist allows discussion of the nuances of a clinical situation, allowing helpful discussion of the risks and benefits, potential harm, or patient factors.[8]

ACR Appropriateness Criteria®

CDS tools have been effectively integrated in the management of pediatric head trauma, and the ACR AC for head injury in children[9] depend upon the clinical PECARN head injury rule. The ACR AC for mild blunt head injury in a child with intermediate risk for clinically important brain injury by PECARN criteria (Table 1.1) indicate that a head CT without IV contrast may be appropriate for initial imaging, but the other listed imaging tests are usually not appropriate. The relative radiation doses of the imaging tests are also given in a graphic manner in this ratings table.

To use the online ACR AC for CDS, from the main page (Box 1.1), choose "Browse Topic" (or create a Login and

Table 1.1　ACR Appropriateness Criteria® Head Trauma-Child. Variant 2: Child. Minor Acute Blunt Head Trauma. Intermediate Risk for Clinically Important Brain Injury per PECARN Criteria. Excluding Suspected Abusive Head Trauma. Initial Imaging

Procedure	Appropriate Category	Relative Radiation Level
CT head without IV contrast	May be appropriate	☢☢☢
Arteriography cerebral	Usually not appropriate	☢☢☢☢
CT head with IV contrast	Usually not appropriate	☢☢☢
CT head without and with IV contrast	Usually not appropriate	☢☢☢☢
CTA head with IV contrast	Usually not appropriate	☢☢☢☢
MRA head without and with IV contrast	Usually not appropriate	○
MRA head without IV contrast	Usually not appropriate	○
MRI head without and with IV contrast	Usually not appropriate	○
MRI head without IV contrast	Usually not appropriate	○
Radiography skull	Usually not appropriate	☢

CT, Computed tomography; *IV,* intravenous; *MRA,* magnetic resonance angiography; *MRI,* magnetic resonance imaging; *PECARN,* Pediatric Emergency Care Applied Research Network.
From https://acsearch.acr.org/docs/3083021/Narrative/. ACR Appropriateness Criteria® content is updated regularly and users should go to the website (https://www.acr.org/Clinical-Resources/ACR-Appropriateness-Criteria®) to access the most current and complete version of the AC.

choose "Search Topics"). After choosing "Browse Topic," choose "Pediatric" (Box 1.2), select "Search" and scroll to "Head Trauma–Child." Choosing the "Narrative and Rating Table" will open a document containing the multiple clinical variants, showing the imaging rating chart for each variant, as seen in Table 1.1. This document also includes a background narrative about that specific AC, including a summary of the literature review, imaging considerations by modality, a discussion of each imaging modality by clinical variant, a summary of recommendations, and a reference list. Other documents that can be chosen include an Evidence Table (summarizes the literature, rates the quality of studies, gives study results) and a Literature Search (shows what searches were performed, including dates, search strategies, and a summary of the literature

review), and many AC include a link to a brief patient-friendly summary of the AC.

Summary

The increasing availability and complexity of imaging technologies can make it difficult for the busy emergency physician to formulate an imaging strategy for every possible presenting clinical scenario, especially in the pediatric patient, for whom it is very important to use an imaging strategy that maximizes clinical benefit while minimizing risk. Evidence-based imaging guidelines, in the form of CDRs, AUC, and clinical pathways, are forms of CDS that serve to guide clinical decision making. Such decision

---

Box 1.1   American College of Radiology Appropriateness Criteria® (ACR AC) Main Page

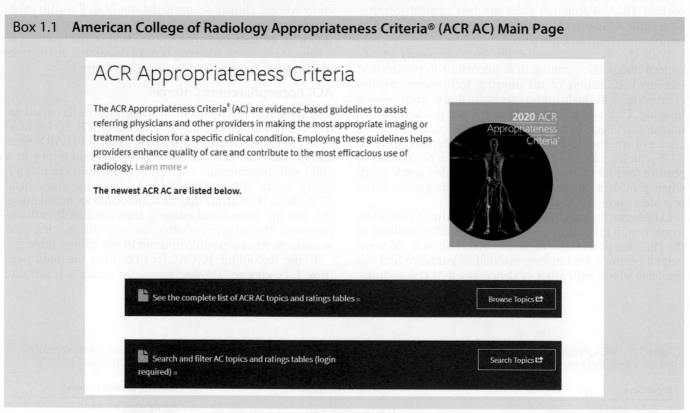

From https://www.acr.org/Clinical-Resources/ACR-Appropriateness-Criteria®.

Box 1.2   American College of Radiology Appropriateness Criteria® (ACR AC) Browse Topic: Pediatric

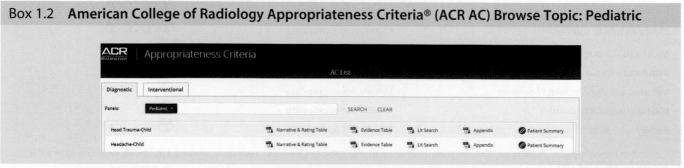

From https://acsearch.acr.org/list.

support can improve the diagnostic yield of imaging, decrease the use of diagnostic tests, and reduce inappropriate variation in practice. CDS mechanisms may be embedded in electronic health information systems and are also available online. One of these is the ACR AC. CDS is best used in conjunction with practitioner clinical judgment and should not replace consultation with a radiologist when necessary.

References

1. Agency for Healthcare Research and Quality Archive. *Understanding Health Care Quality.* 2016. Available at: https://archive.ahrq.gov/consumer/guidetoq/guidetoq4.htm. Accessed August 8, 2020.
2. Medina LS, Blackmore CC. Principles of evidence-based imaging. In: Medina LS, Blackmore CC, eds. *Evidence-Based Imaging: Optimizing Imaging in Patient Care.* New York, NY: Springer; 2006:1-18.
3. Mills AM, Raja AS, Marin JR. Optimizing diagnostic imaging in the emergency department. *Acad Emerg Med.* 2015;22(5):625-631.
4. Marin JR, Mills AM. Developing a research agenda to optimize diagnostic imaging in the emergency department: an executive summary of the 2015 Academic Emergency Medicine Consensus Conference. *Acad Emerg Med.* 2015;22(12):1363-1371.
5. Nigrovic LE, Kuppermann N. Children with minor blunt head trauma presenting to the emergency department. *Pediatrics.* 2019;144(6): e20191495.
6. Schonfeld D, Bressan S, Da Dalt L, et al. Pediatric Emergency Care Applied Research Network head injury clinical prediction rules are reliable in practice. *Arch Dis Child.* 2014;99(5):427-431.
7. Richardson S, Cohen S, Khan S, et al. Higher imaging yield when clinical decision support is used. *J Am Coll Radiol.* 2020;17(4):496-503.
8. Hogan J, Frasso R, Hailu T, et al. Optimizing imaging clinical decision support: perspectives of pediatric emergency department physicians. *J Am Coll Radiol.* 2020;17(2):262-267.
9. Ryan ME, Pruthi S, Desai NK, et al. ACR Appropriateness Criteria® head trauma—child. *J Am Coll Radiol.* 2020;17(5S):S125-S137.

2 · ALARA Principles

DEBRA PENNINGTON, MD, FACR

Exposure to Ionizing Radiation

Exposure to ionizing radiation is a natural consequence of living on Earth. We are exposed to ionizing radiation from the Earth beneath our feet, from the air we breathe, from materials within our own bodies, and from space. Background radiation from natural sources varies by location and is generally greater at higher elevations. For a person in the United States, the estimated average background radiation exposure from natural and manmade sources is approximately 3 mSv/year.[1]

In 1982, natural background radiation contributed most of the public's exposure to ionizing radiation, and the average annual diagnostic medical exposure per person in the United States was estimated to be 0.54 mSv. By 2006, the contribution of radiation exposure from diagnostic medical procedures in the United States had increased by almost six times, to approximately 3 mSv per person per year. This increased medical radiation exposure was largely due to computed tomography (CT) and nuclear medicine procedures. Although CT procedures represented only 15% of diagnostic procedures, CT contributed over half of the cumulative diagnostic procedure dose.[2] At one hospital, although CT accounted for only 15% of the diagnostic radiology procedures, CT contributed approximately 75% of the total effective dose.[3]

Risks of Ionizing Radiation Exposure and ALARA

The primary concern for exposure of patients to ionizing radiation is the risk of cancer induction. Children are considered to be at greater relative risk from radiation exposure than adults are. Children are smaller and incur a greater effective dose per body mass unit than do adults for a given exposure. As children are growing, they have a greater proportion of dividing cells and are considered more sensitive to radiation-induced carcinogenesis.[1] Children also have more life years ahead of them, giving them a longer time to develop the late effects of radiation exposure or to be further exposed to ionizing radiation.[1] There is debate among experts over the risk of cancer induction from medical imaging,[4] but there is agreement that we should act cautiously, assuming risk. Although there are no absolute defined limits for patient radiation exposure, the goal is that radiation exposure from diagnostic imaging should be kept "as low as reasonably achievable" (ALARA).[5]

ALARA: Justification and Optimization

To achieve ALARA goals, a test involving ionizing radiation should be performed only when medically justified and the radiation exposure from a medical test should be kept as low as possible to still achieve a diagnostic result.[6] Justification is the process of ensuring that the examination to be performed is appropriate, with potential benefit to the patient that is greater than the risk presented by the examination. To assist in justification, clinical decision support tools are helpful, including summary recommendations, clinical decision rules, and appropriateness criteria. As part of justification, one considers whether a test is necessary or whether use of an alternative test without exposure to ionizing radiation, such as ultrasound or magnetic resonance imaging, may be diagnostic.

Once an examination is justified, imaging technique is optimized to ensure adherence to ALARA principles. As part of optimization, it is important to tailor technique to patient size while ensuring that the examination is still of diagnostic quality. This applies to all modalities using ionizing radiation. As CT contributes a significant portion of the diagnostic medical radiation dose to individuals and populations, it is important to decrease radiation dose due to CT. There are many mechanisms that can decrease radiation dose due to CT, the first of which is to do only indicated (justified) examinations.

Optimization of CT scanning to decrease dose also includes centering the patient in the CT scanner, using CT automatic exposure control systems, limiting scan length to the area of interest and eliminating multiphase examinations (which are rarely necessary in the pediatric population). More recent CT scanners also use iterative reconstruction technology, in which the computer makes "several passes" through the data, improving signal-to-noise ratio, and improving the quality of images from lower dose scanning.

Most CT equipment manufacturers now provide pediatric-specific technique guidelines or protocols, but pediatric CT protocols are also readily available, such as those provided by the American Association of Physicists in Medicine.[7]

American College of Radiology Dose Index Registry®

For a facility, benchmarking CT dose performance against that of other facilities provides valuable information to guide CT protocol optimization. The American College of Radiology Dose Index Registry (DIR®) was established in 2011 and serves as a tool for quality improvement. Through the DIR, facilities can review dose indices and optimize their CT imaging protocols. Facilities download the DIR program software, which allows them to upload scanning data automatically. This allows the collection of dose index information across facilities but does not collect individual patient doses or identifiable patient data. The facilities receive quarterly feedback through the DIR, which gives them the opportunity to compare their CT practice and dose metrics to those of other facilities, regionally and nationally. In addition, facilities can get online feedback from the DIR at any time.[8]

Image Gently

The Image Gently Alliance is a coalition of health care organizations dedicated to providing safe, high-quality pediatric imaging worldwide, with the primary objective to raise awareness of the need to adjust radiation dose when imaging children. The Image Gently website (www.imagegently. org) can be used as a resource for parents, radiologists, and referring physicians to learn more about imaging studies and radiation exposure in children.[9]

Application of ALARA

Applying ALARA principles can result in a very real change in practice. In a study of application of ALARA guidelines over a period of 6 months, two pediatric radiologists reviewed CT requests for adherence to "justification" and "optimization." Out of 1392 individual anatomic part CT requests, 111 CT requests from 105 pediatric patients were avoided. Thus, 8% of patients were protected from unnecessary radiation exposure by applying ALARA principles.[10]

In the United States, a long-term positive effect of the application of ALARA principles has been demonstrated. The prior upward trend of increasing dose from medical radiation seen from 1980 to 2006 has declined, with the estimated per capita dose in the United States in 2016 lower than in 2006, decreasing from 2.9 mSv in 2006 to 2.3 mSv in 2016.[11]

Summary

Although there is controversy over the degree of risk from exposure to ionizing radiation from medical imaging in children, there is agreement that we should act cautiously, with the goal that radiation exposure from diagnostic imaging should be kept "as low as reasonably achievable" (ALARA). Justification is the process of ensuring that the diagnostic examination to be performed is appropriate, with potential benefit of the examination greater than potential risk. Once an examination is justified, optimization of examination technique is then utilized to ensure adherence to ALARA principles.

References

1. Brody AS, Frush DP, Huda W, et al. Radiation risk to children from computed tomography. *Pediatrics*. 2007;120(3):677-682.
2. Mettler FA, Thomadsen BR, Bhargavan M, et al. Medical radiation exposure in the U.S. in 2006: preliminary results. *Health Phys*. 2008;95(5):502-507.
3. Wiest PW, Locken JA, Heintz PH, et al. CT scanning: a major source of radiation exposure. *Semin Ultrasound CT MR*. 2002;23(5):402-410.
4. Cohen MD. ALARA, Image gently and CT-induced cancer. *Pediatr Radiol*. 2015;45:465-470.
5. Tomà P, Bartoloni A, Salerno S, et al. Protecting sensitive patient groups from imaging using ionizing radiation: effects during pregnancy, in fetal life and childhood. *Radiol Med*. 2019;124(8):736-744.
6. U.S. Food and Drug Administration. *White Paper*: Initiative to Reduce Unnecessary Radiation Exposure from Medical Imaging. June 14, 2019. Accessed August 17, 2020. Available at: https://www.fda.gov/radiation-emitting-products/initiative-reduce-unnecessary-radiation-exposure-medical-imaging/white-paper-initiative-reduce-unnecessary-radiation-exposure-medical-imaging.
7. American Association of Physicists in Medicine. *Pediatric Routine Abdomen and Pelvis CT Protocol*. July 21, 2017. Available at: https://www.aapm.org/pubs/CTProtocols/documents/PediatricRoutineAbdomenPelvisCT.pdf. Accessed August 17, 2020.
8. American College of Radiology website. *Dose Index Registry*. https://nrdrsupport.acr.org/support/solutions/articles/11000028993?_ga=2.238274056.944128003.1604275453-860268161.1563219551. Published August 20, 2018. Accessed August 17, 2020.
9. Image gently. *The Image Gently Alliance*. Available at: https://www.imagegently.org. Published January 22, 2008. Updated 2020. Accessed August 17, 2020.
10. Sodhi KS, Krishna S, Saxena AK, et al. Clinical application of 'Justification' and 'Optimization' principle of ALARA in pediatric CT imaging: "How many children can be protected from unnecessary radiation?" *Eur J Radiol*. 2015;84(9):1752-1757.
11. Mettler FA, Mahesh M, Bhargavan-Chatfield M, et al. Patient exposure from radiologic and nuclear medicine procedures in the United States: procedure volume and effective dose for the period 2006–2016. *Radiology*. 2020;295(2):418-427.

3 Sedation/Anxiolysis for Pediatric Imaging

ROBERT VEZZETTI, MD, FAAP, FACEP

Most pediatric imaging procedures do not require sedation. There are patients, though, who will require some level of sedation in order to obtain a meaningful imaging study. The reasons for sedation are many but include anxiety, painful condition (such as fracture), age of the child (younger children tend to be less cooperative), or study length. Lengthy studies (e.g., extensive magnetic resonance imaging of the brain or spine), studies with painful procedures, children with complex medical conditions in which sedation may be problematic (such as those with cardiac or pulmonary issues), children with tenuous airways or impending airway compromise, or children with medical conditions that the clinician is not familiar or comfortable with should prompt consultation with a pediatric anesthesiologist (or an anesthesiologist who is comfortable and qualified to treat children, including those with complex medical conditions). If such consultation is not available, then consideration should be given to transferring the child to the nearest pediatric facility for the study and further care.

An excellent adjunctive resource to encourage patient cooperation, improve patient comfort, and complete a required imaging study is a child life specialist. Child life specialists use distraction and coping techniques at an age-appropriate level and have been shown to be beneficial in relieving anxiety and increasing cooperation in pediatric patients and to increase family satisfaction with care.[1-3]

The Guidelines for Monitoring and Management of Pediatric Patients Before, During, and After Sedation for Diagnostic and Therapeutic Procedures state that the goals of sedation are as follows[4]:

1. To guard the patient's safety and welfare.
2. To minimize physical discomfort and pain.
3. To control anxiety, minimize psychological trauma, and maximize the potential for amnesia.
4. To modify behavior and/or movement so as to allow the safe completion of the procedure.
5. To return the patient to a state in which discharge from medical/dental supervision is safe, as determined by recognized criteria.

Training and credentialing for pediatric sedation should be held by all personnel involved in the sedation procedure. Appropriate equipment for pediatric patients should be available, keeping in mind that requirements vary from child to child, with age, weight, and underlying medical conditions and usage during the sedation process being given consideration. The American Academy of Pediatrics (AAP), the American Academy of Dentistry, the American College of Emergency Medicine, and the Society of Anesthesiologists have all issued guidelines and recommendations addressing best practices for pediatric sedation outside of the operating room by nonanesthesiologists.[4-7] Continuous monitoring before, during, and after the sedation is indicated; monitoring during sedation should, preferably, be performed by personnel not directly involved in the sedation itself.[4-7] Studies have noted that despite improvement in pediatric sedation practices, there is a persistent rate (although low) of life-threatening events, including apnea, airway obstruction, and laryngospasm.[8]

Patient safety should always be a priority before, during, and after the sedation process. Sedation outside of the operating theater in an emergency department setting is safe and practical, but there are associated risks. Children younger than 6 years of age are particularly at high risk for sedation-related adverse events due to effects on respiratory drive and protective airway reflexes.[4,8] Clinicians should have the clinical skills necessary to rescue patients from an unintended deeper level of sedation, which can occur in the course of the sedation process.[9-11] A study looking at sedation and general anesthesia for pediatric patients undergoing computed tomography or magnetic resonance imaging found the rate of hypoxemia to be 2.9% and that respiratory events were more likely to occur in children with an American Society of Anesthesiologists (ASA) class of III or IV.[12] Prompt recognition of an event and intervention occurred, and no children had sequelae as a result of their respiratory event, highlighting the importance of proper training of sedation personnel and the availability of appropriate equipment. Interestingly, this study also highlighted the problem of inadequate sedation in their study population. The quality of the scans obtained was deemed not optimal in nearly one-third (29%) of patients, the time of sedation to the initiation of the scanning procedure was significantly longer, and some imaging procedures had to be rescheduled, contributing to increased cost and inconvenience to the patients' families due to inadequate patient sedation.[12] The authors proposed the identification of children who are at risk for sedation failure prior to the initiation of sedation and, in these cases, considering general anesthesia for their imaging procedure.[12]

Risk factors for inadequate sedation or failure of sedation include older children, children with higher ASA class, and use of a single agent (benzodiazepines), highlighting that some populations may require general anesthesia.[12] General anesthesia should also be considered in patients with more complex medical conditions (such as congenital heart disease) and in those where the provider is concerned that the patient may be more likely to experience complications from sedation or have inadequate sedation.[12]

Several factors are associated with adverse events and complications from sedation, including inconsistent physiologic monitoring, inadequate presedation evaluation, lack of an independent sedation observer, medication errors, and inadequate recovery procedures.[10] All personnel involved in sedation should have skills in pediatric resuscitation and airway management, specialty-dependent guidelines should be adopted for sedation procedures, and appropriate medications and age-specific equipment should be readily available.[10]

The guidelines promulgated by the AAP and the American College of Emergency Medicine provide general recommendations to help ensure patient safety[4–6]:

1. Appropriate patient selection
2. A responsible guardian (preferably two adults) to accompany the child
3. Appropriate sedation facility, including personnel and equipment to rescue the decompensating child
4. Back-up emergency services, if the sedation is taking place outside of the hospital setting
5. Personnel, medications, and equipment available onsite that is immediately accessible
6. Appropriate documentation, including informed consent outlining the indications, benefits, risks, and alternative options of the sedation procedure
7. Documentation before, during, and after sedation. Weight should be recorded in kilograms and any known drug allergies should be noted.

Proper patient selection for sedation is an important step in ensuring safety and a successful sedation experience. While there is no screening test that has the ability to predict sedation complications, there are resources available to the clinician to help guide the sedation process. The ASA classification can be useful to help select which patients are candidates for sedation.

American Society of Anesthesiologists Classification System:[13]

Class I	A normally healthy patient
Class II	A patient with mild systemic disease (e.g., controlled reactive airway disease)
Class III	A patient with severe systemic disease (e.g., a child who is actively wheezing)
Class IV	A patient with severe systemic disease that is a constant threat to life (e.g., a child with status asthmaticus)
Class V	A moribund patient who is not expected to survive without the operation (e.g., a patient with severe cardiomyopathy requiring heart transplantation)

This classification system is not intended to predict risk per se, but increasing ASA classification has been associated with increased perioperative mortality.[14,15] In the pediatric emergency department setting, an ASA classification of II or higher was associated with a higher incidence of hypoxia.[16] Children who have an ASA classification of III or greater, an anatomy that could potentially complicate sedation (such as Pierre Robin sequence, Prader Willi syndrome, or other craniofacial developmental abnormalities), or any other anatomical or developmental issues should have anesthesiology or subspecialty consultation before sedation.[4,12,17]

It is important that the clinician has a validated, clinically useful method for assessing the quality and depth of sedation for patients undergoing sedation. The AAP, American College of Radiology, and the ASA have adopted four levels of procedural sedation.[4–7,18–20] The Pediatric Sedation State Scale is a widely used measure of the effectiveness and quality of sedation.[21] Parameters such as control of pain, anxiety, movement, and adverse effects were taken into account in the development of this proposed scale. Another useful scale that is simple to apply clinically and has been validated in pediatric patients is the University of Michigan Sedation Scale.[22,23] Other sedation scales used to assess the depth of sedation include the Observer's Assessment of Alertness/Sedation scale, which has been validated in children but has limited ability to differentiate between deeper levels of sedation.[22,24] The Vancouver Sedative Recovery Scale is able to differentiate deeper levels of sedation but is one of the more complex scales available, potentially making clinical application difficult.[22,25]

AAP, ACR, and ASA Levels of Sedation:

SEDATION LEVEL	PATIENT RESPONSE
Minimal	Normal response to verbal commands
Moderate	Purposeful response to verbal commands or light touch
Deep	Difficult to arouse; purposeful response to painful or repeated stimulation
General anesthesia	No response

AAP, American Academy of Pediatrics; *ACR*, American College of Radiology; *ASA*, American Society of Anesthesiologists.

University of Michigan Sedation Scale:

VALUE	PATIENT STATE
0	Awake and alert
1	Minimally sedated: tired/sleepy; appropriate response to verbal conversation and/or sound
2	Moderately sedated: somnolent/sleeping; easily aroused with light tactile stimulation or a simple verbal command
3	Deeply sedated: deep sleep; aroused only with significant physical stimulation
4	Unarousable

Pediatric Sedation Scale (Cravero et al.):[21]

STATE	BEHAVIOR
5	Patient is moving (purposefully or nonpurposefully) in a manner that impedes the proceduralist and requires forceful immobilization. This includes crying or shouting during the procedure, but vocalization is not required. Score is based on movement.
4	Moving during the procedure (awake or sedated) that requires gentle immobilization for positioning. May verbalize some discomfort or stress, but there is no crying or shouting that expresses stress or objection.

STATE	BEHAVIOR
3	Expression of pain or anxiety on face (may verbalize discomfort), but not moving or impeding completion of the procedure. May require help positioning (as with a lumbar puncture) but does not require restraint to stop movement during the procedure.
2	Quiet (asleep or awake), not moving during procedure, and no frown (or brow furrow) indicating pain or anxiety. No verbalization of any complaint.
1	Deeply asleep with normal vital signs, but requiring airway intervention and/or assistance (e.g., central or obstructive apnea, etc.).
0	Sedation associated with abnormal physiologic parameters that require acute intervention (i.e., oxygen saturation <90%, blood pressure 30% lower than baseline, bradycardia receiving therapy)

Much debate has been made on the necessity of nil per os (NPO) status and the ability to engage in sedation. There are NPO guidelines that are used to determine when it is considered safe to administer various levels of sedation and anesthesia in patients undergoing elective procedures.[26,27] The concern is whether the risk for aspiration or other adverse event is increased when administering sedation for radiologic or other procedures when a patient has not been NPO for a given length of time. There has been differing guidance among professional societies addressing NPO status and sedation in a setting that is considered more urgent or emergent.[26,27] A very large study of nearly 140,000 children, conducted by the Pediatric Sedation Research Consortium, examined the relationship of NPO status and aspiration events (defined as an episode of emesis accompanied by a change in respiratory status of the patient or a new radiographic finding).[28] NPO status was known for 107,947 patients, where 25,401 (23.5%) were non—NPO patients. NPO status was defined as no solid food intake for 8 hours, no nonclear fluid intake for at least 6 hours, and no intake of clear liquids for at least 2 hours.[28] Aspiration occurred in 8 of 82,546 NPO patients compared to 2 of 25,401 non—NPO patients. Major complications occurred in 46 of 82,546 NPO patients compared to 15 of 25,401 non—NPO patients.[28] In summary, aspiration was uncommon (<1 event per 10,000 patients) and NPO status for liquids and solids was not an independent predictor of major complications or aspiration. While debate continues regarding sedation and NPO status in the pediatric population and the incidence of aspiration or adverse effects is low, the clinician should consider the indications, urgency, risks, and benefits of sedation for imaging studies.

If the decision is made to utilize sedation in the emergency department or urgent care setting, there are a variety of agents available. Clinicians should be familiar with the indications, benefits, risks, side effects, and pharmacokinetics of whatever agent (or agents) they choose to utilize for sedation and/or anxiolysis. When considering agents, the lowest dose needed with the highest therapeutic index to accomplish imaging should be selected.[4–6] Long-acting agents are rarely indicated for imaging studies and should generally be avoided. If an imaging study is particularly lengthy, such as magnetic resonance imaging of the brain and complete spine, then anesthesiology should be consulted. Options include analgesic agents, sedative-hypnotic (anxiolytic) agents, and agents in their own categories, such as ketamine, propofol, and nitrous oxide.

Once sedation is completed, patients should be monitored (heart rate, respiratory rate, pulse oximetry, and blood pressure) for return to baseline status. Once patients have returned to their baseline mental and ambulatory status, they may be discharged.[29] Discharge instruction appropriate to the agent and level of sedation used should also be provided to the patient's caregiver.

Analgesic Agents

These agents are not commonly used for imaging sedation, but adequate pain control is important to maximize the chances of obtaining a meaningful imaging study. Pain control with appropriate agents is important for fracture imaging. An excellent example of this is imaging supracondylar fractures; a true lateral image is desired to assess the type/degree of the injury (for example, type I, II, or III fractures), which is important for planning appropriate treatment.

MORPHINE

This agent has been found to be as efficacious as fentanyl in the control of pain in pediatric patients.[30] However, like all opioids, morphine can cause respiratory depression and decrease blood pressure through peripheral vasodilation.[31] Morphine is generally not the preferred agent for sedation.[32] This agent should be used cautiously in patients with either airway or cardiovascular compromise. A usual dose is 0.1 mg/kg intravenously.

FENTANYL

Fentanyl is a synthetic opioid with a potency of approximately 100 times that of morphine. This agent has a rapid onset (5 minutes) but a short duration of action (less than 1 hour).[33] Initial intravenous dosing is 1 µg/kg.[34] While these properties make fentanyl a good analgesic option, there are several potential effects associated with its use. These effects are primarily respiratory (hypoxemia, respiratory depression, and apnea), are more likely when fentanyl is combined with another sedative agent, and occur early after administration (5–15 minutes).[34,35]

Chest muscle rigidity (sometimes known colloquially as rigid chest syndrome) is a well-described and feared complication of fentanyl usage but is not common.[36,37] The result of this phenomenon is an inability to ventilate and is a life-threatening complication. While large doses have been associated with this condition (>4 µg/kg), chest wall rigidity has been reported in patients with appropriate intravenous doses, particularly with rapid administration (i.e., a "push" dose).[34,37]

Intranasal fentanyl is being increasingly utilized. This method of delivery is quite advantageous, being effective, easy, painless, and rapid.[38,39] A typical dose is 2 µg/kg, with a maximum of 100 µg per dose, which can be repeated once within 5 minutes if clinically indicated.

Sedative-Hypnotic Agents

ETOMIDATE

Etomidate has a rapid onset of action (less than 30 seconds) and brief duration (usually less than 15 minutes); the usual dose is 0.1–0.3 mg/kg intravenously with 0.05 mg/kg bolus given as clinically indicated.[33,34] This agent has several advantages in addition to its rapid onset, including reducing intracranial pressure and maintaining hemodynamic status.[40] Adverse effects include respiratory depression, vomiting, and nonepileptiform myoclonus.[33,40] Since etomidate inhibits endogenous steroid production, it should not be used in patients with known adrenal insufficiency and should be used with caution in patients with septic shock, since adrenal suppression may be present in patients with this condition. For this reason, etomidate infusions are not recommended.

PROPOFOL

A nonopioid agent that has been used extensively in operative and intensive care settings, propofol has been increasingly used for procedural sedation in emergency departments.[8,41] There are several properties of this agent that make it attractive for sedation use. This agent has a rapid onset of action and recovery (seconds) and lowers intracranial pressure, making its use especially appropriate for neuroimaging of patients with head injury. Propofol may be given as a bolus or as an infusion. A usual starting dose is 100 to 150 µg/kg per minute, with gradual titration of the dose to achieve effect, with a maximum of 200 µg/kg per minute.[33,34,40] If propofol is being used as a bolus, the initial dose is 1 to 2 mg/kg, with additional boluses of 0.5 mg/kg, every 3 to 5 minutes as clinically indicated to maintain sedation.[34,40] However, there are several potentially adverse effects associated with the use of propofol. This agent does not possess analgesic properties, and when analgesia is desired, propofol may be used in combination with other agents that provide analgesia, such as morphine, fentanyl, or ketamine. These combinations may increase the chance for respiratory depression, bradycardia, and hypotension and may also exceed the intended level of sedation.[33,40] One study found that in patients undergoing fracture reduction with propofol and fentanyl, 31% of patients experienced oxygen desaturation and 25% of patients required maneuvers to address respiratory decompensation.[35] Propofol should be used with caution in hypovolemic patients or patients with reduced cardiac function/output; these patients should receive an intravenous fluid bolus prior to being given propofol.[8,33,40] Propofol also causes pain during administration, which may be reduced with the administration of lidocaine (0.5 mg/kg) prior to propofol administration or in combination with another analgesic agent.[33] Adverse effects from propofol use include respiratory depression, apnea, and hypotension (up to 5% of patients)[41,42]; respiratory arrest and cardiac arrest have been reported but are rare.[8,43]

An allergy to eggs has traditionally been a contraindication to propofol use, but studies have shown that propofol has been safely used in patients with a history of egg allergy.[44,45] Propofol infusion syndrome has been described in pediatric patients being cared for in an intensive care setting. This is a constellation of refractory bradycardia in combination with metabolic acidosis, rhabdomyolysis, and hyperlipidemia that progresses to asystole. This syndrome is associated with prolonged propofol infusion or high doses of propofol (>4000 µg/kg/24 hours); it is usually fatal and its exact etiology is unknown.[46,47]

DEXMEDETOMIDINE

This agent is a selective alpha-2-adrenergic receptor agonist. Dexmedetomidine has primarily sedative properties but has some analgesic properties. The main advantage of this agent is excellent sedation with minimal respiratory depression, and dexmedetomidine has been found to be safe in pediatric procedures requiring sedation but not necessarily analgesia.[40] For pediatric patients, doses higher than those used in adult patients are used: 2 to 3 µg/kg intravenous bolus, followed by a 1 to 2 µg/kg/hour infusion.[34,40] Dexmedetomidine has also been found to be effective when given intranasally at doses of 2.5 to 3 µg/kg/dose.[34,48,49] Another advantage of this agent is its use in patients with autism.[40,50] Serious adverse effects, such as laryngospasm, are not common, although 4% of patients receiving this medication had cardiovascular effects (heart rate and blood pressure increases or hypotension); hypertension has been reported in 5% of patients given dexmedetomidine and is associated with younger age, higher doses, and multiple boluses.[50]

MIDAZOLAM

Midazolam is a rapid-acting, short-duration agent that when given intravenously has anxiolytic, amnestic, and muscle relaxant actions. It can be combined with fentanyl to provide moderate sedation; a usual dose is 0.1 mg/kg.[33,34,40] A distinct advantage of midazolam is that there are other routes in which this medication can be given, including oral, sublingual, and intranasal. The preferred method of delivering this medication intranasally is with an atomizer, which produces better absorption and provides better patient comfort when compared to directly instilling the medication. The intranasal dose is higher than the intravenous dose, using 0.2 mg/kg with a maximum of 10 mg per dose.[34,51,52] Adverse effects include respiratory depression and apnea; this risk is increased with coadministration of opioid medications.[33] Paradoxical reactions, such as irritability and aggressive behavior, have been reported.[53] Paradoxical reactions and respiratory depression can be reversed with flumazenil. Flumazenil should be used with caution in patients with a known seizure disorder, as this medication can lower a seizure threshold and precipitate a seizure.

Other Agents

KETAMINE

One of the most commonly used agents for pediatric sedation, this agent produces a dissociative state while at the same time providing both analgesic and sedative effects. Ketamine is a derivative of phencyclidine, more commonly known as PCP, and produces its effects by binding to

N-methyl-d-aspartate (NMDA) receptors. This agent is rapidly acting and has a short duration of action. Ketamine is most often utilized for completion of brief, painful procedures, such as fracture reduction. In addition to excellent and effective sedation and analgesia, ketamine also provides amnesia and immobilization while preserving airway protective reflexes and spontaneous breathing.[33,40] The usual initial intravenous dose of ketamine is 1 to 1.5 mg/kg as a bolus, followed by repeated doses of 0.5 to 1 mg/kg as clinically indicated.[34] Notably, providing initial pain management with an opioid is not a contraindication for procedural sedation with ketamine. Although this does increase the incidence of vomiting and the need for oxygen use, it does not increase the incidence of adverse effects.[54]

Ketamine can be combined with propofol. When ketamine is used in this manner, the dose is reduced to 0.5 mg/kg.[34] A suggested dosing regimen is 0.5 mg/kg of ketamine, followed by 0.5 mg/kg of propofol, with an additional dose of 0.5 mg/kg of propofol given as clinically indicated.[34,55]

Intramuscular (IM) dosing of ketamine is also an option. If ketamine is given through this route, the dose must be increased to achieve effect. A typical IM dose is 4 to 5 mg/kg; if clinically indicated, a second dose of 2 to 4 mg/kg can be given 10 minutes later.[34]

Adverse effects from ketamine typically are vomiting and recovery reactions (irritability, hallucinations, and agitation).[33,40] Although they are the most serious potential complications, laryngospasm and apnea are not commonly seen,[33,40] are usually brief, and can be effectively managed the majority of the time with positive pressure bag-mask ventilation.[34,56] Several large studies have documented adverse effects from ketamine (apnea [<1%], laryngospasm [<1%], and oxygen desaturation [3%]), which are independently associated with young age (<2 years old), intravenous doses greater than an initial dose of 2.5 mg/kg or total dose >5 mg/kg, or coadministration of a benzodiazepine or atropine; vomiting (8%) was associated with older age and high intravenous dosing.[34,57] The IM route of administration is more commonly associated with vomiting and prolonged recovery times.[58] This route does not appear to be associated with increased incidence of laryngospasm, as once thought.[56,59] While ketamine has been shown to cause hypersalivation, routine administration of atropine or glycopyrrolate is not recommended, as the risk of laryngospasm due to hypersalivation is not decreased with these agents in large studies.[60–62] Routine administration of midazolam is also not recommended as a means to mitigate vomiting and/or the emergence reaction sometimes seen with ketamine use.[34,63] Vomiting is the most commonly seen adverse effect from ketamine administration, and some authors recommend routine administration of odansetron for patients undergoing sedation with ketamine.[34,54,64]

Ketamine is contraindicated in patients who are less than 3 months of age or those patients who have had severe emergence reactions in the past.[34] Ketamine is *relatively contraindicated* in patients who have increased intraocular pressure (the evidence for this is debated), increased intracranial pressure (this is a matter of ongoing debate as well), hypertension, and thyroid disease.[34,65]

Intranasal ketamine delivery has recently been investigated and has been found to be effective with few adverse effects, the most common of which was vomiting.[66] As with the intravenous delivery route, routine coadministration of

a benzodiazepine was not supported, as has been reported in previous studies with ketamine in the pediatric population.[66,67] Patients did appear to have a higher incidence of emergence reactions with the intranasal route, but there was no consistent definition of what constituted an emergence reaction.[57,66,68] The perceived satisfaction of the level of sedation with intranasal ketamine for sedation has not been consistent in the literature, and doses have ranged from 2 mg/kg to 9 mg/kg.[68,69] Analgesia has been reported to be satisfactory.[66,70] The superiority of intranasal ketamine versus other agents for sedation has not been proven, however, and studies using intranasal ketamine for fracture reduction are lacking. The lack of rigorous trials on intranasal ketamine use in the pediatric population makes its routine for use for sedation difficult at this time,[66] but there does appear to be promise for use in sedation for brief procedures, such as obtaining an imaging study.

Summary

While sedation or anxiolysis for pediatric radiologic procedures is not always clinically needed, appropriate use of agents for these purposes will allow for patient comfort and minimize motion, resulting in a meaningful radiologic study for management purposes. Clinicians should be familiar with the indications, dosages, and potential adverse effects of whatever agent is chosen, as well as airway rescue techniques should a patient progress to unintended levels of sedation. Properly trained staff familiar with sedation practice and principles will maximize sedation success and minimize complications. The choice of sedation/anxiolytic agent should consider the lowest, most effective dose required to achieve the desired imaging study.

References

1. Sanchez Cristal N, Staab J, Chatham R, et al. Child life reduces distress and pain and improves family satisfaction in the pediatric emergency department. *Clin Pediatr (Phila)*. 2018;57(13):1567-1575.
2. Hall JE, Patel DP, Thomas JW, et al. Certified child life specialists lessen emotional distress of children undergoing laceration repair in the emergency department. *Pediatr Emerg Care*. 2018;34(9):603-606.
3. Tyson ME, Bohl DD, Blickman JG. A randomized controlled trial: child life services in pediatric imaging. *Pediatr Radiol*. 2014;44(11): 1426-1432.
4. Coté CJ, Wilson S, American Academy of Pediatrics; American Academy of Pediatric Dentistry, Work Group on Sedation. Guidelines for monitoring and management of pediatric patients during and after sedation for diagnostic and therapeutic procedures: an update. *Pediatrics*. 2016;138(1):e20161212.
5. Godwin SA, Burton JH, Gerardo CJ, et al; American College of Emergency Physicians. Clinical policy: procedural sedation and analgesia in the emergency department. *Ann Emerg Med*. 2014 Feb;63(2):247-258.
6. American Society of Anesthesiologists Task Force on Sedation and Analgesia by Non-Anesthesiologists. Practice guidelines for sedation and analgesia by non-anesthesiologists. *Anesthesiology*. 2002;96(4):1004-1017.
7. Langhan ML, Mallory M, Hertzog J, et al. Pediatric Sedation Research Consortium. Physiologic monitoring practices during pediatric procedural sedation: a report from the Pediatric Sedation Research Consortium. *Arch Pediatr Adolesc Med*. 2012;166(11):990-998.
8. Cravero JP, Beach ML, Blike GT, et al. Pediatric Sedation Research Consortium. The incidence and nature of adverse events during pediatric sedation/anesthesia with propofol for procedures outside the operating room: a report from the Pediatric Sedation Research Consortium. *Anesth Analg*. 2009;108(3):795-804.

9. Dial S, Silver P, Bock K, Sagy M. Pediatric sedation for procedures titrated to a desired degree of immobility results in unpredictable depth of sedation. *Pediatr Emerg Care*. 2001;17(6):414-420.

10. Coté CJ, Notterman DA, Karl HW, et al. Adverse sedation events in pediatrics: a critical incident analysis of contributing factors. *Pediatrics*. 2000;105(4 Pt 1):805-814.

11. Motas D, McDermott NB, VanSickle T, et al. Depth of consciousness and deep sedation attained in children as administered by nonanes-thesiologists in a children's hospital. *Paediatr Anaesth*. 2004;14(3):256-260.

12. Malviya S, Voepel-Lewis T, Eldevik OP, et al. Sedation and general anaesthesia in children undergoing MRI and CT: adverse events and outcomes. *Br J Anaesth*. 2000;84(6):743-748.

13. American Society of Anesthesiologists. *ASA Physical Status Classification System*. 2011. Available at: http://www.asahq.org/clinical/physicalstatus.htm. Accessed September 22, 2019.

14. Knuf KM, Maani CV, Cummings AK. Clinical agreement in the American Society of Anesthesiologists physical status classification. *Perioper Med (Lond)*. 2018;7:14.

15. Doyle DJ, Garmon EH. *American Society of Anesthesiologists Classification (ASA Class)*. StatPearls [Internet]. Treasure Island, FL: StatPearls Publishing; Jan–May 13, 2019.

16. Caperell K, Pitetti R. Is higher ASA class associated with an increased incidence of adverse events during procedural sedation in a pediatric emergency department? *Pediatr Emerg Care*. 2009;25(10):661-664.

17. Butler MG, Hayes BG, Hathaway MM, et al. Specific genetic diseases at risk for sedation/anesthesia complications. *Anesth Analg*. 2000;91(4):837-855.

18. American Society of Anesthesiologists. *Continuum of depth of sedation; definition of general anesthesia and levels of sedation/analgesia (Approved by ASA House of Delegates on October 13, 1999, and last amended on October 27, 2004)*. Available at: http://www.asahq.org/. Accessed January 16, 2020.

19. Patatas K, Koukkoulli A. The use of sedation in the radiology department. *Clin Radiol*. 2009;64(7):655-663.

20. Macias CG, Chumpitazi CE. Sedation and anesthesia for CT: emerging issues for providing high-quality care. *Pediatr Radiol*. 2011;41(suppl 2):517-522.

21. Cravero JP, Askins N, Sriswasdi P, et al. Validation of the pediatric sedation state scale. *Pediatrics*. 2017;139(5):e20162897.

22. Tobias JD. Sedation of infants and children outside of the operating room. *Curr Opin Anaesthesiol*. 2015;28(4):478-485.

23. Malviya S, Voepel-Lewis T, Tait AR, et al. Depth of sedation in children undergoing computed tomography: validity and reliability of the University of Michigan Sedation Scale (UMSS). *Br J Anaesth*. 2002;88(2):241-245.

24. Chernik DA, Gillings D, Laine H, et al. Validity and reliability of the Observer's Assessment of Alertness/Sedation scale: study with intravenous midazolam. *J Clin Psychopharmacol*. 1990;12(4):244-251.

25. Macnab AJ, Levine M, Glick N, et al. A research tool for measurement of recovery from sedation: the Vancouver Sedative Recovery Scale. *J Pediatr Surg*. 1991;26(11):1263-1267.

26. Green SM, Roback MG, Miner JR, et al. Fasting and emergency department procedural sedation and analgesia: a consensus-based clinical practice advisory. *Ann Emerg Med*. 2007;49(4):454-461.

27. Practice guidelines for preoperative fasting and the use of pharmacologic agents to reduce the risk of pulmonary aspiration: application to healthy patients undergoing elective procedures: an updated report by the American Society of Anesthesiologists Task Force on preoperative fasting and the use of pharmacologic agents to reduce the risk of pulmonary aspiration. *Anesthesiology*. 2017;126(3):376-393.

28. Beach ML, Cohen DM, Gallagher SM, et al. Major adverse events and relationship to nil per os status in pediatric sedation/anesthesia outside the operating room: a report of the Pediatric Sedation Research Consortium. *Anesthesiology*. 2016;124(1):80-88.

29. Doyle L, Colletti JE. Pediatric procedural sedation and analgesia. *Pediatr Clin North Am*. 2006;53(2):279-292.

30. Bendall JC, Simpson PM, Middleton PM. Effectiveness of prehospital morphine, fentanyl, and methoxyflurane in pediatric patients. *Prehosp Emerg Care*. 2011;15(2):158-165.

31. Tobias JD. Sedation and analgesia in paediatric intensive care units: a guide to drug selection and use. *Paediatr Drugs*. 1999;1(2):109-126.

32. Daud YN, Carlson DW. Pediatric sedation. *Pediatr Clin North Am*. 2016;61(4):703-713.

33. Krauss B, Green SM. Procedural sedation and analgesia in children. *Lancet*. 2006;367(9512):766-780.

34. Cravero JP, Roback MG. *Pharmacologic Agents for Pediatric Sedation Outside of the Operating Room*. 2019. Available at: https://www.uptodate.com/contents/pharmacologic-agents-for-pediatric-procedural-sedation-outside-of-the-operating-room. Accessed March 1, 2020.

35. Godambe SA, Eliot V, Matthew D, et al. Comparison of propofol/fentanyl versus ketamine/midazolam for brief orthopedic procedural sedation in a pediatric emergency department. *Pediatrics*. 2003; 112(1 Pt 1):116-123.

36. Fahnenstich H, Steffan J, Kau N, et al. Fentanyl-induced chest wall rigidity and laryngospasm in preterm and term infants. *Crit Care Med*. 2000;28(3):836-839.

37. Dewhirst E, Naguib A, Toias JD. Chest wall rigidity in two infants after low-dose fentanyl administration. *Pediatr Emerg Care*. 2012;28(5):465-468.

38. Mudd S. Intranasal fentanyl in pain management in children: a systemic review of the literature. *J Pediatr Health Care*. 2011;25(5): 316-322.

39. Saunders M, Adelgais K, Nelson D. Use of intranasal fentanyl for the relief of pediatric orthopedic trauma pain. *Acad Emerg Med*. 2010;17(11):1155-1161.

40. Kost S, Roy A. Procedural sedation and analgesia in the pediatric emergency department: a review of sedative pharmacology. *Clin Pediatr Emerg Med*. 2010;11(4):233-243.

41. Vespasiano M, Finkelstein M, Kurachek S. Propofol sedation: intensivists' experience with 7304 cases in a children's hospital. *Pediatrics*. 2007;120(6):e1411-1417.

42. Emrath ET, Stockwell JA, McCracken CE, et al. Provision of deep procedural sedation by a pediatric sedation team at a freestanding imaging center. *Pediatr Radiol*. 2014;44(8):1020-1025.

43. Green SM, Krauss B. Propofol in emergency medicine: pushing the sedation frontier. *Ann Emerg Med*. 2003;42(6):792-797.

44. Asserhoj LL, Mosbech H, Kroigaard M, et al. No evidence for contra-indications to the use of propofol in adults allergic to egg, soy, or peanut. *J Anesth*. 2016 Jan;116(1):77-82.

45. Murphy A, Campbell DE, Baines D, et al. Allergic reactions to propofol in egg-allergic children. *Anesth Analg*. 2011;133(1):140-144.

46. Vasile, VB, Rasulo F, Candiani A, et al. The pathophysiology of propofol infusion syndrome: a simple name for a complex syndrome. *Intensive Care Med*. 2003;29(9):1417-1125.

47. Kam, PC, Cardone D. Propofol infusion syndrome. *Anaesthesia*. 2007;62(7):690-701.

48. Cheung CW, Ng KF, Liu J, et al. Analgesic and sedative effects of intranasal dexmedetomidine in third molar surgery under local anesthesia. *Br J Anaesth*. 2011;107(3):430-437.

49. Neville DN, Hayes KR, Ivan Y, et al. Double blind randomized controlled trial of intranasal dexmedetomidine versus intranasal midazolam as anxiolysis prior to pediatric laceration repair in the emergency department. *Acad Emerg Med*. 2016;23(8):910-917.

50. Sulton C, McCracken C, Simon HK, et al. Pediatric procedural sedation using dexmedetomidine: a report from the Pediatric Sedation Research Consortium. *Hosp Pediatr*. 2016;6(9):536-544.

51. Chiaretti A, Barone G, Rigante D, et al. Intranasal lidocaine and midazolam for procedural sedation in children. *Arch Dis Child*. 2011;96(2):160-163.

52. Wolfe TR, Braude DA. Intranasal medication delivery for children: a brief review and update. *Pediatrics*. 2010;126(3):532-537.

53. Golparvar M, Saghaei M, Sajedi P, et al. Paradoxical reaction following intravenous midazolam premedication in pediatric patients—a randomized placebo controlled trial of ketamine for rapid tranquilization. *Paediatr Anaesth*. 2004;14(11):924-930.

54. Bhatt M, Johnson DW, Chan J, et al. Risk factors for adverse events in emergency department procedural sedation for children. *JAMA Pediatr*. 2017;171(10):957-964.

55. Shah A, Mosdossy G, McLeod S, et al. A blinded, randomized controlled trial to evaluate ketamine/propofol versus ketamine alone for procedural sedation in children. *Ann Emerg Med*. 2011;57(5):425-433.

56. Melendez E, Bachur R. Serious adverse event during procedural sedation with ketamine. *Pediatr Emerg Care*. 2009;25:325.

57. Green SM, Roback MG, Krauss B, et al. Predictors of emesis and recovery agitation with emergency department ketamine sedation: an individual patient data meta-analysis of 8,282 children. *Ann Emerg Med*. 2009;54(2):171-180.

58. Roback MG, Wathen JE, MacKenzie T, et al. A randomized, controlled trial of IV versus IM ketamine for sedation of pediatric patients receiving emergency department orthopedic procedures. *Ann Emerg Med*. 2006;48(5):605-612.

59. Grunwell JR, Rravers C, Stormorkn AG, et al. Pediatric procedural sedation using the combination of ketamine and propofol outside of the emergency department: a report from the Pediatric Sedation Research Consortium. *Pediatr Crit Care Med.* 2017;18(8):e356-e363.
60. Heinz P, Geelhoed GC, Wee C, et al. Is atropine needed with ketamine sedation? A prospective, randomised, double blind study. *Emerg Med J.* 2006;23(3):206-209.
61. Brown L, Christian-Kopp S, Sherwin TS, et al. Adjunctive therapy is unnecessary during ketamine sedation in children. *Acad Emerg Med.* 2008;15(4):314-318.
62. Green SM, Roback MG, Krauss B, and the Emergency Department Ketamine Meta-analysis Study Group. Anticholinergics and ketamine sedation in children: a secondary analysis of atropine versus glycopyrrolate. *Acad Emerg Med.* 2010;17(2):157-162.
63. Wathen JE, Roback MG, MacKenzie T, et al. Does midazolam alter the clinical effects of intravenous ketamine sedation in children? A double-blind, randomized, controlled, emergency department trial. *Ann Emerg Med.* 2000;36(6):579-588.
64. Langston WT, Wathen JE, Roback MG, et al. Effect of odansetron on the incidence of vomiting associated with ketamine sedation in children: a double-blind, randomized, placebo-controlled trial. *Ann Emerg Med.* 2008;52(8):30-34.
65. Green SM, Roback MG, Kennedy RM, et al. Clinical practice guideline for emergency department ketamine dissociative sedation: 2011 update. *Ann Emerg Med.* 2011;57(5):449-461.
66. Poonai N, Canton K, Ali S, et al. Intranasal ketamine for procedural sedation and analgesia in children: a systemic review. *PLoS One.* 2017;12(3):e0173253.
67. Bahetwar SK, Pandey RK, Saksena AK, et al. A comparative evaluation of intranasal midazolam, ketamine, and their combination for sedation of young uncooperative pediatric dental patients: a triple blind randomized crossover trial. *J Clin Pediatr Dent.* 2001;35(4):415-420.
68. Buosenso D, Barone G, Valentini P, et al. Utility of intranasal ketamine and midazolam to perform gastric aspirates in children: a double-blind, placebo controlled, randomized study. *BMC Pediatr.* 2014;14:67.
69. Tse DS, Steele DW, Machan JT, et al. Intranasal ketamine for procedural sedation in pediatric laceration repair: a preliminary report. *Pediatr Emerg Care.* 2012;28(8):767-770.
70. Surendar MN, Pandey RK, Sakensa AK, et al. A comparative evaluation of intranasal dexmedetomidate, midazolam, and ketamine for their sedative and analgesic properties: a triple blind randomized study. *J Clin Pediatr Dent.* 2004;38(3):255-261.

Neonatal

4 My, What a Big Thymus You Have! Neonate/Infant Mediastinal Masses

ROBERT VEZZETTI, MD, FAAP, FACEP

Case Presentation

An 8-month-old male presents with 2 months of cough and intermittent rhinorrhea. He has been seen multiple times by his primary care provider and has been diagnosed at various times with viral upper respiratory tract infection and acute otitis media, for which he has been prescribed oral antibiotics. He has had some intermittent fevers as well, all of which have resolved after several days. There has been no travel or sick contacts, nor has there been any history of choking or concern for foreign body ingestion.

Physical examination reveals a thin but well-appearing and active child. He is afebrile and his vital signs are unremarkable, except for mild tachypnea (65 breaths per minute). There is no rhinorrhea and the oropharynx is clear. His chest demonstrates decreased breath sounds to the upper left chest, but there are no crackles, retractions, grunting, or stridor. He has a normal abdominal examination.

Imaging Considerations

PLAIN RADIOGRAPHY

This imaging modality is the most commonly utilized imaging modality for the neonatal or infant chest.[1] Two views are preferred (anterior-posterior [AP] and lateral) when possible. Plain radiography may suggest the presence of a chest mass, prompting the use of advanced imaging. Ninety percent of chest masses can be visualized by plain radiography.[2]

Plain radiography is the first-line imaging modality when chest masses are suspected.[3] However, this modality may miss small masses, and further imaging is indicated when a mediastinal mass is suspected, since a diagnosis is not usually made by plain radiography alone.[3]

ULTRASOUND (US)

This imaging modality is increasingly used for the evaluation of specific chest conditions. Examples include pneumothorax, pleural effusion, hemothorax, and chest masses.[1] US of the mediastinum is limited, however, in patients above 5 years of age due to poor acoustic windows.[3] The lack of exposure to ionizing radiation, rapidity, availability, and no need for sedation are all advantages of sonography.

COMPUTED TOMOGRAPHY (CT)

This imaging modality is typically utilized when plain radiography is abnormal and further delineation of a suspected chest mass is indicated. CT is also used for surgical planning when indicated.[1] CT is readily available and rapid and usually does not require sedation. CT does include exposure to ionizing radiation, and appropriate pediatric imaging protocols should be utilized to reduce this exposure as much as possible.

CT is often utilized in patients with mediastinal masses. It has been shown to be very accurate for the characterization of masses (such as size and location) and to determine whether there is involvement of adjacent structures.[2-4] CT can differentiate between cystic and solid structures and can evaluate for the presence of calcification, fat, or vascular components.[2] CT findings have been shown to impact management in 65% of cases and have added additional diagnostic information in 82%.[3,4]

MAGNETIC RESONANCE IMAGING (MRI)

As with CT, MRI is used for further anatomic definition and tissue characterization of suspected chest masses. MRI is particularly good at differentiating cystic from solid structures, especially compared to CT.[2,3] MRI may also be used when planning surgical procedures.[1] Availability and the need for sedation are potential disadvantages of MRI.

POSITRON EMISSION TOMOGRAPHY (PET)

PET is not a first-line imaging modality for diagnosing mediastinal masses in pediatric patients. However, PET imaging, including PET-CT or PET-MRI, can be used in staging tumors and monitoring response to therapy.[3,5] Such imaging for children, though, is usually found at tertiary pediatric centers and generally is not widely available.

Imaging Findings

The patient had two-view plain radiography of the chest performed. There is a large rounded opacity in the left mid to upper chest that has a well-defined border laterally and inferiorly. There is mass effect on the lower trachea (displacement to the right) and left mainstem bronchus (displaced inferiorly and medially) (Fig. 4.1).

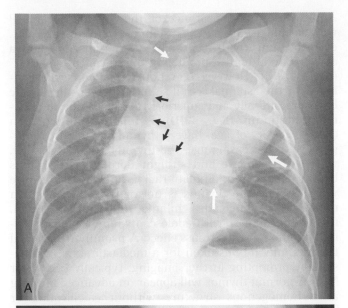

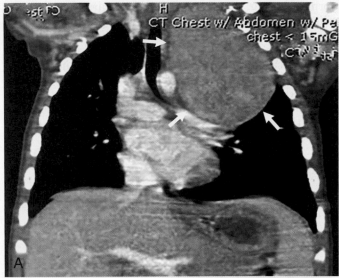

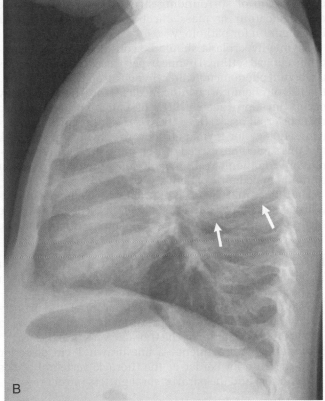

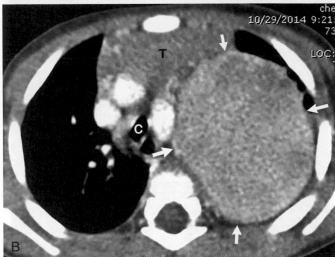

Fig. 4.1 Frontal radiograph (A) of the chest demonstrates a large rounded opacity suggestive of a mediastinal mass in the left mid to upper chest *(white arrows)* with mass effect on the trachea and left mainstem bronchus *(black arrows)*. Lateral view of the chest (B) shows the opacity to be best seen posteriorly *(white arrows)*.

Fig. 4.2 Contrast-enhanced computed tomography (CT) coronal image (A) demonstrates a relatively homogenous, enhancing left mediastinal mass *(white arrows)*. Axial CT image (B) shows an appearance consistent with a mass *(white arrows)* originating in the paraspinal posterior mediastinum and extending into the middle and anterior mediastinum. The mass abuts the normal-appearing thymus *(T)* and causes rightward displacement of normal mediastinal structures, including the carina *(C)*.

Case Conclusion

The patient was admitted with consultation by Pediatric Oncology and Pediatric Surgery. A contrast-enhanced CT scan of the chest was obtained, demonstrating the mass, which appears centered in the posterior left mediastinum but extends to involve the middle and anterior mediastinum

(Fig. 4.2). CT-guided biopsy revealed that the mass was a neuroblastoma. The tumor was determined to be intermediate risk. A metaiodobenzyl guanidine (MIBG) scan, whereby MIBG is absorbed by neuroendocrine cells, making this scan useful in the evaluation of metastasis of neuroendocrine tumors, was negative for metastases. The patient was treated with chemotherapy and subsequent surgical resection of the residual mass.

The most common cause of the appearance of a large mediastinum in neonates and young children is the normal prominence of the thymus. The thymus is important for the development of the immune system during childhood, primarily T cells, which are responsible for regulating cellular immunity, and B cells, which are responsible for regulating humeral immunity. Visualization of the neonatal/childhood (age <5 years) thymus by plain radiography is a normal finding. A normal thymus appears on plain chest radiography as a prominent soft tissue opacity in the anterior mediastinum, sometimes filling the anterior upper chest in young infants.[1] It may be difficult to distinguish from the cardiac silhouette.[6] A feature of the normal thymus often present on plain radiography is the "thymic wave sign," which is undulation of the lateral thymic contour caused by the ribs, since the thymus is soft in texture and abuts the anterior ribs and costal cartilage (Fig. 4.3).[7,8]

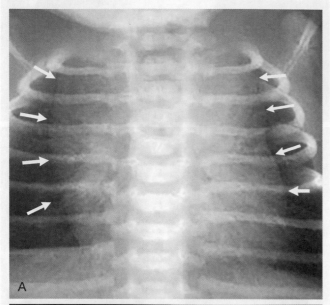

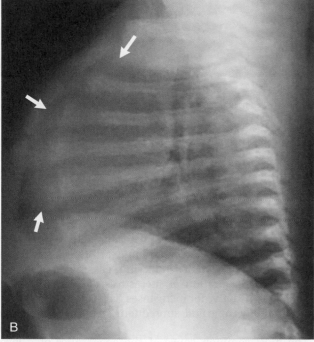

Fig. 4.3 Anterior-posterior (A) and lateral (B) radiographs of the chest show a normal prominent thymus in an infant. Note on the frontal view (A) that the lateral borders of the thymus are indistinguishable from the normal cardiac borders and that the lateral borders of the thymus show undulation, the "thymic wave sign," as the soft thymus abuts the anterior costal cartilages. Also, the thymus is anterior *(white arrows)* on the lateral view (B); therefore, there is no "clear space" in the retrosternal region.

Another normal appearance of the thymus on an AP view is that it can extend asymmetrically to the right, over the lung, with a straight inferior margin, and a convex lateral border, producing the so-called "sail sign" (Fig. 4.4A–C).[7] However, one should not confuse this finding with the "spinnaker-sail sign," in which the thymic lobes are laterally and superiorly displaced due to pneumomediastinum (Fig. 4.4D).[7,8] Infants and children (under 5 years of age) have a thymus with convex margins. With increasing age, the thymus becomes smaller, with more concave and straight borders. The thymus becomes inapparent on plain radiography by the teenage years.[9] While the thymus is normally visible on plain radiography in neonates, infants, and young children, this is not the case with adolescents, and a normal thymus should not cause mass effect. A prominent, normal thymus may be mistaken for a mediastinal mass, occasionally prompting further imaging, typically US, CT, or MRI. A normal thymus will appear on advanced imaging as a homogenous structure without calcification or compression of surrounding structures.[6,9] The presence of calcification or mass effect should prompt further investigation for pathology.

Thymic hyperplasia should be considered in the appropriate clinical setting. Thymic hyperplasia is usually seen as a rebound phenomenon after thymic atrophy due to illness, the use of chemotherapeutic medications (thymic atrophy occurs in approximately 90% of patients), or prolonged corticosteroid use.[6,9] Once there is resolution of the underlying etiology for thymic atrophy, the thymus grows back and this sometimes exceeds the baseline size.[9] While thymomas are commonly seen in adult populations, they are not common in pediatric patients.

The differential diagnosis of pediatric mediastinal masses is broad and can be narrowed based on the location of the suspected mass. The mediastinal compartments of the chest are as follows:[9,10]

1. Anterior compartment—surrounded by the sternum (anteriorly) and anterior margin of the pericardium (posteriorly).
2. Middle compartment—anterior margin of the pericardium and a line drawn approximately 1 cm posterior to the anterior margin of the thoracic vertebral bodies.
3. Posterior compartment—a line drawn 1 cm posterior to the anterior border of the thoracic vertebral bodies (anterior) and the paravertebral gutters (posteriorly).

The differential diagnosis for suspected pediatric chest masses can be narrowed based on location and age:[3,9]

COMPARTMENT	DIFFERENTIAL DIAGNOSIS
Anterior	Thymic masses, germ cell neoplasms, lymphoma, metastatic lymphadenopathy
Middle	Lymphoma, tracheal lesions, esophageal masses, cardiac masses, foregut duplication cysts
Posterior	Peripheral nerve tumors, ganglia tumors, thoracic meningocele

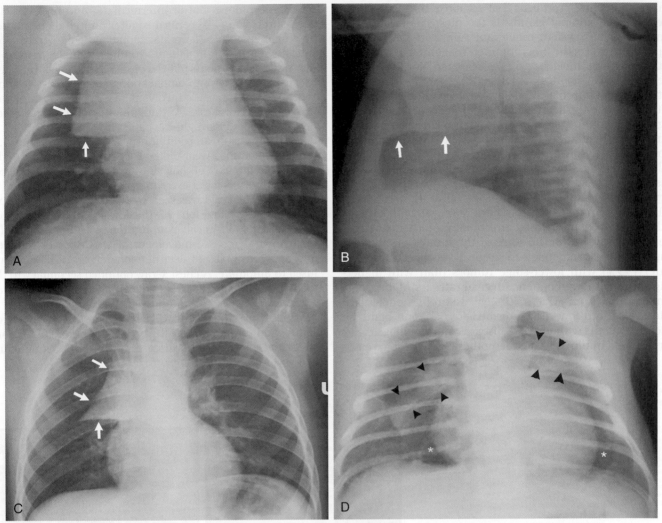

Fig. 4.4 Anterior-posterior view of the chest (A) shows the thymic "sail sign," a normal variation of the appearance of the thymus, with the thymus asymmetrically extending over the right lung, with a straight inferior border *(white arrows)*. Note that the right lateral border of the thymus also shows the undulation of the "thymic wave sign." On the lateral view of the chest (B), the thymus is seen in the anterior chest, also with a straight inferior border *(white arrows)*. (C) Another patient with a normal thymic sail sign *(white arrows)*. The normal thymic sail sign is not the same as the thymic "spinnaker sail" or "angelwing" sign, shown in (D). These latter two terms refer to the appearance of the thymus when it is uplifted superiorly *(black arrowheads)* by a pneumomediastinum *(*)*, as seen in (D).

The location percentage of mediastinal masses in the adult population versus the pediatric population is shown here:[11,12]

LOCATION	ADULT POPULATION	PEDIATRIC POPULATION
Anterior	68	36
Middle	18	12
Posterior	14	52

Lymphoma is the most common cause of anterior mediastinal masses in the pediatric population and represents the third most common malignancy in pediatric patients.[2,6,11] Lymphoma can involve any part of the mediastinum and can infiltrate and enlarge the thymus. The involvement of the thymus in the setting of lymphoma or leukemia usually is due to systemic disease.[6] Pediatric mediastinal masses can be benign, but the majority are malignant. While approximately half of these masses are asymptomatic, systemic symptoms (fever, cough, and malaise are the most common) may be present and are more commonly associated with a malignant process.[2,12]

Pediatric lymphoma may be Hodgkin or non-Hodgkin. Most pediatric lymphomas are non-Hodgkin.[2,11] Patients with non-Hodgkin lymphoma present with nonspecific symptoms, such as cough, stridor, respiratory distress, and superior vena cava obstruction symptoms, as well as constitutional symptoms such as fever, weight loss, night sweats, and lymphadenopathy.[2] Hodgkin lymphoma is more commonly seen in adolescent and young adult patients.

Middle mediastinal masses are often remnants of the foregut and include bronchogenic cysts and esophageal duplication cysts. Treatment is generally surgical.[11]

Posterior mediastinal masses are most often neurogenic in origin, arising from the sympathetic ganglion, intercostal nerves, and paraganglia cells.[11] Neuroblastoma arises from embryonic neural crest cells that comprise the sympathetic ganglion and adrenal glands, is the most common non—central nervous system malignant tumor in the pediatric population, and is the most common malignancy in infancy, with an annual incidence of 700 cases in North America; the mean age at diagnosis is 18 months.[13–15] The majority of patients with neuroblastoma have a retroperitoneal location, but up to one-third are mediastinal. Neuroblastoma is a highly malignant tumor and has often metastasized at presentation.[11] Symptoms and signs associated with neuroblastoma include dyspnea, Horner syndrome (ptosis, miosis, and anhidrosis), vomiting, abdominal distention, and opsoclonus-myoclonus syndrome (in which there are rapid involuntary eye movements).[11,13]

Patients with neuroblastoma are managed with surgery, radiotherapy, chemotherapy, and/or immunotherapy. Treatment is dependent on the stage of the tumor, with higher-stage tumors less amenable to surgical resection. Survival is better (99%) with lower-stage tumors than with higher-stage ones, although patient survival rates for higher-stage tumors range from 50% to 70%.[11,16] Neuroblastoma is also categorized into low-risk, intermediate-risk, and high-risk disease. Patients with low-risk disease can be managed with surgery and minimal to no chemotherapy, or in some cases

observation alone, but in intermediate- and high-risk disease, surgery may be performed after an initial chemotherapy regimen.[13,17,18] Neuroblastoma can demonstrate spontaneous regression in patients younger than 18 months of age, and these patients may be observed provided that there are no life-threatening complications, such as massive hepatomegaly (from hepatic involvement), hepatic dysfunction, or respiratory distress.[18,19] Radiotherapy and immunotherapy are reserved for high-risk patients.[15,20]

For comparison, an additional case is provided in Fig. 4.5.

This patient, a 2-year-old boy, was seen for fussiness, decreased frequency of bowel movements, and decreased movement of his lower extremities, progressing to refusal to ambulate. The child was seen by his pediatrician, who obtained plain radiographs of the lower extremities, which were normal. Physical examination was remarkable for tachypnea, decreased movement of the lower extremities, and apparently absent deep tendon reflexes. The child refused to ambulate. A chest x-ray, obtained secondary to the tachypnea, revealed a large mediastinal mass (see Fig. 4.5a). After subspecialty consultation, the decision was made to obtain further studies with MRI of the chest (see Fig. 4.5b,c), spine, and brain. The MRI revealed enhancing lesions suggestive of metastatic disease in the brain, lungs, and

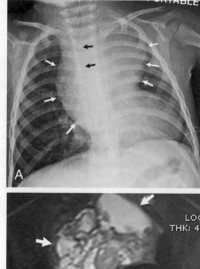
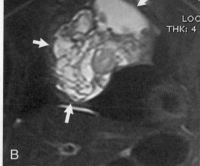
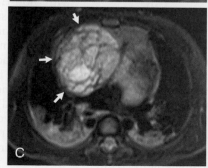
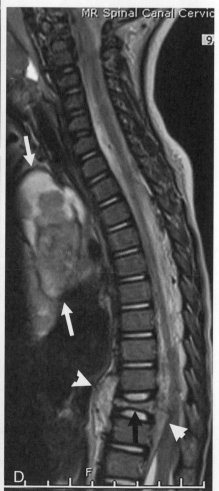

Fig. 4.5 Anterior-posterior view of the chest (A) in a 2-year-old shows enlargement of the mediastinum consistent with a mediastinal mass *(white arrows)* involving the mediastinum bilaterally, with mass effect upon the trachea *(black arrows)*, displacing the trachea toward the patient's right. Coronal (B) and axial (C) T2-weighted magnetic resonance imaging (MRI) images demonstrate a heterogenous cystic and solid mediastinal mass *(white arrows)*, centered in the anterior mediastinum, but the mass extends posteriorly as well, as seen on sagittal imaging *(white arrows)* (D). Sagittal MRI imaging of the spine (D) shows collapse of the T9 vertebral body *(black arrow)*, associated with soft tissue masses anterior and posterior to T9 and adjacent vertebrae *(white arrowheads)*. The posterior intraspinal mass produces a mass effect upon the thoracic spinal cord.

vertebral bodies, with a collapsed T9 vertebral body associated with soft tissue mass anteriorly and posteriorly, the latter with a mass effect on the spinal cord (see Fig. 4.5d). Initial treatment was emergent laminectomy for decompression of the intraspinal mass. Pathologic studies revealed this mass to be a metastatic germ cell tumor. The patient had appropriate chemotherapy and there was resolution of the paravertebral, central nervous system, and pulmonary disease, but the mediastinal mass showed minimal improvement. The chest mass was resected and found to be a benign mature teratoma. The patient completed physical therapy and had a good outcome.

IMAGING PEARLS

1. Plain radiography is the initial imaging modality of choice in patients with mediastinal masses, which are often incidentally discovered when the study is employed during evaluation for other symptoms, such as fever, cough, dyspnea, or chest pain.
2. CT is a secondary imaging modality that has excellent spatial resolution and can help delineate the relationship of a mediastinal mass to surrounding structures. This modality can also be used to plan surgical procedures and can be used to monitor disease progression or treatment response.
3. MRI is a secondary imaging modality that is often utilized to better define the relationship of a mediastinal mass to other structures in the chest, has excellent soft tissue characterization, and can be used to monitor disease progression or treatment response.
4. PET is a secondary and, in some instances, tertiary study that is utilized for tumor staging and to monitor response to treatment.

References

1. Lobo L. The neonatal chest. *Eur J Radiol.* 2006;60(2):152-158.
2. Jaggers J, Balsara K. Mediastinal masses in children. *Semin Thorac Cardiovasc Surg.* 2004;16(3):201-208.
3. Thacker PG, Mahani MG, Amer H, et al. Imaging evaluation of mediastinal masses in children and adults: practical diagnostic approach based on a new classification system. *J Thorac Imaging.* 2015;30(4):247-267.
4. Lee EY. Evaluation of non-vascular mediastinal masses in infants and children: an evidence-based practical approach. *Pediatr Radiol.* 2009;39(suppl 2):S198-S190.
5. Hudson MN, Krasin MJ, Kaste SC. PET imaging in pediatric Hodgkin's lymphoma. *Pediatr Radiol.* 2004;34(3):190-198.
6. Nasseri F, Eftekhari F. Clinical and radiologic review of the normal and abnormal thymus: pearls and pitfalls. *Radiographics.* 2010;39(2):413-428.
7. Alves ND, Sousa M. Images in pediatrics: the thymic sail sign and thymic wave sign. *Eur J Radiol.* 2013;172(1):133.
8. Correia-Pinto J, Henriques-Coelho T. Images in clinical medicine: neonatal pneumomediastinum and the spinnaker-sail sign. *N Engl J Med.* 2010;363(22):2145.
9. Ranganath SH, Lee EY, Restrepo R, et al. Mediastinal masses in children. *AJR Am J Roentgenol.* 2012;198(3):W197-W216.
10. Whitten CR, Khan S, Munneke GJ, et al. A diagnostic approach to mediastinal abnormalities. *Radiographics.* 2007;27(3):657-671.
11. Wright CD. Mediastinal tumors and cysts in the pediatric population. *Thorac Surg Clin.* 2009;19(1):47-61.
12. Takeda S, Miyoshi S, Akashi A, et al. Clinical spectrum of primary mediastinal tumors: a comparison of adult and pediatric populations at a single Japanese institution. *J Surg Oncol.* 2009;83(1):24-30.
13. Sharma R, Mer J, Lion A, et al. Clinical presentation, evaluation, and management of neuroblastoma. *Pediatr Rev.* 2018;39(4):194-203.
14. Siegel DA, King J, Tai E, et al. Cancer incidence rates and trends among children and adolescents in the United States, 2001–2009. *Pediatrics.* 2014;134(4):e945-e955.
15. Matthay KK, Maris JM, Schleiermacher G, et al. Neuroblastoma. *Nat Rev Dis Primers.* 2016;2:16078.
16. Gutierrez JC, Fisher AC, Sola JE, et al. Markedly improving survival of neuroblastoma: a 30 year analysis of 1,646 patients. *Pediatr Surg Int.* 2007;23(7):637-646.
17. Strother DR, London WB, Schmidt ML, et al. Outcome after surgery alone or with restricted use of chemotherapy for patients with low-risk neuroblastoma: results of Children's Oncology Group study P9641. *J Clin Oncol.* 2012 May;39(15):1842-1848.
18. Allen-Roades W, Whittle SB, Rainusso N. Pediatric solid tumors of infancy: an overview. *Pediatr Rev.* 2018;39(2):57-67.
19. Brodeur GM. Spontaneous regression of neuroblastoma. *Cell Tissue Res.* 2018;372(2):277-286.
20. London WB, Castel V, Montclair T, et al. Clinical and biologic features predictive of survival after relapse of neuroblastoma: a report from the International Neuroblastoma Risk Group project. *J Clin Oncol.* 2011;29(24):3286-3292.

5

A Wheezin' We Will Go: Bronchiolitis/Viral Pathology

SUJIT IYER, MD

Case Presentation

A 6-month-old baby with cough, congestion, and fever for 3 days presents to the emergency department with complaints of respiratory distress. Physical examination is significant for a temperature of 102 degrees Fahrenheit, respiratory rate of 55 breaths per minute, pulse oxygen saturation of 92%, and prominent intercostal, subcostal, and suprasternal retractions. On auscultation, there are diffuse crackles and intermittent wheezing heard in all lung fields. Mucous membranes are moist, and the child is still alert and playful despite increased work of breathing.

Imaging Considerations

Several studies have shown that the routine use of radiographs in children with mild bronchiolitis or classic illness may lead to inappropriate antibiotics and is currently not recommended for routine use by pediatric practice guidelines.[1–3] Secondary bacterial pneumonia is an uncommon complication and should be considered in children not having the expected clinical course or those admitted to the intensive care unit (ICU).[4]

Radiographs are most likely to be useful in children with focal findings, severe disease, or signs of complications such as pneumothorax or when history and physical examination point to other causes in the differential diagnosis that may mimic aspects of the bronchiolitis examination (i.e., undiagnosed heart disease, myocarditis, foreign body, etc.).

PLAIN RADIOGRAPHY

The most common radiographic findings in bronchiolitis are either normal radiographs or a combination of findings that often include peribronchial thickening, hyperinflation, and atelectasis. Radiographs are ideal to detect complications such as pneumothorax or bacterial co-infection in children who do not have clinical signs of classic bronchiolitis.

THORACIC ULTRASOUND (US)

Smaller studies have looked at the use of lung US scans in the inpatient settings in correlation with clinical examination findings in investigating for pneumonia. The presence of B lines, subpleural consolidations, and interstitial disease along multiple spaces has been attributed to more severe disease and bacterial pneumonia. However, interrater reliability, operator variability, and lack of validation to differentiate viral versus bacterial disease in these small studies limit the use of US on a broader scale for most cases.[5,6]

Imaging Findings

This child had imaging performed by his primary care provider earlier in the day. A two-view chest radiograph study is shown. There are bilateral patchy and streaky perihilar opacities, diffuse interstitial prominence, and central airway thickening. There is no focal infiltrate or effusion, including the retrocardiac space (Figs. 5.1 and 5.2). Similar imaging findings for a different child with bronchiolitis are also shown (Figs. 5.3 and 5.4).

Case Conclusion

The patient was suctioned in the emergency department and observed while feeding on pulse oximetry. There was moderate improvement in work of breathing after suctioning, and the child's oxygen saturations improved to >92% while feeding and with activity. The child was discharged home to follow-up with the primary care provider in 1 to 2 days with the explanation that the peak of illness would likely continue for the next 72 hours.

Bronchiolitis is the leading cause of hospitalization in infants and young children. The peak incidence is in children between 2 and 6 months of age.[7] The classic clinical course includes an initial 1- to 3-day period of upper respiratory symptoms highlighted by rhinorrhea and nasal congestion. On days 3 to 6, lower respiratory tract symptoms begin to peak, with prominent crackles and/or wheezing in addition to tachypnea and signs of respiratory distress. A viral etiology is seen in the vast majority of cases and can include many different viruses dependent on the season, with respiratory syncytial virus being the most common cause.

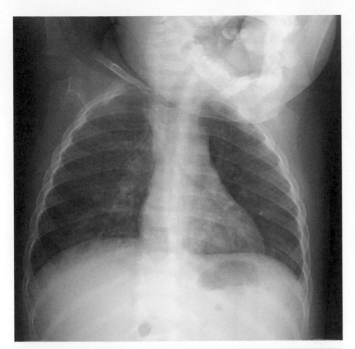

Fig. 5.1 Anterior-posterior view of the chest demonstrates increased streaky interstitial lung markings in the parahilar regions with bronchial wall thickening.

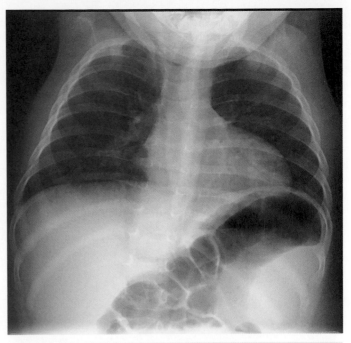

Fig. 5.3 Plain radiograph of another patient with bronchiolitis. There are streaky opacities commonly seen with lower viral respiratory tract infection.

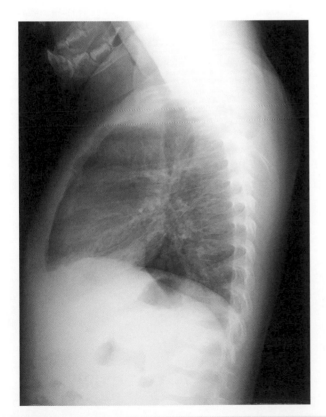

Fig. 5.2 Lateral view of the chest shows increased interstitial lung markings centrally.

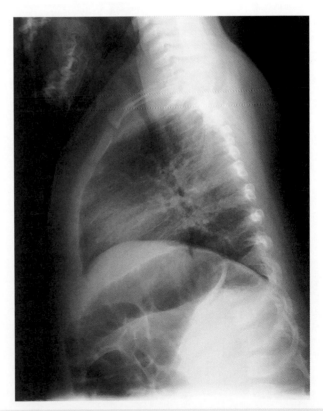

Fig. 5.4 Lateral projection again demonstrating streaky opacities consistent with a viral process.

IMAGING PEARLS

1. Plain chest radiography is rarely indicated for classic viral bronchiolitis. Expected findings of lower respiratory tract disease in bronchiolitis may lead to overprescription of antibiotics.
2. Chest radiograph should be considered when clinical examination and story do not correlate with classic disease and other conditions or complications are a consideration.
3. Children with severe bronchiolitis requiring ICU admission are a different cohort that may warrant a higher rate of chest radiographs.
4. Thoracic ultrasound still has limited utility in providing additional information to guide clinical management of bronchiolitis.

References

1. Swingler GH, Hussey GD, Zwarenstein M. Randomised controlled trial of clinical outcome after chest radiograph in ambulatory acute lower-respiratory infection in children. *Lancet.* 1998;351(9100):404-408.
2. Schuh S, Lalani A, Allen U, et al. Evaluation of the utility of radiography in acute bronchiolitis. *J Pediatr.* 2007;150(4):429-433.
3. Ralston SL, Lieberthal AS, Meissner HC, et al. Clinical practice guideline: the diagnosis, management, and prevention of bronchiolitis. *Pediatrics.* 2014;134(5):e1474-e1502.
4. Thorburn K, Harigopal S, Reddy V, et al. High incidence of pulmonary bacterial co-infection in children with severe respiratory syncytial virus (RSV) bronchiolitis. *Thorax.* 2006;61(7):611-615.
5. Basile V, Di Mauro A, Scalini E, et al. Lung ultrasound: a useful tool in diagnosis and management of bronchiolitis. *BMC Pediatr.* 2015;15:63.
6. Biagi C, Pierantoni L, Baldazzi M, et al. Lung ultrasound for the diagnosis of pneumonia in children with acute bronchiolitis. *BMC Pulm Med.* 2018;18(1):191.
7. Shay DK, Holman RC, Newman RD, et al. Bronchiolitis-associated hospitalizations among US children, 1980–1996. *JAMA.* 1999;282(15):1440-1446.

6 Twisting the Night Away: Malrotation

ROBERT VEZZETTI, MD, FAAP, FACEP

Case Presentation

A 5-day-old male infant presents with decreased feeding and activity for the past 24 hours. The parents report emesis that initially looked like infant formula but over the past 12 hours has become "yellow-green" and the last several episodes have been "green." The emesis has occurred whenever the child attempts to feed, which was typically every 3 hours, but the parents have been attempting to feed more frequently (every hour or so) because they feel the child is not "keeping anything down." There has been no fever, cough, congestion, rhinorrhea, or reported/known trauma. The child had initially been fussy and appeared "uncomfortable."

The child's physical examination reveals an ill-appearing, afebrile child. His heart rate is 116 beats per minute, respiratory rate is 20 breaths per minute, and oxygen saturations are 96% on room air. He has a sunken anterior fontanelle, dry mucous membranes, and dry skin without lesions. His skin turgor is poor with delayed capillary refill. There is no appreciable heart murmur and his lungs are clear. His abdominal examination demonstrates generalized distention with no obvious hepatosplenomegaly and the abdomen appears to be tense.

Imaging Considerations

Emesis in the neonate has causes that range from benign to life-threatening, and history and physical examination can help to determine the need for imaging. Bilious emesis can indicate a surgical emergency and, while imaging is desirable, rapid treatment of the patient and prompt surgical consultation should not be delayed in these patients, especially if they appear ill or are in extremis.

PLAIN RADIOGRAPHY

Plain abdominal radiography is a readily available imaging modality and can provide the clinician with an overall view of the bowel gas pattern, as well as the presence of pneumoperitoneum. This is a first-line imaging modality when intestinal pathology is suspected, such as bowel obstruction, and may demonstrate gaseous distention of the stomach and proximal duodenum when a volvulus is present. However, children with malrotation often have a normal bowel gas pattern.[1]

FLUOROSCOPY

Upper gastrointestinal series (UGI) is the imaging study of choice for the diagnosis of malrotation.[1-6] UGI has a sensitivity of 93% to 100% for malrotation,[1,7] and studies have found a positive predictive value of 90%.[3] Patients with malrotation will have an abnormal position of the duodenojejunal junction and there are a variety of abnormal positions that are associated with malrotation. If Ladd bands are present, abnormal duodenal configuration may be noted, and if there is midgut volvulus, a corkscrew pattern and possible obstruction of the duodenum may be seen.[1,2,6,8] The reported sensitivity of UGI for detecting volvulus is 79%.[5,7] Anatomic variants can interfere with proper interpretation of a UGI series and special attention should be given to proper technique to ensure a meaningful study.[4,5,7] This imaging test should be performed and interpreted by a pediatric radiologist or a radiologist experienced in pediatric fluoroscopy. If this expertise is not available, the clinician should arrange transfer of the patient to a facility that has this capability.

ULTRASOUND (US)

The role that US plays in the diagnosis of intestinal malrotation and volvulus is a matter of debate. While large studies are lacking, there is evidence to suggest that ultrasonography is useful in detecting malrotation. A finding described as suggestive of malrotation is inversion of the usual relationship of the superior mesenteric artery (SMA) and the superior mesenteric vein (SMV). Although some have reported this SMA/SMV inversion to be sensitive in detecting malrotation, both false-positive and false-negative results in studies have been reported.[1,2] An abnormal relationship between the SMA and the third segment of the duodenum on US has also been utilized to detect malrotation, and the presence of a "whirlpool sign" (a swirling appearance of the mesentery and SMV around the SMA) is suggestive of volvulus.[1,2,9-11] This latter finding should prompt either confirmatory UGI or surgical consultation.[1,2,10,11] When combining these three sonographic features (inversion of the SMA and SMV, the whirlpool sign, and an intraperitoneal transverse duodenum), Zhou et al. found a sensitivity of 100% and specificity of 97.8%, noting that the study included 70 children with a mean age of 31 days.[9] The prospect of utilizing US as a means to identifying malrotation is an exciting one, but additional study is needed before this modality is considered as a first-line test or as a replacement to a UGI. Also, US examination for these vascular and intestinal relationships is operator dependent and likely to have greatest utility in facilities with dedicated pediatric sonographers and pediatric imagers, rather than in a general community setting.

COMPUTED TOMOGRAPHY

This modality is not a first-line imaging test and is typically not employed when investigating malrotation or volvulus. It can differentiate between malrotation and nonrotation and may detect malrotation when the study is employed for other clinical reasons.[1]

MAGNETIC RESONANCE IMAGING (MRI)

MRI is not a first-line imaging modality when assessing for the presence of intestinal malrotation but can detect this condition. In a pediatric study of MRI compared to UGI, the authors found that if four specific anatomic criteria were met by MRI, then intestinal rotation could be considered normal.[12] While MRI has the potential to avoid ionizing radiation exposure, it is not the gold standard at this time and, if performed, is an ancillary study.

Imaging Findings

The child was thought not to be stable enough to undergo a UGI. Plain bedside radiography was obtained, as initial resuscitation began and the patient was intubated. Postintubation imaging, including one-view chest imaging and two-view abdominal imaging, was provided. There was a large pneumoperitoneum; the tip of the endotracheal tube was seen just above the carina but retracted into the midthoracic trachea and there was a nasogastric tube in the stomach (Figs. 6.1 and 6.2).

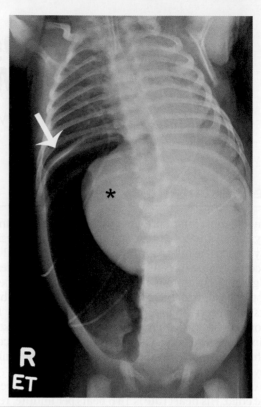

Fig. 6.2 Left lateral decubitus view again shows a large pneumoperitoneum, outlining the right hemidiaphragm *(arrow)* and outlining the liver *(asterisk)*. The endotracheal tube has retracted into the midthoracic trachea.

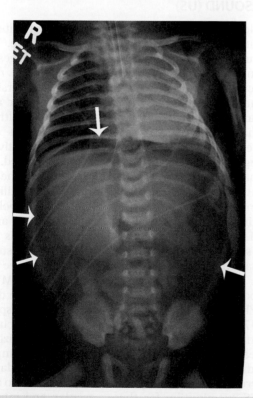

Fig. 6.1 Post-intubation frontal view of the chest and abdomen. A large pneumoperitoneum is seen as an abnormal lucency filling the entire abdomen and pelvis *(white arrows)*. The increased opacity of the left lung is consistent with atelectasis related to low endotracheal tip position, tip just above the carina.

Case Conclusion

Pediatric Surgery was emergently consulted and the child was taken to the operating room. The child was found to have intestinal malrotation with subsequent necrosis and perforation of the greater curvature of the stomach, necessitating a partial gastrectomy. As treatment for malrotation, a Ladd procedure was performed; an appendectomy was also performed. The child had a complicated course and remained in the neonatal intensive care unit for 3 months, during which time he was cared for by multiple pediatric subspecialists prior to recovery and discharge.

Intestinal malrotation is a congenital anomaly that occurs in approximately 1 in 500 to 2000 live births.[1,3,12] Most (90%) cases of malrotation present with symptoms in the first year of life, and 75% present under 1 month of age.[1,4] In malrotation, the lack of proper fixation of the bowel predisposes the intestines to twist around the SMA and SMV, leading to life-threatening volvulus and ischemia. Bilious emesis is a common presenting symptom, but patient presentations also include nonbilious emesis, abdominal pain, and shock.[1] Older children may present with more subtle symptoms and may have partial obstruction and chronic or intermittent volvulus.[1,5]

There are several congenital conditions that are associated with malrotation, including trisomies 13, 18, and 21, Cornelia de Lange syndrome, and Eagle-Barret syndrome.[1] Infants born with congenital diaphragmatic hernia, gastroschisis, biliary atresia, duodenal atresia, genitourinary abnormalities, and omphalocele also have increased rates of malrotation.[1,2]

Rapid identification of intestinal malrotation or midgut volvulus is important, and these children can appear quite ill. Definitive treatment is the Ladd procedure (first described in 1936 by Dr. W.E. Ladd), which is counterclockwise detorsion of the bowel, division of Ladd bands, widening of the small intestine mesentery, and reorientation of the small bowel on the right and the cecum and colon on the left.[1,13]

IMAGING PEARLS

1. UGI is the imaging modality of choice to diagnose malrotation with or without volvulus.
2. Plain radiography can be useful in the patient with emesis, allowing for the evaluation of the bowel gas pattern and pneumoperitoneum.
3. CT and MRI are not first-line modalities for the evaluation of malrotation with or without volvulus.
4. Do not delay resuscitation and pediatric surgical consultation in ill-appearing patients in order to obtain imaging. While imaging is desirable, malrotation with volvulus can be life-threatening and needs emergent management.

References

1. Marine MB, Karmazyn B. Imaging of malrotation in the neonate. *Semin Ultrasound CT MR.* 2014;35(6):555-570.
2. Orzech N, Navarro OM, Langer JC. Is ultrasonography a good screening test for intestinal malrotation? *J Pediatr Surg.* 2006;41(5):1005-1009.
3. Birajdar S, Rao SC, Bettenay F. Role of upper gastrointestinal contrast studies for suspected malrotation in neonatal population. *J Paediatr Child Health.* 2017;53(7):644-649.
4. Stouse PJ. Disorders of intestinal rotation and fixation ("malrotation"). *Pediatr Radiol.* 2004;34(11):837-851.
5. Applegate KE, Anderson JM, Klatte EC. Intestinal malrotation in children: a problem-solving approach to the upper gastrointestinal series. *Radiographics.* 2006;26(5):1485-1500.
6. Laurence NC, Pollock AN. Malrotation with midgut volvulus. *Pediatr Emerg Care.* 2012;28(1):87-89.
7. Sizemore AW, Rabbani KZ, Ladd A, et al. Diagnostic performance of the upper gastrointestinal series in the evaluation of children with clinically suspected malrotation. *Pediatr Radiol.* 2008;38(5):518-528.
8. Ortiz-Neira CL. The corkscrew sign: midgut volvulus. *Radiology.* 2007;242(1):315-316.
9. Zhou LY, Li SR, Wang W, et al. Usefulness of sonography in evaluating children suspected of malrotation: comparison with an upper gastrointestinal contrast study. *J Ultrasound Med.* 2015;34(10):1825-1832.
10. Chao HC, Kong MS, Chen JY, et al. Sonographic feature related to volvulus in neonatal intestinal malrotation. *J Ultrasound Med.* 2000;19(6):371-376.
11. Esposito F, Vitale V, Noviello D, et al. Ultrasonographic diagnosis of midgut volvulus with malrotation in children. *J Pediatr Gastroenterol Nutr.* 2014;59(6):786-788.
12. Fay JS, Chernyak V, Taragin BH. Identifying intestinal malrotation on magnetic resonance examinations ordered for unrelated indications. *Pediatr Radiol.* 2017;47(11):1477-1482.
13. Ladd WE. Surgical disease of the alimentary tract in infants. *N Engl J Med.* 1936 215;705-709.

7 Double Bubble... Double Trouble! Duodenal Obstruction

ROBERT VEZZETTI, MD, FAAP, FACEP

Case Presentation

A 4-day-old patient presents to the emergency department with forceful emesis associated with every feed. The emesis is described as nonbloody, slightly green in color. The child has decreased feeding and activity over the past 24 hours. There has been no fever, diarrhea, cough, or congestion. There is no report of trauma. The child was the product of an uncomplicated term spontaneous vaginal delivery and the mother had good prenatal care. The parents state that the child has had emesis since 12 hours of life but were told that this was due to "formula allergy" and the child was switched to a soy formula. The emesis has continued.

The patient's physical examination reveals a quiet child in no apparent distress. There is no fever; the patient has a heart rate of 190 beats per minute, respiratory rate of 35 breaths per minute, blood pressure of 80/40 mm Hg, and pulse oximetry of 100% on room air. The child has had a 20% weight loss compared to the documented birth weight. The anterior fontanel is slightly sunken and the mucous membranes are dry. There is no heart murmur and the lungs are clear. The abdomen is nondistended and there is no hepatosplenomegaly. There does not appear to be any obvious tenderness.

You decide to ask the mother to feed the child. She does so, and several minutes later, there is obvious bilious emesis.

Imaging Considerations

PLAIN RADIOGRAPHY

Plain radiography is a typical first-line imaging modality in neonates with emesis, particularly if the emesis is bilious, although over the age of 2 days, upper gastrointestinal series (UGI) is also a first-line imaging study in order to evaluate for malrotation (Table 7.1). On plain radiography, the bowel gas pattern may be assessed for evidence of obstruction as well as the presence of free air. However, plain radiography may be nonspecific or unrevealing.[1,2] The "double bubble" sign may be present and indicates duodenal obstruction, classically duodenal atresia, but it is not entirely specific for this entity. A double bubble sign may also be associated with malrotation, duodenal web, duodenal stenosis, and annular pancreas, and these entities may coexist.[3,4] The true or classic "double bubble" appearance is produced by air-filled dilated proximal duodenum and stomach, usually associated with lack of bowel gas more distally.[3,5] Visualizing a "double bubble" on plain radiography and a lack of distal bowel gas suggests duodenal obstruction, and further investigation and/or pediatric surgical consultation is indicated.

UPPER GASTROINTESTINAL SERIES

Many authors and the American College of Radiology appropriateness guidelines (Table 7.1) advocate that the presence of a classic "double bubble" (two gas bubbles, the second bubble large and round, to the right of the spine) in a newborn, especially 2 days old or younger, on plain radiography should prompt surgical consultation, and further workup is not indicated,[1,6] since duodenal obstruction with duodenal dilatation indicates a surgical lesion. However, if a double bubble appearance is seen in an infant with associated prematurity or other congenital anomalies such as congenital heart disease that will delay surgery, then UGI may be indicated to evaluate whether an emergent indication for surgery such as malrotation is present. UGI is also employed when the etiology of the emesis is not clear, such as when a classic double bubble sign is not present. Duodenal obstruction may be suggested on a UGI when a dilated proximal duodenum and duodenal obstruction to passage of contrast on UGI are seen.[7] Expertise in the performance and interpretation of this imaging test is required to produce a meaningful study.

ULTRASOUND (US)

Polyhydramnios is present in roughly 80% of patients with duodenal atresia.[1,3,8,9] The combination of polyhydramnios, a dilated stomach, and a dilated duodenal bulb on prenatal US is suggestive of duodenal obstruction, most commonly duodenal atresia, but this may be difficult to visualize.[1] Other causes of duodenal obstruction, such as annular pancreas, may be seen with US.[1,10,11] US is useful to evaluate upper gastrointestinal tract anatomy in infants with esophageal atresia and suspected duodenal obstruction, as plain radiography has limited utility and UGI cannot be performed with a discontinuous esophagus. US can be utilized to evaluate for malrotation and volvulus, using the position of the transverse duodenum, mesenteric vessel orientation (superior mesenteric artery and vein), and the whirlpool sign seen with volvulus (see chapter on Malrotation)[1,11–13] US may also be used when evaluating an infant with non-bilious emesis and concern for pyloric stenosis.

Table 7.1   American College of Radiology Appropriateness Criteria:® Vomiting in Infants*

Procedure	Appropriateness Category	Relative Radiation Level
Variant 1	**Vomiting within the first 2 days after birth. Poor feeding or no passage of meconium. Initial imaging.**	
Radiography abdomen	Usually appropriate	☢☢
US abdomen (UGI tract)	Usually not appropriate	O
Fluoroscopy contrast enema	Usually not appropriate	☢☢☢☢
Fluoroscopy upper GI series	Usually not appropriate	☢☢☢
Nuclear medicine gastroesophageal reflux scan	Usually not appropriate	☢☢☢
Variant 2	**Vomiting within the first 2 days after birth. Radiographs show classic double bubble or triple bubble with little or no gas distally (suspected proximal bowel obstruction or atresia). Next imaging study.**	
Fluoroscopy upper GI series	May be appropriate	☢☢☢
US abdomen (UGI tract)	Usually not appropriate	O
Fluoroscopy contrast enema	Usually not appropriate	☢☢☢☢
Nuclear medicine gastroesophageal reflux scan	Usually not appropriate	☢☢☢
Variant 4	**Bilious vomiting within the first 2 days after birth. Radiographs show a nonclassic double bubble with gas in the distal small bowel, or few distended bowel loops, or a normal bowel gas pattern. Next imaging study.**	
Fluoroscopy upper GI series	Usually appropriate	☢☢☢
US abdomen (UGI tract)	May be appropriate	O
Fluoroscopy contrast enema	Usually not appropriate	☢☢☢☢
Nuclear medicine gastroesophageal reflux scan	Usually not appropriate	☢☢☢
Variant 5	**Bilious vomiting in an infant older than 2 days (suspected malrotation). Initial imaging.**	
Fluoroscopy upper GI series	Usually appropriate	☢☢☢
US abdomen (UGI tract)	May be appropriate	O
Radiography abdomen	May be appropriate (disagreement)	☢☢
Fluoroscopy contrast enema	Usually not appropriate	☢☢☢☢
Nuclear medicine gastroesophageal reflux scan	Usually not appropriate	☢☢☢

Adapted from the Expert Panel on Pediatric Imaging. Alazraki AL, Rigsby CK, Iyer RS, et al. American College of Radiology ACR Appropriateness Criteria®
vomiting in infants. https://acsearch.acr.org/docs/69445/Narrative/
*ACR Appropriateness Criteria® content is updated regularly and users should go to the website (https://www.acr.org/Clinical-Resources/ACR-Appropriateness-Criteria)
   to access the most current and complete version of the Appropriateness Criteria®.
GI, Gastrointestinal; *UGI*, upper gastrointestinal series; *US*, ultrasound.

COMPUTED TOMOGRAPHY (CT)

This modality is not a first-line imaging modality in infants with emesis or suspected duodenal obstruction.

MAGNETIC RESONANCE IMAGING (MRI)

This modality is not a first-line imaging modality in infants with emesis or suspected duodenal obstruction.

Imaging Findings

Plain abdominal radiography was obtained (two views—supine and left lateral decubitus). There was abnormal gas distention of the stomach and the proximal duodenum, without gas noted elsewhere within the intestines. No free air was noted. This is consistent with a "double bubble" configuration (Figs. 7.1 and 7.2).

Case Conclusion

Pediatric surgery was consulted. While there was suspicion for duodenal atresia, this infant was 4 days old and did not have emesis reported with the first feed, and a UGI series was recommended. This was obtained, and selected images are provided here. UGI demonstrated a patent pyloric channel with contrast immediately emptying into a very dilated duodenal bulb. However, no contrast emptied from the duodenal bulb into the descending duodenum and beyond. The duodenal bulb remained distended throughout the exam. The findings are consistent with complete duodenal obstruction distal to the duodenal bulb (Figs. 7.3 and 7.4).

The patient was taken to the operating suite and found to have an annular pancreas, collapsed distal duodenum, and a duodenal web just distal to the annular pancreas. There was also note of a near obstructing Meckel diverticulum. The patient underwent a duodenoduodenostomy and resection of the Meckel diverticulum. This procedure was

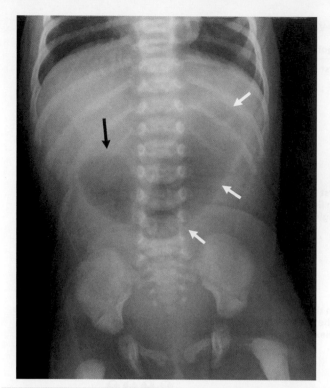

Fig. 7.1 Abdominal radiography demonstrates an abnormal gas pattern, with gas seen in the stomach *(white arrows)* and in a very dilated duodenum *(black arrow)*, the latter on the patient's right, to the right of the spine. These findings are that of a true, classic "double bubble." On this supine view, gas is seen in both the stomach and duodenum.

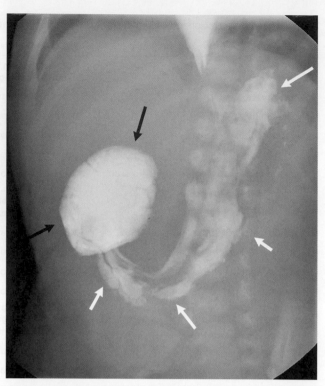

Fig. 7.3 Upper gastrointestinal series shows contrast to empty from the stomach *(white arrows)* into the dilated proximal duodenum *(black arrows)*. No contrast is seen to empty from the proximal duodenum into the mid to distal duodenum or beyond. These findings are consistent with complete duodenal obstruction at a level just distal to the duodenal bulb.

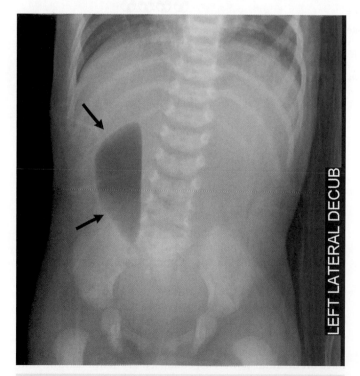

Fig. 7.2 On this left lateral decubitus view, gas has moved into the dilated duodenum *(black arrows)*, with an air fluid level in the duodenum. No gas is seen in the intestines beyond the dilated proximal duodenum, and no free air is noted.

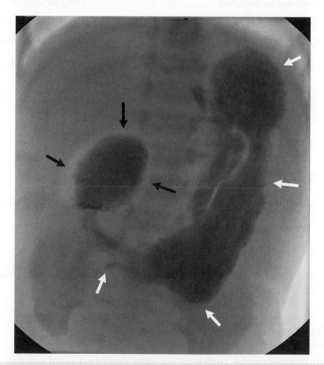

Fig. 7.4 Upper gastrointestinal series shows contrast to empty from the stomach *(white arrows)* into the dilated proximal duodenum *(black arrows)*. No contrast is seen to empty from the proximal duodenum into the mid to distal duodenum or beyond. These findings are consistent with complete duodenal obstruction at a level just distal to the duodenal bulb.

tolerated well. A thorough evaluation for any coexisting medical conditions, including cardiac, was performed and none were found.

Vomiting in the pediatric patient has a variety of etiologies. Vomiting can be categorized as:[14]

1. Acute—The cause of acute vomiting may be due to infectious causes (such as viral gastroenteritis), surgical causes (such as bowel obstruction, intestinal malrotation, testicular or ovarian torsion, and appendicitis), metabolic causes (inborn errors of metabolism), intracranial causes (hemorrhage, hydrocephalus, or mass), traumatic causes, ingested foreign body, migraines, or food-protein allergies.
2. Chronic—Chronic vomiting is defined as emesis in a timeframe of days to weeks, is rarely voluminous, and is rarely associated with dehydration. Causes to consider include gastroesophageal reflux disease, food allergies, or gallbladder disease.
3. Cyclic—Cyclic vomiting is characterized by acute periods of emesis interspersed with asymptomatic periods. Cyclic vomiting tends to be stereotypical and repetitive. Causes include cyclic vomiting syndrome, which is a migraine variant.

The age of the child is extremely useful in constructing a differential diagnosis. Common causes of emesis in the neonatal period (0 to 30 days) include the following:

Acute vomiting: Hirschsprung disease, intestinal atresia, malrotation, pyloric stenosis, food-protein-induced enterocolitis syndrome, viral illness.
Chronic vomiting: gastroesophageal reflux disease, metabolic syndromes; cyclic, gastroesophageal reflux disease, metabolic disease.[14]

While the color of emesis is not pathognomonic of any particular disease process, the presence of bile (yellow or green) should prompt immediate evaluation, as this may indicate a bowel obstruction, most emergent being malrotation with volvulus.[14] Emesis that contains bright red blood can be indicative of an active bleeding process, swallowed maternal blood, or bleeding from the nose, whereas dark blood can be indicative of a slower bleed that may be seen in gastritis.[14]

While vomiting is often associated with a gastric or intestinal process, one should not overlook the possibility of a neurologic origin. Signs of a neurologic process include increasing head circumference, visual disturbances, focal neurologic findings on physical examination, and gait disturbances; inborn errors of metabolism may also be associated with mental status changes.[14]

Annular pancreas is a well-documented cause of intestinal obstruction in pediatric patients. The incidence has been reported to be 1 in 1000 births and results from incomplete rotation of the pancreatic bud, resulting in a ring of tissue surrounding the second portion of the duodenum. Symptoms depend on the degree of encirclement: the patient may be asymptomatic or may have nonspecific symptoms or duodenal obstruction.[1,15] Presentation may be during early infancy, primarily in the neonatal period.[10,16] Chromosomal anomalies are associated with annular pancreas, as well as Meckel diverticulum.[1,16] The character of the emesis in patients with annular pancreas is often nonbilious, and the obstruction tends to be incomplete. One study found nonbilious emesis in 94% of patients with annular pancreas, as opposed to bilious

emesis rates of 80% to 90% in patients with other etiologies of duodenal obstruction.[16,17]

Management of annular pancreas involves consultation with pediatric surgery; a duodenoduodenostomy is the surgical procedure of choice. Long-term survival rates are very good and over the last several decades have improved dramatically (up to 100% in some series).[16,17]

Duodenal atresia represents one-half of congenital bowel obstructions, with an incidence of approximately 1 in 5000 to 10,000 births, and may be associated with chromosomal and other congenital anomalies, including cardiac anomalies, the VATER (Vertebral anomalies, Anal atresia, Cardiac anomalies, Tracheoesophageal fistula, Renal anomalies) association, as well as malrotation. Duodenal atresia is often associated with polyhydramnios in utero, and many patients with duodenal atresia are born prematurely.[1,3,9,18] The exact cause of duodenal atresia is not known, but there are various theories proposed. While typically isolated, familial cases have been reported.[19] The presentation of duodenal atresia may be nonspecific. The most common symptom is emesis, which is usually bilious due to obstruction distal to the ampulla of Vater. Abdominal distention is not commonly seen.[1] The timing of emesis with duodenal obstruction is often dependent on the underlying cause of the obstruction. For example, duodenal atresia usually presents with emesis within hours of initiating feeding, whereas partial duodenal obstruction may present later.[1]

The management of duodenal atresia involves consultation with a pediatric surgeon. Gastric decompression and appropriate fluid resuscitation should be performed as clinically indicated. Definitive management is surgical repair, and as with annular pancreas, the procedure of choice is duodenoduodenostomy. Survival rates are very good, approximately 90%; mortality is usually related to comorbidities from associated anomalies or ultrashort gut syndrome.[1,3,18]

IMAGING PEARLS

1. Plain radiography is employed as a first-line imaging modality in patients, particularly infants, with emesis in which an abdominal surgical cause is suspected.
2. The presence of a "double bubble" is suggestive of a duodenal obstruction. An infant with a "double bubble" sign on plain abdominal radiography who has bilious emesis requires pediatric surgical consultation, and further imaging may or may not be indicated. This can be determined by the pediatric surgeon.
3. A UGI series is the next recommended imaging test in infants with suspected duodenal obstruction in whom further imaging has been deemed necessary. A UGI series can help determine if immediate operative intervention (such as with malrotation and volvulus) or if urgent elective surgery (such as with duodenal atresia) is indicated.
4. US can be useful in the prenatal period to detect signs of duodenal obstruction. In the postnatal period, while US is excellent at detecting pyloric stenosis, it is less useful in detecting duodenal obstruction or malrotation/volvulus.
5. CT and MRI are not first-line imaging modalities used to evaluate neonates/infants with emesis.

References

1. Brinkley MF, Tracy ET, Maxfield CM. Congenital duodenal obstruction: causes and imaging approach. *Pediatr Radiol.* 2016;46(8):1084-1095.
2. Maxfield CM, Bartz BH, Shaffer JL. A pattern-based approach to bowel obstruction in the newborn. *Pediatr Radiol.* 2013;43(3): 318-329.
3. Morris G, Kennedy Jr A, Cochran W. Small bowel congenital anomalies: a review and update. *Curr Gastroenterol Rep.* 2016;18(4):16.
4. Thurkal C, Freedman SD. Annular pancreas. In: *Up To Date.* 2020. Accessed March 9, 2020.
5. Correia-Pinto J, Ribeiro A. Congenital duodenal obstruction and double-bubble sign. *N Engl J Med.* 2014;371(11): e16.
6. Traubici J. The double bubble sign. *Radiology.* 2001 Aug;220(2): 463-464.
7. Benya EC. Pancreas and biliary system: imaging of developmental anomalies and diseases unique to children. *Radiol Clin North Am.* 2002;40(6):1355-1362.
8. Pauer HU, Viereck V, Krauss V, et al. Incidence of fetal malformations in pregnancies complicated by oligo- and polyhydramnios. *Arch Gynecol Obstet.* 2003;268(1):52-56.
9. Poki HO, Holland AJ, Pitkin J. Double bubble, double trouble. *Pediatr Surg Int.* 2005;21(6):428-431.
10. McCollum MO, Jamieson DH, Webber EM. Annular pancreas and duodenal stenosis. *J Pediatr Surg.* 2002;37(12):1776-1777.
11. Schmidt H, Abolmaali N, Vogl TJ. Double bubble sign. *Eur Radiol.* 2002;12(7):1849-1853.
12. Yousefzadeh DK. The position of the duodenojejunal junction: the wrong horse to bet on in diagnosing or excluding malrotation. *Pediatr Radiol.* 2009;39(suppl 2):S172-S177.
13. Menten R, Reding R, Godding V, et al. Sonographic assessment of the retroperitoneal position of the third portion of the duodenum: an indicator of normal intestinal rotation. *Pediatr Radiol.* 2012;42(8):941-945.
14. Shields TM, Lightdale JR. Vomiting in children. *Pediatr Rev.* 2018;39(7): 342-358.
15. Zyromski NJ, Sandoval JA, Pitt HA, et al. Annular pancreas: dramatic differences between children and adults. *J Am Coll Surg.* 2008;206(5): 1019-1025.
16. Jimenez JC, Emil S, Podnos Y, et al. Annular pancreas in children: a recent decade's experience. *J Pediatr Surg.* 2004;39(11):1654-1657.
17. Sencan A, Mir E, Gunsar C, et al. Symptomatic annular pancreas in newborns. *Med Sci Monit.* 2002;8(6):434-437.
18. Escobar MA, Ladd AP, Grosfeld JL, et al. Duodenal atresia and stenosis: long-term follow-up over 30 years. *J Pediatr Surg.* 2004;39(6): 867-871.
19. Gahukamble DB, Khamage AS, Shaheen AQ. Duodenal atresia: its occurrence in siblings. *J Pediatr Surg.* 1994;29(12):1599-1600.

8 Cyanotic and Acyanotic Congenital Heart Disease

ROBERT VEZZETTI, MD, FAAP, FACEP

Case Presentation

A 12-hour-old infant presents "looking blue" and with poor feeding per the mother. The child was delivered at home and the mother had no prenatal care. She describes her pregnancy as uneventful. The physical examination reveals an overall well-appearing infant who is afebrile. There is a heart rate of 150 beats per minute, a respiratory rate of 60 breaths per minute, a blood pressure of 68/48 mm Hg, and a pulse oximetry reading of 85% on room air. The lungs are clear. The cardiac examination demonstrates regular rate and rhythm with a harsh III/VI systolic ejection murmur that is difficult to localize in the chest. Capillary refill is approximately 2–3 seconds with 2+ pulses in all extremities.

Intravenous access is difficult to obtain and umbilical artery catheters are placed. An umbilical vein catheter was unable to be placed. Intravenous fluids are ordered, blood is drawn for laboratory tests, antibiotics are ordered, and prostaglandin is ordered to the bedside. Oxygen was administered.

Imaging Considerations

PLAIN RADIOGRAPHY

Chest radiography (chest x-ray [CXR]) is utilized as first-line imaging in patients with congenital heart disease (CHD) or in patients ultimately diagnosed with this condition, since the initial symptoms of CHD may mimic respiratory pathology (i.e., tachypnea, hypoxia, crackles, retractions, wheezing). Chest radiography has been found to have a low sensitivity for structural heart disease (26%–59%), a negative predictive value of 46%–52%, and a lower sensitivity in premature infants, less than 35 weeks' gestation.[1] The use of chest radiography as a routine screening test for CHD is not supported, and patients with unremarkable radiography in the clinical context of suspected CHD should have echocardiography.[1] The performance of CXR in the detection of cardiac enlargement in pediatric patients has been compared to a gold standard of cardiac enlargement by echocardiography. CXR was found to have high specificity and negative predictive value (92.3% and 91.1%, respectively) for cardiac enlargement, but low sensitivity and positive predictive value (58.8% and 62.5%, respectively).[2] The identification of cardiomegaly by plain chest radiography in adults has also been shown to have low sensitivity (40%) but high specificity (91%).[3] The cardiothoracic ratio has been used as a marker for cardiac size in adult and pediatric patients; in adult patients, a cardiothoracic ratio greater than 0.55 has been shown to correlate with an increased risk of death.[4]

Plain chest radiography, however, does have value. Causes of respiratory distress, such as pneumonia or pneumothorax, can be detected by this modality. Additionally, ionizing radiation exposure is minimal, sedation is not required, and radiographic imaging is rapid and readily available.

COMPUTED TOMOGRAPHY (CT)

This noninvasive modality is useful to image vascular and extracardiac structures, especially those with limited visualization on echocardiography.[5,6] CT angiography has been utilized to visualize cardiac anatomy, the coronary arteries, and other vascular structures.[7] CT angiography is very useful in evaluating major arteries and veins, the aortic arch, and vascular rings.[5] The relationship of vascular and airway structures can also be evaluated.[5,6] Compared to cardiac magnetic resonance imaging (MRI), CT angiography has superior spatial resolution (allowing for more detailed visualization of small vessels), is preferred when there are airway or pulmonary abnormalities, and may be used in patients in whom MRI may be contraindicated, such as patients with a pacemaker, internal defibrillator, or aneurysm clip.[7]

CT does involve exposure to ionizing radiation and use of intravenous contrast material. While sedation is generally not necessary, it may at times be needed. CT is a readily available modality and can rapidly produce useful images for diagnosis and management, but CT for CHD should be performed and interpreted by those with expertise in pediatric CT imaging for CHD to obtain a diagnostic study and a meaningful interpretation.

MAGNETIC RESONANCE IMAGING

MRI and magnetic resonance angiography (MRA) have proven to be excellent imaging modalities for patients with CHD, in both preoperative and postoperative patients. MRI can be utilized to assess anatomy and physiologic function and has the ability to assess for multiple conditions, including tetralogy of Fallot (TOF), transposition of the great vessels, single ventricle physiology, cardiac tumors, myocarditis, and cardiomyopathies.[5,6,8–10] Not all cardiac MRI studies require intravenous contrast. Gadolinium-based contrast agents are the typical contrast agents utilized. Contrast enhancement facilitates visualization of vascular structures and allows performance of cardiac function and perfusion studies.[5] In patients with cardiomyopathies, right ventricular dysplasia, and myocarditis, contrast-enhanced MRI studies can be used to detect scarring or fibrosis.[5,11]

One disadvantage of cardiac MRI is the length of time needed to complete a study, and breath holds or sedation may be required. Some young infants may not require sedation, as they may be swaddled.[5,9,12]

ULTRASOUND (US)

Echocardiography continues to be a first-line imaging modality in pediatric patients with suspected CHD. Excellent visualization of cardiac structure, anatomy, and function can be achieved with echocardiography.[5,13] Echocardiography can be utilized to diagnose structural cardiac disease and plan for operative repair and to clinically follow patients.[5]

Imaging Findings

A single frontal view plain radiograph of the chest is obtained. There is cardiomegaly with normal pulmonary vascularity by chest radiograph. The lungs do not show focal consolidation or pneumothorax (Fig. 8.1).

Case Conclusion

The child was somewhat responsive to oxygen administration and the oxygen saturations improved. The laboratory tests were not suggestive of infection, but antibiotics were administered due to the lack of prenatal care and the possibility of sepsis. While consideration was given to a metabolic syndrome as the cause of the patient's symptoms, a cardiac etiology was also considered. An emergent echocardiogram was performed, showing anatomy consistent with TOF with an absent pulmonary valve. The patient was

admitted to the pediatric cardiac intensive care unit and consultation with pediatric cardiology and pediatric cardiothoracic surgery was obtained. Appropriate management was provided and the patient was able to be discharged from the hospital with close monitoring and follow-up. At 4 months of age, the patient had CT angiography performed, and selected images are provided here. This study demonstrates findings consistent with TOF with absent pulmonary valve, including marked dilatation of the right and left main pulmonary arteries (Fig. 8.2). Although pulmonary artery dilatation is not a common feature of TOF, it is a characteristic finding of TOF with absent pulmonary valve, due to chronic pulmonary regurgitation. CT also demonstrates an aortic coarctation just beyond the origin of the left subclavian artery (Fig. 8.3).

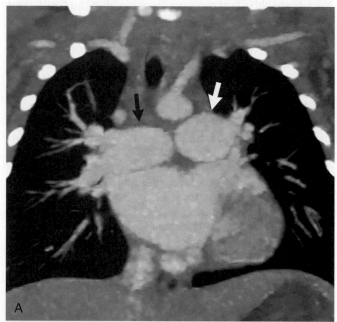

A

B

Fig. 8.2 Coronal (A) and axial (B) images from a computed tomography angiogram of the chest demonstrate marked enlargement of the right *(black arrows)* and left *(white arrows)* main pulmonary arteries. In patients such as this with tetralogy of Fallot with absent pulmonary valve, the central pulmonary arteries are enlarged due to severe pulmonary regurgitation.

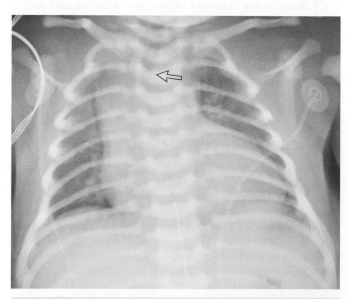

Fig. 8.1 One view (anterior-posterior) of the chest demonstrates mild cardiomegaly with normal pulmonary vascularity by plain radiograph. There is a left-sided aortic arch, the evidence of this is the bowing of the trachea toward the right *(open arrow)*, away from the side of the aortic arch. The cardiac apex is also left sided.

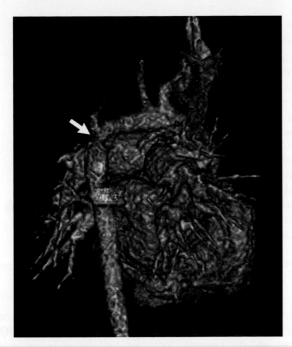

Fig. 8.3 Three-dimensional reconstruction of the computed tomography angiography study demonstrates focal constriction *(arrow)* of the proximal descending aorta, consistent with aortic coarctation.

partial pressure of oxygen (PaO_2) will not rise above 100 mm Hg (and usually remains less than 60 mm Hg).[15,16]

Another useful physical examination tool that may be implemented to ascertain if there is coarctation of the aorta or an interrupted aortic arch is the measurement of the blood pressure in the four extremities. A difference of more than 20 mm Hg between upper and lower extremity blood pressures suggests an aortic obstructive lesion between the arterial supply of the upper and lower extremities, including aortic coarctation or an interrupted aortic arch.[15,16]

Prostaglandin is an essential medication used to maintain the patency of the ductus arteriosus. Since infants with ductal-dependent heart lesions can decompensate quickly, it is essential to maintain ductal patency to stabilize the child until a definitive diagnosis can be made. Prostaglandin E1 (alprostadil) is used for this purpose in pediatric patients.[17] These substances dilate the smooth muscle of the ductus arteriosus and can be delivered through intravenous or intraosseous routes. In infants with suspected ductal-dependent CHD, initiation of prostaglandin should not be delayed. The dose is titrated to effect; one should see improvement in oxygenation (75%–85%) and pulses.[17] Potential side effects of prostaglandin administration include apnea and fever (very commonly seen); hypotension, tachycardia, lower seizure threshold, hypothermia, and cardiac arrest have been reported but are very rare.[17] The clinician should anticipate these potential adverse effects and address them appropriately.

In 2011, the Routine Universal Screening Program was implemented in the majority of states in the United States and the District of Columbia to screen newborns for critical CHD prior to discharge from the hospital.[15,18] The purpose of this program is to screen newborns for critical CHD typically discovered in the newborn period, such as critical coarctation of the aorta, TOF, truncus arteriosus, tricuspid atresia, total anomalous pulmonary venous return (TAPVR), pulmonary atresia, and transposition of the great vessels, among others, although a failed screen may also indicate a pulmonary process, such as pulmonary hypertension.[15] This screen is easily accomplished with pulse oximetry, noting differences between the extremities, and is performed after 24–48 hours of age. Infants with a failed screen should have chest radiography, an electrocardiogram (ECG), and echocardiography.[15,19] A significant percentage of infants, though, will be discharged from the hospital with undiagnosed CHD.[17]

At 6 months of age, the patient underwent repair of the cardiac defects. He was hospitalized for several weeks but did well.

The incidence of CHD is approximately 4–10 in 1000 live births.[5,14,15] The diagnosis of CHD in pediatric patients can be challenging. The presenting symptoms may mimic a variety of conditions, including viral upper respiratory infection, metabolic illness, dehydration, pneumonia, and sepsis. A history of cyanosis, increased work of breathing, and sweating or rapid tiring with feeding are concerning for a cardiac lesion. Tachypnea and hepatomegaly are signs of CHD but are not immediately present, nor present in all cases of CHD. Attention should be given to palpation of the femoral pulses. Weak or absent femoral pulses suggest coarctation of the aorta or an interrupted aortic arch.

The hyperoxia test has been used as a quick method to discern whether hypoxia in a neonate is cardiac or pulmonary in origin. The test is performed by providing 100% oxygen for at least 10 minutes. No improvement with this maneuver suggests cardiac disease; in an abnormal (positive) test, the

Cyanotic Congenital Heart Disease:

LESION	CLINICAL SIGNS	INITIAL DIAGNOSIS	MANAGEMENT
Tetralogy of Fallot VSD Overriding aorta RV outflow obstruction RV hypertrophy	Harsh pulmonary ejection murmur "Tet" spells	Echocardiogram "Tet" spells CXR—"boot"-shaped heart—not sensitive or specific; concave main pulmonary artery segment Decreased pulmonary circulation	"Tet" Spell: Calming maneuvers/O_2 IV fluids Morphine Surgical repair
Transposition of the great vessels	Cyanosis (usually early) Usually no murmur	Echocardiogram CXR—narrow superior mediastinal silhouette "egg on a string"	Surgical repair
Truncus arteriosus	Pulmonary overcirculation Loud systolic murmur	Echocardiogram CXR—pulmonary overcirculation	Diuresis Fluid restriction Surgical repair

Continued

Cyanotic Congenital Heart Disease:—cont'd

LESION	CLINICAL SIGNS	INITIAL DIAGNOSIS	MANAGEMENT
TAPVR	Cyanosis (usually early) Respiratory distress Pulmonary overload	Echocardiogram CXR—overcirculation or pulmonary venous hypertension, if severe heart failure, "whiteout" of lung fields, cardiac silhouette variable size according to type; snowman mediastinum (supracardiac TAPVR)	Surgical emergency
Hypoplastic left heart syndrome	Cyanosis as the PDA closes Poor urine output Poor pulses Mottling Respiratory distress	Echocardiography CXR—pulmonary vascular congestion Congestive heart failure Possible cardiomegaly	Initial stabilization (prostaglandin E1) Staged palliative repair

Reproduced with permission from Puri K, Allen HD, Qureshi AM. Congenital heart disease. *Pediatr Rev.* 2017 Oct;38(10):471–486.

CXR, chest x-ray; *IV*, intravenous; *PDA*, patent ductus arteriosus; *RV*, right ventricle; *TAPVR*, total anomalous pulmonary venous return; *VSD*, ventricular septal defect.

TETRALOGY OF FALLOT

TOF is the most common form of cyanotic CHD.[15] "Tet spells" are cycles of cyanosis that are associated with stress or illness. During these times, agitation or crying will increase pulmonary vascular resistance and heart rate, increasing pulmonary outflow obstruction and producing cyanotic episodes. Management of these episodes includes keeping the patient calm, administering intravenous fluids, providing oxygen in as comfortable a manner as possible ("blow by" oxygen administration, for example), and administering morphine.[15] Definitive treatment is surgical correction of heart defects, which has replaced palliative procedures, such as the Blalock-Taussig shunt. Surgical repair is usually accomplished between 3 and 11 months, usually around 6 months of age.[20] Postrepair complications include right ventricular dilation owing to postsurgical pulmonary regurgitation and the development of arrythmias, which can lead to sudden death.[15,21]

TRANSPOSITION OF THE GREAT ARTERIES (TGA)

TGA is the second most common form of cyanotic CHD.[15] TGA commonly will reveal itself during the first week of life. In this cardiac defect, the aorta arises from the right ventricle and the pulmonary artery from the left ventricle. There is usually a patent foramen ovale or atrial septal defect (ASD) that allows for blood mixing.[15] Most cases of TGA will be apparent in the first 12 hours of life, but this may be delayed if there is a ventricular septal defect (VSD).[15] Definitive management in these patients is operative repair, switching the vessels to their normal ventricular connection.[22] Postrepair complications include regurgitation of the aortic valve (>75%), supravalvar pulmonary stenosis (>75%), and coronary artery disease; up to 30% of patients require repeat surgical intervention at some point.[15,23] Like patients with TOF, these patients are followed by cardiology for the remainder of their lives.

TRUNCUS ARTERIOSUS

This cardiac defect presents early in the neonatal period. It is due to incomplete or failed division of the embryologic common truncus arteriosus into the aorta and pulmonary artery, producing pulmonary overcirculation. A VSD is nearly always present. Truncus arteriosus is associated with the deletion of 22q11.2 (DiGeorge syndrome or velocardial facial syndrome) in one-third of patients with these genetic conditions.[15] Initial management of these patients is diuresis and fluid restriction with repair performed typically within the first 2 weeks of life.[15,24]

TOTAL ANOMALOUS PULMONARY VENOUS RETURN (TAPVR)

This is an uncommon cardiac defect. Anomalous pulmonary venous return can be partial (at least one pulmonary vein returns to the left atrium) or total (no pulmonary veins return directly to the left atrium). A patent foramen ovale and/or ASD are usually present, and there is right atrial hypertension and mixing of oxygenated pulmonary venous blood with deoxygenated systemic venous blood returning to the heart.[15]

TAPVR can be obstructed or nonobstructed, depending on the anatomic arrangement of the returning veins. Obstructed anatomy leads to pulmonary venous hypertension and pulmonary edema (and this can lead to pulmonary arterial hypertension) and will manifest clinically with cyanosis and respiratory distress; nonobstructive anatomy can present more subtly with a delay in respiratory distress but cyanosis is present.[15] Administration of oxygen does not produce clinical improvement, and prostaglandin may cause worsening due to shunting of more blood at the level of the ductus arteriosus.[15] Obstructed TAPVR is a surgical emergency; nonobstructed cases may be followed closely by a pediatric cardiologist and pediatric cardiothoracic surgeon with plan for repair urgently at a later date.[15] After surgical repair, recurrence of pulmonary obstruction is around 15%.[15,25] Symptoms of recurrence of pulmonary obstruction include dyspnea, tachypnea, and wheezing.

HYPOPLASTIC LEFT HEART SYNDROME (HLHS)

This lesion has severe mitral and aortic valve stenosis or atresia, resulting in hypoplasia of the left ventricle and ascending aorta. HLHS is ductal dependent: systemic blood flow is dependent on a patent ductus arteriosus (PDA) remaining open. The natural closure of the ductus arteriosus after birth can lead to acute, life-threatening shock. Maintaining the patency of the ductus by administering prostaglandin is critical for initial stabilization of these patients and is life-saving. Surgery for HLHS is a staged palliative procedure. The palliative procedure is a single ventricle repair: the larger, functional right ventricle is converted to pump to the systemic circulation, and systemic venous return is directed to the pulmonary arteries, without an intervening ventricle. This is accomplished through staged repairs:

Stage I (Norwood procedure)—This is usually performed within the first 1–2 weeks of life. The right ventricle is converted to the systemic ventricle by disconnecting the main pulmonary artery from the right and left pulmonary arteries and creating a neoaorta, with anastomosis of the main pulmonary artery to the existing aorta, using a homograft patch to augment the proximal aorta. Blood supply to the pulmonary arteries is also supplied from the systemic circulation, using either a modified Blalock-Taussig shunt from the subclavian artery or a Sano shunt from the ventricle, to the pulmonary arteries. An ASD is also created.[15] Notably, there is mixing of oxygenated and deoxygenated blood after this procedure; this will produce "normal" oxygen saturations of usually 75%–85%, although this can be lower or higher depending on the amount of pulmonary blood flow.[15] A murmur should be heard when auscultating the chest in these patients.

Stage II (hemi-Fontan or Glenn)—Anastomosis of the superior vena cava to the pulmonary artery (pulmonary arterial system) and takedown of the Blalock-Taussig shunt are the next steps of this three-step process and is known as the Glenn procedure. The timing of this stage depends on the clinical status and symptoms that would indicate outgrowing of the stage I repair, such as decreasing oxygen saturations. Most commonly, this stage is performed around 4–6 months of age.[15] However, after this stage, oxygen saturations are usually in the 80%–85% range, owing to continued mixing of oxygenated and deoxygenated blood.

Stage III (Fontan)—The last stage in this process is the connection of the inferior vena cava (IVC) to the pulmonary arterial system, preventing the mixing of oxygenated and deoxygenated blood, termed the Fontan procedure. As with the Glenn procedure, the timing of this stage depends on clinical signs and symptoms that the patient is outgrowing their Glenn (oxygen saturation trending downward). This usually occurs around 2–4 years of age.[15] After the Fontan procedure, oxygen saturations in these patients should be approximately 95%.[15]

After single ventricle palliative repair, patients are at risk of developing right-sided heart failure or systemic heart failure,[15] given the fact they are dependent on single ventricle physiology. Signs of heart failure include tachypnea, edema, chronic cough, decreasing oral intake, and decreased activity. Long-term complications include increased risk for thromboembolism, protein losing enteropathy and plastic bronchitis (also a protein-losing pathology), and liver fibrosis.

Evaluation for pulmonary embolus (PE) in a post-Fontan patient—As these patients are at increased risk of thromboembolism, it is important to note that CT angiogram for PE or nuclear medicine perfusion scan must be performed with alterations to contrast injection technique and alteration of timing of scanning for CT, and the interpreting radiologist must have knowledge of the postrepair anatomy and hemodynamics for proper scanning protocol determination and interpretation. This avoids misinterpretation of unopacified blood from the IVC in the pulmonary arteries as PE when only upper or lower extremity injection is used. There should either be simultaneous contrast injection into the upper and lower extremity veins for nuclear medicine perfusion scan or CT pulmonary angiogram, with early and delayed scanning of the chest for CT; alternatively, there can be injection of a single extremity vein, with delayed equilibrium phase imaging of the chest for CT.[26] Alternatives for imaging include MRI and catheter pulmonary angiogram. Also, it is important to note that a temporary, "retrievable" IVC filter may be irretrievable in a post-Fontan patient, as some filters are exclusively retrievable by a jugular approach, and the filter may therefore be unable to be removed with post-Fontan venous anatomy. When evaluating a post-Fontan patient for thrombotic complications, especially PE, and especially if treatment or prophylaxis for PE is considered, consultation with the patient's cardiologist or cardiac surgeon is recommended, as is consultation with the interventional radiologist, including discussion of post-Fontan anatomy, prior to ordering IVC filter placement.

Acyanotic Congenital Heart Disease:

LESION	CLINICAL SIGNS	DIAGNOSIS	MANAGEMENT
Ventricular septal defect	Pansystolic murmur Pulmonary overcirculation	Echocardiogram CXR—cardiomegaly, pulmonary overcirculation ECG (ventricular hypertrophy)	Diuretics (if indicated) Nutritional support Surgical repair if indicated, some close spontaneously
ASD	Pulmonic murmur Fixed split S_2 CHF (with associated lesions)	Echocardiogram CXR—right atrium/ventricle enlargement, pulmonary overcirculation	Surgical repair if indicated Some close spontaneously

Continued

Acyanotic Congenital Heart Disease:—cont'd

LESION	CLINICAL SIGNS	DIAGNOSIS	MANAGEMENT
Aortic (AS) or pulmonary (PS) valve stenosis	Systolic ejection murmur	Echocardiogram ECG (ventricular hypertrophy) CXR—Poststenotic dilatation of ascending aorta (AS) or main and left main pulmonary arteries (PS)	Balloon valvuloplasty Surgical valvotomy Valve replacement surgery Surgical autograft
Coarctation of the aorta	Poor lower extremity pulses Shock mimicking sepsis Gradient difference between upper and lower extremity BP Harsh murmur over the back	Echocardiogram, CTA, MRI/MRA CXR—"3" sign of proximal descending aorta, collateral vessel effects, including rib notching (after age 6) of inferior 3rd–8th ribs	Initial stabilization (prostaglandin E1) Surgical repair

VSD and ASD lesions may not be detectable on plain chest radiography but are readily detected by echocardiography.
Reproduced with permission from Puri K, Allen HD, Qureshi AM. Congenital heart disease. *Pediatr Rev.* 2017 Oct;38(10):471–486.
ASD, Atrial septal defect; *CHF,* congestive heart failure; *CTA,* computed tomography angiography; *CXR,* chest x-ray; *ECG,* electrocardiogram; *MRA,* magnetic resonance angiography; *MRI,* magnetic resonance imaging; *VSD,* ventricular septal defect.

VENTRICULAR SEPTAL DEFECT

This is the most common CHD, accounting for up to 60% of cases, and most are perimembranous.[15] Initially, patients may be asymptomatic, but a pansystolic murmur may be heard as the pulmonary vascular resistance decreases and left to right shunting develops. Patients with a hemodynamically significant VSD may present with congestive heart failure due to pulmonary overload.[15] Many of these lesions will close on their own. Patients with a significant VSD (failure to thrive or evidence of left ventricular or atrial enlargement) may be managed with appropriate diuretics and nutritional support. For symptomatic patients with a persistent VSD, repair is accomplished with a surgical patch or, in some cases, using cardiac catheterization techniques.

ATRIAL SEPTAL DEFECT

These cardiac defects account for approximately 10% of CHD.[15] There are various types of ASD, but secundum ASD is the most common.[15,27] The presence of an ASD causes left to right shunting of blood, increasing the diastolic volume in the right ventricle, leading to dilation. If there are other associated cardiac lesions, congestive heart failure may be present. A secundum ASD is repaired surgically with direct closure or a patch, which is usually done around 3–4 years of age.[15,28]

ATRIOVENTRICULAR (AV) SEPTAL DEFECTS

These defects are also known as AV canal defects and are very commonly seen in patients with Down syndrome, seen in up to 50% of patients.[15] These patients will have cardiac murmurs and may present in congestive heart failure in some cases; failure to thrive may also be seen.[15] As with a VSD, diuretics and nutritional management play an early role. Surgical repair usually is accomplished at 3–4 months of age, depending on the presence of congestive heart failure, in which case repair may be undertaken earlier.[15]

VALVULAR STENOSIS

Aortic and pulmonary valve stenosis account for approximately 10% of CHDs.[15] In addition to obstruction of blood flow, there may be associated regurgitation. Management depends on the degree of stenosis. Patients with critical

stenosis require balloon valvuloplasty in the newborn period.[15,26] Definitive repair, though, is dependent on valve gradient measurement guidelines.[15,26] Patients who had valvuloplasty for critical stenosis require reintervention approximately 50% of the time and approximately 30% of the time for noncritical stenosis.[15,29]

COARCTATION OF THE AORTA

Coarctation results from narrowing of the aorta and, in extreme cases, interruption of the aortic arch. The majority of patients with coarctation have an associated VSD.[15] While blood pressure difference and unequal femoral pulses are classically described, older patients with noncritical coarctation may not have a significant blood pressure difference due to the formation of collateral circulation.[18] Patients with critical coarctation require initiation of prostaglandin while awaiting surgical repair. Definitive management is surgical in most infants, but older children may be candidates for balloon angioplasty and stent placement in the catheterization laboratory.[15]

A comparison case is provided here:

A 3-year-old girl presented with a murmur on physical examination, without cyanosis. Chest radiography demonstrated cardiomegaly, increased pulmonary blood flow, and an enlarged main pulmonary artery segment (Figs. 8.4 and 8.5). Echocardiogram was performed and showed an ASD and a PDA.

IMAGING PEARLS

1. Plain radiography is a first-line imaging modality in patients with suspected cardiac disease but is not sensitive or specific. However, it is useful to evaluate for pulmonary conditions, such as pneumonia, pneumothorax, and pulmonary edema.
2. There are times when plain radiography may suggest a cardiac lesion. However, if plain radiographs are unremarkable and there is suspicion for a cardiac lesion, echocardiography should be performed.
3. Echocardiography is indicated in patients with suspected cardiac defects.
4. Advanced imaging, such as CT angiography, and cardiac MRI are complementary modalities to echocardiography.

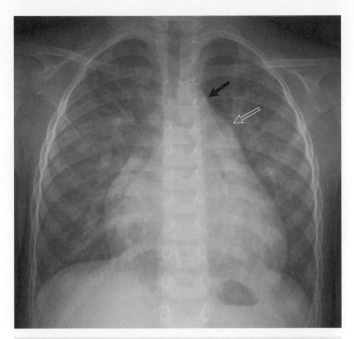

Fig. 8.4 Frontal view of the chest in a 3-year-old with a murmur demonstrates cardiomegaly and prominent pulmonary vessels consistent with increased pulmonary blood flow. There is a left-sided aortic arch *(black arrow)* and an enlarged main pulmonary artery *(open white arrow)*. Echocardiogram demonstrated an atrial septal defect and a patent ductus arteriosus, both acyanotic left to right shunt lesions contributing to increased pulmonary blood flow.

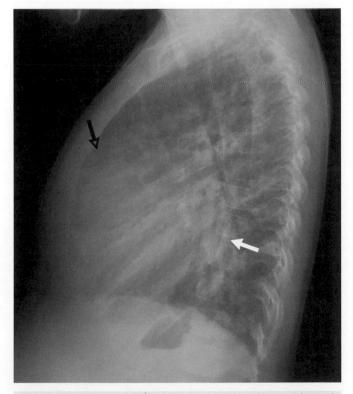

Fig. 8.5 Lateral view of the chest in a 3-year-old with an atrial septal defect and a patent ductus arteriosus shows cardiomegaly and increased pulmonary blood flow. The enlargement of the right heart is seen anteriorly *(open black arrow)* and cardiomegaly causes the posterior heart border to extend abnormally far posteriorly, to overlie the spine *(white arrow)*.

References

1. Fonseca B, Chang RK, Senac M, et al. Chest radiography and evaluation of the neonate for congenital heart disease. *Pediatr Cardiol.* 2005;26(4):361-372.
2. Satou GM, Lacro RV, Chung T, et al. Heart size on chest x-ray as a predictor of cardiac enlargement by echocardiography in children. *Pediatr Cardiol.* 2001;22(3):218-222.
3. McKee JL, Ferrier K. Is cardiomegaly on chest radiograph representative of true cardiomegaly: a cross-sectional observational study comparing cardiac size on chest radiograph to that on echocardiography. *N Z Med J.* 2017;130(1464):57-63.
4. Grotenhuis HB, Zhiou C, Tomlinson G, et al. Cardiothoracic ratio on chest radiograph in pediatric heart disease: how does it correlate with heart volumes at magnetic resonance imaging? *Pediatr Radiol.* 2015;45(11):1616-1623.
5. Opfer E, Shah S. Advances in pediatric cardiovascular imaging. *Mo Med.* 2018;115(4):354-360.
6. Mortensen KH, Tann O. Computed tomography in paediatric heart disease. *Br J Radiol.* 2018;91(1092):20180201.
7. Siripornpitak S, Pornkul R, Khowsathit P, et al. Cardiac CT angiography in children with congenital heart disease. *Eur J Radiol.* 2013;82(7):1067-1082.
8. Ntsinjana HN, Hughes ML, Taylor AM. The role of cardiovascular magnetic resonance in pediatric congenital heart disease. *J Cardiovasc Magn Reson.* 2011;13(1):51.
9. Kellenberger CJ, Yoo SJ, Büchel ER. Cardiovascular MR imaging in neonates and infants with congenital heart disease. *Radiographics.* 2007;27(1):5-18.
10. Dillman JR, Hernandez RJ. Role of CT in the evaluation of congenital cardiovascular disease in children. *AJR Am J Roentgenol.* 2009;192:1219-1231.
11. Franco A, Javidi S, Ruehm SG. Delayed myocardial enhancement in cardiac magnetic resonance imaging. *J Radiol Case Rep.* 2015;9(6):6-18.
12. Windram J, Grosse-Wortmann L, Shariat M, et al. Cardiovascular MRI without sedation or general anesthesia using a feed-and-sleep technique in neonates and infants. *Pediatr Radiol.* 2012;42(2):183-187.
13. Lai WW, Geva T, Shirali GS, et al. Guidelines and standards for performance of a pediatric echocardiogram: a report from the Task Force of the Pediatric Council of the American Society of Echocardiography. *J Am Soc Echocardiogr.* 2006 ;19(12):1413-1430.
14. Marelli AJ, Mackie AS, Ionescu-Ittu R, et al. Congenital heart disease in the general population: changing prevalence and age distribution. *Circulation.* 2007;115(2):163-172.
15. Puri K, Allen HD, Qureshi AM. Congenital heart disease. *Pediatr Rev.* 2017;38(10):471-486.
16. Hashim MJ, Guillet R. Common issues in the care of sick neonates. *Am Fam Physician.* 2002;66(9):1685-1692.
17. Singh Y, Mikrou P. Use of prostaglandins in duct-dependent congenital heart conditions. *Arch Dis Child Educ Pract Ed.* 2018;103(3):137-140.
18. Oster ME, Aucott SW, Glidewell J, et al. Lessons learned from newborn screening for critical congenital heart defects. *Pediatrics.* 2016;137(5):e20154573.
19. Mahle WT, Newburger JW, Matherne GP, et al; American Heart Association Congenital Heart Defects Committee of the Council on Cardiovascular Disease in the Young, Council on Cardiovascular Nursing, and Interdisciplinary Council on Quality of Care and Outcomes Research; American Academy of Pediatrics Section on Cardiology and Cardiac Surgery; Committee on Fetus and Newborn. Role of pulse oximetry in examining newborns for congenital heart disease: a scientific statement from the AHA and AAP. *Pediatrics.* 2009;124(2):823-836.
20. Van Arsdell GS, Maharaj GS, Tom, J, et al. What is the optimal age of repair of tetralogy of Fallot? *Circulation.* 2000;102(19 suppl 3):123-129.
21. Valente AM, Gauvreau K, Assenza GE, et al. Rationale and design of an International Multicenter Registry of patients with repaired tetralogy of Fallot to define risk factors for late adverse outcomes: the INDICATOR cohort. *Pediatr Cardiol.* 2013;34(1):95-104.
22. Villafañe J, Lantin-Hermoso MR, Bhatt AB, et al; American College of Cardiology's Adult Congenital and Pediatric Cardiology Council. D-transposition of the great arteries: the current era of the arterial switch operation. *J Am Coll Cardiol.* 2014;64(5):498-511.

23. Michalak KW, Moll JA, Sobczak-Budlewska K, et al. Reoperations and catheter interventions in patients with transposition of the great arteries after the arterial switch operation. *Eur J Cardiothorac Surg.* 2017;51(1):34-42.

24. Naimo PS, Fricke TA, Yong MS, et al. Outcomes of truncus arteriosus repair in children: 35 years of experience from a single institution. *Semin Thorac Cardiovasc Surg.* 2016;28(2):500-511.

25. Husain SA, Maldonado E, Rasch D, et al. Total anomalous pulmonary venous connection: factors associated with mortality and recurrent pulmonary venous obstruction. *Ann Thorac Surg.* 2012;94(3):825-831.

26. Mahani MA, Argawal PP, Rigsby CK, et al. CT for assessment of thrombosis and pulmonary embolism in multiple stages of single-ventricle palliation: challenges and suggested protocols. *Radiographics.* 2016;36(5):1273-1284.

27. Feltes TF, Bacha E, Beekman RH III, et al; American Heart Association Congenital Cardiac Defects Committee of the Council on Cardiovascular Disease in the Young; Council on Clinical Cardiology; Council on Cardiovascular Radiology and Intervention; American Heart Association. Indications for cardiac catheterization and intervention in pediatric cardiac disease: a scientific statement from the American Heart Association. *Circulation.* 2011;123(22): 2607-2652.

28. Knepp MD, Rocchini AP, Lloyd TR, et al. Long-term follow up of secundum atrial septal defect closure with the Amplatzer septal occluder. *Congenit Heart Dis.* 2010;5(1):32-37.

29. Pedra CA, Sidhu R, McCrindle BW, et al. Outcomes after balloon dilation of congenital aortic stenosis in children and adolescents. *Cardiol Young.* 2004;14(3):315-321.

9 More Than Constipation: Failure to Pass Meconium

ROBERT VEZZETTI, MD, FAAP, FACEP

Case Presentation

A 2-day-old patient is referred to the emergency department for failure to pass meconium. He was born at home and had prenatal care, although this was not consistent, as the mother had missed some of her appointments. The delivery was at term (38 weeks gestation), vaginal, and apparently uncomplicated. The infant was vigorous and did not require resuscitation other than standard drying and stimulation. The mother's serologies were negative. He has been breastfeeding for 10–15 minutes' total time, approximately every 2–3 hours. He appears to feed well. He has had some small voids.

Physical examination reveals an afebrile, vigorous child. Heart rate is 150 beats per minute, respiratory rate is 30 breaths per minute, and a blood pressure is 75/50 mm Hg. He has an overall normal examination, but there is abdominal fullness. There is no hepatosplenomegaly, apparent tenderness, or discoloration of the abdomen. He has a patent anus and appears to have decreased rectal tone with digital rectal examination.

Imaging Considerations

PLAIN RADIOGRAPHY

Plain radiography is an excellent first-line imaging modality in patients where a bowel obstruction, either mechanical or functional, is suspected. It is the initial imaging modality typically used in the evaluation of patients with suspected meconium ileus or meconium plug syndrome.[1] In patients with suspected Hirschsprung disease, radiographs of the abdomen may demonstrate marked gaseous distension of the colon with an undilated rectum with a transition zone in-between.[1,2] This modality has the advantage of detecting free air and calcifications and evaluating bowel gas patterns.

CONTRAST ENEMA

After initial plain radiography is performed, contrast enema with water-soluble iodinated contrast is the imaging modality of choice for further evaluation of the newborn with failure to pass meconium and/or abdominal distension and dilated bowel loops suggestive of lower gastrointestinal obstruction. Water-soluble enema can be therapeutic for meconium ileus and immature left colon syndrome (also called small left colon syndrome or meconium plug syndrome).[1] An enema for this indication should only be performed by a pediatric radiologist or a radiologist otherwise experienced in neonatal fluoroscopy, as there is a risk of bowel perforation.

COMPUTED TOMOGRAPHY (CT)

In neonates with failure to pass meconium and suspected bowel obstruction, CT is not utilized.

ULTRASOUND (US)

Prenatal sonography can show findings of gastrointestinal obstruction, including findings suggestive of meconium ileus and Hirschsprung disease. However, ultrasound is generally not utilized as a first-line study in the evaluation of newborns with failure to pass meconium.

Imaging Findings

The history of delayed passage of meconium was concerning in this child. Plain abdominal radiography was obtained. These images demonstrated a very abnormal bowel gas pattern, with dilated bowel loops suggestive of a distal small bowel or proximal colonic obstruction, very suspicious for meconium ileus considering the mottled soap bubble-like appearance of gas in the right abdomen (Fig. 9.1).

Case Conclusion

The child was admitted to the neonatal intensive care unit; multiple subspecialists, including pediatric surgery, pediatric gastroenterology, and medical genetics, were consulted. The patient underwent a contrast enema, which demonstrated a nondilated and patent, but empty, colon, with reflux of contrast into nondilated distal ileum, without meconium in the visualized distal ileum. As differential considerations included total colonic Hirschsprung disease, a rectal biopsy was performed, revealing no ganglion cells in the rectum. Further evaluation showed no ganglion cells in the colon, or ileum. At surgery, the transition zone was in the distal jejunum/proximal ileum. This was consistent with long-segment Hirschsprung disease. A distal jejunostomy was created with a total abdominal colectomy and ileal resection, as well as a Hartmann pouch of the rectum; the child ultimately had a pull-through procedure. He has had a difficult clinical course, with several admissions for enterocolitis and dehydration. The child underwent genetic testing and was found to have a genetic profile consistent with long-segment Hirschsprung disease.

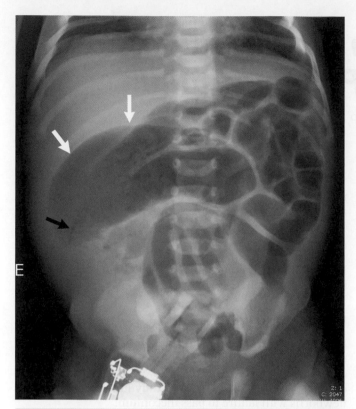

Fig. 9.1 Supine view of the abdomen demonstrates tubular, dilated, gas-filled bowel loops throughout most of the abdomen, with a markedly distended bowel loop in the right upper quadrant *(white arrows)*. It is difficult to distinguish the small bowel from the colon in a neonate, but the appearance suggests a distal small bowel or proximal colonic obstruction. The appearance is suspicious for meconium ileus considering the mottled bubbly appearance of gas in the right abdomen, which appears to be gas contained in intraluminal contents *(black arrow)*.

When a neonate fails to pass meconium, cystic fibrosis with meconium ileus, Hirschsprung disease, and meconium plug syndrome should be considered as possible etiologies, but metabolic disorders (thyroid disease), genetic disorders (Down syndrome), and intestinal disorders (e.g., intestinal atresia) are also in the differential diagnosis. Meconium ileus is a functional obstruction at the level of the terminal ileum that is caused by inspissated meconium.[3-6] Immature left colon syndrome (small left colon or meconium plug syndrome) is a benign cause of functional large bowel obstruction in the neonatal period that presents with delayed passage of meconium. A water-soluble contrast enema is often needed for resolution, although meconium plug syndrome can resolve on its own.[1,7] In most cases, after the therapeutic effect of the enema, there are no further issues.[1]

Imaging in meconium ileus will demonstrate a normal-length, small-caliber colon (microcolon), with inspissated meconium in the terminal ileum, and dilation of the small bowel proximal to the obstruction.[1] In patients with immature left colon syndrome, the descending colon and rectosigmoid are normal in caliber, with transition to dilated more proximal colon at the splenic flexure, and scattered pellets of meconium are seen in the colon. Almost all patients with meconium ileus will be found to have cystic

fibrosis, and repeat enemas may be necessary to treat meconium ileus. If enemas fail to relieve the obstruction, surgical management may become necessary.

Contrast enema is also the diagnostic imaging modality of choice in patients with suspected Hirschsprung disease. Findings consistent with Hirschsprung disease on enema include a normal caliber rectum and colon distal to the transition between the normally innervated colon and the more distal aganglionic segment. Bowel proximal to the transition is dilated. Rarely, Hirschsprung disease can involve the entire colon or the small bowel. Retention of contrast in the bowel 24 hours after the enema on the delayed radiograph can be seen with Hirschsprung disease or other motility disorders.[1]

Hirschsprung disease was first described in 1886. The etiology of Hirschsprung disease is due to both cellular and genetic factors, with an incidence of 1 in 5000 births.[8] Early arrest of the migration of neural-crest—derived neuroblasts to the developing intestine leads to an agangliotic segment.[1,6,8,9] This impedes the propagation of peristaltic waves due to the absence of parasympathetic intrinsic ganglion cells, causing functional obstruction.[8,10] There are multiple genetic factors that influence the development of Hirschsprung disease, and having siblings with a history of Hirschsprung disease is associated with an increased risk of the condition in subsequent children.[8,11] The majority of patients are diagnosed in the neonatal period (90%), but diagnosis may be delayed and can present outside of the neonatal period as chronic constipation.[6,8,12] In addition to delayed meconium passage, feeding intolerance, vomiting, and abdominal distention are also presenting symptoms; abdominal distention and emesis are particularly common symptoms in children with Hirschsprung disease.[8] Infants with fever, diarrhea, and abdominal distention should be carefully evaluated for Hirschsprung-associated enterocolitis, which, if not recognized and appropriately treated with fluid resuscitation, antibiotics, and emergent surgical consultation, can progress to toxic megacolon, which has a high mortality.[8,13]

The diagnosis of Hirschsprung disease can be confirmed by several methods. Initial testing is accomplished with contrast enema, anorectal manometry, and either full-thickness rectal biopsy or rectal suction biopsy. The sensitivity and specificity for Hirschsprung disease have been reported to be 65%–80% and 61%–100%, respectively, for contrast enema; 75%–100% and 85%–97%, respectively, for anal manometry; and 90%–100% for surgical diagnosis.[2,8,14]

The management of Hirschsprung disease should begin with a thorough history and physical examination. If there are signs of Hirschsprung-associated enterocolitis (fever, diarrhea, and abdominal distention), aggressive resuscitation, antibiotics, and prompt surgical consultation are indicated; this entity can occur both before and after repair and can be fatal.[6,15] Surgical repair of Hirschsprung disease has traditionally involved a several-staged repair, but one-stage transanal laparoscopic pull-through techniques have been developed and utilized as well.[6,8,16–18] Outcomes are generally good. Patients with long-segment disease and those with Down syndrome tend to have poorer outcomes.[6] Postoperative complications include early complications (wound infection, wound dehiscence, and bowel obstruction) and late complications (bowel obstruction, stricture, incontinence, and enterocolitis), but there is clinical overlap between the two.[6,8]

IMAGING PEARLS

1. Plain abdominal radiography is a good choice as an initial imaging modality in neonates with failure to pass meconium normally.
2. After plain radiography is performed, water-soluble contrast enema is the imaging modality of choice in newborns with failure to pass meconium and suspected bowel obstruction. Water-soluble enema can also be therapeutic for meconium ileus and immature left colon syndrome. This test is useful for the diagnosis of Hirschsprung disease but may be normal in some cases. Additional testing (rectal biopsy or anal manometry) may be indicated if there is a high index of suspicion for this etiology.

References

1. Carroll AG, Kavanagh RG, Ni Leidhin C, et al. Comparative effectiveness of imaging modalities for the diagnosis of intestinal obstruction in neonates and infants: a critically appraised topic. *Acad Radiol.* 2016;23(5):559-568.
2. De Lorijn F, Kremer LC, Reitsma JB, et al. Diagnostic tests in Hirschsprung disease: a systematic review. *J Pediatr Gastroenterol Nutr.* 2006;42(5):496-505.
3. Karimi A, Gorter RR, Sleeboom C, et al. Issues in the management of simple and complex meconium ileus. *Pediatr Surg Int.* 2011;27(9):963-968.
4. Gorter RR, Karimi A, Sleeboom C, et al. Clinical and genetic characteristics of meconium ileus in newborns with and without cystic fibrosis. *J Pediatr Gastroenterol Nutr.* 2010;50(5):569-572.
5. Wood KE. Meconium ileus in a neonate with cystic fibrosis. *N Engl J Med.* 2018;378(12):1142.
6. Langer JC. Hirschsprung disease. *Curr Opin Pediatr.* 2013;25(3):368-374.
7. Cuenca AG, Ali AS, Kays DW, et al. "Pulling the plug"—management of meconium plug syndrome in neonates. *J Surg Res.* 2012;15:175(2):e43-e46.
8. Haricharan RN, Georgeson KE. Hirschsprung disease. *Semin Pediatr Surg.* 2008;17(4):266-275.
9. Tam PK, Garcia-Barcelo M. Molecular genetics of Hirschsprung's disease. *Semin Pediatr Surg.* 2004;13(4):236-248.
10. Swenson O. Hirschsprung's disease: a review. *Pediatrics.* 2002;109(5):914-918.
11. Amiel J, Sproat-Emison E, Garcia-Barcelo M, et al. Hirschsprung disease, associated syndromes and genetics: a review. *J Med Genet.* 2008;45(1):1-14.
12. Singh SJ, Croaker GD, Manglick P, et al. Hirschsprung's disease: the Australian Paediatric Surveillance Unit's experience. *Pediatr Surg Int.* 2003;19(4):247-250.
13. Teitelbaum DH, Cilley RE, Sherman NJ, et al. A decade of experience with the primary pull-through for Hirschsprung disease in the newborn period: a multicenter analysis of outcomes. *Ann Surg.* 2000;232(3):372-380.
14. De Lorijn F, Reitsma JB, Voskuijl WP, et al. Diagnosis of Hirschsprung's disease: a prospective, comparative accuracy study of common tests. *J Pediatr.* 2005;146(6):787-792.
15. Gosain A, Frykman PK, Cowles RA, et al., and the American Pediatric Surgical Association Hirschsprung Disease Interest Group. Guidelines for the diagnosis and management of Hirschsprung-associated enterocolitis. *Pediatr Surg Int.* 2017;33(5):517-521.
16. Somme S, Langer JC. Primary versus staged pull-through for the treatment of Hirschsprung disease. *Semin Pediatr Surg.* 2004;13(4):249-255.
17. Yamataka A, Kobayashi H, Hirai S, et al. Laparoscopy-assisted transanal pull-through at the time of suction rectal biopsy: a new approach to treating selected cases of Hirschsprung disease. *J Pediatr Surg.* 2006;41(12):2052-2055.
18. Georgeson KE, Robertson DJ. Laparoscopic-assisted approaches for the definitive surgery for Hirschsprung's disease. *Semin Pediatr Surg.* 2004;13(4):256-262.

10 | *Rumbly in the Tumbly: Pneumatosis Intestinalis and Necrotizing Enterocolitis*

ROBERT VEZZETTI, MD, FAAP, FACEP

Case Presentation

A 10-day-old infant presents to the emergency department with 1 day of fussiness, decreased oral intake, decreased urine output, and three grossly bloody stools. There has been no fever, cough, congestion, vomiting, or rash. The child is breastfed exclusively and the mother denies she has had cracked nipples or bleeding from the breast. She has noted the child is feeding less vigorously today.

The child was born vaginally at 34 weeks and spent 4 days in the hospital to observe feeding and required blow by oxygenation for 24 hours. The mother had excellent prenatal care. Prior to hospital discharge, the patient had normal feeding and stooling.

The child is afebrile with a heart rate of 170 beats per minute, a respiratory rate of 30 breaths per minute, and a pulse oxygenation saturation of 98% on room air. While not in obvious distress, the child is fussy during the examination but otherwise remains quiet, which the parents state is not typical. The physical examination is unremarkable, except for mild abdominal distention without obvious tenderness; rectal examination shows a patent anus and is guaiac positive. Right after the rectal examination, she passes a loose, grossly bloody stool.

Imaging Considerations

Pneumatosis discovered on radiography is a sign, rather than a specific diagnosis, which can be associated with either benign or potentially life-threatening conditions.[1]

PLAIN RADIOGRAPHY

Plain radiography is the first-line imaging modality employed in many instances when bowel pathology is a concern. Pneumatosis, portal venous gas and free intraperitoneal air can be detected on abdominal radiographs. Initial imaging should include a supine and cross-table, horizontal view. Although a left lateral decubitus view is preferred, the cross-table view is often obtained in the supine position in ill-appearing infants to minimize movement.[2] Attention should be paid to intraluminal, intramural, portal venous, and free intraperitoneal gas visualized with abdominal radiography.[2-6] In infants with a clinical history and examination compatible with necrotizing enterocolitis (NEC), the finding of pneumatosis intestinalis with or without portal venous gas should prompt concern for this entity.[7] Pneumoperitoneum can be demonstrated by plain radiography, appearing as an unusual and at times oblong central lucency on the anteroposterior view and can often be more easily seen on a left lateral decubitus view.[7] While abdominal radiography may not be sensitive enough to detect pneumatosis early in its course,[1,7] it does remain the initial imaging modality of choice.[2,8]

COMPUTED TOMOGRAPHY (CT)

CT is not a first-line imaging study but has been shown to be more sensitive at detecting pneumatosis intestinalis and portal venous gas compared to plain radiography.[1,4,6] CT may also demonstrate bowel wall thickening, free fluid, and peri-intestinal soft-tissue stranding, which are associated with a serious underlying process.[1] This imaging test may be useful if the diagnosis is uncertain or there is suspicion for complex disease or deteriorating clinical status.[4,5]

Both plain abdominal radiography and CT are useful to help distinguish so-called pseudo-pneumatosis intestinalis (which is gas trapped in feces or against the mucosal surface) from true pneumatosis based on the location, pattern, and distribution of the observed gas.[1] Features suggestive of true pneumatosis include portal or mesenteric venous gas, intramural gas superior to a gas-fluid level, continuous gas outlining the bowel wall, and dissecting gas in the bowel wall edge.[1]

ULTRASOUND (US)

US has become an imaging modality of interest for use in patients with pneumatosis and suspected NEC. Among infants with NEC, US is a useful adjunct to plain radiography of the abdomen.[2,8,9] In addition to identifying free air, pneumatosis, and portal venous gas, US can detect ascites and bowel wall thickening, and Doppler examination can detect bowel wall ischemia, helping assess for bowel viability.[2,8,9] Highly concerning sonographic findings in infants with NEC include free air, absent bowel peristalsis, absent bowel wall perfusion, and complex ascites.[8] US of the bowel in infants is personnel dependent, requiring experienced sonographers and experienced pediatric imagers to obtain and interpret these studies.

Imaging Findings

An abdominal radiograph was obtained and demonstrates a nonobstructive bowel gas pattern, with a mottled appearance of gas over the lateral left lower quadrant suggestive of pneumatosis, and a small lucency over the right upper abdomen concerning for possible free air (Fig. 10.1). A lateral decubitus film was then obtained, demonstrating an irregular lucency over the nondependent abdomen adjacent to the distended bowel suggesting free air (Fig. 10.2).

Case Conclusion

The child was placed on intravenous antibiotics and bowel rest and admitted to the hospital for treatment and observation. Serial examinations and close radiographic follow-up were ensured. The patient's examination improved and follow-up imaging demonstrated resolution of the previously identified findings. She did not require surgical intervention.

Pneumatosis intestinalis is gas in the bowel wall.[4,5,10] This may be an incidental finding on plain abdominal radiography but may also be associated with more serious processes, such as infection or trauma.[11] The exact mechanism that produces pneumatosis is not clear, but there are

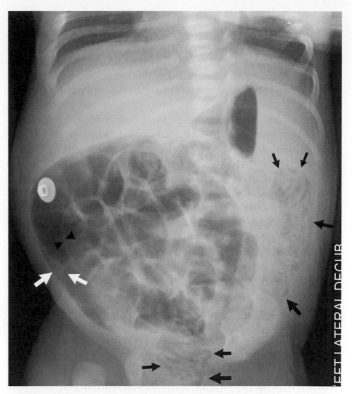

Fig. 10.2 A left lateral decubitus radiograph confirms free intraperitoneal air: seen as a triangle of gas between the right colon and the abdominal wall *(white arrows)* and as a Rigler sign, where both sides of the wall of a bowel loop are outlined by air *(black arrowheads)*. As gas in the lumen has cleared from bowel loops in the left abdomen, left-sided pneumatosis is better visualized, with extensive linear and curvilinear arcs of gas seen in the bowel wall of the left colon and rectum *(black arrows)*.

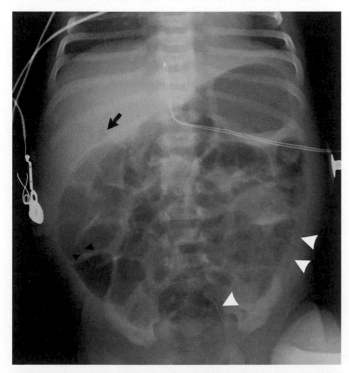

Fig. 10.1 Supine abdomen radiograph demonstrates a mottled appearance of gas over the lateral left lower quadrant, with bubbly and linear lucencies paralleling the bowel wall of the descending colon and the left side of the rectum, consistent with pneumatosis *(white arrowheads)*. An unusual small lucency *(black arrow)* projects in the right upper quadrant just superior to bowel loops and is suspicious for free intraperitoneal air. In addition, a Rigler sign, where both sides of the wall of a bowel loop are outlined by air, is seen in bowel loops in the right abdomen *(black arrowheads)*, a finding indicative of free intraperitoneal air.

multiple theories addressing this formation process.[5] Clinical presentation may include abdominal pain, fever, vomiting, diarrhea, abdominal distention, and signs of sepsis, but pneumatosis may be asymptomatic.[1,5,12]

Pneumatosis intestinalis can be associated with ischemic and nonischemic processes, and both have been well described in the literature. Nonischemic processes include bacterial overgrowth (for example, in immunocompromised or immunosuppressed patients undergoing treatment with steroids or chemotherapy) and inflammatory bowel disease. In the former case, there is bacterial penetration of the bowel mucosa and production of intramural gas; in the latter, there is mucosal ulceration, allowing gas to penetrate the bowel wall.[4,5,10,11,13] Ischemic processes can be present during infection, such as with NEC or enteritis, in which intramural gas is produced by necrosis of the bowel wall due to bacterial fermentation activity.[5,11,13,14] Pneumatosis has been associated with trauma,[5,13–15] intussusception, and volvulus,[4,5] and rarely after laparoscopic surgery including appendectomy.[6] A broad differential should be considered when pneumatosis intestinalis is encountered.

Pediatric pneumatosis intestinalis outside of the neonatal period has been reported in the literature and has been described as benign in many cases.[4,5,10,13,14] Several theories have been postulated as to the underlying pathology leading to pneumatosis in the older age group.[4] Pneumatosis has been described in patients with underlying medical conditions, including pulmonary disease, immunocompromise, congenital heart disease, and short gut syndrome, with some cases being recurrent.[4] Another study examining patients outside of the neonatal period (age greater than 30 days) found pneumatosis not only in patients with chronic illness but also in healthy children.[16] In this series, pneumatosis was caused by noninfectious colitis (32%), acute enteric infection or toxin (27%), bowel ischemia (20%), and gastrointestinal dysmotility (17%). The majority (78%) of cases resolved with medical management; however, portal venous gas and low serum bicarbonate were associated with poor outcomes.[16] A case report of a child with corticosteroid dependence due to chronic medical illness was reported to have pneumatosis intestinalis without portal venous gas; he was managed medically, with a good outcome.[10]

Pneumatosis intestinalis from blunt abdominal trauma, while rare, can occur.[3,13–15] Mucosal tearing produced from sudden bowel compression allows gas to enter the intramural space; this causes a disruption in the blood supply of the bowel, producing dissection of gas into the bowel wall.[13–15] The presence of portal venous gas may also be associated with abdominal trauma; due to an acute change in pressure, gas penetrates submucosal veins and travels to the portal venous system.[13,14,17] It is important to note that while the presence of gas in the bowel wall implies mucosal injury, it does not necessarily mean necrosis in this setting.[14,17] If pneumatosis intestinalis, with or without portal venous gas, is present on radiography, the clinician should consider traumatic causes, particularly if there is no history, physical examination findings, or laboratory values to suggest another source, such as an infectious process. Bowel necrosis as a result of blunt abdominal trauma and subsequent clinical deterioration in a premature infant with pneumatosis intestinalis and extensive portal venous gas, eventually leading to death, has been reported in the literature.[15] Blunt abdominal injury is a leading cause of death due to nonaccidental trauma in the pediatric population and can present as an isolated finding; the lack of apparent signs of physical abuse (bruising, swelling, pain) or intra-abdominal injuries (solid organ lacerations or intestinal hematomas) should not dissuade the clinician from considering nonaccidental trauma as a potential etiology when pneumatosis is discovered on radiography.[14]

In the neonatal period, pneumatosis intestinalis with or without portal venous gas is seen as a sign of NEC, an extremely grave condition with a mortality rate of up to 30%.[5,18,19] NEC is commonly seen in premature infants, with the risk decreasing with increasing age and weight,[14,19,20] but can be seen in full-term infants.[13] NEC is thought to be due to intestinal immaturity, leading to a predisposition for endothelial disruption and special properties of the newborn intestinal response to stressful physiologic situations.[14,15] Low birth weight is the most commonly reported risk factor for NEC, but small for gestational age, assisted ventilation, sepsis, hypotension, and prolonged rupture of membranes have also been reported risk factors.[18,19] Infants affected with NEC have been shown to have an increased incidence of adverse neurodevelopmental outcomes, intestinal strictures, short gut syndrome, and growth delay.[19,21] Clinical signs of NEC include temperature instability, poor feeding, lethargy, apnea, hypotension, abdominal distention, bloody stools, and signs of sepsis.[7] Bacterial species found in association with NEC include *Escherichia coli*, *Klebsiella pneumoniae*, *Proteus mirabilis*, *Enterobacter cloacae*, *Clostridium perfringens*, and *Pseudomonas aeruginosa*.[7]

Management of pneumatosis depends on history, physical examination, and the suspected underlying etiology. The management of NEC in the neonatal period consists of broad-spectrum antibiotics, bowel rest, intravenous fluids, and ionotropic support.[7,19,22] Surgical intervention is usually indicated if there is suspicion of necrosis, regardless of etiology.[3,5,23] This is often the case with NEC that is failing medical management, as up to 50% of infants with NEC require surgery and the need for surgery is linked to a higher mortality rate.[7,19] Pneumatosis thought not to require surgical intervention can be managed medically with close observation, including bowel rest, bowel decompression, and antimicrobial therapy as clinically indicated.[4–7,10,11,13,24] Since it can be difficult to distinguish the two radiographically, history and clinical examination are paramount when interpreting radiographic findings[11] and planning a course of management.

IMAGING PEARLS

1. The significance of finding pneumatosis on any imaging study should be evaluated in the context of the patient's history and physical examination.
2. Plain radiography is the initial imaging modality of choice to detect pneumatosis as well as portal venous and free intraperitoneal gas. Radiography obtained early in the course of development of pneumatosis may not reveal any abnormalities, so follow-up imaging, when clinically indicated, is appropriate. This modality is low in ionizing radiation relative to CT, readily available, and relatively inexpensive.
3. CT is better at detecting pneumatosis than plain radiography, particularly early in development of pneumatosis. However, it is not typically a first-line imaging modality. It may be indicated if the diagnosis is uncertain or there is suspicion for complex disease or deteriorating clinical status. This modality does employ significantly more ionizing radiation than plain radiography does.
4. The use of US to detect pneumatosis intestinalis and other sites of abdominal gas has been increasing. Studies utilizing US in the detection and management of NEC show this modality to have promise. The advantages of US include the ability to detect fluid and help assess bowel viability. Some sonographic findings in infants with NEC have shown to help predict prognosis as well.

References

1. Wang JH, Furlan A, Kayla DA, et al. Pneumatosis intestinalis versus pseudo-pneumatosis: review of CT findings and differentiation. *Insights Imaging.* 2011;2(1):85-92.
2. Epelman M, Daneman A, Navarro OM, et al. Necrotizing enterocolitis: review of state-of-the-art imaging findings with pathologic correlation. *Radiographics.* 2007;27(2):285-305.
3. Koutouzis T, Lee J. Blunt abdominal trauma resulting in pneumatosis intestinalis in an infant. *Ann Emerg Med.* 2000;36(6):619-621.
4. Fenton LZ, Buonomo C. Benign pneumatosis in children. *Pediatr Radiol.* 2000;30(11):786-793.
5. Nellihela L, Mutalib M, Thompson D, et al. Management of pneumatosis intestinalis in children over the age of 6 months: a conservative approach. *Arch Dis Child.* 2018;103(4):352-355.

6. Vendryes C, Hunter CJ, Harlan SR, et al. Pneumatosis intestinalis after laparoscopic appendectomy: case report and review of the literature. *J Pediatr Surg.* 2011;46(11):e21-e24.

7. Rich BS, Dolgin SE. Necrotizing enterocolitis. *Pediatr Rev.* 2017;38(12):552-559.

8. Cuna AC, Reddy N, Robinson AL, et al. Bowel ultrasound for predicting surgical management of necrotizing enterocolitis: a systematic review and meta-analysis. *Pediatr Radiol.* 2018;48(5):658-666.

9. Bohnhorst B. Usefulness of abdominal ultrasound in diagnosing necrotising enterocolitis. *Arch Dis Child Fetal Neonatal Ed.* 2013;98(5):F445-F450.

10. Cruz AT, Naik-Mathuria BJ, Bisset GS. Pneumatosis intestinalis in a corticosteroid-dependent child. *J Emerg Med.* 2015;48(5):607-608.

11. George S, Cook JV. Pneumatosis intestinalis. *J Pediatr.* 2014; 165(3):637.

12. St Peter SD, Abbas MA, Kelly KA. The spectrum of pneumatosis intestinalis. *Arch Surg.* 2003;138(1):68-75.

13. Jona JZ. Benign pneumatosis intestinalis coli after blunt trauma to the abdomen in a child. *J Pediatr Surg.* 2000;35(7):1109-1111.

14. Deutsch SA, Christian CW. Pneumatosis intestinalis due to child abuse. *Pediatr Emerg Care.* 2019;35(2):e32-e33.

15. Ergaz Z, Arad I, Simanovsky N. Portal venous gas following trauma in a preterm infant. *Fetal Pediatr Pathol.* 2006;25(3):147-150.

16. Kurbegov AC, Sondheimer JM. Pneumatosis intestinalis in non-neonatal pediatric patients. *Pediatrics.* 2001;108(2):402-406.

17. Gurland B, Dolgin SE, Shlasko E, et al. Pneumatosis intestinalis and portal vein gas after blunt abdominal trauma. *J Pediatr Surg.* 1998; 33(8):1309-1311.

18. Samuels N, van de Graaf RA, de Jonge RCJ, et al. Risk factors for necrotizing enterocolitis in neonates: a systematic review of prognostic studies. *BMC Pediatr.* 2017;17(1):105.

19. Niño DF, Sodhi CP, Hackam DJ. Necrotizing enterocolitis: new insights into pathogenesis and mechanisms. *Nat Rev Gastroenterol Hepatol.* 2016;13(10):590-600.

20. Short SS, Papillon S, Berel D, et al. Late onset of necrotizing enterocolitis in the full-term infant is associated with increased mortality: results from a two-center analysis. *J Pediatr Surg.* 2014; 49(6):950-953.

21. Adams-Chapman I. Necrotizing enterocolitis and neurodevelopmental outcome. *Clin Perinatol.* 2018;45(3):453-466.

22. Papillon S, Castle SL, Gayer CP, et al. Necrotizing enterocolitis: contemporary management and outcomes. *Adv Pediatr.* 2013;60: 263-279.

23. Pear BL. Pneumatosis intestinalis: a review. *Radiology.* 1998;207(1): 13-19.

24. Chew SJ, Victor RS, Gopagondanahalli KR, et al. Pneumatosis intestinalis in a preterm infant: should we treat all intestinal pneumatosis as necrotising enterocolitis? *BMJ Case Rep.* 2018;2018:bcr2018224356.

Cardiac

11 *Matters of the Heart: Pericarditis*

TIM RUTTAN, MD

Case Presentation

A 13-year-old male presents to the emergency department (ED) with 2 weeks of chest pain. He describes the pain as sharp and constant, worsening over the past week. Two weeks ago, the patient had fever to 102 degrees Fahrenheit and cough. He then developed sharp frontal chest pain that he described as "stabbing." The pain worsened when lying down. He was seen by his primary care provider and at that time had a chest radiograph and electrocardiogram (ECG) that were reported to be normal. He was diagnosed with a viral infection and prescribed symptomatic care. His fevers have resolved but the chest pain has worsened. He denies vomiting, abdominal pain, back pain, difficulty breathing, or trauma.

Physical examination reveals unremarkable vital signs other than mild tachycardia (heart rate of 110 beats per minute with a blood pressure of 110/70 mm Hg). He has slightly distant heart sounds and there appears to be a friction rub without a discernable murmur. His lungs are clear. An ECG is obtained, demonstrating low voltage throughout with no other acute abnormalities.

Imaging Considerations

The choice of imaging modalities will depend on the clinical presentation, but when pericarditis is suspected, it will typically begin with plain chest radiography and may be followed by bedside ultrasound (US), echocardiogram, cardiac computed tomography (CT), or cardiac magnetic resonance imaging (MRI).

PLAIN RADIOGRAPHY

Chest imaging may be normal in many patients with early or mild cases of pericarditis. In addition to helping to identify other etiologies of chest pain or fever in patients with potential pericarditis, findings can include cardiomegaly (most often due to a pericardial effusion referred to as a "water bottle sign"). Associated findings may also include pleural effusion, pulmonary edema, lung infiltrates, or an enlarged mediastinum.[1,2] A pericardial effusion may distort the cardiac silhouette, but often, chest radiography appears unremarkable.[3] Plain radiography is also useful to detect other causes of chest pain, such as pneumothorax, rib fractures, pleural effusion, and pneumonia. This modality is readily available, rapid, and exposes the patient to minimal ionizing radiation.

CARDIAC US/ECHOCARDIOGRAPHY

Transthoracic echocardiography is an excellent imaging modality for patients with a suspected cardiac process, including pericarditis. This modality can detect pericardial effusion, assess cardiac function, and be useful to distinguish between pericarditis and myocarditis (in which cardiac dysfunction is usually present).[3]

If possible, a point of care cardiac US should be performed on all suspected cases of pericarditis to evaluate for pericardial effusion and signs of cardiac tamponade, since this modality is highly sensitive and specific (96% and 98%, respectively) for pericardial effusion.[1] In particular, bedside imaging is critical in ill-appearing or hypotensive patients, where early identification of an effusion and tamponade physiology can guide management and resuscitation including pericardiocentesis.[1] Echocardiography by Pediatric Cardiology can help to identify smaller effusions, especially in patients who do not present in more advanced disease states.

CARDIAC CT

This imaging modality may be used in patients with chronic or constrictive pericarditis but is not indicated in the acute period of illness.[1,3]

CARDIAC MRI

Cardiac MRI is not typically indicated in the ED setting or in the acute course, but if the diagnosis is uncertain or additional complications such as constrictive pericarditis, complex effusion, and myocardial involvement are considered, these can be identified through the use of MRI.[1-3]

Imaging Findings

This patient had a bedside point-of-care US (POCUS) performed in the ED, which revealed grossly normal cardiac function but the presence of a pericardial effusion. Pediatric Cardiology was consulted. Since he was deemed stable for a more confirmatory study, the decision was made to perform cardiac MRI. Select images from this study are provided. There is a moderate pericardial effusion noted, with thickened and enhancing pericardium, but the study was otherwise unremarkable (Figs. 11.1–11.3).

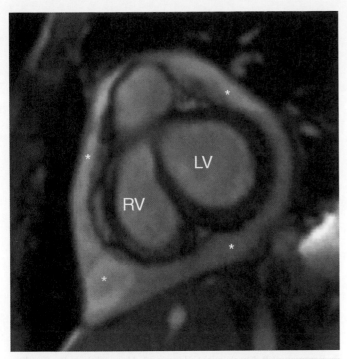

Fig. 11.1 Steady-state free precession short-axis image from a cardiac magnetic resonance image demonstrates high signal pericardial effusion *(asterisks)* surrounding the heart. The left ventricle *(LV)* and right ventricle *(RV)* are also shown. (Image courtesy of Karen Hasbani, MD, Pediatric Cardiologist at DCMC.)

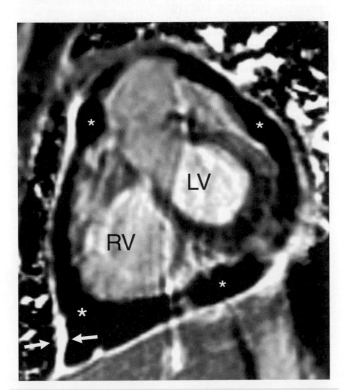

Fig. 11.2 Short-axis contrast-enhanced cardiac magnetic resonance image shows low signal pericardial effusion *(asterisks)* to surround the heart. The pericardium is thickened and enhancing (between *arrows*). The left ventricle *(LV)* and right ventricle *(RV)* are also shown. (Image courtesy of Karen Hasbani, MD, Pediatric Cardiologist at DCMC.)

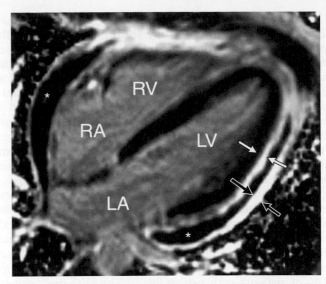

Fig. 11.3 Four-chamber contrast-enhanced cardiac magnetic resonance image shows thickened and enhancing visceral (between *small white arrows*) and parietal (between *large open arrows*) pericardium, consistent with pericarditis. Pericardial effusion *(asterisks)* is low signal on this sequence. The left atrium *(LA)*, left ventricle *(LV)*, right atrium *(RA)*, and right ventricle *(RV)* are also shown. (Image courtesy of Karen Hasbani, MD, Pediatric Cardiologist at DCMC.)

Case Conclusion

The patient was admitted to the hospital for clinical monitoring due to the moderate-size pericardial effusion and for initiation of nonsteroidal antiinflammatory drug (NSAID) medications. He clinically deteriorated 24 hours later and became hypotensive (blood pressure 80/40 mm Hg). Emergent pericardiocentesis was performed, with an improvement in his symptoms postprocedure. Bacterial culture results from the obtained fluid were negative, but viral studies revealed the presence of Coxsackie virus. The patient recovered uneventfully.

Chest pain is a frequent complaint in pediatric patients, and serious diagnoses are rare in children compared to the adult population.[1] Pericarditis is a process that affects the layers overlying the heart. There are two of these layers that have a thin layer of intervening fluid for lubrication that also serves as a barrier to protect the heart from a variety of inflammatory, rheumatologic, infectious, and neoplastic illnesses.[2-5] Pericarditis is the most common form of pericardial disease and has many etiologies, including infectious (viral or postviral are the most common causes), autoimmune, metabolic, traumatic (including postoperative), and neoplastic processes.[1,2,5] Adolescent patients commonly have a viral etiology, and bacterial (*Streptococcus* or *Staphlococcus*) etiology is more common in patients younger than 2 years of age.[3,4] Postpericardiotomy syndrome is a phenomena seen in patients who have had cardiac surgery. In this entity, a pericardial effusion develops following the procedure.[3] While the development of a pericardial effusion (which may lead to pericardial tamponade in some cases) is common in pericarditis, pericardial effusion is not always present and pericarditis can exist without an effusion.[3]

Chest pain is a presenting symptom of pericarditis. Classically, this pain is improved by sitting and worsens with coughing or placing the patient in a supine position; these patients may resist lying down.[2-5] Fever and tachycardia may be present. A common historical finding is report of a recent or current viral infection.[1-3] While physical examination findings may not be remarkable, auscultation of the chest may reveal a precordial friction rub; in cases of a large pericardial effusion, muffled heart tones may be present as well.[3] Notably, though, there is a wide clinical spectrum with which these patients may present, from mild illness or discomfort to life-threatening shock and vascular collapse.

The diagnosis of pericarditis can be difficult. Laboratory testing, ECG, and use of imaging studies are all utilized to assist in making the diagnosis. Laboratory tests include white blood cell counts and inflammatory markers (C-reactive protein and erythrocyte sedimentation rate), which may be elevated but are nonspecific.[1-3] Troponin elevation may be seen in up to 30% of patients with pericarditis.[1,3] The ECG may acutely demonstrate diffuse ST-segment elevation in the precordial leads, without T-wave inversion, and PR-interval depression. Most patients will have an abnormal ECG.[1,3]

NSAIDs are a mainstay of pericarditis treatment. Consultation with a pediatric cardiologist is recommended, especially early in the course of illness.[1] Colchicine has been used as well to help reduce the rate of recurrence.[1,6] The use of corticosteroids is generally not indicated and in some studies has been associated with recurrence of pericarditis.[1,3] However, low-dose corticosteroids (0.25–0.5 mg/kg/day) have been used for pericarditis refractory to NSAIDS or in cases due to an underlying immune process, but there is a lack of large randomized studies in the pediatric population.[1,3,6] Routine antimicrobial therapy is not indicated but may be utilized if a specific pathogen is identified.[1] If a large pericardial effusion is present or there are signs of tamponade, pericardiocentesis is therapeutic and may help to determine the etiology of the effusion.[1,3,7] Engaging in strenuous physical activity should be avoided until the patient is symptom free, inflammatory markers have normalized, and the echocardiogram and ECG are normal.[3,8]

The majority of pediatric patients with pericarditis have a self-limited, benign course. Death is rare but is higher in those cases with a bacterial etiology.[3] Patients who have constrictive pericarditis, while very rare, have a worse prognosis.[3] Recurrence of pericarditis is reported to be around 10%.[3,7]

IMAGING PEARLS

1. Chest radiography is the first-line imaging test of choice for patients with suspected pericarditis but may be normal in the majority of patients.
2. Echocardiography should be strongly considered in all patients with suspected pericarditis and helps to identify pericardial effusion and tamponade as well as assess cardiac function. A patient who is critically ill should have, if available, immediate beside cardiac US, as this can be used to guide life-saving immediate management.
3. Advanced imaging modalities, such as cardiac CT or cardiac MRI, are not indicated in the acute setting and are utilized when the diagnosis is in question, for suspected complications, and for recurrent pericarditis.

References

1. Durani Y, Giordano K, Goudie BW. Myocarditis and pericarditis in children. *Pediatr Clin North Am.* 2010;57(6):1281-1303.
2. Bergmann KR, Kharbanda A, Haveman L. Myocarditis and pericarditis in the pediatric patient: validated management strategies. *Pediatr Emerg Med Pract.* 2015;12(7):1-22.
3. Tunuguntla H, Jeewa A, Denfield SW. Acute myocarditis and pericarditis in children. *Pediatr Rev.* 2019;40(1):14-25.
4. Mangus CW, Fatusin O, Ngo TL. Acute-onset chest pain in a 17-year-old female adolescent with systemic lupus erythematosus. *Pediatr Emerg Care.* 2017;33(5):346-349.
5. Lim FF, Chang HM, Lue KH, et al. Pneumococcal pneumonia complicating purulent pericarditis in a previously healthy girl: a rare yet possible fatal complication in the antibiotic era. *Pediatr Emerg Care.* 2011;27(8):751-753.
6. Imazio M, Brucato A, Pluymaekers N, et al. Recurrent pericarditis in children and adolescents: a multicentre cohort study. *J Cardiovasc Med (Hagerstown).* 2016;17(9):707-712.
7. Shakti D, Hehn R, Gauvreau K, et al. Idiopathic pericarditis and pericardial effusion in children: contemporary epidemiology and management. *J Am Heart Assoc.* 2014;3(6):e001483.
8. Adler Y, Charron P, Imazio M, et al; ESC Scientific Document Group. 2015 ESC guidelines for the diagnosis and management of pericardial diseases: the Task Force for the Diagnosis and Management of Pericardial Diseases of the European Society of Cardiology (ESC) Endorsed by: the European Association for Cardio-Thoracic Surgery (EACTS). *Eur Heart J.* 2015;36(42):2921-2964.

12 · A Bit of a Mix-up: Right-sided Aortic Arch

ROBERT VEZZETTI, MD, FAAP, FACEP

Case Presentation

A 7-week-old male presents with difficulty breathing while feeding for 1 day. The child is formula fed 3 ounces every 3–4 hours, but over the past 2–3 days, he has been feeding every 4 hours and not completing the 3 ounces. One day ago, he developed increased work of breathing while feeding and "turned pale for several seconds" according to the parents. There was no associated tonic-clonic activity with this event and the child did not stop breathing. This continued with most of the feeds during the day but otherwise there were no other concerns. On the day of presentation, he "turned blue for a few seconds" while feeding. With these episodes, the mother reports nasal congestion and copious oral secretions (with some formula) that she has been suctioning with a bulb syringe. There has been no fever, vomiting, diarrhea, rash, or known trauma, and the child is reported otherwise to be at his baseline.

The child recently arrived from Central America. The parents report the child has not had problems with breathing or feeding in the past and has "been healthy." There was little prenatal care but the mother was told the child "had a heart problem" on a prenatal ultrasound, but she did not understand what the issue was and was told "nothing could be done." Aside from this, the parents report no other concerns or problems. They have not yet been to a local pediatrician.

The physical examination reveals an overall well-appearing, vigorous child who is in no acute distress. He is afebrile with a heart rate of 170 beats per minute, respiratory rate of 45 breaths per minute, and a pulse oximetry reading of 100% on room air. He has a completely normal examination; his cardiac examination demonstrates no heart murmur, rub, or click; he has equal pulses throughout and is well perfused.

Imaging Considerations

PLAIN RADIOGRAPHY AND FLUOROSCOPY

Chest radiography is often employed as a first-line resource in patients when there is concern for a cardiopulmonary process. In interpreting the chest radiograph, attention should be given to the side of the cardiac apex, the aortic arch, and the stomach bubble. In young infants and children, the aortic arch may not be directly visible, but its position is inferred by the appearance of the trachea. There is a mild mass effect upon the trachea from the side of the aortic arch, and the trachea mildly deviates or buckles away from the side of the aortic arch on a frontal view of the chest. If

the position of the aortic arch is difficult to determine on chest radiograph, chest fluoroscopy can be utilized to determine aortic arch positioning. A fluoroscopic esophagram using barium contrast is useful in the evaluation for vascular rings and slings, in which developmental anomalies of the aortic arch and pulmonary artery can produce a mass effect upon the esophagus and trachea. A contrast esophagram performed for the evaluation of vascular anatomy should be performed by a practitioner experienced in pediatric imaging.

ECHOCARDIOGRAPHY (ECHO)

For suspected cardiac disease and aortic arch anomalies, echo is employed. Anatomy and function can be demonstrated. If very complex anatomy is discovered, and especially if aortic anatomy is not well delineated on echo, this may prompt the use of additional advanced imaging, such as computed tomography (CT) or magnetic resonance imaging (MRI). Echo is resource dependent; expertise in the performance and interpretation of pediatric echo is needed to obtain a meaningful study and interpretation. Additionally, availability may restrict immediate or routine use in an emergent setting.

COMPUTED TOMOGRAPHY

This imaging modality is used as a secondary study when either plain radiography or echo is abnormal or inconclusive. CT angiography has been found to be useful to further delineate aortic arch anatomy.[1,2] The decision for CT utilization may be made after subspecialty consultation or in hospitalized patients undergoing further evaluation. Contrast-enhanced CT angiography of the chest is especially useful in the evaluation for aortic abnormalities, including aortic arch anomalies and aortic coarctation, as well as to evaluate pulmonary artery anatomy and systemic to pulmonary collateral vessels. Pediatric imaging expertise is necessary for the performance and interpretation of CT angiography for pediatric cardiovascular disease.

MAGNETIC RESONANCE IMAGING

This modality is also typically obtained after initial imaging, such as chest radiography or an echocardiogram. MRI has the advantage of providing excellent anatomic detail and can be used to evaluate anomalies of the aortic arch, aortic coarctation, pulmonary artery anatomy, and cardiac anatomy and function.[2] As with CT, subspecialty consultation should be considered before utilizing this imaging test.

While MRI has the advantage of a lack of ionizing radiation, the length of time to complete the study often requires sedation in infants and young children. Pediatric imaging expertise is necessary for the performance and interpretation of pediatric cardiovascular MRI and magnetic resonance angiography.

Imaging Findings

The history of an unknown heart problem, coupled with the development of decreased feeding and color change, prompted concerns for a worsening cardiac condition, although the physical examination was not concerning. A two-view chest x-ray series was obtained. This demonstrated a right-sided aortic arch with a cardiothymic silhouette that is in the upper range of normal in size (Fig. 12.1).

Case Conclusion

An electrocardiogram was obtained and was normal. Pediatric Cardiology was consulted. An echocardiogram (not provided) was performed and demonstrated an aortic arch that appeared to be right sided without intracardiac abnormalities. The aortic arch branching pattern was not clearly defined but there appeared to be a vessel arising from the descending aorta, suggesting the presence of an aberrant left subclavian artery and potential vascular ring; there was good biventricular systolic function.

The echocardiogram findings prompted obtaining a contrast-enhanced CT angiogram of the chest in order to better visualize the patient's vascular anatomy. This study demonstrated a right aortic arch with an atretic left proximal subclavian artery (right aortic arch with isolation of the left subclavian artery) (Fig. 12.2), with no vascular ring.

Pediatric Cardiothoracic Surgery was consulted and no surgical intervention was recommended. An upper

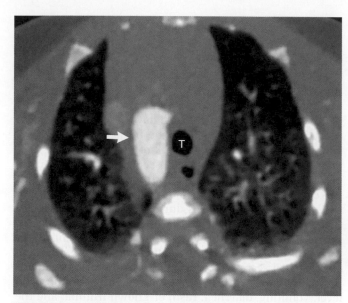

Fig. 12.2 Axial image from a computed tomography angiogram of the chest demonstrates the transverse aortic arch *(arrow)* to course to the right of the trachea *(T)*, consistent with a right-sided aortic arch.

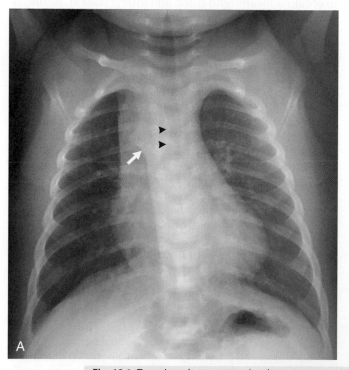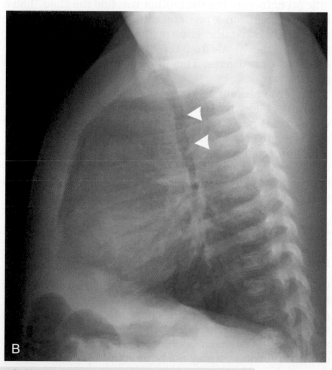

Fig. 12.1 Two-view chest x-ray series demonstrates a right-sided aortic arch. Frontal view (A) shows a right-sided aortic arch *(white arrow)*, a mild impression upon the right side of the lower trachea *(black arrowheads)*, and mild deviation of the lower trachea to the left; these tracheal findings confirm the presence of a right-sided aortic arch. Lateral view (B) of the chest shows the air-filled trachea to have a normal appearance *(white arrowheads)*.

gastrointestinal series was obtained, which included evaluation of the esophagus, and demonstrated gastroesophageal reflux but no vascular mass effect upon the esophagus. The child was monitored carefully and was discharged with close monitoring and follow-up.

A right-sided aortic arch is a variant of aortic anatomy in which the aortic arch crosses over the right bronchus and courses to the right of the trachea. It is present in up to 0.1% of pregnancies.[3–6] This condition can be diagnosed prenatally, occasionally as early as 12 weeks' gestation.[5] A right-sided aortic arch can be associated with congenital cardiac disease, including truncus arteriosus, tricuspid atresia, pulmonary atresia, and ventricular septal defect.[3,7–9] However, a right-sided aortic arch can be an incidental finding that is asymptomatic.[3,7–9] A right-sided aortic arch can also be associated with a vascular ring, which produces a mass effect upon the esophagus and trachea, and can produce symptoms of respiratory distress or dysphagia.[3,9,10] A double aortic arch is the most common complete, symptomatic vascular ring, and may appear as a double aortic arch or as a right-sided aortic arch on chest radiography. A right-sided aortic arch has been associated with DiGeorge syndrome (chromosome 22 q11 deletion), with a prevalence of 8%–24%.[3,8,9] One study found cardiac anomalies, including a right-sided aortic arch, vascular rings (formed with the right-sided arch), and multiple cardiac anatomic variations, in 75%–80% of patients with chromosome 22 q11 deletion.[11]

There are several types of right-sided aortic arches based on the pattern of branching of arch vessels:

- Right-sided aortic arch with aberrant left subclavian artery.
- Right-sided aortic arch with mirror image branching.
- Right-sided aortic arch with isolation of the left subclavian artery.

A right-sided aortic arch with an aberrant left subclavian artery is the most common right aortic arch variant.[12–14] This anomaly is often asymptomatic and is usually an incidental finding on imaging; however, a complete vascular ring may be formed and cause esophageal (usually seen in adult populations) or tracheal compression (more commonly seen in pediatric populations).[12,13] If this is the case, symptoms such as wheezing and chronic cough may be present. There are two types of this anomaly. In one, the aberrant left subclavian artery arises from a portion of the left dorsal aorta persisting as a retroesophageal diverticulum (diverticulum of Kommerell); this variant is usually not associated with congenital cardiac anomalies but is the second most common cause of a vascular ring.[12–14] The other, less common type has the aberrant left subclavian artery not associated with a retroesophageal diverticulum. While a vascular ring is not formed in these patients, this variant is often associated with other cardiac anomalies, particularly tetralogy of Fallot and truncus arteriosus.[12–14]

A right-sided aortic arch with mirror branching pattern is the second most common right-sided aortic arch anomaly and is almost always associated with congenital heart disease (up to 98% of cases), including tetralogy of Fallot, truncus arteriosus, tricuspid atresia, and transposition of the great vessels, although a vascular ring is usually not present.[12]

Right aortic arch with isolation of the left subclavian artery, as seen in this patient, is a rare entity. In this anomaly, an arch vessel arises from the pulmonary artery via the ductus arteriosus or ligamentum arteriosum without a connection to the aorta.[12] It is associated with congenital heart disease in over 50% of cases, most commonly tetralogy of Fallot.[12]

The management of a right-sided aortic arch is dependent on whether the patient is symptomatic and what other associated anomalies might be present. Patients with symptomatic vascular rings are candidates for surgical treatment.[3,7] Consultation with pediatric cardiology and pediatric cardiothoracic surgery is appropriate.

Infants may present with esophageal or airway compression symptoms later, during the first 2 years of life, and should be followed carefully for development of breathing or feeding difficulties.[15] Some authors recommend assessment for esophageal atresia in infants with prenatally diagnosed right-sided aortic arch prior to initiation of feeding.[15]

IMAGING PEARLS

1. Plain radiography is the initial imaging modality of choice in patients with suspected cardiovascular or pulmonary disease.
2. Echo is an excellent imaging modality used to evaluate cardiac anatomy and function. This modality requires expertise in technique and interpretation.
3. CT with contrast-enhanced angiography is a follow-up imaging modality that can confirm and delineate aortic arch anatomy and, if indicated, is useful for surgical planning. The decision to employ this modality is often made after consultation with a pediatric cardiologist.
4. MRI is also a follow-up imaging modality that, like CT, can be used to confirm and better delineate aortic arch anatomy. However, availability and the need for sedation may be limiting factors.

References

1. Soleimantabar H, Sabouri S, Khedmat L, et al. Assessment of CT angiographic findings in comparison with echocardiography findings of chest among patients with aortic arch anomalies. *Monaldi Arch Chest Dis.* 2019;89(3): doi:10.4081/monaldi.2019.1120.
2. Boxt LM. Magnetic resonance and computed tomographic evaluation of congenital heart disease. *J Magn Reson Imaging.* 2004;19(6): 827-847.
3. Razon Y, Berant M, Fogelman R, et al. Prenatal diagnosis and outcome of right aortic arch without significant intracardiac anomaly. *J Am Soc Echocardiogr.* 2014;27(12):1352-1358.
4. Achiron R, Rotstein Z, Heggesh J, et al. Anomalies of the fetal aortic arch: a novel sonographic approach to in-utero diagnosis. *Ultrasound Obstet Gynecol.* 2002;20(6):553-557.
5. Zidere V, Tsapakis EG, Huggon IC, et al. Right aortic arch in the fetus. *Ultrasound Obstet Gynecol.* 2006;28(7):876-881.
6. Arazińska A, Polguj M, Szymczyk K, et al. Right aortic arch analysis—anatomical variant or serious vascular defect? *BMC Cardiovasc Disord.* 2017;17(1):102.
7. Glew D, Hartnell GG. The right aortic arch revisited. *Clin Radiol.* 1991;43(5):305-307.
8. Bronshtein M, Blumenfeld Z, Naroditsky I, et al. Outcome of a right aortic arch diagnosed in utero. *Prenat Diagn.* 2016;36(2): 194-196.
9. Mogra R, Kesby G, Sholler G, et al. Identification and management of fetal isolated right-sided aortic arch in an unselected population. *Ultrasound Obstet Gynecol.* 2016;48(6):739-743.

10. McElhinney DB, Hoydu AK, Gaynor JW, et al. Patterns of right aortic arch and mirror-image branching of the brachiocephalic vessels without associated anomalies. *Pediatr Cardiol*. 2001;22(4):285-291.
11. McElhinney DB, McDonald-McGinn D, Zackai EH, et al. Cardiovascular anomalies in patients diagnosed with a chromosome 22q11 deletion beyond 6 months of age. *Pediatrics*. 2001;108(6):E104.
12. Hanneman K, Newman B, Chan F. Congenital variants and anomalies of the aortic arch. *Radiographics*. 2017;37(1):32-51.
13. Türkvatan A, Büyükbayraktar FG, Olçer T, et al. Congenital anomalies of the aortic arch: evaluation with the use of multidetector computed tomography. *Korean J Radiol*. 2009;10(2):176-184.
14. Backer CL, Mavroudis C. Congenital heart surgery nomenclature and database project: patent ductus arteriosus, coarctation of the aorta, interrupted aortic arch. *Ann Thorac Surg*. 2000;69(suppl 4):S298-S307.
15. D'Antonio F, Khalil A, Zidere V, et al. Fetuses with right aortic arch: a multicenter cohort study and meta-analysis. *Ultrasound Obstet Gynecol*. 2016;47(4):423-432.

13 You're Surrounded: Vascular Ring/Sling

ROBERT VEZZETTI, MD, FAAP, FACEP

Case Presentation

A 2-year-old female presents to the emergency department with wheezing and cough. The family states that she has had mild fever to 100.1 degrees Fahrenheit for the past 2 days. There has been no vomiting or diarrhea. She has been taking oral fluids well and is otherwise behaving at her baseline. Her physical examination reveals a well-appearing child in no respiratory distress. She has nasal congestion and some inspiratory wheezing at the upper lung fields.

The parents state they are frustrated and "want something for the cough and wheezing," which has been intermittently present "as long as they can remember" and seems to get worse when the child has upper respiratory infections. They have seen their primary care provider multiple times for these symptoms and have been told the child has reactive airway disease. Albuterol was prescribed, but the family states that this medication is not helping the child's wheezing. Multiple courses of oral steroids have been prescribed and the child has been given a fluticasone inhaler but this too has had no impact on her symptoms.

Imaging Considerations

PLAIN RADIOGRAPHY

Two-view chest radiography (anteroposterior [AP] and lateral views) is the first-line imaging modality in patients with respiratory symptoms and serves as a helpful screening examination for vascular rings. On AP views, one should evaluate the relationship of the aorta relative to the trachea, determining the side of the aortic arch, and one should evaluate for tracheal narrowing on the lateral view, which may suggest compression from a vascular ring or sling.[1–5] A right-sided aortic arch may be associated with a variety of cardiac lesions (up to 50% of patients), including persistent truncus arteriosus, pulmonary atresia with ventricular septal defect, and tetralogy of Fallot.[3] Anomalies of the aortic arch and the resulting aortic arch branching pattern and position of the ductus arteriosus will determine whether the vasculature forms a complete vascular ring, producing clinical symptoms.[3] Two branching patterns of a right-sided aortic arch, a retroesophageal aberrant left subclavian artery (65%) and mirror-image branching (35%), can be seen, with the mirror-image branching type more commonly associated with congenital heart disease.[3] A left-sided aortic arch with a an aberrant right subclavian artery may also be associated with congenital heart disease, but this configuration will form an incomplete vascular ring, thus producing fewer clinical symptoms compared to a right-sided arch configuration.

Findings suspicious for a vascular ring on AP images include a right-sided aortic arch, abnormal tracheal indentation, and a right descending aorta, whereas lateral radiographic findings include increased retrotracheal opacity, tracheal narrowing, and anterior tracheal bowing.[5,6] If a double aortic arch is present, the aorta may not be easily visualized.[1,2] Unilateral hyperinflation of the right lung, tracheal narrowing, and an atypical orientation of main bronchi suggest a pulmonary artery sling.[3] Chest radiography has the advantage of availability, rapidity, and minimal ionizing radiation exposure. However, more advanced imaging techniques become necessary if an abnormality is suspected.

BARIUM ESOPHAGOGRAPHY

Barium esophagram has historically been utilized to evaluate for suspected vascular rings.[1–4] An esophagram is useful in that it demonstrates relatively characteristic extrinsic impressions on the esophagus from anomalous vessels that contribute to a vascular ring. The presence of a double aortic arch may be seen with bilateral aortic arch and posterior crossing vessel indentations upon the esophagus. With other vascular rings, depending on the location and orientation of the vascular ring, different degrees of esophageal indentation may be seen.[1,3] Barium esophagography can also be used to evaluate other etiologies of feeding difficulties, such as gastroesophageal reflux and tracheoesophageal anomalies. This modality, however, requires expertise in performance of the study and interpretation of imaging results and includes exposure to ionizing radiation. Availability may be institution dependent. While the diagnosis of a vascular ring can be made with this modality, barium esophagography does not directly visualize the vascular ring and additional imaging is usually required.[1] A well-performed negative barium esophagram can exclude a vascular ring, with the exception of an aberrant innominate artery.[2,7] Abnormal barium esophagography should be followed by either computed tomography (CT) or magnetic resonance imaging (MRI). These cross-sectional imaging modalities will provide direct imaging of the vasculature, which is critical in determining if a surgical lesion is present and for planning appropriate operative repair.

COMPUTED TOMOGRAPHY

CT angiography with intravenous contrast is an excellent imaging modality to identify vascular anomalies of the aortic arch and pulmonary arteries and can depict resulting vascular rings.[1,2,3,6] CT is often obtained as part of the presurgical planning process.

MAGNETIC RESONANCE IMAGING/MAGNETIC RESONANCE ANGIOGRAPHY (MRA)

This imaging modality is very useful for imaging mediastinal vascular structures and can provide anatomic information with or without the use of intravenous contrast. MRI and MRA are also used as part of presurgical planning.[1,3,8]

CT VERSUS MRI

CT and MRI have the same sensitivity for detecting vascular rings.[3] CT has the advantage of availability, rapidity, and not requiring sedation in most cases. This modality also has excellent spatial resolution and multiplanar and three-dimensional reconstruction capabilities, can be used for virtual bronchoscopy, and can evaluate the vasculature, airways, and, to some degree, the esophagus.[3,6] CT angiography involves the use of ionizing radiation and intravenous contrast material. MRI can visualize the relationship of the vasculature and trachea very well, in addition to detecting airway anomalies, and can also provide evaluation of the heart and any associated anomalies; intravenous contrast agents are not always utilized for MRI and their use may be institution dependent.[2,3,8] MRI, though, is limited by the need for sedation and availability, which may be institution dependent.

Which modality, CT or MRI, is employed may be dependent on the previously-mentioned factors, in addition to subspecialty preference. Consultation with pediatric cardiology or cardiothoracic surgery and pediatric radiology prior to obtaining advanced imaging is appropriate.

ULTRASOUND (US)

Patients with a diagnosis of vascular ring should have echocardiography, since 12% of patients with a vascular ring have associated congenital heart disease.[2] Prenatal US has been reported to be useful in screening for vascular rings. Once a vascular ring is suspected, detailed attention may be provided to the relationship of the aortic arches, ductal arches, and the trachea.[3,9–13] Postnatal US can be used to identify the laterality of the aortic arch and aortic branching patterns.[4,13] US has the advantage of lacking ionizing radiation, lacking the need for sedation, and general availability. However, ultrasonography is less effective at visualization for vascular anomalies in older patients (due to a decreasing size of the thymic acoustic window with increasing age).[4,6]

Imaging Findings

The patient has an acute illness that is consistent with a viral infection. However, due to the history of chronic wheezing and cough, the decision was made to obtain plain radiography of the chest. These images are provided here. The trachea normally buckles away from the side of the aortic arch. There is leftward tracheal deviation consistent with a right aortic arch. There is no focal consolidation or effusion; the heart size and pulmonary vascularity are normal (Fig. 13.1).

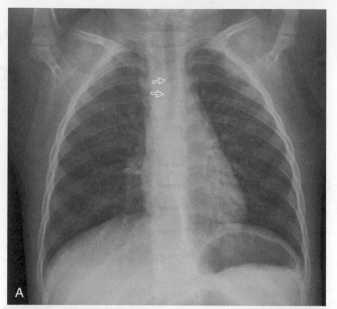

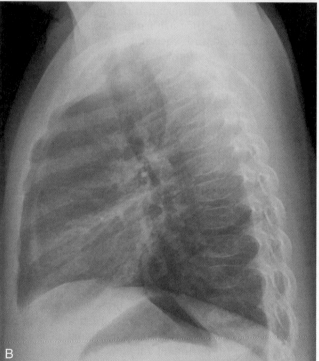

Fig. 13.1 Frontal (A) and lateral (B) views of the chest demonstrate a right-sided aortic arch, which produces a mild mass effect on the right side of the trachea on the frontal view *(white arrows)*, with a subtle tracheal deviation to the left, away from the aortic arch. The lateral view is normal.

Case Conclusion

The patient had barium esophagography performed, after discussion with Pediatric Cardiothoracic Surgery. Selected images are provided here. Fluoroscopic evaluation during ingestion of barium demonstrates a prominent posterior esophageal impression suggestive of an aberrant left subclavian artery in this patient with right-sided aortic arch (Figs. 13.2 and 13.3).

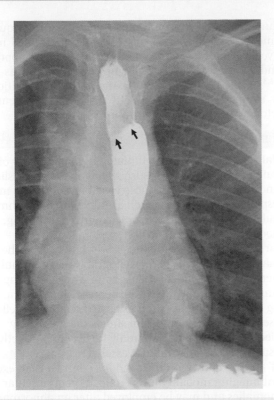

Fig. 13.2 Frontal view from a barium esophagram demonstrates an obliquely-oriented lucency across the upper thoracic esophagus *(arrows)*, consistent with mass effect from a crossing vessel. In this patient with a right-sided aortic arch, the appearance is suggestive of an aberrant left subclavian artery, arising from the right-sided aorta, and crossing behind the esophagus.

Following the esophagram, the decision was made to obtain CT angiography for confirmation and for potential operative repair planning. Selected images are provided here. The aortic arch has the following branching pattern: left common carotid, right common carotid, right subclavian, followed by the left aberrant subclavian artery, which arises from the right-sided aorta and crosses the mediastinum posterior to the esophagus. The tracheal airway courses through this region without significant focal narrowing, indicating this is likely a "loose" ring (Figs. 13.4 and 13.5).

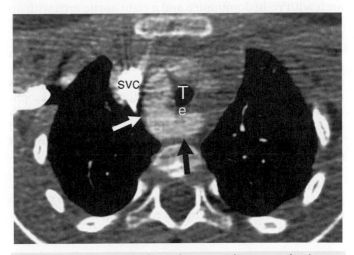

Fig. 13.4 Axial contrast-enhanced computed tomography image demonstrates a right-sided aortic arch *(white arrow)*, and an aberrant left aberrant subclavian artery *(black arrow)* arises from a diverticulum of Kommerell *(black arrow)* from the right-sided aorta. Vessels encircle the trachea *(T)* and the location of the esophagus *(e)* without significant tracheal compression. The superior vena cava is also labeled *(SVC)*.

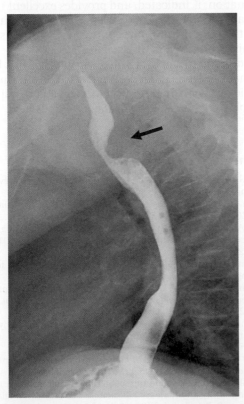

Fig. 13.3 Lateral view from a barium esophagram demonstrates a prominent extrinsic posterior esophageal impression *(arrow)*, consistent with a crossing vessel, likely an aberrant left subclavian artery.

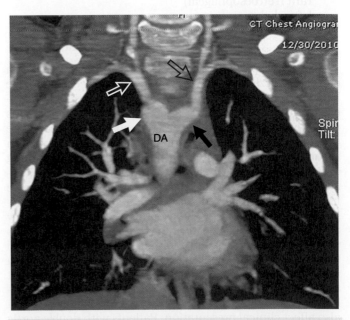

Fig. 13.5 Coronal reconstructed image from a contrast-enhanced computed tomography scan demonstrates a right-sided aortic arch *(white arrow)* and descending aorta *(DA)*. The aberrant left subclavian artery *(black open arrow)* arises from the right-sided aorta from a diverticulum of Kommerell *(black arrow)*. The right subclavian artery *(open white arrow)* arises more proximally from the aortic arch.

The patient underwent operative repair of the ring without incident and recovered uneventfully. Her previous wheezing resolved.

Vascular rings represent approximately 1% of congenital cardiovascular abnormalities and can cause compression of the trachea, esophagus, or both.[3] Most vascular rings present within the first few months of life.[3] The development of a vascular ring (including a double aortic arch) depends on the persistence, involution, or regression of the embryonal aortic arches, and a variety of anatomic variants are possible.[2,3] Common anatomic arrangements leading to a complete vascular ring include a double aortic arch with right dominance and a right aortic arch with an aberrant retroesophageal left subclavian artery and a left ligamentum arteriosum (remnant of the ductus arteriosus).[2,14] While pulmonary artery slings (anomalous origin of the left pulmonary artery from the right pulmonary artery) are the least common anomaly, the anomalous pulmonary artery courses between the trachea and esophagus and pulmonary slings are often associated with tracheal stenosis.[2,3] Other conditions may be associated with vascular rings, including renal and tracheobronchial conditions and chromosomal aberrations, such as chromosome 22q11 deletion.[3,15]

Vascular rings can be classified as complete or incomplete; the International Congenital Heart Surgery Nomenclature and Database Committee has proposed a classification system:[3,16]

COMPLETE VASCULAR RING	INCOMPLETE VASCULAR RING
Double aortic arch	Innominate artery compression syndrome
Right aortic arch, aberrant (retroesophageal) left subclavian artery	Pulmonary artery sling
	Left aortic arch, aberrant right subclavian artery

Classically, patients with a vascular ring present with cough, wheezing, and noisy breathing; the cough may be barky.[2,3] Patients may have symptoms suggestive of gastroesophageal reflux (GERD) and dysphagia; some patients may have a GERD diagnosis or a diagnosis of asthma before the ring is detected.[2,3,17] Pulmonary artery slings have been reported to be associated with apparent life-threatening events now termed brief resolved unexplained event.[2] Recurrent upper respiratory infections and failure to thrive have also been reported with a pulmonary sling.[3] The degree of compression of the esophagus and/or trachea by anomalous vessels can determine the age of presentation as well as the severity; patients with a double aortic arch tend to present in the newborn or early infancy periods, with more severe clinical symptoms, whereas those rings that are less compressive may not become apparent until childhood or even adulthood.[3,17] The type of vascular ring can also affect clinical presentation. Patients with double aortic arch have been found to present principally with respiratory symptoms secondary to tracheal compression, whereas patients with anomalies that result in esophageal compression, such as an aberrant subclavian artery, tend to present with primarily gastrointestinal symptoms.[18]

Management of a symptomatic vascular ring requiring treatment is operative. Repair is usually performed in the first year of life in symptomatic patients.[6] The approach depends on the nature of the ring (or sling) and its location.[2,3] While the majority of patients have resolution of their symptoms, approximately 5% develop recurrent symptoms and require reoperation.[2]

IMAGING PEARLS

1. Plain radiography is the initial imaging modality of choice for patients with suspected vascular ring/sling. Since the symptoms of these vascular anomalies mimic respiratory conditions, such as infection and asthma, and may present with chronic cough or wheezing, this modality is a reasonable first step.

2. Barium esophagography has traditionally been the next imaging modality if plain radiography is abnormal or if there is strong clinical suspicion of a vascular ring/sling. This modality also has the advantage of evaluating other conditions, such as gastroesophageal reflux disease, but an esophagram shows the secondary effects of the vascular anomaly rather than directly visualizing the anomalous vessels.

3. CT angiography with intravenous contrast is an excellent imaging modality for visualization of vascular anomalies and may be employed after an abnormal chest radiograph or barium esophagram. Like MRI, CT angiography demonstrates the relationship between the vascular ring and the trachea and bronchi.

4. MRI angiography is also excellent at evaluating the vasculature. MRI has the added benefit of cardiac evaluation, if indicated, and provides excellent visualization of the relationship between the trachea and the ring. Intravenous contrast is not always required, but is often utilized.

5. The decision to employ CT angiography or MRA is based on multiple factors. It is reasonable to consult a pediatric cardiologist or cardiothoracic surgeon and a pediatric radiologist when advanced imaging is indicated.

References

1. Lowe G, Donaldson JS, Backer CL. Vascular rings: 10-year review of imaging. *Radiographics.* 1991;11(4):637-646.
2. Backer CL, Monge MC, Popescu AR, et al. Vascular rings. *Semin Pediatr Surg.* 2016;25(3):166-175.
3. Licari A, Manca E, Rispoli GA, et al. Congenital vascular rings: a clinical challenge for the pediatrician. *Pediatr Pulmonol.* 2015;50(5):511-524.
4. Hernanz-Schulman M. Vascular rings: a practical approach to imaging diagnosis. *Pediatr Radiol.* 2005;35(5):961-979.
5. Pickhardt PJ, Siegel MJ, Gutierrez FR. Vascular rings in symptomatic children: frequency of chest radiographic findings. *Radiology.* 1997;203(2):423-426.
6. Etesami M, Ashwath R, Kanne J, et al. Computed tomography in the evaluation of vascular rings and slings. *Insights Imaging.* 2014;5(4):507-521.
7. Backer CL, Mavroudis C, Rigsby CK, et al. Trends in vascular surgery. *J Thorac Cardiovasc Surg.* 2005;129(6):1339-1347.
8. Griel GF, Kramer U, Dammann F, et al. Diagnosis of vascular rings and slings using an interleaved 3D double-slab FISP MR angiography technique. *Pediatr Radiol.* 2005;35(4):396-401.
9. Amirav I, Rotschild M, Bar-Yishay E. Pulmonary function tests leading to the diagnosis of vascular ring in an infant. *Pediatr Pulmonol.* 2003;35(1):62-66.

10. Avni FE, Cos T, Cassart M, et al. Evolution of fetal ultrasonography. *Eur Radiol.* 2007;17(2):419-431.

11. Li S, Luo G, Norwitz ER, et al. Prenatal diagnosis of congenital vascular rings and slings: sonographic features and prenatal outcome in 81 consecutive cases. *Prenat Diagn.* 2011;31(4):334-346.

12. Turan S, Turan OM, Maisel P, et al. Three-dimensional sonography in the prenatal diagnosis of aortic arch abnormalities. *J Clin Ultrasound.* 2009;37(5):253-257.

13. Young AA, Hornberger LK, Haberer K, et al. Prenatal detection, comorbidities, and management of vascular rings. *Am J Cardiol.* 2019;123(10):1703-1708.

14. Ishak A, Le Soufe P, Schultz A. Vascular ring: unmasked. *J Paediatr Child Health.* 2017;53(5):502-506.

15. McElhinney DB, Clark BJ, Weinberg PM, et al. Association of chromosomal 22q11 deletion with isolated anomalies of aortic arch laterality and branching. *J Am Coll Cardiol.* 2001;37(8):2114-2119.

16. Backer CL, Mavroudis C. Congenital heart surgery nomenclature and database project: vascular rings, tracheal stenosis, pectus excavatum. *Ann Thorac Surg.* 2000;69(suppl 4):S308-S318.

17. Fernandez-Valls M, Arnaiz J, Lui D, et al. Double aortic arch presents with dysphagia as initial symptom. *J Am Coll Cardiol.* 2012;60(12):1114.

18. Shah RK, Mora BN, Bacha E, et al. The presentation and management of vascular rings: an otolaryngology perspective. *Int J Pediatr Otorhinolaryngol.* 2007;71(1):57-62.

SECTION 3

Gastroenterology

14 *Twisting Tubes: Gastrostomy Tube Issues*

ROBERT VEZZETTI, MD, FAAP, FACEP

Case Presentation

A 7-month-old male with a history of prematurity (27 weeks' gestation) presents with a gastrostomy button that fell out approximately 3 hours prior to arrival. The child has had the gastrostomy button for 3 months. The mother tells you that the button "slipped out" during the child's feeding. She attempted to replace the button but was unsuccessful. The child was seen at an outside facility, who attempted to replace the button through the existing stoma. This was done with great difficulty and there was a small amount of bleeding noted postinsertion. There are no other symptoms or concerns.

The child's physical examination is unremarkable and his vital signs are appropriate for his age. There is a stoma noted, which has some minimal granulation tissue but no erythema, edema, discharge, or bleeding. There is no abdominal distention or apparent tenderness.

Imaging Considerations

Imaging may be used to confirm the position of a gastrostomy button that has been replaced in the emergent or urgent setting. Improper placement of a gastrostomy tube (G-tube) can result in gastric perforation, false tract formation, and peritonitis.[1] However, complication rates following gastrostomy tube replacement in the emergency department are low and are often associated with replacing the tube through an immature tract or changing from one tube type to another.[2-4] According to the literature, a confirmatory contrast study of a replaced gastrostomy button may not be routinely indicated; however, at the author's institution, we do routinely perform such a test, using water-soluble contrast injection and plain radiography, according to institution protocol. If the button was difficult to place or there is any concern about button position following placement, then confirmatory radiography should be obtained. Higher confirmatory imaging rates are found in patients undergoing gastrostomy replacement who had significantly higher rates of immature tracts, difficult G-tube replacement, and stomal stenosis.[2] Clinical signs of proper placement include aspiration of gastric contents through the G-tube (although this is not always considered reliable).[1,5,6]

PLAIN RADIOGRAPHY

This modality has been traditionally utilized to confirm proper placement of a gastrostomy button. Water-soluble contrast is instilled through the gastrostomy button and several images are taken to document the passage of contrast into the stomach and exclude contrast leakage outside of the stomach, and the examination usually shows contrast emptying into the small intestine.

Sample protocol for gastrotomy tube placement confirmation[a]:

1. A gastrotomy tube is placed.
2. Two views of the abdomen are obtained (anteroposterior [AP] supine and left lateral decubitus views). Images are shown to the radiologist to confirm that it is okay to instill contrast.
3. Then 10 mL of water-soluble contrast is injected into the gastrotomy tube, followed by 10 mL of sterile normal saline (at our institution, we use 10 mL of Omnipaque 240 [GE Healthcare, Marlborough, MA, USA], but other water-soluble contrast agents can be used).
4. Two views of the abdomen are obtained after water-soluble contrast injection (AP supine and lateral views).

ULTRASOUND (US)

Replacing a dislodged gastrostomy button in a pediatric patient using point-of-care US (POCUS) guidance has been described.[1,7] The transducer is placed in a transverse orientation below the stoma with the probe marker toward the operator's left and the stoma at approximately the midpoint of the transducer, taking care to identify the stomach and surrounding landmarks prior to tube insertion.[1] Confirmatory contrast abdominal radiography follows, demonstrating proper tube placement.[1] US has the advantage of lack of ionizing radiation, portability, and rapidity of placement; however, the use of radiography to confirm placement does include radiation exposure. While the number of reported cases using US for gastrostomy button placement is not large, POCUS may have a place in gastrostomy tube replacement procedures.

COMPUTED TOMOGRAPHY (CT)

CT has been shown to be useful to help guide placement of gastrotomy tubes. This has been demonstrated in general populations and is often utilized in patients that have complex anatomic conditions or when placement by endoscopy or fluoroscopy has been either unsuccessful or is clinically contraindicated.[8] This imaging modality allows for detailed visualization of the surrounding anatomy and can detect

---

[a]Protocol courtesy of Gael Lonergan, MD (Pediatric Radiology, Dell Children's Medical Center of Central Texas, Austin, TX).

complications from gastrotomy tube placement that may not be evident from plain radiography or contrast studies. CT may show pneumoperitoneum and peritonitis caused by intraperitoneal leakage, or gastric or colonic perforation.[9] CT can demonstrate an aberrant gastrostomy tube course, such as a tube traversing the colon between the stomach and abdominal wall. However, routine use of CT imaging after gastrostomy tube replacement is not indicated.

Imaging Findings

The decision was made to obtain plain abdominal radiography with water-soluble contrast injection to confirm the position of the gastrostomy button, since there was reported difficulty in placing the tube. Precontrast images of the abdomen show the gastrostomy tube in the left upper quadrant in the expected vicinity of the stomach (Fig. 14.1). However, after injection of contrast through the button, two additional views of the abdomen showed contrast in the peritoneal cavity outlining bowel loops, and no contrast was seen within the stomach lumen or intestine. This is consistent with the extraluminal location of the gastrostomy tube with contrast spilling into the peritoneal cavity (Fig. 14.2).

Case Conclusion

Given the imaging results, the Pediatric Surgery team elected to take the child to the operating room for surgical placement of the button under laparoscopic guidance. During the procedure, no iatrogenic injury was noted. A gastrostomy button was placed without difficulty and functionality was confirmed. Repeat imaging was obtained after the procedure and feeds were started, which the child tolerated well.

For comparison, images of a properly positioned gastrostomy tube are provided (Figs. 14.3 and 14.4). These images demonstrate normal filling of the stomach and proximal small bowel after administration of water-soluble contrast. There is no contrast extravasation.

The use of gastrostomy tubes has been increasing in the pediatric population.[1] Gastrostomy buttons are placed for a variety of reasons, including nutritional support, mitigation of aspiration risk, bypassing an obstruction, medication delivery, and improvement in quality of life for both patients and caregivers.[5,10] Pediatric gastrostomy tubes can be a percutaneous gastrostomy tube (PEG tube), a long gastrostomy tube, or a low-profile tube (commonly called a "button"). The most commonly encountered button is the MIC-KEY button (Avanos Medical Devices, Alpharetta, GA).[5] PEG and long gastrostomy tubes are placed with a surgical or pull-through technique; these tubes can be converted to a low-profile button after 8 weeks.[5]

Complications following initial gastrostomy tube placement are seen bimodally[5,11,12]:

Early—These occur less than 7 days after placement and include pneumoperitoneum, pneumomediastinum, peritonitis, wound dehiscence, tube malposition, bleeding, wound infection, ileus, pain, and feeding intolerance.

Late—These occur greater than 7 days after placement and include granulation tissue formation, tube dislodgement,

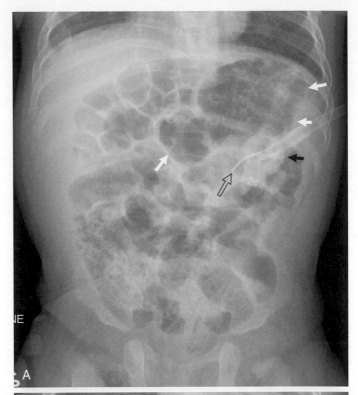

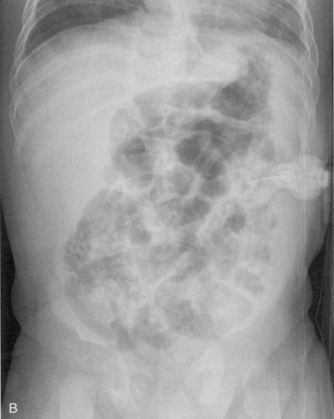

Fig. 14.1 Precontrast scout anteroposterior supine (A) and left lateral decubitus (B) views of the abdomen show the external portion of the gastrostomy tube button *(black arrow)* over the left upper quadrant, the internal tip *(open black arrow)* of the tube overlying the inferior aspect of the stomach. In (A), gas in the stomach is denoted by *white arrows*. The bowel gas pattern is normal and the left lateral decubitus view (B) shows no free air.

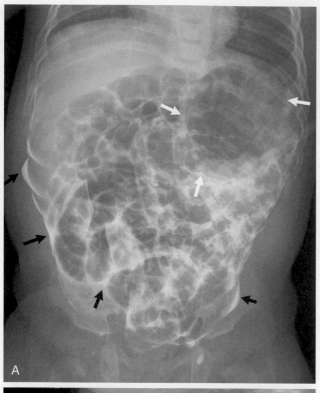

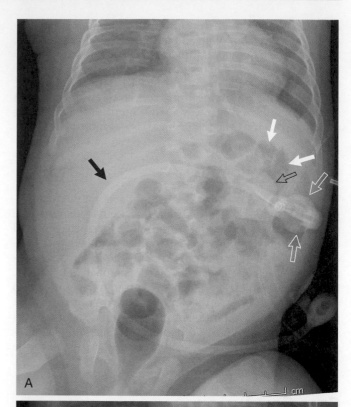

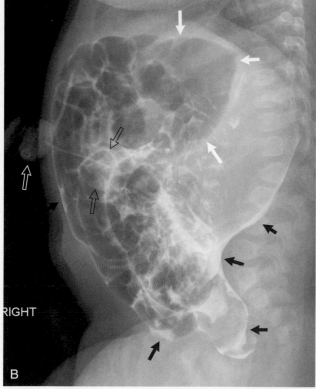

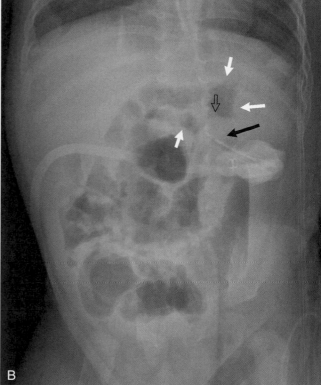

Fig. 14.2 Contrast study demonstrating a gastrostomy tube outside of the gastric lumen. Anteroposterior supine (A) and lateral (B) views of the abdomen after injection of nonionic water-soluble contrast through the gastrostomy tube button demonstrate free spillage of contrast in the peritoneal cavity *(black arrows)*. Contrast outlines the peritoneal spaces and surrounds bowel loops. No intraluminal contrast is seen within the stomach *(white arrows)* or small bowel. On the lateral view (B), the external gastrostomy button is denoted by an *open white arrow* and the internal gastrostomy tube and retention balloon are denoted by *open black arrows*.

Fig. 14.3 Precontrast scout images of a recently replaced and properly positioned gastrostomy tube. Precontrast anteroposterior supine view (A) shows the gastrostomy tube with external button *(open white arrows)* over the left upper quadrant, and the internal retention balloon *(open black arrow)* is outlined by gas in the stomach *(white arrows)*. The *black arrow* points to the external tubing used to access the button. Left lateral decubitus view (B) shows no free intraperitoneal gas. The internal portion of the gastrotomy tube is denoted by the *black arrow*; the retention balloon *(open black arrow)* is partially outlined by gas in the stomach lumen *(white arrows)*.

drainage around the tube, skin breakdown, cellulitis, fistula formation, and buried bumper syndrome (which occurs due to excessive pulling on the tube or a large change in body habitus, causing the balloon to be pulled into the submucosa of the gastric wall, leading to pain and sometimes peritonitis; surgical intervention is required to manage this complication). Granulation tissue formation and dislodgement are the most commonly reported complications.

Leaking around gastrostomy tubes is a common reason to seek care. A typical cause is underinflation of the balloon, but the balloon may also be broken, necessitating replacement of the tube.[5] Leakage around the tube may cause skin irritation, which can be mitigated with a barrier cream, such as Calmoseptine (Calmoseptine, Inc., Huntington Beach, CA). If there is concern for a candida infection, then a topical antifungal, such as nystatin, can be applied.[5] If cellulitis is suspected, then antibiotics (oral or intravenous) appropriate to the child's clinical condition should be initiated. Blocked tubes are also seen, and instillation of crushed tablets is a common cause.[5] Flushing the blocked tube with warm saline using the syringe that comes with the gastrostomy button kit may clear the clog; soft drinks or bicarbonate or phosphate-containing drinks generally should not be utilized.[5] Granulation tissue often forms at the stoma site, which may bleed. Application of silver nitrate using silver nitrate sticks or triamcinolone cream will help with this issue.[5] It is important to attempt to limit the application of silver nitrate to the granulation tissue and not the surrounding skin. After application of silver nitrate, the granulation tissue should be covered with gauze.[5]

The literature has reported that 65% of patients experience dislodgement of their tube within 5 years of placement.[2,6,12] If a PEG or long gastrostomy tube has become dislodged, subspecialty consultation (usually the specialist or specialty service who placed the tube) is often indicated, as there are internal retaining devices (in the case of a PEG tube there is an internal bumper and in the case of a long gastrostomy tube there is a balloon) and both have an external retaining device,[5,10] potentially complicating simple bedside replacement by an emergency physician. These devices can also be replaced by a radiologist under fluoroscopic guidance if necessary.[5] However, long tubes that have been in place for more than 8 weeks and have had the extrinsic fixation device removed can be replaced by an emergency physician.[5] Low-profile gastrostomy buttons are commonly replaced by physicians in the emergent setting, with a very low rate of complications.[6] However, if the button has been in place for less than 6 to 8 weeks or the stoma is difficult to visualize, then subspecialty consultation is recommended.[5] It is important to note that the stoma site will begin to close within 1 to 6 hours once the gastrostomy tube has been dislodged.[5] If a button cannot be replaced, the clinician should insert a Foley catheter one size larger, if possible, to keep the stoma open until a definitive button can be placed.[5] Gastrojejunal (GJ) tubes are usually placed under fluoroscopic guidance, and if a GJ tube becomes dislodged, it should be replaced under fluoroscopic guidance by a qualified radiologist.

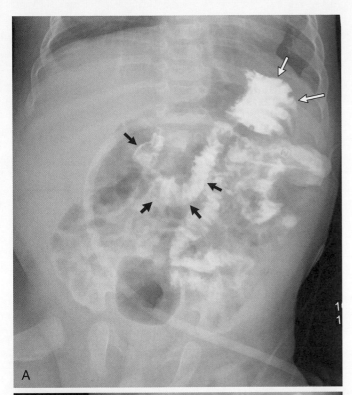
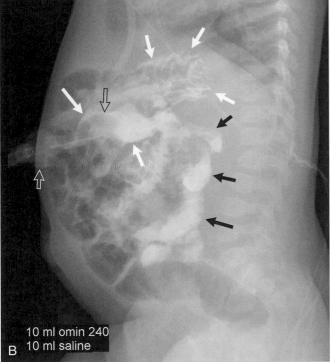

Fig. 14.4 Contrast study of a recently replaced and properly positioned gastrostomy tube. After instillation of 10 mL of water-soluble contrast, followed by 10 mL of sterile saline, anteroposterior supine (A) and lateral (B) views were obtained. Contrast is seen in the gastric lumen *(white arrows)* and has emptied into small bowel loops *(black arrows)*. In part B, the retention balloon *(open black arrow)* of the gastrostomy tube is outlined by contrast in the gastric lumen. The external button is denoted by an *open white arrow*.

3. Schrag SP, Sharma R, Jaik NP, et al. Complications related to percutaneous endoscopic gastrostomy (PEG) tubes. A comprehensive clinical review. *J Gastrointestin Liver Dis.* 2007;16(4):407-418.
4. McQuaid KR, Little TE. Two fatal complications related to gastrostomy "button" placement. *Gastrointest Endosc.* 1992;38(5):601-603.
5. Fuchs S. Gastrostomy tubes: care and feeding. *Pediatr Emerg Care.* 2017;33(12):787-791.
6. Saavedra H, Losek JD, Shanley L, et al. Gastrostomy tube-related complaints in the pediatric emergency department: identifying opportunities for improvement. *Pediatr Emerg Care.* 2009;25(11):728-732.
7. Wu TS, Leech SJ, Rosenberg M, et al. Ultrasound can accurately guide gastrostomy tube replacement and confirm proper tube placement at the bedside. *J Emerg Med.* 2009;36(3):280-284.
8. Brown S, McHugh K, Ledermann S, Pierro A. CT findings in gastrocolic fistula following percutaneous endoscopic gastrostomy. *Pediatr Radiol.* 2007;37(2):229-231.
9. Zissin R, Konikoff F, Gayer G. CT findings of iatrogenic complications following gastrointestinal endoluminal procedures. *Semin Ultrasound CT MR.* 2006;27(2):126-138.
10. Heuschkel RB, Gottrand F, Devarajan K, et al. ESPGHAN position paper on management of percutaneous endoscopic gastrostomy in children and adolescents. *J Pediatr Gastroenterol Nutr.* 2015;60(1):131-141.
11. Zamakhshary M, Jamal M, Blair GK, et al. Laparoscopic vs percutaneous endoscopic gastrostomy tube insertion: a new pediatric gold standard? *J Pediatr Surg.* 2005;40(5):859-862.
12. Naiditch JA, Lautz T, Barsness KA. Postoperative complications in children undergoing gastrostomy tube placement. *J Laparoendosc Adv Surg Tech A.* 2010;20(9):781-785.

1. Radiographic confirmation after gastrostomy tube/button replacement may not be routinely indicated, but there are circumstances where confirmatory radiography should be obtained. There are no standard guidelines for the use of confirmatory radiography after gastrostomy tube/button replacement.
2. Plain radiography of the abdomen using water-soluble contrast may be performed to confirm proper tube placement.
3. Point-of-care ultrasound (POCUS) has been utilized to assist in, and confirm, gastrostomy tube placement. This does require expertise in abdominal US technique.
4. Computed tomography may be utilized to evaluate for complications of G-tube placement, such as an aberrant course of the tube, and has the advantage of demonstrating detailed anatomy, but it is not a first-line imaging modality for gastrostomy tube replacement.

References

1. Myatt TC, Medak AJ, Lam SHF. Use of point-of-care ultrasound to guide pediatric gastrostomy tube replacement in the emergency department. *Pediatr Emerg Care.* 2018;34(2):145-148.
2. Showalter CD, Kerrey B, Spellman-Kennebeck S, et al. Gastrostomy tube replacement in a pediatric ED: frequency of complications and impact of confirmatory imaging. *Am J Emerg Med.* 2012;30(8):1501-1506.

15 Not Movin': Pediatric Bowel Obstruction

ROBERT VEZZETTI, MD, FAAP, FACEP

Case Presentation

A 2-year-old male with a medical history of Hirschsprung disease requiring colectomy and ileo-anal pullthrough presents with multiple episodes of nonbilious emesis and no stool output over the past 24 hours. The mother states that she has noted that the child has had increased abdominal girth over the past 48 hours and has become fussy. He has had decreased oral intake. There has been no fever, cough, congestion, or diarrhea.

Shortly after birth, he underwent colectomy and ileostomy (which was taken down several months prior to his acute presentation). He has a chronic dysmotility disorder and is followed closely by Pediatric Gastroenterology. The mother has tried rectal dilatation and Miralax at home, per the child's usual regimen when there is decreased stool output, without success. She has also noted no passage of flatus.

Physical examination reveals an interactive, non–toxic appearing, but visibly uncomfortable, child. He is afebrile. He has a heart rate of 130 beats per minute, respiratory rate of 24 breaths per minute, blood pressure of 93/54 mm Hg, and pulse oximetry of 99% on room air. His examination is remarkable for a moderately distended abdomen that does not appear to be tender. There is no organomegaly. Digital rectal examination results in an explosion of liquid, brown, nonbloody stool.

Imaging Considerations

The location of the suspected obstruction will help the clinician determine which imaging modality to employ.

PLAIN RADIOGRAPHY

This modality is often a first-line test and is rapidly available, requiring minimal exposure to ionizing radiation. Plain radiography can assist in the identification of the level of obstruction and can help guide the clinician in choosing more advanced imaging modalities, if indicated.[1,2] Bowel gas patterns can be associated with various pathologies: the "double bubble" sign of duodenal atresia, the "triple bubble" sign of proximal jejunal atresia, various abnormal patterns associated with meconium ileus, multiple air-filled loops of bowel with a lack of rectal gas in the infant with Hirschsprung disease, distended stomach in some infants with pyloric stenosis, radio-opaque foreign bodies, and a soft tissue mass effect on the right and lack of colonic air in some infants with intussusception.[3] Perforation and free air can also be demonstrated. This is a primary value of plain abdominal radiography, but plain radiographs may vary and may even be normal in some pathologies, such as malrotation and volvulus.[4]

ULTRASOUND

Ultrasound is a first-line imaging modality for several causes of intestinal obstruction in pediatric patients, such as pyloric stenosis, intussusception, and pediatric appendicitis.[1,3] The usefulness of ultrasound to detect malrotation has been investigated. In this technique, the relationship of the superior mesenteric artery (SMA) and the superior mesenteric vein (SMV) is evaluated. The SMA is normally to the left of the SMV. When the SMV is to the left of the SMA, the relationship of the vessels is inverted. It has been suggested that if this relationship is abnormal, the patient should undergo an upper gastrointestinal series (UGI) to confirm the presence or absence of malrotation.[4–6] A study examining this relationship reported a false-positive rate of 21% (abnormal ultrasound and normal UGI) and a false-negative rate of 2% (normal ultrasound and abnormal UGI).[4,7] Another series found an abnormal relationship between these structures to have a sensitivity and specificity of 67% to 100% and 75% to 83% for malrotaion.[8] Therefore, SMA/SMV inversion as a solitary finding is not highly sensitive or specific for malrotation. Additional sonographic signs that improve the value of ultrasound for malrotation include the "whirlpool sign," where the mesentery and mesenteric vessels are wrapped around the SMA and SMV,[4] and evaluation of whether the transverse duodenum is in a normal retroperitoneal position. When these two additional signs are evaluated in addition to SMA/SMV inversion, the sensitivity of ultrasound for malrotation is markedly improved, with one study showing a sensitivity of 100% and a specificity of over 97% in the detection of malrotation.[9] However, such an examination requires significant pediatric sonographic imaging expertise to perform and interpret and would find greatest utility in a facility with dedicated pediatric sonography.

UPPER GASTROINTESTINAL SERIES

This is the diagnostic test of choice in patients with suspected malrotation with or without volvulus as a cause of intestinal obstruction.[2] False-positive and false-negative test results do occur, reported to be up to 15% and up to 6%, respectively,[4,10] so proper technique and expertise in imaging interpretation are essential to provide meaningful and accurate results.

COMPUTED TOMOGRAPHY (CT)

While not a typical first-line imaging test in children with suspected bowel obstruction, CT is useful at detecting such pathology. The pediatric literature is not as prolific compared to the adult literature investigating the use of CT in the diagnosis of intestinal obstruction. However, one study looking at small bowel obstruction reported a sensitivity of 87% and a specificity of 86% for detecting small bowel obstruction in pediatric patients (especially those over the age of 2 years); these percentages included patients with adynamic ileus, since this may be difficult to distinguish from bowel obstruction on CT.[11] CT is also useful in detecting the level of obstruction (comparable to adult studies) in most patients (86%) but was not as useful in determining the cause of obstruction (54%).[11] CT may be employed as a secondary test if other imaging modalities are equivocal or there is concern for a complex intra-abdominal process.

Imaging Findings

Plain radiography of the abdomen was obtained. These images demonstrated dilated small bowel loops in the upper abdomen without evidence of free air (Figs. 15.1 and 15.2).

Case Conclusion

Pediatric Surgery and Pediatric Gastroenterology were both consulted and the child was admitted to the pediatric

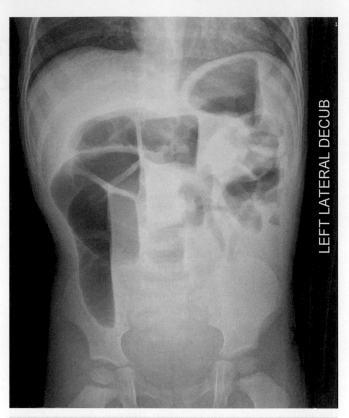

Fig. 15.2 Left lateral decubitus view of the abdomen demonstrating dilated small bowel loops with air fluid levels, without evidence of free air; there is no rectal gas.

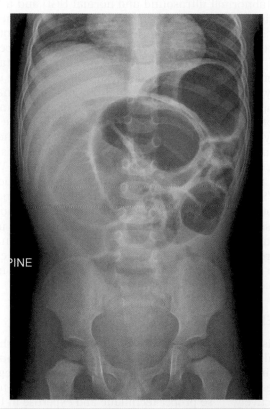

Fig. 15.1 Supine AP view of the abdomen demonstrating dilated small bowel loops in the upper abdomen; there is no rectal gas.

hospitalist service for management of the obstruction. During his first hospital day, he underwent rectal dilatation and an SMOG (saline, mineral oil, glycerine) enema with a return of a very large amount of liquid stool. He improved after rectal dilatation and was ultimately discharged home.

Pediatric bowel obstruction has many causes and may present with a variety of symptoms, including acute abdominal pain, fussiness, vomiting, and shock, as well as having a more chronic presentation, as may be the case with partial or recurring episodes of obstruction. A thorough history and physical examination can guide the clinician in the investigation of a bowel obstruction as well as management. It may be helpful to think of the etiologies of neonatal and pediatric bowel obstruction by potential underlying causes. These include congenital, infective, traumatic, inflammatory, and neoplastic, among others. Consider the age of the patient, as certain causes of bowel obstruction occur more frequently in particular age groups.

Pediatric bowel obstruction has many causes and is associated with significant morbidity and mortality if these conditions are not detected and managed in a timely manner. As in adults, appendicitis and postoperative adhesions are causes of bowel obstruction in children. Children also experience bowel obstruction due to congenital and other pathologies not generally seen in adults. Causes of bowel obstruction in children also include the following:

Intestinal Atresia

This is the most common cause of congenital intestinal obstruction and represents a large portion of neonatal obstruction cases.[1] While mortality for this condition was significant (up to 90%), this has declined to around 10%.[1] Duodenal atresia (often associated with an annular pancreas) and jejunoileal atresia can be seen in this age group and present as bilious emesis. The classic appearance of a "double bubble" on plain radiography suggests duodenal atresia.[1,2] Whether an imaging evaluation is indicated varies by suspected etiology and level of obstruction but, if indicated, should be performed by a pediatric radiologist or an imager with significant pediatric experience. Fluid resuscitation and surgical management are indicated for these patients.

Pyloric Stenosis

Typically seen in the first 3–6 weeks of life, this is the most common cause of gastric outlet obstruction in this age group.[1] A typical history consists of repeated episodes of nonbilious, "projectile" emesis with feeding. The often-cited electrolyte abnormalities include a hypochloremic, hypokalemic metabolic alkalosis. First-line imaging evaluation is a pyloric ultrasound. Fluid resuscitation, correction of metabolic derangements, and surgical consultation are cornerstones of management.

Malrotation With or Without Volvulus

The majority of pediatric patients with malrotation with or without volvulus will present in the first month of life, although this entity may present in older children, including teenagers.[1,12] First-line imaging evaluation is a fluoroscopic UGI series. Prompt recognition and surgical management are imperative in order to avoid significant morbidity and mortality associated with this condition.

Meconium Ileus

While not commonly encountered in the emergency department, meconium ileus is significant due to its association with cystic fibrosis and pancreatic dysfunction. Children with cystic fibrosis may also have distal intestinal obstruction syndrome, constipation, megacolon, and rectal prolapse.[1] Meconium ileus presents in the neonatal period, in the first couple days of life. Uncomplicated cases of meconium ileus are managed with supportive care and hyperosmolar enema; complicated cases should have pediatric surgical consultation and are usually managed with operative resection/anatamoses.[1]

Intussusception

This is the most common cause of infant bowel obstruction and is usually found in children under the age of 6 years old.[1] The underlying etiology of intussusception varies by age group: Infants and young children usually have "idiopathic" intussusceptions, with a lead point of inflamed intestinal lymphoid tissue, whereas older children often have a true lead point, such as a polyp, Meckel diverticulum or neoplastic process.[1] First-line imaging for intussusception is ultrasound evaluation, but treatment for idiopathic intussusception is generally accomplished with an air enema.[1] Children in extremis require fluid resuscitation, especially prior to any radiologic study or surgical intervention; these patients may require a pediatric surgical consult, particularly if the patient has had prolonged symptoms or there are signs of peritonitis.[1]

Hirschsprung Disease

In a patient with a history of delayed passage of meconium during the immediate postpartum period who presents with signs of bowel obstruction, the clinician should consider Hirschsprung disease as a possible etiology. This entity can be associated with other underlying medical conditions, such as Down syndrome. Imaging evaluation is performed with a water-soluble contrast enema. Until a patient is able to undergo surgical correction, bowel washouts are utilized in an attempt to keep the bowel decompressed.[1]

Intestinal Strictures

As a consequence of abdominal trauma, intestinal strictures have been reported and should be considered in a patient with a history of intestinal perforation or previous abdominal surgery.[1,13] Children with a history of blunt abdominal trauma who present with signs of bowel obstruction may have strictures or adhesions.[13] Children with inflammatory bowel disease can also develop intestinal strictures and inflammatory masses involving affected portions of the bowel, both producing signs of bowel obstruction.[1] Children with Crohn disease may require surgical intervention performed in cases of stricturing.[14] Management involves consultation with pediatric surgery and pediatric gastroenterology for patients with complications from underlying inflammatory bowel disease.

Foreign Body Ingestions

The literature is replete with all manner of foreign bodies producing intestinal obstruction; children with pica or a history of developmental delay are at particular risk for foreign body ingestion.[15–19] Plain radiography is the first-line imaging modality. Management depends on the type, quantity, and location of the foreign body and may be made in consultation with pediatric surgery and/or pediatric gastroenterology.

Intestinal Tumors

Intestinal tumors are not common in children, but when present as a cause of intestinal obstruction, lymphoma is the dominant pathology.[1] Management is directed at the underlying etiology of the tumor.

Omphalomesenteric Remnants

A Meckel diverticulum can cause intestinal obstruction[1,20] and is a common congenital malformation of the gastrointestinal tract.[20] Bowel obstruction is a common complication of Meckel diverticulum and can produce obstruction due to intussusception, adhesions, or volvulus.[20] These complications can be detected with CT. Management includes consultation with pediatric surgery for surgical correction.

Several illustrative cases are provided here:

Figs. 15.3 and 15.4 show a 10-year-old female who presented with 1 day of rapidly progressive abdominal pain and distention, as well as emesis. Plain radiography of the abdomen demonstrated marked colonic distention. Pediatric Gastroenterology was consulted and the child was taken to the endoscopy suite, at which time a sigmoid volvulus identified and reduced successfully. Interestingly, this was the child's third occurrence. Pediatric Surgery was consulted and the child was then taken to the operating suite for sigmoidectomy.

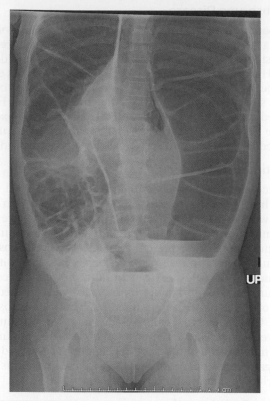

Fig. 15.3 Upright AP view of the abdomen demonstrating marked colonic distention.

Figs. 15.5 and 15.6 show a 10-year-old child who swallowed several magnets 2 days prior to evaluation, then several more 1 day prior to evaluation. She did not tell anyone of the ingestion secondary to not wanting to get into trouble. She presented with one episode of nonbilious/nonbloody emesis and generalized abdominal pain. Imaging revealed findings of early or partial small bowel obstruction with scattered "string of pearls" air-fluid levels and organized dilated loops of small bowel. There are four radio-opaque foreign bodies consistent with the history of swallowing magnets, which appear to be stuck together. Due to her symptoms, Pediatric Surgery was consulted and the patient was taken to the operating suite for laparoscopic removal. During this procedure, the small bowel was found to be dilated and four microperforations were discovered. She had an uneventful recovery.

Figs. 15.7 and 15.8 show a 15-month-old child who presented with symptoms suggestive of intussusception. Plain radiography prior to an ultrasound demonstrated small bowel obstruction. Ultrasound confirmed intussusception. The child underwent an air enema procedure for reduction, which was partially successful. Pediatric Surgery was consulted and the child required operative reduction. Twenty-four hours later, symptoms of intussusception returned and he required repeat operative reduction. No pathologic lead point was identified. After the second reduction, he did well.

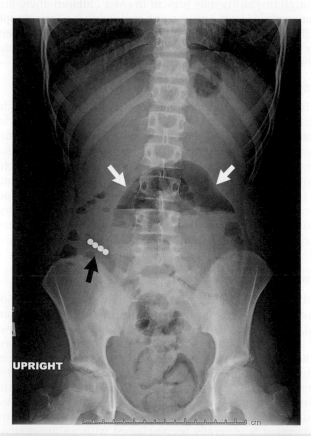

Fig. 15.5 Upright AP view of the abdomen demonstrating early or partial small bowel obstruction with organized dilated loops of small bowel with air fluid levels in the mid abdomen *(white arrows)*, but there is still colonic gas present. There are four radio-opaque metallic foreign bodies consistent with ingested magnets, which appear to be stuck together *(black arrow)*.

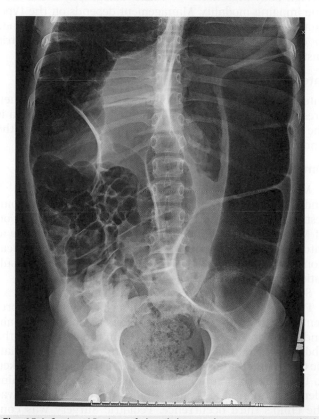

Fig. 15.4 Supine AP view of the abdomen demonstrating marked colonic distention.

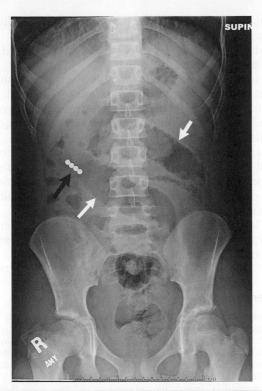

Fig. 15.6 Supine AP view of the abdomen demonstrating early or partial small bowel obstruction with organized dilated loops of small bowel in the mid abdomen *(white arrows)*, but there is still colonic gas present. There are four radio-opaque metallic foreign bodies consistent with ingested magnets, which appear to be stuck together *(black arrow)*.

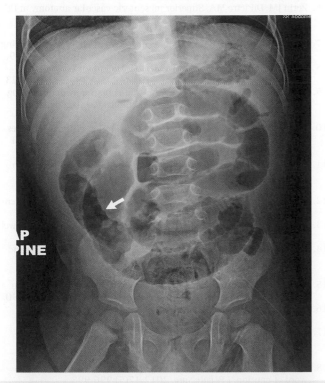

Fig. 15.7 Supine anteroposterior view demonstrates abnormal tubular dilated gas-filled small bowel throughout much of the abdomen, with very little gas in the colon, consistent with small bowel obstruction. Small bowel fold thickening in the right abdomen suggests bowel wall edema *(arrow)*.

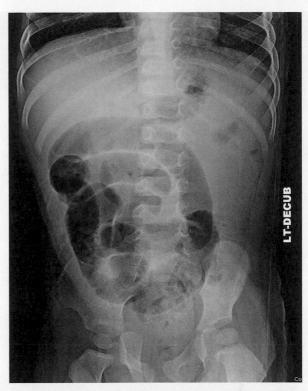

Fig. 15.8 Left lateral decubitus view demonstrates abnormal tubular dilated gas-filled small bowel throughout much of the abdomen, with very little gas in the colon, consistent with small bowel obstruction.

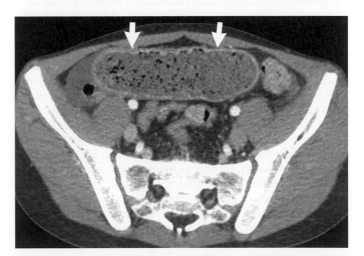

Fig. 15.9 Axial contrast-enhanced computed tomography (CT) image demonstrates a dilated small bowel loop containing stool-like material *(arrows)* in the pelvis. Small bowel does not normally contain stool-like material, except occasionally in the distal-most ileum. This appearance of dilated small bowel containing stool-like material on CT is a finding suggestive of small bowel obstruction. At surgery, this patient had a Meckel diverticulum as the cause of small bowel obstruction.

Fig. 15.9 shows a selected CT image of an 11-year-old male who presented with emesis and acute abdominal pain. He initially had an abdominal ultrasound for appendicitis that was equivocal. Pediatric Surgery was consulted and recommended CT scanning. An intravenous (IV) contrast-enhanced CT scan was obtained showing abnormal dilatation of the small bowel to the mid ileum and dilated distal small bowel

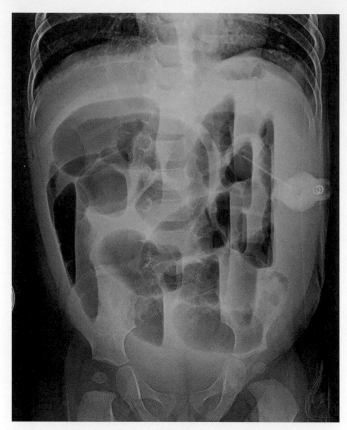

Fig. 15.10 Left lateral decubitus view of the abdomen demonstrating long air-fluid levels within several dilated small bowel loops, a pattern consistent with small bowel obstruction. A gastrotomy tube is present in the left upper quadrant.

loops containing stool-like material, findings suggesting small bowel obstruction. He was taken to the operating suite and was found to have a Meckel diverticulum as the source of his obstruction. This was resected and the patient did well.

Fig. 15.10 shows a child with a history of complex medical issues, including a Cri du Chat syndrome, gastrostomy, and a Ladd procedure, who presented with emesis and abdominal distention. He was quite ill-appearing and required fluid resuscitation. Plain abdominal radiography was obtained (a selected view is provided here), demonstrating long air-fluid levels within several dilated small bowel loops and no significant colonic gas, consistent with small bowel obstruction. Due to his complexity, as well as previous abdominal surgical procedures, Pediatric Surgery was consulted and the child was taken to the operating suite for exploratory laparotomy. He was found to have multiple sites of bowel adhesion, as well as small bowel perforations. He underwent resection of a portion of the small bowel and had a very difficult postoperative course. Ultimately, after several weeks in the hospital (including the pediatric intensive care unit), he was able to be discharged.

IMAGING PEARLS

1. In suspected bowel obstruction, plain radiography is a good first-line imaging choice. In infants/young children (<8 years of age), anterior-posterior supine and left lateral decubitus views and in older children upright and flat views can be obtained, if possible.

Plain radiography has the advantage of availability and rapidity and can help determine the level of obstruction, the presence of free air, and the need for more advanced imaging.

2. US is an excellent imaging modality when intussusception, appendicitis, or pyloric stenosis is suspected. While ultrasound is usually readily available, expertise in ultrasound technique and interpretation is required to have a clinical useful study.

3. UGI series is the imaging modality of choice when malrotation, with or without volvulus, is suspected. Expertise in pediatric fluoroscopy and interpretation is needed and this study is not always readily available at a nonpediatric facility.

4. CT is usually reserved for equivocal cases or if complex intraabdominal pathology is suspected. IV contrast should be utilized.

References

1. Hajivassiliou CA. Intestinal obstruction in neonatal/pediatric surgery. *Semin Pediatr Surg.* 2003;12(3):241-253.
2. Carroll AG, Kavanagh RG, Leidhin CN, et al. Comparative effectiveness of imaging modalities for the diagnosis of intestinal obstruction in neonates and infants: a critically appraised topic. *Acad Radiol.* 2016;23(5):559-568.
3. Maclennan AC. Investigation in vomiting children. *Semin Pediatr Surg.* 2003;12(4):220-228.
4. Applegate KE. Evidence-based diagnosis of malrotation and volvulus. *Pediatr Radiol.* 2009;39(suppl 2):S161-S163.
5. Weinberger E, Winters WD, Liddell RM, et al. Sonographic diagnosis of intestinal malrotation in infants: importance of the relative positions of the superior mesenteric vein and artery. *AJR Am J Roentgenol.* 1992;159(4):825-828.
6. Zerin JM, DiPietro MA. Superior mesenteric vascular anatomy at US in patients with surgically proved malrotation of the midgut. *Radiology.* 1992;183(3):693-694.
7. Ozrech N, Navarro OM, Langer JC. Is ultrasonography a good screening test for intestinal malrotation? *J Pediatr Surg.* 2006;41(5):1005-1009.
8. Dulfor D, Daleat MH, Dassonville M, et al. Midgut malrotation, the reliability of sonographic diagnosis. *Pediatr Radiol.* 1992;22(1):21-23.
9. Zhou L, Li S, Wang W, et al. Usefulness of sonography in evaluating children suspected of malrotation. *J Ultrasound Med.* 2015;34: 1825-1832.
10. Applegate KE, Anderson JA, Klatte E. Malrotation of the gastrointestinal tract: a problem solving approach to performing the upper GI series. *Radiographics.* 2006;26:1485-1500.
11. Jabra AA, Eng J, Zaleski CG, et al. CT of small-bowel obstruction in children. Sensitivity and specificity. *AJR Am J Roentgenol.* 2001;177(2):431-436
12. Pelcio M, Haywood Y. Midgut volvulus: an unusual case of adolescent abdominal pain. *Am J Emerg Med.* 1994;12:167-171.
13. Jones VS, Soundappan SV, Cohen RC, et al. Posttraumatic small bowel obstruction in children. *J Pediatr Surg.* 2007;42(8):1386-1388.
14. Rinawi F, Assa A, Hartman C, et al. Incidence of bowel surgery and associated risk factors in pediatric-onset Crohn's disease. *Inflamm Bowel Dis.* 2016;22(12):2917-2923.
15. Serour F, Witzling M, Frenkel-Laufer D, et al. Intestinal obstruction in an autistic adolescent. *Pediatr Emerg Care.* 2008;24(10):688-690.
16. Alfonzo MJ, Baum CR. Magnetic foreign body ingestions. *Pediatr Emerg Care.* 2016;32(10):698-702.
17. Quintana JF, Walker RN, McGeehan A. Child with small bowel obstruction and perforation secondary to ileal bezoar. *Pediatr Emerg Care.* 2008;24(2):99-101.
18. Stringle G, Parker M, McCoy E. Vinyl glove ingestion in children: a word of caution. *J Pediatr Surg.* 2012;47(5):996-998.
19. Retter J, Neff W, Singer MV. Small bowel obstruction produced by a phytobezoar. *Clin Gastroenterol Hepatol.* 2008;6(1):A20.
20. Choi SY, Hong SS, Park HJ, et al. The many faces of Meckel's diverticulum and its complications. *J Med Imaging Radiat Oncol.* 2017;61(2):225-231.

16 *Screaming Fits: Intussusception*

TINA CHU, MD

Case Presentation

A 15-month-old boy is brought into the emergency department by his parents for inconsolable crying for the last 6 hours. He has been crying and refusing to feed and has had nonbloody, nonbilious emesis twice. He is afebrile and his other vital signs are heart rate in the 160s beats per minute, respiratory rate of 30 breaths per minute, blood pressure of 107/89 mm Hg, and an oxygen saturation of 98% on room air. He is asleep and does not wake up except to grimace during his abdominal examination. There are no deformities, corneal abrasions, and other abnormalities on the rest of his examination.

Imaging Considerations

Imaging modalities largely depend on institutional practices, the availability of fluoroscopy and ultrasound (US), and the experience and preference of the providers managing the patient. A prompt surgical consult is warranted in children with obvious signs of peritonitis as operative management is required. For children who are not in extremis, several imaging choices are available to clinicians.

PLAIN RADIOGRAPHY

A two-view study (anterior-posterior and upright or preferably left lateral decubitus) is preferred to look for signs of obstruction (dilated bowel loops, air fluid levels) or for bowel perforation (free air), especially prior to any attempted enema reduction or surgical intervention. However, given the reported low sensitivity (48%) and specificity (21%) of plain film for intussusception in pediatric patients, abdominal radiographs in general should not to be used exclusively to exclude the diagnosis of intussusception.[1] Left lateral decubitus views are favored over upright views in young children at greatest risk for intussusception. On upright views, gas moves superiorly, with decreased gas in the cecum and distal colon, which can cause spurious concern for intussusception.[2] On left lateral decubitus views, colonic gas moves into the cecum and right colon, the area of greatest concern with suspected intussusception.[2] Findings, which depend on the duration of symptoms and degree of associated complications, that suggest abnormality include:

- Other signs of obstruction: proximal bowel dilation with distal paucity of gas (Figs. 16.1 and 16.2).
- Right upper quadrant findings of an elongated or rounded mass (see Fig. 16.1), obscured liver margin, or a focal paucity of gas.
- Target sign superimposed over the right kidney, with central fat within a rounded area of mass effect.[3]

- Meniscus sign: a rounded soft-tissue mass (the intussusceptum) protruding into the gas-filled transverse colon can be seen on plain radiography, but the equivalent is well seen on an included image from an air enema (Fig. 16.3A).

ABDOMINAL US

US has a 98% to 100% sensitivity and 88% to 100% specificity for diagnosing intussusception and a negative predictive value approaching 100%.[4] This makes it the preferred method of choice for diagnosis. The lack of ionizing radiation and the rapidity of the scanning time make this modality ideal in the pediatric population. However, US for intussusception may not be readily available at nonpediatric centers as familiarity with this technique may be lacking, and experience and expertise are needed to obtain and interpret imaging. US may also be used as the guiding imaging modality during hydrostatic reduction of intussusception and to identify underlying pathology such as polyps or other lead points not readily detected by fluoroscopy.[4] Findings on US that suggest intussusception include the following:

- Target sign (or bull's-eye or doughnut sign) showing the different intestinal layers of concentric bowel loops, represented by alternating echogenic and hypoechogenic bands, seen on scanning transversely through an intussusception (Fig. 16.4).
- Pseudokidney, in which the appearance of the intussuscepted segment of bowel resembles a kidney, seen on longitudinal scanning.
- Crescent in a doughnut sign, a variation of the target sign, referring to an echogenic asymmetric crescent inside the target, created by mesenteric fat pulled into the intussusception with the leading edge of the intussusceptum, the inner loop of bowel in the intussusception (Fig. 16.4).

COMPUTED TOMOGRAPHY (CT) SCANS

Intussusception can be visualized on CT. However, a CT scan is not necessary for the diagnosis or management of intussusception and is not recommended as an initial diagnostic modality.

FLUOROSCOPY

A hydrostatic (liquid) or air enema is the standard treatment for both diagnosis and management of ileocolic intussusception in stable children with no evidence of bowel perforation. Both can be performed without sedation or general anesthesia and have an 80% to 95% success rate.[5-7] The technique chosen depends on institutional practices and the radiologist's preference. Air or a water-soluble medium (saline for US or iodinated contrast for fluoroscopy) is introduced

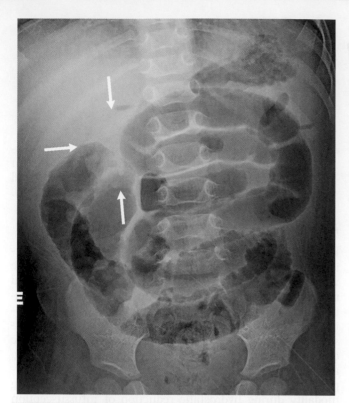

Fig. 16.1 Anterior-posterior view demonstrating abnormal bowel gas pattern with a paucity of gas in the colon. Tubular, dilated, gas-filled loops of small bowel are consistent with small bowel obstruction. There is a subtle mass effect suggesting an intussusception in the right upper quadrant (arrows).

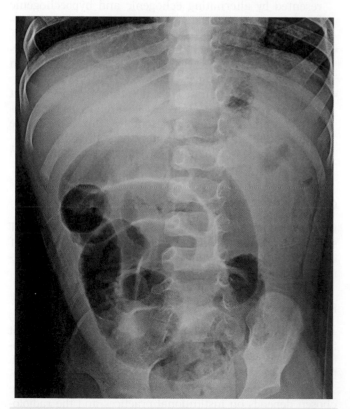

Fig. 16.2 Left lateral decubitus view demonstrating small bowel obstruction, scattered air fluid levels, and no free air.

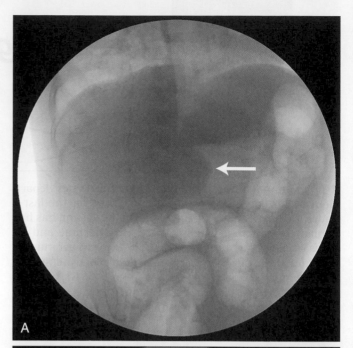

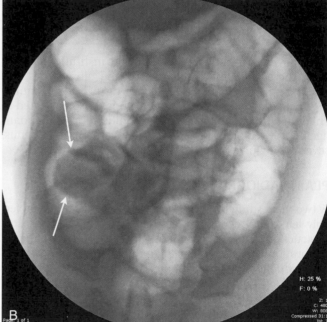

Fig. 16.3 Selected images of air enema reduction. (A) Intussusception (arrow) encountered in the mid transverse colon. (B) Residual filling defect of an intussusception (arrows) in the air-filled cecum, consistent with partial reduction. The intussusception was subsequently completely reduced.

through the rectum and this retrograde pressure is used to reduce the ileocolic intussusception. There have been reports of more successful rates of reductions with air (83%) as compared to hydrostatic reductions (70%).[7] There is a less than 1% risk of tension pneumoperitoneum with air enema reductions, and failures/complications are associated with younger children (less than 6 months), prolonged duration of symptoms (over 48 hours), or evidence of small bowel obstruction.[8–11] However, these factors are not contraindications to the performance of a therapeutic enema reduction.

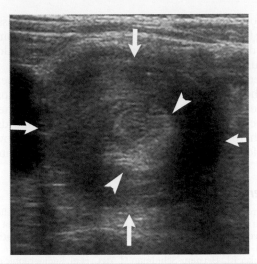

Fig. 16.4 Ultrasound demonstrating the target or doughnut sign of an intussusception *(arrows)* imaged in cross-section (transverse). Crescent in doughnut sign *(arrowheads)* is an echogenic crescent of mesenteric fat within the intussusception.

Image Findings

Suspecting intussusception, plain radiography was obtained while preparations were made to proceed to abdominal US. There is abnormal tubular dilated gas-filled small bowel throughout much of the abdomen, with the appearance suggesting bowel wall edema of the dilated small bowel in the right abdomen. There is a paucity of colonic gas and no free air is noted (Figs. 16.1 and 16.2).

The US study demonstrates an intussusception in the right abdomen extending into the right upper quadrant (Fig. 16.4).

For comparison, another case is presented here. A 4-year-old child presented with abdominal pain and emesis for the past week, developing bloody stools during the last day of his illness. Plain radiography demonstrated a soft tissue mass effect on the left side of the abdomen (Figs. 16.5 and 16.6). The US (Fig. 16.7) revealed an intussusception extending from the left upper quadrant to the left lower quadrant. There was a rounded soft tissue mass with a stalk along the inferior aspect of the intussusception, concerning for a polyp. Because of the suspected lead point seen on US, initially, a water-soluble contrast enema was performed. The intussusception was incompletely reduced, and additional reduction attempts with air were performed. Despite multiple attempts, reduction was not successful. This child required operative intervention. At the time of surgery, a polyp was discovered, likely serving as the lead point for the child's colocolic intussusception. Biopsy later determined this was a juvenile polyp.

Case Conclusion

The child underwent successful reduction of his intussusception by air enema (Figs. 16.3A,B) and was admitted to the hospital for further monitoring. He was discharged the next day after tolerating oral fluids.

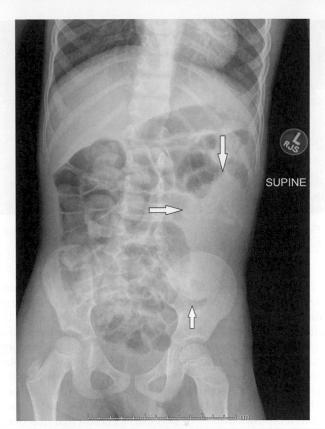

Fig. 16.5 Anterior-posterior view demonstrating mass effect, with localized absence of bowel gas, in the left abdomen *(arrows)*.

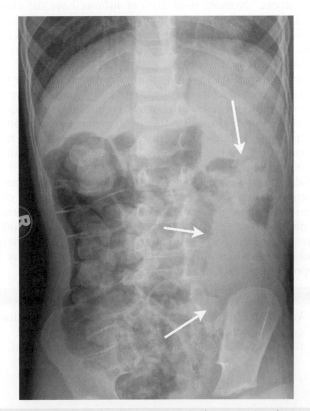

Fig. 16.6 Left lateral decubitus view again demonstrating the mass effect in the left abdomen *(arrows)*.

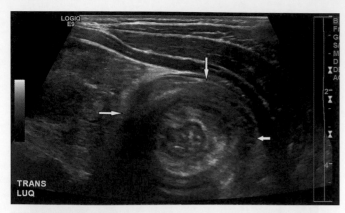

Fig. 16.7 Ultrasound demonstrating the target or doughnut sign of intussusception *(arrows)* in the left colon.

Inconsolability in infants is a common pediatric complaint. Ear infections, oral ulcers, corneal abrasions, or hair tourniquets are easily ruled out by physical examination. In the setting of fussiness, lethargy, vomiting, and abdominal pain, one must consider intussusception. This most commonly occurs in the 3 months to 12 months age range.[12] Intussusception occurs when a proximal segment of the bowel (intussusceptum) is telescoped into the lumen of the distal segment of bowel (intussuscipiens) and fails to reduce, instead enlarging as it is pulled distally by peristalsis. Persistent intussusception leads to venous and lymphatic congestion, with resulting ischemia of the bowel wall and mesentery, intestinal wall edema, pain, and the eventual sloughing of mucosal wall and hemorrhage, which can present clinically as "currant red jelly stools." Notably, only 20% of infants have the classic triad of episodic abdominal pain, vomiting, and bloody stools.[12] The majority of intussusception in children is ileocolic (up to 90% of cases),[13] but the condition can occur anywhere along the bowel.

Ileo-colic intussusception requires reduction, and the majority of cases are successfully treated with enema (often air is employed). Unsuccessful or partial reductions may require surgical intervention, although delayed repeat reduction attempts may be made at the discretion of the pediatric radiologist and pediatric surgeon while monitoring the patient carefully for any signs of clinical decompensation. Short small bowel to small bowel intussusception (e.g., jejuno-jejunal or ileo-ileal) generally self-reduces. Whether children are discharged immediately after successful reduction or observed for a period of time is controversial, but studies have suggested that in uncomplicated patients, discharge and careful observation after successful reduction may be appropriate.[14–17]

IMAGING PEARLS

1. When imaging is indicated for evaluation of intussusception, the initial modality of choice is abdominal ultrasound, targeted to evaluate for intussusception.

2. Two-view abdominal radiography is helpful in assessing for complications such as obstruction, free air, or for determining an alternate diagnosis but should not be used to exclude intussusception.
3. Enema reduction is the gold standard for treatment if there is no evidence of perforated bowel. In most cases, air- or water-soluble iodinated contrast enema is performed depending on institutional standards.
4. If there is clinical or radiographic evidence of bowel perforation, then surgical management is indicated.

References

1. Carroll AG, Kavanagh RG, Ni Leidhin C, et al. Comparative effectiveness of imaging modalities for the diagnosis and treatment of intussusception: a critically appraised topic. *Acad Radiol.* 2017;24(5):521-529.
2. Hooker RL, Hernanz-Schulman M, Yu C, et al. Radiographic evaluation of intussusception: utility of left-side-down decubitus view. *Radiology.* 2008;248(3):987-994.
3. Ratcliffe JF, Fong S, Cheong I, O'Connell P. Plain film diagnosis of intussusception: prevalence of the target sign. *AJR Am J Roentgenol.* 1992;158(3):619-621.
4. Hryhorczuk AL, Storuse PJ. Validation of US as first-line diagnostic test for assessment of pediatric ileocolic intussusception. *Pediatr Radiol.* 2009;39(10):1075-1079.
5. Stein-Wexler R, O'Connor R, Daldrup-Link H, et al. Current methods for reducing intussusception: survey results. *Pediatr Radiol.* 2015;45(5):667-674.
6. Flaum V, Schneider A, Gomes Ferreira C, et al. Twenty years' experience for reduction of ileocolic intussusceptions by saline enema under sonography control. *J Pediatr Surg.* 2016;51(1):179-182.
7. Hadidi AT, El Shal N. Childhood intussusception: a comparative study of nonsurgical management. *J Pediatr Surg.* 1999;34(2):304-307.
8. Sadigh G, Zou KH, Razavi SA, et al. Meta-analysis of air versus liquid enema for intussusception reduction in children. *AJR Am J Roentgenol.* 2015;205(5):W542-W549.
9. Daneman A, Navarro O. Intussusception. Part 2: an update on the evolution of management. *Pediatr Radiol.* 2004;34(2):97-108.
10. Reijnen JA, Festen C, van Roosmalen RP. Intussusception: factors related to treatment. *Arch Dis Child.* 1990;65(8):871-873.
11. Fallon SC, Lopez ME, Zhang W, et al. Risk factor for surgery in pediatric intussusception in the era of pneumatic reduction. *J Pediatr Surg.* 2013;48(5):1032-1036.
12. Shaw KN, Bachur RG. *Fleisher and Ludwig's Textbook of Pediatric Emergency Medicine.* 7th ed. Philadelphia: Lippincott Williams & Wilkins; 2016:1317-1319.
13. Mandeville K, Chien M, Willyerd FA, et al. Intussusception: clinical presentations and imaging characteristics. *Pediatr Emerg Care.* 2012;28(9):842-844.
14. Whitehouse JS, Gourlay DM, Winthrop AL, et al. Is it safe to discharge intussusception patients after successful hydrostatic reduction? *J Pediatr Surg.* 2010;45(6):1182-1186.
15. Gilmore AW, Reed M, Tenenbein M, et al. Management of childhood intussusception after reduction by enema. *Am J Emerg Med.* 2011;29(9):1136-1140.
16. Bajaj L, Roback MG. Postreduction management of intussusception in a children's hospital emergency department. *Pediatrics.* 2003;112(6 Pt 1):1302-1307.
17. Gray MP, Li SH, Hoffmann RG, et al. Recurrence rates after intussusception enema reduction: a meta-analysis. *Pediatrics.* 2014;134(1):110-119.

17 *My Tummy! Appendicitis*

ROBERT VEZZETTI, MD, FAAP, FACEP

Case Presentation

A 10-year-old male presents with 2 days of initially intermittent, now constant, abdominal pain. He states that the pain started on the right side of his abdomen and was crampy in quality, although now has become more sharp. The pain has now localized to the right lower quadrant, although he complains of radiation to the umbilicus and the right upper quadrant. He has not had documented fever but his mother states he has "felt warm" and has reported nausea, but no vomiting, diarrhea, dysuria, or back pain. There is no history of trauma.

His examination reveals a somewhat uncomfortable-appearing child with a temperature of 100.1 degrees Fahrenheit, a heart rate of 105 beats per minute, respiratory rate of 18 breaths per minute, and blood pressure of 100/65 mm Hg. He has tenderness to the right lower quadrant and periumbilical areas, with mild voluntary guarding and rebound to the right lower quadrant. He has no hepatosplenomegaly. He has no scrotal or testicular tenderness or edema. You ask him to ambulate, which he does with some discomfort on the right side. Laboratory evaluation shows a white blood cell count (WBC) of 10 Thou/cc mm with 75% neutrophils and 20% lymphocytes. His urinalysis is normal, except for a specific gravity of >1.030.

Imaging Considerations

While the diagnosis of appendicitis is ultimately made by a surgeon in the operative suite, imaging plays an important role in determining which patients may require operative intervention. However, equally important is which patients do not require imaging to make the diagnosis of appendicitis. This is based on clinical suspicion, including specific history and physical examination findings. The decision whether to ultimately obtain imaging may be institution dependent and may be influenced by such factors as availability of pediatric surgical consultation and imaging resources. Even in dedicated pediatric emergency departments, there is variation in initial imaging choice, which is influenced by variation in hospital resources.[1]

There are well-validated appendicitis scoring systems that can be used to determine the probability of appendicitis in the pediatric patient, such as the Pediatric Appendicitis Score.[2–4] There are also recently proposed scoring systems that have utilized new biomarkers in addition to traditional laboratory testing to assist the clinician in determining which patents are at low risk for appendicitis.[5] Patients with a score suggestive of appendicitis may not need imaging; evaluation by a surgeon prior to imaging in these cases may be appropriate.

LIMITED ABDOMINAL ULTRASONOGRAPHY (US)

US has become the initial imaging test of choice for the evaluation of pediatric appendicitis. The American College of Radiology Appropriateness Criteria for Right Lower Quadrant Pain-Suspected Appendicitis and the American College of Emergency Physicians both promulgate ultrasound as the initial imaging modality in pediatric patients.[6,7] This modality is noninvasive, utilizes no ionizing radiation exposure, is readily available at pediatric centers, and is increasing in use. The reliability of ultrasound in detecting appendicitis has been well documented, with reported sensitivities of around 90%[8] and specificities of 95% when the appendix is clearly visualized.[9] This modality is operator dependent, and skill in pediatric ultrasound is necessary for identification of the appendix and interpretation of the images. A child may not be cooperative for the study, potentially making it difficult to obtain meaningful images. The implementation of a training program at nonpediatric facilities focusing on language, the developmental level of a child, and interaction techniques can make for a productive experience.[10]

Diagnostic criteria exist for the identification of appendicitis by ultrasound. An appendiceal diameter of greater than 7 mm,[11–13] a single wall thickness of greater than 2 mm, noncompressibility of the appendix, and the presence of a sonographic "target sign," with a fluid-filled lumen are each direct indications of appendicitis.[8,14] An appendicolith, if present, may be identified. The diameter of the appendix as a sole criterion for detecting appendicitis is not recommended.[13] A negative examination for appendicitis can be either an examination with complete visualization of a normal appearing appendix or an examination with a partially or nonvisualized appendix, with adequate visualization of other right lower quadrant structures and no secondary signs suggestive of appendicitis.[11] Ultrasound may also demonstrate an alternative diagnosis as a cause of the presenting symptoms, such as genitourinary or gastrointestinal tract pathology. Ultrasound results can be equivocal or nondiagnostic. Adequate visualization can be impaired by inadequate compression due to pain or obesity, overlying gas, and retrocecal location of the appendix. If ultrasound is inconclusive and there are indirect findings suggestive of appendicitis, such as surrounding free fluid, and increased echogenicity of mesenteric fat,[14] or a clinical appendicitis score suggestive of appendicitis, then secondary imaging options (such as computed tomography [CT] or magnetic resonance imaging [MRI]) or, in some instances, surgical consultation should be considered. Conversely, lack of these findings with an equivocal ultrasound may warrant observation of the patient with strict return precautions and reevaluation within 24 hours.[6]

COMPUTED TOMOGRAPHY

CT has proven to be an excellent imaging modality for diagnosing appendicitis, with reported sensitivities of 93% or greater and specificities of 92% or greater.[6,15] CT also can depict other etiologies of abdominal pain, such as colitis, bowel obstruction, ovarian pathology, and urinary calculi, as well as bladder and kidney infection. Anatomical variation of appendix location, as seen with a retrocecal appendix, can also be visualized. Intravenous (IV) contrast is recommended for this study.[11] Although most normal appendices measure 7 mm or less in diameter on CT, a normal appendix can measure greater in diameter. Therefore, diameter should be used cautiously as a diagnostic criterion for appendicitis on CT.[13] As with ultrasound, one should consider other signs of an inflammatory process, such as appendiceal wall thickening, hyperenhancement, periappendiceal inflammation, phlegmon, or abscess.[11]

The current trend and suggested best practice favor CT as a secondary study in suspected uncomplicated appendicitis,[16] with CT considered in patients where the diagnosis of appendicitis is clinically suspected but ultrasound imaging is equivocal or nondiagnostic. However, in facilities where ultrasound is not routinely used to diagnose appendicitis, CT is an acceptable alternative imaging strategy, especially if pediatric surgical consultation is not available. CT is also appropriate in cases where there are suspected intraabdominal complications, such as perforation and abscess. Of course, this modality exposes the patient to ionizing radiation and IV placement is required. Sedation is rarely needed since CT is rapid. If CT imaging is employed, the lowest dose of ionizing radiation needed to achieve visualization and a meaningful study should be used.

MAGNETIC RESONANCE IMAGING

MRI has recently been considered as an imaging modality to investigate pediatric appendicitis. Protocols vary and there is no accepted standard protocol for evaluating pediatric appendicitis, but most utilize a rapid-sequence technique and contrast is not always employed, as gadolinium has not been shown to increase diagnostic accuracy in detecting appendicitis.[17,18] Reported sensitivity and specificity rates in the pediatric population are approximately 96%.[18,19] Findings reported to be consistent with appendicitis include an appendiceal diameter greater than 7 mm, periappendiceal fat infiltration, and restricted diffusion of the appendiceal wall.[17]

MRI has the added advantage of not exposing the patient to ionizing radiation. This, and the apparent accuracy of MRI, makes this an attractive alternative to US and CT imaging. However, this modality is not always readily available, potentially requires sedation for optimal imaging in younger patients, may not be cost-effective at this time, and requires expertise at interpreting a pediatric study. Studies have demonstrated that, in children older than 5 years of age, this modality can be utilized without the need for sedation.[17,20,21] At this time, most MRIs of appendicitis have been performed in dedicated pediatric facilities; however, a recent study showed magnetic resonance (MR) to be clinically effective when used in a stepwise ultrasound to MR algorithm for imaging for appendicitis in a nonpediatric

hospital, with interpretation by nonpediatric radiologists. This study also reported the capability to decrease the MRI examination time for children to 11 minutes.[22]

Imaging Findings

This child had graded compression limited abdominal ultrasound imaging of his right lower quadrant. There is a noncompressible, blind-ending tubular structure that measures 10 mm in diameter. Hyperemia is present with some free fluid surrounding the structure. There is no appendicolith (Fig. 17.1). The tip of the appendix is seen with surrounding edema and hyperemia (Fig. 17.2). For comparison, the findings of acute appendicitis on IV-contrast CT from another patient are provided (Fig. 17.3).

Case Conclusion

The child had a Pediatric Appendicitis Score of 6 (equivocal for appendicitis). A limited abdominal ultrasound was performed and the appendix was identified. The imaging findings

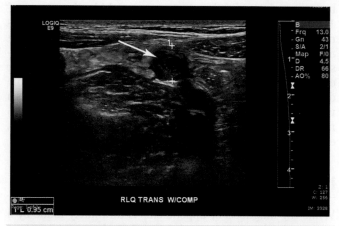

Fig. 17.1 Ultrasound image of appendicitis. A transverse image of a fluid-filled structure *(arrow)* measuring 10 mm with surrounding free fluid. This is a classic "target sign."

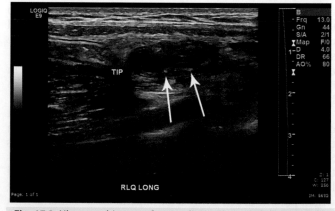

Fig. 17.2 Ultrasound image of appendicitis. The tip of the appendix can be seen, with loss of the usual definition of appendiceal wall structure *(arrows)*.

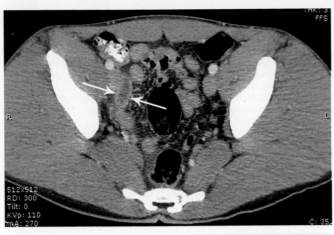

Fig. 17.3 Axial contrast-enhanced CT image shows a fluid-filled structure that is 1.2 cm in diameter (transverse) with wall enhancement *(arrows)* consistent with appendicitis. There is no perforation or associated abscess.

were consistent with acute appendicitis without perforation. Surgical consultation was obtained and the child was taken for appendectomy; findings during laparoscopic surgery were consistent with appendicitis. The procedure was completed without complication and the child was discharged from the hospital the next day.

The etiology of pediatric appendicitis is unknown, but multiple mechanisms have been proposed, including genetic (family history) and infectious etiologies.[23] Interestingly, appendicitis has shown seasonal variation.[24] Laparoscopic appendectomy is the currently preferred surgical approach, with the traditional open appendectomy approach declining.[23,25] At many children's centers, laparoscopic appendectomy has become an outpatient procedure.[23,26]

Recently, the adult surgical literature has examined antibiotic-only management of appendicitis. Several studies have shown that while antibiotic-only management has fewer complications, there is a high rate of recurrence compared to appendectomy.[23,27,28] This treatment option in the pediatric population has been examined, but large controlled studies are lacking and short- and long-term failure rates in children are not well known at this time.[29–31]

IMAGING PEARLS

1. Not all pediatric patients with suspected appendicitis need imaging. In some patients, historical and physical examination findings may strongly suggest appendicitis and surgical consultation may be appropriate prior to, or instead of, imaging.
2. Ultrasound should be the initial imaging test in pediatric patients suspected of appendicitis; however, this modality is highly operator dependent. At institutions where appendix ultrasound is not available, CT may be used as an initial imaging modality.
3. Ultrasound with failure to visualize the appendix has value. Patients with imaging findings that do not confirm appendicitis in the context of a patient with a low probability of appendicitis (i.e., by clinical scoring system) can be observed carefully with serial examinations (on an outpatient or inpatient basis) and strict return precautions with timely follow-up.

4. CT may be indicated in cases where the diagnosis of appendicitis is not clear, such as after equivocal appendix ultrasound results, or if there are suspected intra-abdominal complications.
5. MRI has emerged as a useful alternative to CT when ultrasound is nondiagnostic and the diagnosis of appendicitis is in question.

References

1. Fullerton K, Depinet H, Iyer S, et al. Association of hospital resources and imaging choice for appendicitis in pediatric emergency departments. *Acad Emerg Med.* 2017;24(4):400-409.
2. Samuel M. The pediatric appendicitis score. *J Pediatr Surg.* 2002;37(6):877-881.
3. Schneider C, Kharbanda A, Bachur R. Evaluating appendicitis scoring systems using a prospective pediatric cohort. *Ann Emerg Med.* 2007;49(6):778-784.
4. Bhatt M, Joseph L, Ducharme FM, Dougherty G, et al. Prospective validation of the pediatric appendicitis score in a Canadian pediatric emergency department. *Acad Emerg Med.* 2009;16(7):591-596.
5. Benito J, Fernandez S, Gendive M, et al. A new clinical score to identify children at low risk for appendicitis. *Am J Emerg Med.* 2020;38(3):554-561. doi:10.1016/j.ajem.2019.05.050.
6. Howell JM, Eddy OL, Lukens TW, et al. Clinical policy: critical issues in the evaluation and management of emergency department patients with suspected appendicitis. *Ann Emerg Med.* 2010;55(1):71-116.
7. Koberlein GC, Trout AT, Rigsby CK, et al. *Expert Panel on Pediatric Imaging: ACR Appropriateness Criteria – Suspected Appendicitis.* 2018. https://www.acsearch.acr.org/docs/3105874/narrative. Accessed September 1, 2019.
8. Kessler N, Cyteval C, Gallix B, et al. Appendicitis: evaluation of sensitivity, specificity, and predictive values of US, Doppler US, and laboratory findings. *Radiology.* 2004;230(2):472-478.
9. Mittal MK, Dayan PS, Macias CG, et al. Performance of ultrasound in the diagnosis of appendicitis in children in a multi-center cohort. *Acad Emerg Med.* 2013;20(7):697-702.
10. Baron M, Joslin S, Kim JS, et al. Enhancing the imaging experience for pediatric patients. *Radiol Manage.* 2016;38(3):31-34.
11. Swenson DW, Ayala RS, Sams C, et al. Practical imaging strategies for appendicitis in children. *AJR Am J Roentgenol.* 2018;211:901-909.
12. Goldin AB, Khanna P, Thapa M, et al. Revised ultrasound criteria for appendicitis in children improve diagnostic accuracy. *Pediatr Radiol.* 2011;41(8):993-999.
13. Orschein ES, Trout AT. Appendiceal diameter: CT versus sonographic measurements. *Pediatr Radiol.* 2016;46(3):316-321.
14. Gerhard, Adam EJ, Nielsen MB, et al. How to diagnose acute appendicitis: ultrasound first. *Insights Imaging.* 2016;7(2):255-263.
15. Doria AS, Moineddin R, Kellenberger CJ, et al. US or CT for diagnosis of appendicitis in children and adults? A meta-analysis. *Radiology.* 2006;241(1):83-94.
16. Bachur RG, Hennelly K, Callahan MJ, et al. Advanced radiologic imaging for pediatric appendicitis, 2005-2009: trends and outcomes. *J Pediatr.* 2012;160(6):1034-1038.
17. Mittal MK. Appendicitis: role of MRI. *Pediatr Emerg Care.* 2019;35(1):63-66.
18. Duke E, Kalb B, Arif-Tiwari H, et al. A systematic review and meta-analysis of diagnostic performance of MRI for evaluation of acute appendicitis. *AJR Am J Roentgenol.* 2016;203(3):508-517.
19. Moore MM, Kulaylat AN, Hollenbeck CS, et al. Magnetic resonance imaging in pediatric appendicitis: a systematic review. *Pediatr Radiol.* 2016;46(6):928-939.
20. Aspelund G, Fingeret A, Gross E, et al. Ultrasonography/MRI versus CT for diagnosing appendicitis. *Pediatrics.* 2014;133(4):586-593.
21. Johnson AK, Filippi CG, Andrew T, et al. Ultrafast 3-T MRI in the evaluation of children with acute lower abdominal pain for the detection of appendicitis. *AJR Am J Roentgenol.* 2012;198(6):1424-1430.

22. Covelli JD, Madireddi SP, May LA, et al. MRI for pediatric appendicitis in an adult-focused general hospital: a clinical effectiveness study—challenges and lessons learned. *AJR Am J Roentgenol.* 2019;212: 180-187.

23. Rentea RM, St Peter SD, Snyder CL. Pediatric appendicitis: state of the art review. *Pediatr Surg Int.* 2017;33(3):269-283.

24. Deng Y, Chang DC, Zhang Y, et al. Seasonal and day of the week variations of perforated appendicitis in US children. *Pediatr Surg Int.* 2010;26(7):691-696.

25. Jen HC, Shew SB. Laparoscopic versus open appendectomy in children: outcomes comparison based on a statewide analysis. *J Surg Res.* 2010;161(1):13-17.

26. Al-Omran M, Mamdani M, McLeod RS. Epidemiologic features of acute appendicitis in Ontario, Canada. *Can J Surg.* 2003;46(4):263-268.

27. Styrud J, Eriksson S, Nilsson I, et al. Appendectomy versus antibiotic treatment in acute appendicitis. a prospective multicenter randomized controlled trial. *World J Surg.* 2006;30(6):1033-1037.

28. Vons C, Barry C, Maitre S, et al. Amoxicillin plus clavulanic acid versus appendicectomy for treatment of acute uncomplicated appendicitis: an open-label, non-inferiority, randomised controlled trial. *Lancet.* 2011;377(9777):1573-1579.

29. Svensson JF, Patkova B, Almström M, et al. Nonoperative treatment with antibiotics versus surgery for acute nonperforated appendicitis in children. *Ann Surg.* 2015;261(1):67-71.

30. Steiner Z, Buklan G, Stackievicz R, et al. A role for conservative antibiotic treatment in early appendicitis in children. *J Pediatr Surg.* 2015;50(9):1566-1568.

31. Hartwich J, Luks FI, Watson-Smith D, et al. Nonoperative treatment of acute appendicitis in children: a feasibility study. *J Pediatr Surg.* 2016;51(1):111-116.

18

It's Not In to Be Thin: SMA Syndrome

ROBERT VEZZETTI, MD, FAAP, FACEP

Case Presentation

A 14-year-old male is brought to the emergency department with severe diffuse abdominal pain. He has had multiple episodes of nonbloody but bilious emesis accompanying the pain. There has been no fever, diarrhea, or trauma. There are no sick contacts or travel. He has had decreased oral intake of both solids and fluids due to nausea over the past 5 days. Notably, his weight is 30.7 kg and height is 177 cm (body mass index of 9.6 kg/m^2).

Physical examination reveals a miserable appearing afebrile child lying in a fetal position in obvious discomfort. His vital signs are a heart rate of 130 beats per minute, respiratory rate of 30 breaths per minute, and a blood pressure of 127/80 mm Hg. Noticeably, the child is quite thin and appears malnourished. He is difficult to examine but he indicates that he has diffuse abdominal pain that you are unable to localize and his abdomen appears to be distended.

As you consider imaging options, his mother tells you that the child has a history of "liver problems" and was "a preemie, but did not stay in the NICU for more than a few weeks." She is unable to elaborate further on this bit of history.

Imaging Considerations

Pediatric abdominal pain is one of the most common symptoms encountered in the emergency department. Most of these children have a benign or self-limited cause, such as a viral illness or constipation. A thorough history and physical examination will often assist the clinician in determining the etiology of abdominal pain, and not all children require imaging.

Abdominal imaging should be considered in any child in whom a potentially complex surgical condition is a concern (such as appendicitis with abscess) or in whom bowel obstruction is suspected or when a diagnosis is in question and imaging will help clarify a clinical situation. This child has thin body habitus and signs of bowel obstruction.

There are several options available to the clinician.

PLAIN RADIOGRAPHY

A readily available imaging modality with minimal ionizing radiation exposure, plain radiography can be useful in the pediatric patient with acute abdominal pain. Sedation is not required. Assessment of the bowel gas pattern is easily accomplished and an abnormal pattern can suggest a bowel obstruction. The presence of free air can be noted, if present, suggesting bowel perforation. Bowel wall thickening may also be seen, suggesting edema, which may be secondary to an inflammatory process, such as enteritis or colitis. Radio-opaque foreign bodies that are at high risk for producing perforation or obstruction, such as sharp objects or magnets, may be a source of abdominal pain in pediatric patients and can be easily identified.

A two-view series of the abdomen (anterior-posterior [AP] supine and left lateral decubitus views in young children, typically less than 8 years old, or AP supine and upright views in older children) is preferable to assess the bowel gas pattern and to assess for the presence of free air, bowel obstruction, and radio-opaque foreign bodies. A horizontal beam radiograph (AP upright or left side down decubitus views) is necessary to evaluate for free intraperitoneal air. On an upright view, to adequately evaluate for free air, the diaphragms must be included. On a left lateral decubitus view, the right lateral abdomen must be fully included. If an upright or left lateral decubitus view cannot be obtained, a cross-table lateral view of the abdomen, with the patient supine, may be utilized. There may be situations where a two-view abdominal series is not possible and an AP view will have to suffice.

COMPUTED TOMOGRAPHY (CT)

CT of the abdomen is useful in the evaluation of abdominal pain in the pediatric population. CT imaging depicts a wide range of causes of abdominal pain, including inflammatory (colitis, enteritis), infectious (abscess, pyelonephritis), surgical (bowel obstruction, appendicitis, intussusception, hernia), renal calculi, and traumatic injuries. CT is generally readily available and rapid; pediatric patients rarely require sedation to obtain a quality study. Ionizing radiation is a concern, and ALARA (as low as reasonably achievable) principles should be applied when choosing to make use of CT imaging. For conditions well evaluated by sonography, such as intussusception or appendicitis, ultrasound (US) is preferred as the first-line imaging test. Oral contrast for CT scanning is generally not indicated in the acute setting.[1] For suspected renal calculus disease, CT imaging is performed without intravenous (IV) contrast. For most other suspected causes of abdominal pain, IV contrast is indicated. If there is any question regarding the use of IV contrast, consultation with the radiologist is recommended. Placing an IV in the pediatric patient can be traumatic; if time allows, a topical anesthetic, such as topical lidocaine (4%), can help make IV placement smoother.

ULTRASOUND

This imaging modality is commonly used in pediatric patients with abdominal pain, particularly when appendicitis is suspected. US is also the first-line imaging test for suspected intussusception, biliary tract disease including cholecystitis, and gynecologic, testicular, and urinary tract pathologies. The availability, rapidity of the study, and lack of ionizing radiation exposure are attractive attributes of sonography.

Imaging Findings

This child had plain radiographic imaging initially performed. The child was unable to cooperate for a two-view abdominal radiograph examination, despite pain medications; thus, a one-view (AP) radiograph was obtained (Fig. 18.1). There is no obvious evidence of bowel obstruction, but there is a paucity of intestinal gas (a nonspecific finding), with appearance that is suspicious for fluid distension of the stomach.

UPPER GASTROINTESTINAL (UGI) SERIES

While not commonly obtained in the emergency department, the clinician should always remember this is a useful test. UGI series is useful in evaluating the esophagus, stomach, and duodenum.[2] Using fluoroscopy, barium is given to the patient, either orally or by nasogastric tube if the patient is uncooperative or unable to drink the contrast. Images are obtained during the real-time examination under fluoroscopy. A small bowel follow-through may also be performed to image the remaining small bowel. A UGI series is

useful in identifying malrotation/volvulus, pyloric stenosis (although not the preferred first-line imaging test), and small bowel obstruction, including superior mesenteric artery (SMA) syndrome. With a distended stomach upon presentation, it is helpful to empty the stomach using a nasogastric tube, and the tube may then be used to administer the barium in a controlled manner.

Case Conclusion

The patient continued to have significant pain and a CT scan with IV contrast was obtained. The stomach and proximal to mid-duodenum are markedly distended and fluid filled (Fig. 18.2). These images suggest duodenal obstruction. A UGI series was obtained, which showed gastric distension, proximal duodenal distension, and delayed passage of contrast across the transverse portion of the duodenum. There was a vertically oriented extrinsic indentation across the transverse duodenum (Fig. 18.3A–D), consistent with extrinsic compression by the SMA. Beyond this indentation at the level of the SMA, contrast-filled small bowel loops are not dilated. A diagnosis of SMA syndrome was made.

SMA syndrome is due to compression of the transverse portion of the duodenum between the aorta and the SMA. This compression occurs from a reduction of the angle between the SMA and the aorta, often secondary to a lack of intraperitoneal fat.[3-7] This angle is usually between 38 and 65 degrees.[5] SMA syndrome can be seen with trauma, anorexia, and surgical procedures.[3-7] Abdominal pain, emesis, early satiety, and lack of weight gain are common presenting symptoms.[3-7]

Treatment is usually conservative, consisting of fluid resuscitation, bowel rest, total parenteral nutrition, and enteric feeding with a nasojejunal tube inserted past the obstruction.[3-7] Surgical options have been advocated as

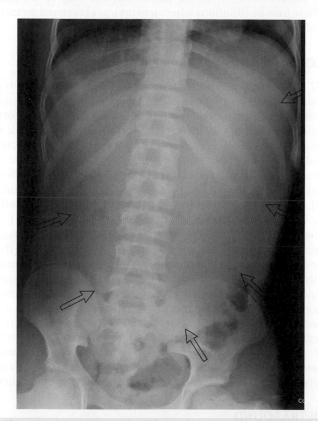

Fig. 18.1 Anterior-posterior abdominal radiograph demonstrates a paucity of intestinal gas and an appearance suggesting a fluid distended stomach *(arrows)*.

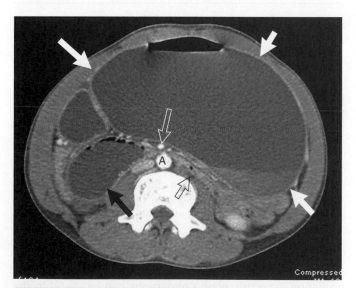

Fig. 18.2 Axial computed tomography image with intravenous contrast demonstrates fluid distension of the stomach *(white arrows)* and of the proximal transverse duodenum *(black arrow)*. The duodenum passes between the aorta *(A)* and the superior mesenteric artery (SMA) *(open white arrow)*. Distal to passage between the aorta and the SMA, the transverse duodenum is collapsed and nondilated *(open black arrow)*.

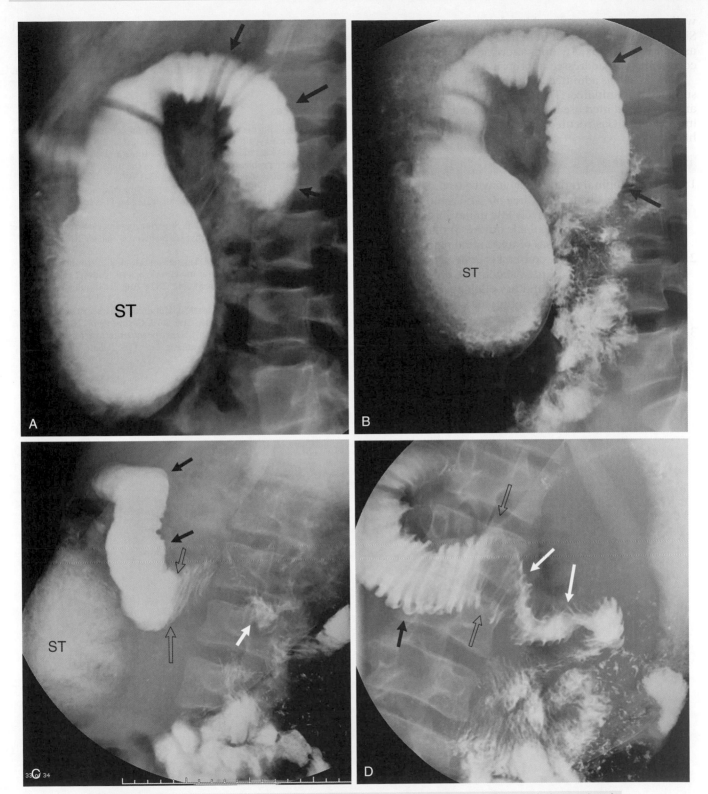

Fig. 18.3 A upper gastrointestinal series demonstrates distension of the proximal duodenum (black arrows), and to and fro peristalsis was seen in the proximal duodenum. There was delayed, intermittent passage of contrast from the dilated proximal duodenum into nondilated distal transverse duodenum (white arrows), through the site of narrowing at the extrinsic impression of the superior mesenteric artery upon the duodenum (open black arrows). The contrast-filled distal stomach is also seen (ST).

well and are often employed in adult patients with chronic SMA syndrome.[3-7] In all patients, psychiatric issues, such as depression, anxiety, and anorexia nervosa, should be considered and addressed appropriately if present.

This child was admitted to the hospital, where nutritional support was initiated. This patient's symptoms improved and his weight increased. Subspecialty consultation, including Pediatric Gastroenterology and Psychiatry, assisted in his recovery.

IMAGING PEARLS

1. Plain abdominal radiography may be useful in assessing for bowel obstruction, free air, and radio-opaque foreign bodies. It is relatively low in ionizing radiation exposure and widely available but has limited diagnostic utility in many causes of abdominal pain.
2. Abdominal CT with IV contrast is indicated when there is potential for serious intra-abdominal processes, such as an abscess, an inflammatory etiology is suspected, or the etiology of the child's symptoms is unclear and CT imaging is needed to direct appropriate therapy.
3. Oral contrast for CT imaging is seldom indicated in acute presentations of abdominal pain. Consultation with pediatric radiology or pediatric surgery may be helpful if oral contrast is desired.
4. A UGI can be a useful imaging modality when proximal bowel obstruction is a concern, especially when malrotation and volvulus are differential considerations. This test is typically obtained after subspecialty consultation.

References

1. Kessner R, Barnes S, Halpern P, et al. CT for acute abdominal pain—is oral contrast really required? *Acad Radiol.* 2017;24(7): 840-845.
2. Applegate KE, Anderson JM, Klatte EC. Intestinal malrotation in children: a problem-solving approach to the upper gastrointestinal series. *Radiographics.* 2006;26(5):1485-1500.
3. Merrett ND, Wilson RB, Cosman P, et al. Superior mesenteric artery syndrome: diagnosis and treatment strategies. *J Gastrointest Surg.* 2009;13(2):287-292.
4. Unal B, Aktas A, Kemal G, et al. Superior mesenteric artery syndrome: CT and ultrasonography findings. *Diagn Interv Radiol.* 2005;11(2): 90-95.
5. Russell EA, Braverman RM, Vasudevan SA, et al. A traumatic quinceañera: acute superior mesenteric artery syndrome in an adolescent girl. *Pediatr Emerg Care.* 2018 Aug 20. [Epub ahead of print].
6. Sato H, Tanaka T. Acute gastric dilatation due to a superior mesenteric artery syndrome: an autopsy case. *BMC Gastroenterol.* 2014;14:37.
7. Kurbegov A, Grabb B, Bealer J. Superior mesenteric artery syndrome in a 16-year-old with bilious emesis. *Curr Opin Pediatr.* 2010;22(5): 664-667.

You Ate What? Swallowed Foreign Bodies

GUYON HILL, MD and GREG HAND, MD

Case Presentation

A 4-year-old male presents to the emergency department after his parents witnessed the ingestion of a coin. His mother states that he grabbed one out of her purse that was lying on the ground nearby. The patient is resting comfortably in the room, in no acute distress. His lungs are clear to auscultation, there is no stridor, and he is managing his secretions. His vitals are all within normal limits.

Imaging Considerations

PLAIN RADIOGRAPHY

Anteroposterior and lateral x-rays of the neck, chest, and abdomen should be the initial diagnostic choice when there is concern for foreign body ingestion.[1,2] This recommendation is regardless of whether the object is thought to be radiolucent or if symptoms indicate a particular location of the foreign body. Radiography will help determine the size, location, and shape of radiopaque foreign bodies and the management plan. Although radiolucent objects may not be seen on plain radiographs, there are secondary signs such as relative radiolucency, air fluid levels, free air, air trapping in lung, bowel obstruction, or soft tissue swelling that can be appreciated.[2]

COMPUTED TOMOGRAPHY (CT)

A CT scan should be considered for further evaluation of foreign body ingestion when no foreign body is found on radiographs and the child is exhibiting symptoms such as difficulty breathing, wheezing, or inability to tolerate secretions, or if the likely ingestion has high-risk characteristics (such as a large object [≥25 mm in diameter or >5 cm in length]), concern for radiolucent foreign object ingestion, or a history of esophageal strictures. Although a small radiolucent foreign body could still potentially be missed, CT has been shown to be highly effective at identifying ingested foreign bodies. CT has also been found to be useful in identifying perforation, abscess formation, inflammation, peritonitis, and other complications from foreign body impaction.[1,3]

UPPER GASTROINTESTINAL SERIES (UGI)

UGI is another useful option for foreign body ingestion, including radiolucent objects that might not appear on plain radiographs. The use of barium is not recommended due to the potential for obscuration if endoscopy is performed afterward. A water-soluble contrast should be used instead.

POINT-OF-CARE ULTRASOUND (US)

There have been multiple cases of point-of-care US being used in the identification of foreign body ingestions in children.[4,5] The use of this modality is operator dependent, but US can be especially useful in the identification and localization of radiolucent foreign bodies. It not only provides a nonionizing radiation option but also can be done at the bedside. Foreign bodies are usually visualized as hyperechoic structures with posterior shadowing.

MAGNETIC RESONANCE IMAGING (MRI)

MRI can also be used to evaluate for the ingestion of radiolucent foreign bodies and subsequent complications. As with CT, this additional imaging is not warranted if the patient is asymptomatic and the object is not known to have any high-risk characteristics. MRI is contraindicated in the case of any metallic foreign body.

Imaging Findings

Plain radiography was obtained and demonstrated a metallic, flat, disk-shaped foreign body in the distal thoracic esophagus, likely a coin (Figs. 19.1 and 19.2).

Case Conclusion

The patient was admitted for observation and serial x-rays. The coin spontaneously passed into the stomach without complication and the patient was discharged home with outpatient follow-up.

Children are notorious for placing objects in their mouths. While many of these objects pass without any symptoms or perhaps awareness of the parents, they can, on occasion, become impacted in the gastrointestinal (GI) tract and cause serious complications. Children may present completely asymptomatic with a parent or witness claiming they saw a possible ingestion. When evaluating these patients in the emergency department, it is vital to determine if an ingestion occurred, what was ingested, and where the object is located and assess the potential risk to the child.

An impaction in the esophagus generally requires the most urgent management. Anatomic sites of narrowing in the esophagus that are most common for impaction include the level of the aortic arch as well as the upper (level of thoracic inlet) and lower esophageal sphincters. Patients with an esophageal foreign body can present with vomiting, pooling

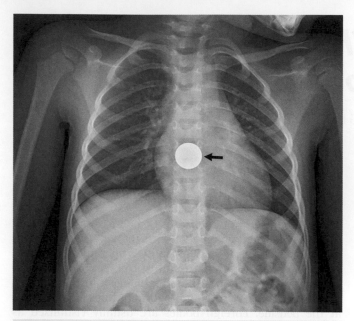

Fig. 19.1 Anteroposterior plain radiography demonstrates a metallic round disk-shaped foreign body *(arrow)* in the mid to distal thoracic esophagus, appearance consistent with a coin.

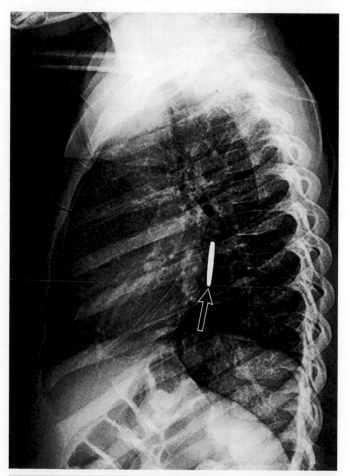

Fig. 19.2 On the lateral view the edge of the foreign body is symmetric *(open white arrow)*, consistent with a coin. Button (disk) batteries have an asymmetric, beveled edge.

of secretions, refusal to eat, dysphagia, chest pain, or respiratory symptoms such as stridor or wheezing or they can be asymptomatic. Management is based on the object ingested and the degree of symptoms. Button batteries, sharp objects, multiple magnets, and large objects causing complete obstruction will require emergent removal by endoscopy. In contrast, small, round, or inert objects not causing significant symptoms can be observed for up to 24 hours from time of ingestion to see if they spontaneously pass into the stomach.[1]

The vast majority of foreign bodies that pass spontaneously into the stomach will continue their journey through the GI tract without complication. These can generally be managed conservatively with serial radiographs as an outpatient until the object has passed. Certain objects may still need removal depending on their size and shape.

COINS

Coins are the most common foreign body ingested by pediatric patients.[6] Due to their radiopaque nature, they are usually found on plain radiography. Anteroposterior (AP) and lateral radiographic views of the neck, chest, and abdomen, to include from the nasopharynx to the anus, should be obtained. Management will be based on the location and size of the coin.

In cases where the location of trachea versus esophagus is in question, using two views to localize the foreign body with respect to the tracheal air column is most useful. Traditional teaching has held that coins in the trachea tend to orient themselves in a sagittal plain while coins in the esophagus tend to orient themselves in the coronal plane. This was described as due to vocal cord sagittal orientation and the C-shaped cartilaginous rings of trachea that would cause coins to align sagittally, along the larger anteroposterior diameter, if in the trachea.[7] However, this is not supported in the literature: Coins are most likely to be lodged in the esophagus, and although coins most commonly align in a coronal plane in the esophagus, a coin in the esophagus may be sagittally oriented, especially in older children.[7,8]

BUTTON BATTERIES

Button batteries pose a unique risk when ingested due to their ability to cause severe caustic injury to the esophagus within a few hours of ingestion.[10] The number of such battery ingestions has increased as they have become more available.

The type of battery can be identified from the battery code on the packaging if available. The first two numbers in a four-digit code give the diameter in millimeters. The last two numbers in the four-digit code give the height in tenth of a millimeter. For help in identification and management of battery ingestion, call the National Battery Ingestion hotline at 800-498-8666.

Prehospital Management[9,11–13]

Do Not Induce Emesis

Assume lithium battery ingestion unless otherwise known
Administer honey (10 mL every 10 minutes, up to six doses) IF:
- Child >12 months of age
- Child can swallow
- Honey immediately available
Hearing aid battery not ingested

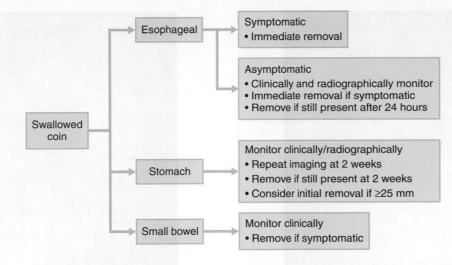

Ingested Coin Management Guideline.[1,9] Approximately 30% of all coins found in the esophagus will spontaneously pass into the stomach. A US quarter is 24 mm in size.

It is very important to distinguish between a button battery that requires emergent removal and a benign coin that may pass spontaneously. Two distinguishing characteristics of a button battery on radiography that can help differentiate a battery from a coin are the halo sign and step-off edge. When a button battery is visualized "en face" on a radiograph (usually on the AP view in the esophagus), there will be a lucent second ring seen along the outer edge giving the appearance of a halo (Figs. 19.3A and 19.4A,B). A coin will not have the lucent second ring. When a button battery is viewed in profile (usually on the lateral view in the esophagus), there is a step-off between the anode and cathode side of the battery (Figs. 19.3B and 19.5A,B), as opposed to the symmetrical edge of a coin (see Fig. 19.2).[14]

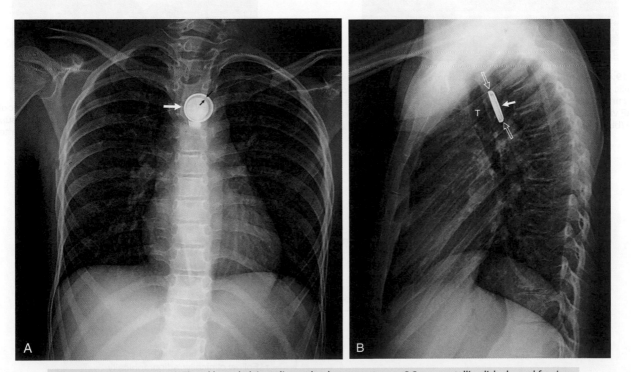

Fig. 19.3 Anteroposterior (AP) and lateral plain radiography demonstrates a <2.3-cm, metallic, disk-shaped foreign body *(white arrows)* with a halo sign on the AP view (A; *black arrows*) and beveled, peripheral edges (B) *(open white arrows)*, that is lodged within the proximal thoracic esophagus, consistent with an ingested button battery. Note that the tracheal air column *(T)* is anterior to the location of the foreign body, and there is no mass effect on the trachea and no soft tissue swelling between the esophageal foreign body and the trachea.

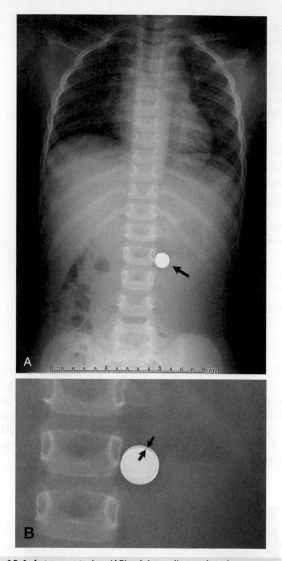

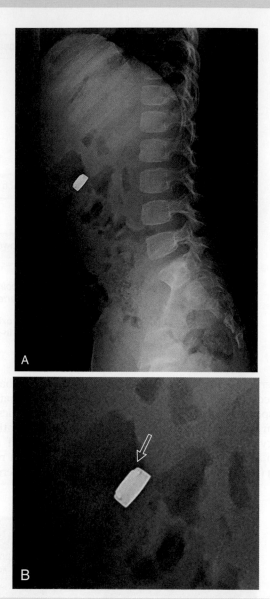

Fig. 19.4 Anteroposterior (AP) plain radiography demonstrates a metallic object with typical shape of a small disk battery *(arrow)* projecting in the left upper quadrant, likely in the stomach. (B) Note on the AP view that there is a thin lucent halo sign *(black arrows)*, a sign of a disk/button battery.

Fig. 19.5 Lateral view plain radiography demonstrates a metallic object with typical shape of a small disk battery (A, *black arrow*). The superior edge is beveled (B, *open white arrow*), a sign of a disk/button battery.

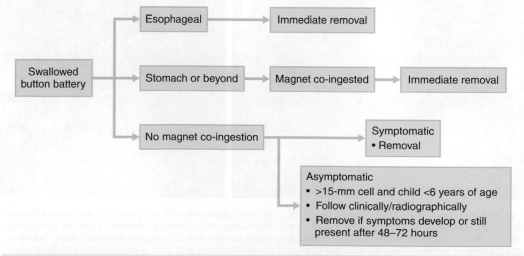

Ingested Button Battery Management Guideline: ≤12 years of age OR > 12 years of age and battery > 12 mm.[9,11–13]

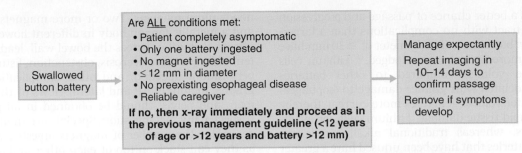

Are **ALL** conditions met:
- Patient completely asymptomatic
- Only one battery ingested
- No magnet ingested
- ≤ 12 mm in diameter
- No preexisting esophageal disease
- Reliable caregiver

If no, then x-ray immediately and proceed as in the previous management guideline (<12 years of age or >12 years and battery >12 mm)

Swallowed button battery →

Manage expectantly

Repeat imaging in 10–14 days to confirm passage

Remove if symptoms develop

Ingested Button Battery Management Guideline > 12 years of age and battery < 12 mm.[9,11–13]

An infant experienced a choking episode while playing on a carpet. Physical examination revealed a child in moderate respiratory distress and drooling. Plain radiography revealed two stacked circular metallic foreign bodies within the neck posterior to the subglottic airway, consistent with location in the esophagus (Figs. 19.6 and 19.7). While the objects may resemble a single button battery (especially on the lateral view), closer inspection reveals this to be two stacked coins, with two adjacent symmetrical edges on the lateral view. Emergent endoscopic removal was performed.

Diameter and Voltage of Button Batteries

The diameter of an ingested button battery will impact the likelihood that a battery will pass through the esophagus and into the stomach and beyond. A battery with a diameter

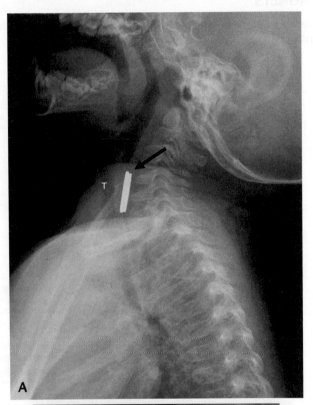

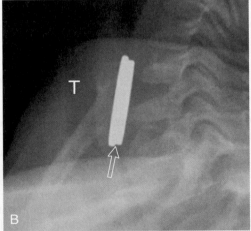

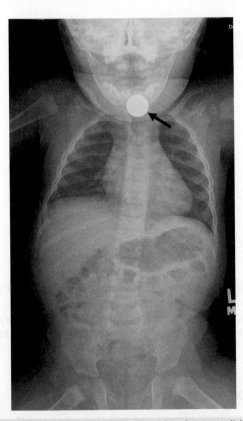

Fig. 19.6 Anteroposterior plain radiography shows a disk-shaped metallic foreign body *(black arrow)* in the lower neck, which appears to be one object on the frontal view and on the lateral view (Fig. 19.7A) is posterior to the subglottic trachea *(T)*, consistent with esophageal positioning.

Fig. 19.7 Lateral view (A) plain radiography shows a disk-shaped metallic foreign body *(black arrow)* posterior to the subglottic trachea *(T)*, consistent with esophageal positioning. Although the appearance mimics a button battery, closer inspection (B) shows an appearance consistent with two adjacent stacked coins *(open white arrow)*; the more posterior coin has a smaller diameter.

of <12 mm has a better chance of passage and progression through the GI tract with no complications than a larger-diameter battery; batteries with a diameter of ≥20 mm have been shown to more likely become lodged.[16] Lithium cells have twice the voltage compared to other batteries and are also associated with greater damage to esophageal tissues.[16] A greater voltage generates more current, thereby causing more rapid tissue damage. Lithium cells, for example, are 3 volts, whereas traditional alkaline cells are 1.5 volts.[16,17] Batteries that have been unused have a greater potential for tissue damage due to their discharge state.[17]

MAGNETS

The ingestion of high-powered magnets poses another unique risk. These are also known as rare-earth or neodymium magnets. Two or more magnets or a magnet and a metallic foreign body in different bowel lumens can attract each other across the bowel wall, leading to the potential for pressure necrosis, obstruction, fistula formation, perforation, infection, and other complications.[18] Radiographs, including AP and lateral views of the neck, abdomen, and pelvis, should be obtained in all patients with suspected magnet ingestion. Special care should be taken to determine the number of magnets ingested when possible as they can stack on top of each other and appear as one magnet on radiographs. Although magnets may align with one another on a radiograph, the aligned magnets can be in different bowel loops. Even one high-powered magnet ingested can cause serious complications if another metal object is ingested or if the magnet attracts to metal on clothing or elsewhere outside the body.

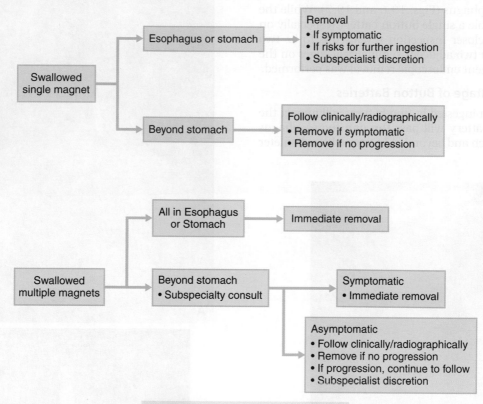

Ingested Magnet Management Guideline.[9,18]

A 9-year-old patient ingested a magnetic bracelet on a dare. He presented to the emergency department 24 hours after the ingestion with complaints of abdominal pain. Plain radiography was obtained and demonstrated a metallic bracelet seen in the right lower abdomen without obstruction (Fig. 19.8). The patient was admitted for serial examinations and radiography. Repeat imaging demonstrated the ingested magnetic bracelet now projecting in the left lower quadrant (Fig. 19.9). His pain resolved and the patient was discharged with close follow-up but did not see his primary care provider as planned. He presented to the emergency department several days later with severe abdominal pain and vomiting. Imaging demonstrated an abnormal bowel gas pattern, with air fluid levels in dilatated small bowel, suggestive of early or partial small bowel obstruction, and the magnets remained in the left lower quadrant (Fig. 19.10). Pediatric Surgery was consulted and the patient was taken to the operating room, where a bowel fistula was encountered associated with the magnets seen on radiography. The magnets were removed and the fistula was repaired.

LONG OR SHARP OBJECTS

Long and blunt objects can fail to transit the stomach or become impacted in the small intestine, necessitating surgical intervention. Sharp objects perforating the esophagus can cause neck pain and swelling, pneumomediastinum, or crepitus.

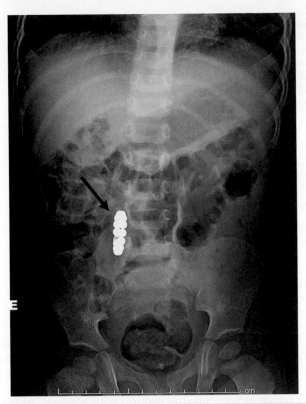

Fig. 19.8 Abdominal radiography demonstrates a bracelet-like configuration of metallic ball magnets *(arrow)* in the right lower abdomen, without evidence of bowel obstruction.

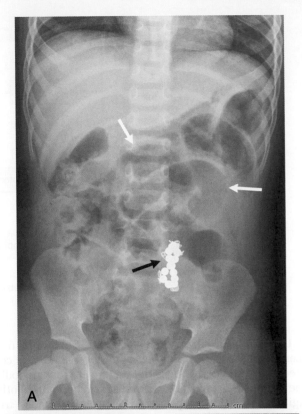

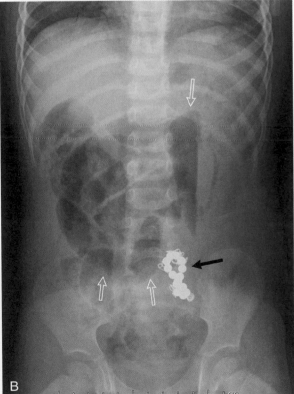

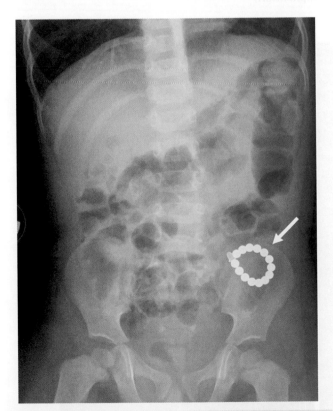

Fig. 19.9 The follow-up image shows that the objects *(arrow)* have progressed, in a similar configuration, into the left lower quadrant, but bowel gas pattern remains normal.

Fig. 19.10 Follow-up supine (A) and left lateral decubitus (B) abdominal radiographic views several days later show that the magnets maintain relationship to one another but have not progressed from the left lower quadrant *(black arrows)*. There is interval development of dilatation of gas-filled small bowel loops *(white arrows)*, with air fluid levels on the decubitus view *(open white arrows)*, and decreased gas in the colon. Appearance is consistent with an early or partial small bowel obstruction.

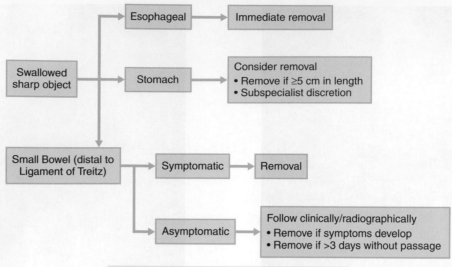

Swallowed sharp object → Esophageal → Immediate removal

Swallowed sharp object → Stomach → Consider removal
• Remove if ≥5 cm in length
• Subspecialist discretion

Swallowed sharp object → Small Bowel (distal to Ligament of Treitz) → Symptomatic → Removal

Small Bowel (distal to Ligament of Treitz) → Asymptomatic → Follow clinically/radiographically
• Remove if symptoms develop
• Remove if >3 days without passage

Ingested Sharp Object Management Guideline.[10,19,20]

If there is high suspicion for a foreign body but none is seen on radiographs, further evaluation should be conducted due to the risk of missing radiolucent foreign bodies. If the patient is asymptomatic and suspicion is high, other imaging modalities such as CT, UGI, or US can be used to identify foreign body ingestions. Symptomatic patients warrant immediate consultation.

A child was with her parents in their garage when she told them she "ate something" and complained of throat pain, which resolved after the child arrived in the emergency department. Imaging demonstrated a foreign object consistent with a swallowed screw (Fig. 19.11). She was monitored at home and did well.

A teenager was "playing around with a pencil" in their mouth when it was accidentally swallowed. Plain radiography demonstrated a faint object consistent with a pencil (Fig. 19.12), which was removed endoscopically without complication.

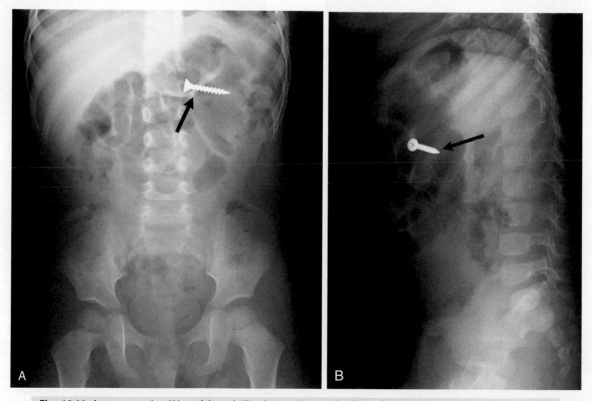

Fig. 19.11 Anteroposterior (A) and lateral (B) plain radiographic views demonstrating a <3.4 cm in length, radiopaque, metallic screw *(arrows)*, with position most consistent with location within the stomach.

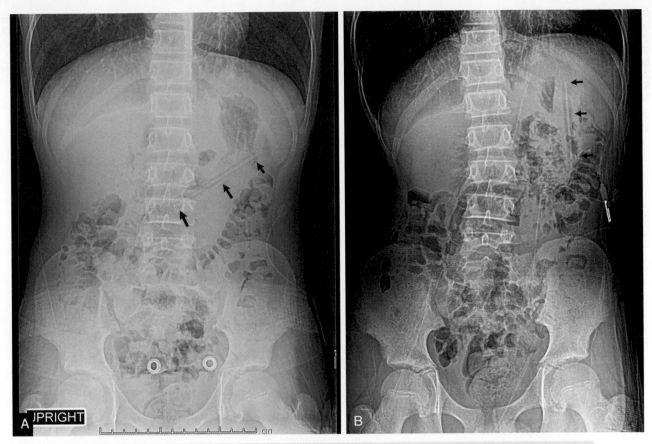

Fig. 19.12 Anteroposterior (A) and left lateral decubitus (B) radiographic views of the abdomen demonstrate an approximately 9–10-cm linear foreign body *(arrows)* in the left upper quadrant, most consistent with foreign body position within the stomach. The foreign body has a radiolucent periphery (wood) and a mildly radiopaque core, consistent with the history of pencil ingestion. The bowel gas pattern is normal, with no evidence of free intraperitoneal gas.

IMAGING PEARLS

1. Initial diagnostic imaging should consist of plain radiographs of the neck, chest, and abdomen in both AP and lateral projections. This will allow for visualization of the majority of foreign bodies. Images should include the entire GI tract, from the nasopharynx to the anus.
2. If there is high suspicion of dangerous foreign body ingestion and no foreign body is found on initial radiographs, a CT scan should be performed for further evaluation.
3. Water-soluble contrast should be used with UGI in case of perforation.
4. Point-of-care US can be a useful tool in the initial evaluation of foreign body ingestion that does not use ionizing radiation.
5. Look for evidence of a halo sign and edge step-off when looking to distinguish between button battery ingestion and coin ingestion.

References

1. Uyemura MC. Foreign body ingestion in children. *Am Fam Physician.* 2005;72(2):287-291.
2. Arana A, Hauser B, Hachimi-Idrissi S, et al. Management of ingested foreign bodies in childhood and review of the literature. *Eur J Pediatr.* 2001;160(8):468-472.
3. Kazam JK, Coll D, Maltz C. Computed tomography scan for the diagnosis of esophageal foreign body. *Am J Emerg Med.* 2005;23(7):897-898.
4. Salmon M, Doniger SJ. Ingested foreign bodies: a case series demonstrating a novel application of point-of-care ultrasonography in children. *Pediatr Emerg Care.* 2013;29(7):870-873.
5. Shiu-Cheung Chan S, Russell M, Ho-Fung VM. Not all radiopaque foreign bodies shadow on ultrasound: unexpected sonographic appearance of a radiopaque magnet. *Ultrasound Q.* 2014;30(4):306-309.
6. Waltzman ML. Management of esophageal coins. *Curr Opin Pediatr.* 2006;18(5):571-574.
7. Rahmani SH, Faridaalaee G, Dehkharghani MZ, et al. Coin ingestion in an 8-year-old child; an atypical presentation. *Emerg Med Trauma Care J.* 2019 EMTCJ-100018.
8. Raney LH, Losek JD. Child with esophageal coin and atypical radiograph. *J Emerg Med.* 2018;34(1):63-66.
9. Kramer RE, Lerner DG, Lin T, et al. Management of ingested foreign bodies in children: a clinical report of the NASPGHAN Endoscopy Committee. *J Pediatr Gastroenterol Nutr.* 2015;60(4):562-574.
10. Soto PH, Reid NE, Litovitz TL. Time to perforation for button batteries lodged in the esophagus. *Am J Emerg Med.* 2019;37(5):805-809.
11. National Capital Poison Center. *National Capital Poison Center Button Battery Ingestion Triage and Treatment Guideline.* Available at: https://www.poison.org/battery/guideline. Accessed September 1, 2019.
12. Litovitz T, Whitaker N, Clark L, et al. Emerging battery-ingestion hazard: clinical implications. *Pediatrics.* 2010;125(6):1168-1177.
13. Pugmire BS, Lin TK, Pentiuk S, et al. Imaging button battery ingestions and insertions in children: a 15-year single-center review. *Pediatr Radiol.* 2017;47(2):178-185.
14. Semple T, Calder AD, Ramaswamy M, et al. Button battery ingestion in children—a potentially catastrophic event of which all radiologists must be aware. *Br J Radiol.* 2018;91(1081):20160781.

15. Hussain SZ, Bousvaros A, Gilger M, et al. Management of ingested magnets in children. *J Pediatr Gastroenterol Nutr.* 2012;55(3): 239-242.
16. Varga Á, Kovács T, Saxena AK. Analysis of complications after button battery ingestion in children. *Pediatr Emerg Care.* 2018;34(6):443-446.
17. Krom H, Visser M, Hulst JM, et al. Serious complications after button battery ingestion in children. *Eur J Pediatr.* 2018;177(7):1063-1070.
18. Liu S, de Blacam C, Lim FY, et al. Magnetic foreign body ingestions leading to duodenocolonic fistula. *J Pediatr Gastroenterol Nutr.* 2005; 41(5):670-672.
19. Velitchkov NG, Grigorov GI, Losanoff JE, et al. Ingested foreign bodies of the gastrointestinal tract: retrospective analysis of 542 cases. *World J Surg.* 1996;20(8):1001-1005.
20. Wyllie R. Foreign bodies in the gastrointestinal tract. *Curr Opin Pediatr.* 2006;18(5):563- 564.

20 Right Out of 'The Exorcist': Pyloric Stenosis

ROBERT VEZZETTI, MD, FAAP, FACEP

Case Presentation

A 3-week-old male presents with nonbilious, nonbloody emesis for the past 1.5 weeks. Initially there were two to three episodes per day, occasionally with feeding, but this has increased to emesis with every feed. The parents report that the emesis is "forceful" and afterward the child appears to want to eat again. He has had decreased urine output over the past 24 hours. There has been no fever, diarrhea, or known trauma. He has been increasingly fussy for the past several days. He has an unremarkable medical history and was born "full term."

Physical examination reveals an afebrile child with a heart rate of 130 beats per minute, respiratory rate of 40 breaths per minute, and a blood pressure of 84/60 mm Hg. The baby is fussy but consoles as he eagerly takes a pacifier. Mucous membranes are slightly dry, but the physical examination is otherwise normal

Imaging Considerations

PLAIN RADIOGRAPHY

Plain abdominal radiography is not particularly useful for the diagnosis of pyloric stenosis. However, if obtained, gastric distention may be seen or perhaps mass impression of the thickened pyloric muscle on an air-filled gastric antrum may be noted.[1,2]

ULTRASOUND (US)

US is the imaging modality of choice in children with suspected pyloric stenosis. This modality is readily available and there is no exposure to ionizing radiation. Criteria that suggest the diagnosis of pyloric stenosis in full-term infants are as follows[1-4]:

1. Muscle thickness greater than 3 mm.
2. Channel length greater than 16–18 mm.

US has a diagnostic sensitivity and specificity of 89% and 100%, respectively.[4] The passage of gastric contents in real time can help aid with the diagnosis of pyloric stenosis in this group.[2] An interesting phenomenon is that of pylorospasm, a common cause of gastric outlet obstruction in neonates; this is managed conservatively, but close follow-up is indicated.[1,5,6] Infants with equivocal results should be followed closely as well, with repeat imaging as clinically indicated.[6]

UPPER GASTROINTESTINAL SERIES (UGI)

This modality was traditionally used to diagnose pyloric stenosis and has the ability to detect other conditions that may mimic pyloric stenosis, such as gastroesophageal reflux.[1,3] A UGI has a sensitivity and specificity for pyloric stenosis reported to be 96% and 100%, respectively.[6] This test does require expertise in the technique of administering oral contrast and interpreting the results. UGI series includes exposure to ionizing radiation, and this exposure can be increased due to increased fluoroscopic observation times necessitated by the delay in gastric emptying in patients with pyloric stenosis.[1]

COMPUTED TOMOGRAPHY (CT)

Computed tomography of the abdomen is not indicated to diagnose pyloric stenosis.

Imaging Findings

Given the history and physical examination, an abdominal US was obtained. There is abnormal circumferential muscular wall thickening of the antropyloric region, with a single-wall thickness of 4.4 mm, a channel length of 19 mm, with mass effect upon the gastric antrum and duodenum bulb (Figs. 20.1 and 20.2).

Case Conclusion

Pediatric Surgery was consulted. The child had bloodwork done, demonstrating a potassium level of 2.5 mmol/L, a chloride level of 90 mmol/L, and a CO_2 level of 35 mmol/L. Fluid resuscitation with 20 cc/kg of normal saline was given as a bolus, followed by rehydration. The child's electrolytes normalized and he was taken to the operating suite for pyloromyotomy. He recovered uneventfully and was discharged from the hospital on postoperative day 2.

Pyloric stenosis is a common cause of emesis in the neonatal period, with an incidence of 1 to 4 per 1000 births, and is more common in males and in firstborn children.[3,4] The exact etiology of this condition remains unknown. There does appear to be familial clustering.[4] Proposed theories include molecular and nerve cell conditions, resulting in poor pylorus muscle innervation.[3,7,8] Interestingly, this innervation returns to normal in the months following surgery.[3,7]

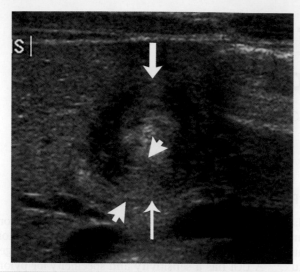

Fig. 20.1 Transverse ultrasound image through the antropyloric region shows a rounded, target-like appearance *(arrows)* of the hypertrophied pylorus in pyloric stenosis. The *short arrows* outline the single-wall thickness of the hypertrophic pyloric muscle and is what is measured for pyloric muscular thickness.

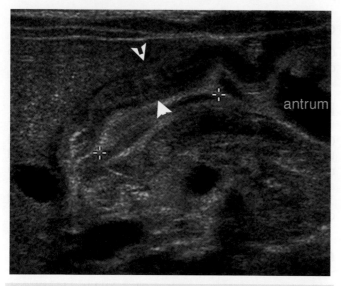

Fig. 20.2 Longitudinal ultrasound image through the antropyloric region in pyloric stenosis. The gastric antrum is fluid filled. The pyloric region shows elongated, circumferential muscular wall thickening, with single-wall thickness of the anterior muscular wall outlined by *arrowheads.*

The clinical presentation of pyloric stenosis follows a classic pattern: A previously well infant develops progressively worsening nonbilious, nonbloody, forceful (often described as projectile) emesis. Age at presentation varies from 2 weeks to 8 weeks, with peak presentation in the 3- to 5-week age range. Premature infants tend to present earlier compared to term infants.[3,4] Most infants are not ill-appearing, although as symptoms continue, dehydration and decreased

activity develop. Infants are generally hungry after the emesis.

The clinician should also consider a broad differential diagnosis in the neonate with emesis. It may be difficult to diagnose pyloric stenosis immediately, since many other entities can produce similar symptoms. These include gastroesophageal reflux and overfeeding, surgical causes (such as malrotation, volvulus, and bowel obstructions), infection, metabolic disorders, neurologic etiologies (hydrocephalus), and injuries form nonaccidental trauma. A thorough history and physical examination can usually assist the clinician in determining the most likely etiology of the emesis and which, if any, diagnostic tests are indicated, including imaging. The clinician should make every effort to determine if the emesis is bilious or not, as bilious emesis in a neonate is a surgical emergency until proven otherwise, suggesting malrotation with or without volvulus, and requires immediate evaluation.

The classic physical examination finding in an infant with pyloric stenosis is palpation of the enlarged pyloric muscle, described as feeling a small mass, much like an "olive." This mass is pathognomonic for pyloric stenosis.[4] It is common not to feel this mass early in the course of the illness, but it does become more detectable as symptoms worsen and dehydration progresses.[9] If the condition is detected early enough, a mass may never be palpable.[9] If a clinician suspects pyloric stenosis, consultation with a pediatric surgeon prior to obtaining imaging is appropriate. If the consulting surgeon is comfortable diagnosing pyloric stenosis by physical examination alone, this reduces the need for radiographic studies and is cost-effective.[3,10] Imaging is often employed to make the diagnosis, particularly given the availability of US.

Electrolyte abnormalities are associated with pyloric stenosis, and measuring serum electrolytes, especially in a clinically dehydrated child, can be useful. These abnormalities include the classic hypokalemic, hypochloremic metabolic alkalosis and, if these metabolic derangements are present, can suggest the diagnosis.[3] Correction of this state is important prior to surgery, and following electrolytes that were initially abnormal to age-appropriate values can guide resuscitation. These values do not have to completely normalize for an infant to undergo surgical repair; individual institutions may have guidelines suggesting when the infant can undergo surgery.[3] Infants with severe metabolic abnormalities should, after resuscitation with intravenous fluids, have their electrolytes corrected slowly.[3]

An infant diagnosed with pyloric stenosis requires consultation with a pediatric surgeon or a qualified general surgeon who is well versed in treating this condition, as treatment for pyloric stenosis is a pyloromyotomy. While a traditional abdominal surgical approach may be employed, a laparoscopic technique has been successfully used and has demonstrated superior outcomes.[3,8,11–13] The long-term effects of the condition and its repair are minimal, with generally no long-term sequelae.[3,14] Recurrent pyloric stenosis is extremely rare and is felt to be a clinical entity separate from incomplete pyloromyotomy and may represent a de novo process.[8] The treatment of recurrent pyloric stenosis is surgical.

IMAGING PEARLS

1. Infants with history and physical examination findings consistent with pyloric stenosis require prompt surgical consultation and may not need imaging.
2. If there is concern for bowel obstruction, plain radiography may be helpful.
3. If imaging is desired, US is the preferred imaging modality for pyloric stenosis.
4. CT of the abdomen is not indicated in infants with suspected pyloric stenosis. However, if there is concern for an intracranial process or complex abdominal pathology, this modality may be employed.

References

1. Raske ME, Dempsey ME, Dillman JR, et al. ACR appropriateness criteria vomiting in infants up to 3 months of age. *J Am Coll Radiol.* 2015;12(9):915-922.
2. Rao P. Neonatal gastrointestinal imaging. *Eur J Radiol.* 2006;60(2):171-186.
3. Letton Jr RW. Pyloric stenosis. *Pediatr Ann.* 2001;30(12):745-750.
4. Dinkevich E, Ozuah PO. Pyloric stenosis. *Pediatr Rev.* 2000;21(7):249-250.
5. Cohen HL, Blumer SL, Zucconi WB. The sonographic double-track sign: not pathognomonic for hypertrophic pyloric stenosis; can be seen in pylorospasm. *J Ultrasound Med.* 2004;23(5):641-646.
6. Hernanz-Schulman M. Pyloric stenosis: role of imaging. *Pediatr Radiol.* 2009;39(suppl 2):S134-S139.
7. Kobayashi H, Wester T, Puri P. Age-related changes in innervation in hypertrophic pyloric stenosis. *J Pediatr Surg.* 1997;32(12):1704-1707.
8. Hendricks CM, Edgerton CA, Lesher AP. Recurrent pyloric stenosis. *Am Surg.* 2018;84(9):e354-e356.
9. Bakal U, Sarac M, Aydin M. et al. Recent changes in the features of hypertrophic pyloric stenosis. *Pediatr Int.* 2016;58(5):369-371.
10. White MC, Langer JC, Don S, et al. Sensitivity and cost minimization analysis of radiology versus olive palpation for the diagnosis of hypertrophic pyloric stenosis. *J Pediatr Surg.* 1998;33(6):913-917.
11. Bufo AJ, Merry C, Shah R, et al. Laparoscopic pyloromyotomy: a safer technique. *Pediatr Surg Int.* 1998;13(4):240-242.
12. Costanzo CM, Vinocur C, Berman L. Postoperative outcomes of open versus laparoscopic pyloromyotomy for hypertrophic pyloric stenosis. *J Surg Res.* 2018;224:240-244.
13. Taghavi K, Powell E, Patel B, et al. The treatment of pyloric stenosis: evolution in practice. *J Paediatr Child Health.* 2017;53(11):1105-1110.
14. Keys C, Johnson C, Teague W, et al. One hundred years of pyloric stenosis in the Royal Hospital for Sick Children Edinburgh. *J Pediatr Surg.* 2015;50(2):280-284.

SECTION 4

Genitourinary

21 Twists and Turns: Testicular Torsion

WINNIE WHITAKER, MD, FAAP

Case Presentation

A 15-year-old male presents with left scrotal pain and swelling for the past 5 hours. He states that he was jumping on a trampoline just prior to presentation and afterward, he experienced his symptoms. He denies genital trauma. He has not had fever, back pain, dysuria, hematuria, penile discharge, abdominal pain, or vomiting. He denies being sexually active.

Physical examination reveals a well-appearing pleasant adolescent in some discomfort. He is afebrile but he is mildly tachycardic with a heart rate of 110 beats per minute; his respiratory rate is 16 breaths per minute; his blood pressure is 125/65 mm Hg. He has a nontender abdominal examination without rebound, guarding, or masses. His genital examination demonstrates a Tanner IV male, without obvious erythema or masses. There are no signs of trauma. He has tenderness to the left epididymis and to the left scrotum in general. The testicles feel normal but he has pain with examination of the left side and the left testicle appears to lie slightly higher than the right. There is mild left scrotal swelling. He is circumcised. There is no discharge from the penis. There are no lesions.

Imaging Considerations

PLAIN RADIOGRAPHY

While plain radiography of the abdomen may be utilized in cases of abdominal pain, it is not indicated as a first-line imaging study in patients who have suspected testicular pathology.

ULTRASOUND (US)

Readily available and without ionizing radiation exposure, US is an excellent means by which to visualize the scrotum and its contents. It is the imaging modality of choice across all age groups when ruling out testicular torsion, particularly duplex examination including color and spectral Doppler sonography, with sensitivity and specificity both approaching 100%.[1] US can also detect other entities that may mimic symptoms of testicular torsion, including epididymo-orchitis, hydroceles, varicoceles, and testicular masses.

A high-frequency transducer is used to scan the testicle in its entirety in both the transverse and longitudinal planes. Gray-scale and color Doppler images should be obtained. Both venous and arterial flow may be compromised. A lack of normal arterial blood flow is suspicious for testicular torsion; however, the phenomenon can be partial or intermittent, and

the presence of normal or decreased Doppler arterial flow cannot completely rule it out. A sonographic finding that is definitive for testicular torsion is the "whirlpool sign," in which there is an abrupt change in the course of the spermatic cord with a spiral twist at the external inguinal ring or in the scrotal sac.[2] A "torsion knot" may also be seen by US, in which redundant, tortuous spermatic cord twists, often around a small, reactive hydrocele. Normally, the testes have a vertical lie. A horizontal lie, or bell clapper deformity, can occur from abnormal attachment of the tunica vaginalis and is associated with intermittent testicular torsion. A US demonstrating horizontal or oblique lie, especially in the setting of diminished or absent intratesticular flow, is concerning for testicular torsion.[3]

US is the diagnostic imaging modality of choice for all patients when testicular torsion is suspected, but the presence of vascular flow by Doppler alone cannot be exclusively relied upon to exclude this condition in patients whose symptoms and examination are consistent with testicular torsion. The clinician should also consider the history, clinical examination, and other US findings when interpreting sonography results, and if overall suspicion is high, emergent urological consultation is warranted.

COMPUTED TOMOGRAPHY (CT)

CT scan is generally not indicated in the work-up of testicular torsion. However, there is literature suggesting that perfusion CT scanning may be considered as a secondary method of diagnosing testicular torsion in indeterminate cases.[4] It should not be utilized as a first-line imaging modality due to radiation exposure.

MAGNETIC RESONANCE IMAGING (MRI)

While also not a first-line imaging modality for patients with testicular pain, MRI is considered to be highly sensitive for testicular torsion. Specifically, the dynamic contrast-enhanced (DCE)–subtraction technique can demonstrate changes in testicular perfusion by assessing testicular contrast enhancement.[5] MRI, however, is not a practical choice to diagnose testicular torsion given its limited availability, length of study, and cost.

SCROTAL SCINTIGRAPHY

Scrotal scintigraphy is a nuclear study in which a radioisotope is used to demonstrate testicular blood flow. Although it used to be widely utilized starting in 1971, it has been replaced by ultrasonography, which is readily available and does not require exposure to ionizing radiation. Scintigraphy may still play a role when testicular torsion has not been ruled out and US is inconclusive.[6]

NEAR-INFRARED SPECTROSCOPY (NIRS)

NIRS has been proposed as a potentially useful modality in ruling out testicular torsion because it is noninvasive, portable, easily accessible for bedside use, and easy to interpret. It uses light transmission and absorption to measure tissue oxygen saturation in superficial body layers up to several centimeters deep. In testicular torsion, the affected testicle is predicted to have significantly lower tissue oxygen saturation than the unaffected contralateral testicle. Although promising in theory, there is not enough evidence to support routine use of NIRS in the work-up of testicular torsion.[7,8]

Imaging Findings

The patient had grayscale and color and spectral Doppler ultrasonography performed. Selected images from that study are noted here. While the right epididymis and testis are normal in appearance and have normal color and spectral arterial flow, the left testis is heterogeneous and slightly hyperechoic. There is no demonstrable Doppler flow to this testis. These findings are highly suggestive of left testicular torsion (Figs. 21.1–21.3).

Case Conclusion

Pediatric Urology was consulted and the patient was taken to the operating room for definitive management. During surgery, the left testicle was noted to be torsed with three

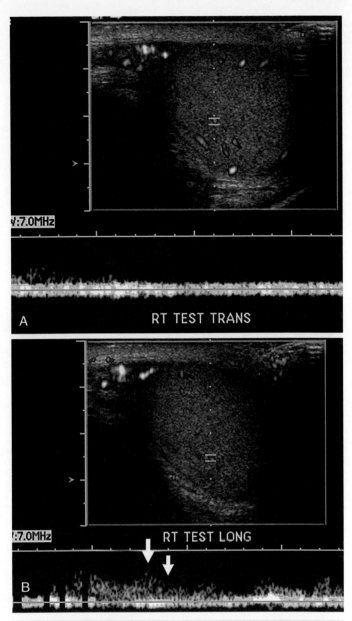

Fig. 21.2 Normal Doppler imaging of the right testis. Transverse (A) and longitudinal (B) Doppler images of the right testis demonstrate color flow in the right testis, with a normal-appearing arterial spectral Doppler tracing *(white arrows)*.

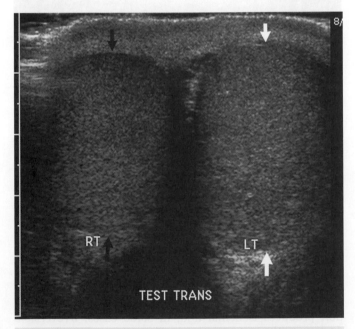

Fig. 21.1 Transverse ultrasound image of both testes shows the left testis *(white arrows)* to be enlarged and to show a mildly heterogenous echotexture and increased echogenicity as compared to the right testis *(black arrows)*.

360-degree turns of the spermatic cord, proximal to the epididymis. The testicle was dark purple in color and was wrapped in warm saline-soaked gauze while the right scrotum was explored. During this exploration, the right testicle appeared healthy but there was a bell clapper deformity and an orchiopexy was performed. Once this was done, the left testicle appeared to have restored color and was placed back into the scrotum. The patient recovered uneventfully.

A comparison case demonstrates a patient with a US consistent with left testicular torsion (Figs. 21.4–21.6). This 12-year-old patient presented with a 2-day history of abdominal pain, scrotal pain, and left scrotal swelling. Selected images from a scrotal US demonstrate a lack of arterial flow in the left testis, consistent with torsion. Unfortunately, the testicle was unable to be salvaged.

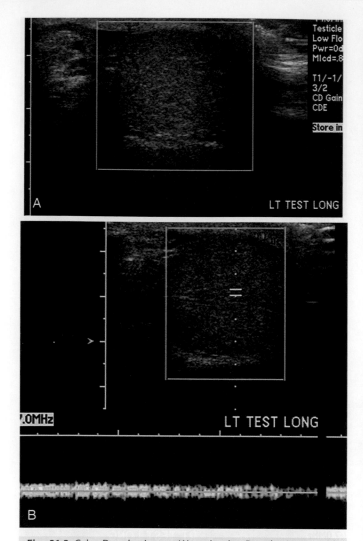

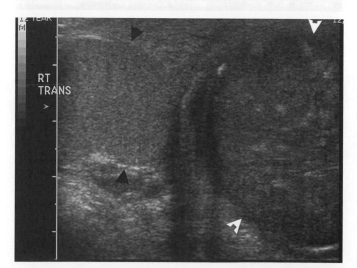

Fig. 21.3 Color Doppler image (A) and color Doppler image with spectral tracing (B) show no detectable color Doppler flow and no detectable spectral blood flow tracings in the left testis. These findings are consistent with left testicular torsion.

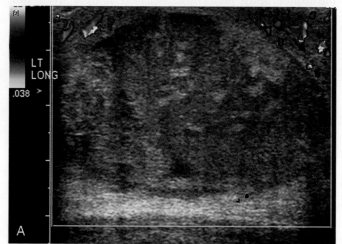

Fig. 21.4 Transverse ultrasound image of both testes shows the left testis *(white arrowheads)* to be enlarged and to demonstrate abnormal, heterogeneous echotexture as compared to the normal-appearing right testis *(black arrowheads)*.

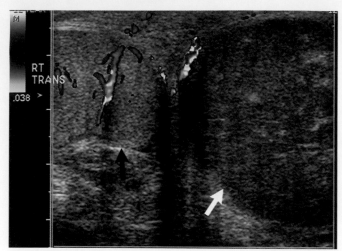

Fig. 21.5 Transverse color Doppler image showing color indicating blood flow in the right testis *(black arrow)*, with a lack of color Doppler flow in the left testis *(white arrow)*.

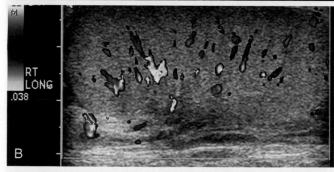

Fig. 21.6 Longitudinal color Doppler images demonstrate abnormal heterogeneous echotexture of the left testis, with no color Doppler flow (A). Color Doppler flow is well demonstrated in the right testis (B). Findings are consistent with left testicular torsion.

Testicular torsion occurs when there is sudden twisting of the spermatic cord in the scrotum. This emergent condition produces ischemia and, in some cases, irreversible damage to the involved testicle. The estimated incidence of this condition is 5 in 100,000 males, with prepubertal and adolescent males the most commonly affected group.[8,9] There is a bimodal distribution of testicular torsion, in the first year of life and in early adolescence.[1] Torsion can occur within the tunica vaginalis (intravaginal torsion) or associated with the tunica vaginalis (extravaginal torsion).[9,10] The majority of cases outside the neonatal period are intravaginal; extravaginal torsion is usually seen within the neonatal period and is associated with generally poor outcomes.[9] The most common anatomic defect leading to intravaginal torsion is the so-called "bell clapper deformity." The etiology of this anatomic condition is a high insertion point of the tunica vaginalis, preventing full descent of the testicle into the scrotum and allowing free rotation of the testis and spermatic cord, which can rotate impressively (from 180 degrees to greater than 720 degrees).[9]

Acute onset of severe scrotal pain is the classic presenting symptom of testicular torsion. Inguinal or lower quadrant abdominal pain, scrotal swelling, and nausea/vomiting may also be presenting symptoms. The TWIST score was developed to diagnose testicular torsion in pediatric patients[11]:

SYMPTOM/FINDING	POINTS
Testicular swelling	2
Testicular hardness	2
Absent cremasteric reflex	1
Nausea/vomiting	1
High riding testis	1

Retrospective validation has found a positive predictive value of 100% in patients with scores >5 and 100% negative predictive value in patients with scores <2.

Testicular torsion is managed by surgical correction (orchiopexy). While imaging is valuable to determining if there is indeed a torsion, patients with a history and clinical examination consistent with torsion should have immediate urologic consultation; surgical management should not be delayed by imaging, which could prolong ischemia and lead to an unfavorable outcome.[9] The duration of symptoms has been shown to be a significant prognostic factor in favorable (or unfavorable) outcomes. Ideally, patients with testicular torsion outside of the neonatal period should be managed as quickly as possible without transfer to a pediatric facility if a general urologist, an anesthesiologist, and adequate operative facilities are available, although many times, pediatric patients with torsion are transferred to pediatric facilities.[9,12–15]

The use of a manual detorsion maneuver as a temporizing measure prior to orchiopexy has been utilized. This technique is performed by a medial to lateral twisting of the affected testis (the "open book" technique), since torsion occurs by rotating in a lateral to medial manner along the axis of the spermatic cord.[9,10] However, torsion can occur in any direction, the degree of torsion can vary (there can be multiple twists), and a manual detorsion may be incomplete.[9,15] As with imaging, manual detorsion maneuvers should not delay operative intervention, and the standard of care for testicular torsion remains surgical exploration and orchiopexy.[9]

IMAGING PEARLS

1. A clinical history and examination consistent with testicular torsion should prompt immediate surgical consultation and does not always require imaging.

2. Since imaging is often utilized, scrotal US with Doppler imaging is the first-line imaging testing in patients with suspected testicular torsion. Easy availability, lack of ionizing radiation, and excellent ability to visualize the vascular flow to the testes make this an ideal modality.

3. US sensitivity is extremely high (approaching 100%), but testicular Doppler sonography can be operator dependent. Arterial blood flow alone, as detected by Doppler, is not always sufficient to exclude testicular torsion. The clinician should consider all findings on US when determining if torsion is present.

4. When US is indeterminate for testicular torsion, other imaging modalities such as perfusion CT, MRI, or scrotal scintigraphy may be considered as adjunct tests. However, lack of availability, time needed to obtain imaging, cost, and exposure to ionizing radiation must be taken into consideration.

References

1. Liang T, Metcalfe P, Sevcik W, et al. Retrospective review of diagnosis and treatment in children presenting to the pediatric department with acute scrotum. *AJR Am J Roentgenol.* 2013;200(5):W444-W449.
2. McDowall J, Adam A, Gerber L, et al. The ultrasonographic "whirlpool sign" in testicular torsion: valuable tool or waste of valuable time? A systematic review and meta-analysis. *Emerg Radiol.* 2018;25(3):281-292.
3. Bandarkar AN, Blask AR. Testicular torsion with preserved flow: key sonographic features and value-added approach to diagnosis. *Pediatr Radiol.* 2018;48(5):735-744.
4. Ovali GY, Yilmaz O, Tarhan S, et al. Perfusion CT evaluation in experimentally induced testicular torsion. *Can Urol Assoc J.* 2009;3(5):383-386.
5. Watanabe Y, Nagayama M, Okumura A, et al. MR imaging of testicular torsion: features of testicular hemorrhagic necrosis and clinical outcomes. *J Magn Reson Imaging.* 2007;26(1):100-108.
6. Paltiel HJ, Connolly LP, Atala A, et al. Acute scrotal symptoms in boys with an indeterminate clinical presentation: comparison of color Doppler sonography and scintigraphy. *Radiology.* 1998;207(1):223-231.
7. Laher A, Swart M, Honiball J, et al. Near-infrared spectroscopy in the diagnosis of testicular torsion: valuable modality or waste of valuable time? A systematic review. *ANZ J Surg.* 2020;90(5):708-714. doi:10.1111/ans.15402.
8. Osumah TS, Jimbo M, Granberg CF, et al. Frontiers in pediatric testicular torsion: an integrated review of prevailing trends and management outcomes. *J Pediatr Urol.* 2018;14(5):394-401.
9. Zhao LC, Lautz TB, Meeks JJ, et al. Pediatric testicular torsion epidemiology using a national database: incidence, risk of orchiectomy and possible measures toward improving the quality of care. *J Urol.* 2011;186(5):2009-2013.
10. Sharp VJ, Kiera K, Arien AM. Testicular torsion: diagnosis, evaluation, and management. *Am Fam Physician.* 2013;88(12):835-840.
11. Barbosa JA, Tiseo BC, Barayan GA, et al. Development and initial validation of a scoring system to diagnose testicular torsion in children. *J Urol.* 2013;189(5):1859-1864.
12. Preece J, Ching C, Yackey K, et al. Indicators and outcomes of transfer to tertiary pediatric hospitals for patients with testicular torsion. *J Pediatr Urol.* 2017;13(4):388.e1-388.e6.
13. Bayne CE, Gomella PT, DiBianco JM, et al. Testicular torsion presentation trends before and after pediatric urology subspecialty certification. *J Urol.* 2017;197(2):507-515.
14. Hussman DA. Who should be taking care of adolescent testicular torsion? *J Urol.* 2017;197(2):282-283.
15. Yecies T, Bandari J, Schneck F, et al. Direction of rotation in testicular torsion and identification of predictors of testicular salvage. *Urology.* 2018;114:163-166.

That Looks Painful: Hydrocele

ROBERT VEZZETTI, MD, FAAP, FACEP

Case Presentation

A 4-month-old male presents with bilateral scrotal swelling. Per the mother, this has been present since 1 month of age but has worsened over the past week and she has noted that the right side of the scrotum appears darker than normal. The mother also states that there has been mild congestion and cough for the past week and today the child developed a fever to 102.5 degrees Fahrenheit. There have been no other symptoms, including vomiting, diarrhea, rash, or fussiness. He has been drinking well. His physical examination reveals a temperature of 101 degrees Fahrenheit, a respiratory rate of 30 breaths per minute, and a heart rate of 120 beats per minute. He is very well appearing and in no distress. He has mild nasal congestion with normal tympanic membranes. His lungs are clear. His abdominal examination is unremarkable; there is no apparent tenderness, masses, or hepatosplenomegaly. His genital examination shows an uncircumcised male with the scrotum markedly enlarged bilaterally making the examination difficult. There is no erythema; there are no palpable masses; there is induration but no palpable fluctuance. Transillumination of the scrotum reveals probable fluid.

Imaging Considerations

Pediatric scrotal complaints can be acute or chronic, involving the testicle or extratesticular structures. Common etiologies of acute scrotal pain or swelling include traumatic (i.e., scrotal hematoma or testicular rupture), infectious (epididymitis or epididymo-orchitis, cellulitis), and vascular (testicular torsion or torsion of an appendix testis) causes. Included in this acute group is scrotal wall edema, which may be due to insect bites/stings or be associated with Henloch-Schönlein purpura, often as a first sign of this disease process.[1,2] Another finding that may be seen in pediatric patients is testicular microlithiasis. These arise from calcifications in the seminiferous tubules, and their clinical significance is not entirely certain. While often idiopathic, microlithiasis can be associated with certain congenital syndromes, such as Down syndrome and Kleinfelter syndrome.[3] They were once considered to place patients at risk for testicular cancer, but this association has been questioned, especially in asymptomatic patients.[1-4] While no standardized protocols exist for cancer surveillance risk,[4] the finding of scrotal microlithiasis should prompt referral to Pediatric Urology for ongoing surveillance.

Chronic scrotal complaints in the pediatric population are usually congenital and include hydroceles and undescended testes. Undescended testes, termed cryptorchidism, are an important finding. The testes may be located anywhere along the path where testicles descend, but the inguinal canal is the most common location; they appear as asymmetric, small, and hypoechoic compared to normal testis.[1] Finding undescended testes should prompt referral to Pediatric Urology, as they do pose a risk for testicular cancer.[1,2,5,6]

Neonatal scrotal swelling is most often due to congenital hydrocele, but other etiologies, such as inguinal hernias (more commonly seen in premature infants[7]), scrotal hematomas (associated with high birth weight, trauma, and bleeding diasthasis[8]), neoplasm (rare—either germ cell tumors or stromal tumors), and testicular torsion (occurs most often in utero[9]) have all been reported.[10]

ULTRASOUND

Ultrasound is the preferred imaging modality to evaluate acute and chronic scrotal complaints in the pediatric population. The excellent resolution, lack of ionizing radiation, and Doppler capabilities make this modality an ideal imaging choice to identify important anatomical landmarks, such as the epididymis, spermatic cord, and testes, as well as visualizing the inguinal canal.[1] Doppler imaging is excellent for visualizing blood flow to the testis and surrounding structures.[4,11] Expertise in the performance and interpretation of pediatric scrotal ultrasound is required for accurate diagnosis and appropriate treatment.

Imaging Findings

The child had ultrasonography with color-flow duplex Doppler performed of the testes and scrotal contents. Selected images are provided. There are bilateral, large, simple hydroceles (Fig. 22.1); the testes are normal in echotexture and location. Duplex Doppler demonstrates normal waveforms with normal amplitude, indicating normal blood flow to the testes (Figs. 22.2 and 22.3). There is no evidence of testicular torsion.

Case Conclusion

The child was referred to Pediatric Urology for outpatient evaluation and management, since imaging revealed no signs of torsion, hernia, or other acute surgical or infectious processes. The child's urinalysis was normal; the fever was attributed to a viral upper respiratory infection.

Pediatric hydroceles are due to excessive fluid accumulation in the tunica vaginalis. They are the most common cause of painless scrotal swelling in the pediatric population.[5,12]

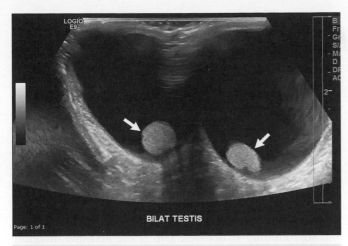

Fig. 22.1 On transverse ultrasound image of the scrotum, the testes are seen as soft tissue structures *(arrows)* surrounded by hydrocele fluid.

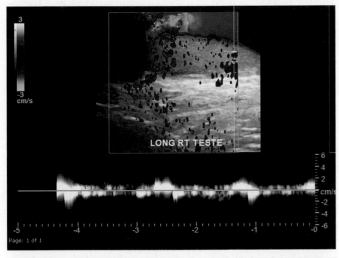

Fig. 22.2 Longitudinal duplex Doppler sonography of the right testicle demonstrates color Doppler blood flow and both arterial and venous tracings.

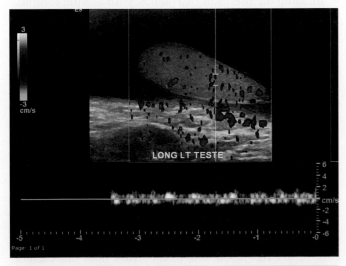

Fig. 22.3 Longitudinal duplex Doppler sonography of the left testicle demonstrates color Doppler blood flow and both arterial and venous tracings.

In infants and young children, hydroceles are most often congenital, due to fluid remaining after closure of the processus vaginalis or may be due to a processus vaginalis that remains patent, allowing flow of peritoneal fluid into the scrotal sac due to continued communication with the abdominal cavity.[5,12] Inguinoscrotal (a closed processus vaginalis at the internal inguinal ring and the hydrocele extending from this location into the scrotum) and abdominoscrotal (quite rare—the hydrocele extends into the peritoneal cavity) hydroceles have also been described.[13,14] Older children may acquire a hydrocele, usually due to trauma, infection, testicular torsion, or (less commonly) masses.[5,12]

Ultrasound is the imaging modality of choice to evaluate hydroceles. Ultrasound findings consistent with hydrocele include scrotal fluid that is typically anechoic.[3,12] Hydroceles due to infection will demonstrate septations.[3]

Treatment for hydroceles depends on the age of the child and the history surrounding the detection of the hydrocele. With congenital hydroceles, the majority will resolve by 2 years of life.[5] Hydroceles that persist beyond this age, those that are found in older children, and those associated with significant scrotal trauma or surgical conditions (such as masses or testicular torsion) should be promptly referred to pediatric urology.

IMAGING PEARLS

1. Ultrasound is the imaging modality of choice with scrotal complaints in the pediatric population.
2. Scrotal ultrasound should be performed with Doppler imaging to visualize blood flow to the testes and surrounding tissues.

References

1. Rebik K, Wagner JM, Middleton W. Scrotal ultrasound. *Radiol Clin North Am.* 2019;57(3):635-648.
2. Winter TC, Kim B, Lowrance WT, et al. Testicular microlithiasis: what should you recommend? *AJR Am J Roentgenol.* 2016;206:1164-1169.
3. Delaney LR, Karmazyn B. Ultrasound of the pediatric scrotum. *Semin Ultrasound CT MR.* 2013;34(3):248-756.
4. Alkhori NA, Barth RA. Pediatric scrotal ultrasound: review and update. *Pediatr Radiol.* 2017;47(9):1125-1133.
5. Aso C, Enriquez G, Fite M, et al. Gray-scale and color Doppler sonography of scrotal disorders in children: an update. *Radiographics.* 2005;25(5): 1197-1214.
6. Kolon TF, Herndon CD, Baker LA, et al. Evaluation and treatment of cryptorchidism: AUA guideline. *J Urol.* 2014;192(2):337-345.
7. Lao OB, Fitzgibbons Jr RJ, Cusick RA. Pediatric inguinal hernias, hydroceles, and undescended testicles. *Surg Clin North Am.* 2012; 92(3):487-504.
8. Diamond DA, Borer JG, Peters CA, et al. Neonatal scrotal haematoma: mimicker of neonatal testicular torsion. *BJU Int.* 2003;91:675-677.
9. Kaye JD, Levitt SB, Friedman SC, et al. Neonatal torsion: a 14-year experience and proposed algorithm for management. *J Urol.* 2008; 179(6):2377-2383.
10. Basta AM, Courtier J, Phelps A, et al. Scrotal swelling in the neonate. *J Ultrasound Med.* 2015;34(3):495-505.
11. Lemini R, Guanà R, Tommasoni N, et al. Predictivity of clinical findings and Doppler ultrasound in pediatric acute scrotum. *Urol J.* 2016;13(4):2779-2783.
12. Schmitz K, Snyder K, Geldermann D, et al. The large pediatric scrotum: ultrasound technique and differential considerations. *Ultrasound Q.* 2014;30(2):119-134.
13. Costantino E, Ganesan GS, Plaire JC. Abdominoscrotal hydrocele in an infant boy. *BMJ Case Rep.* 2017; 2017:1-4.
14. Karthikeyan VS, Sistla SC, Ram D, et al. Giant inguinoscrotal hernia—report of a rare case with literature review. *Int Surg.* 2014;99(5):560-564.

23 *Unusually Painful: Ovarian Torsion*

ROBERT VEZZETTI, MD, FAAP, FACEP

Case Presentation

A 13-year-old female presents with acute onset of right lower quadrant pain for the past 4 hours. She states that she has been in her usual, normal state of health and was "just walking down the street" when she experienced the pain, which was accompanied by nausea and she has had three episodes of nonbilious/nonbloody emesis. She states that after the emesis, she feels "a little better" but the pain has persisted. She denies fever, diarrhea, or trauma. She denies being sexually active and there is no history of vaginal bleeding or discharge. She began her menses 2 years ago and has had occasional cramping with her menstrual cycle; her last menstrual period was 2 weeks ago.

Physical examination reveals a slightly uncomfortable-appearing patient, complaining of abdominal pain, mostly in the right lower quadrant. She is afebrile, and aside from mild tachycardia (a heart rate of 120 beats per minute), the vital signs are unremarkable. She has mild tenderness to palpation of the right lower quadrant and suprapubic areas; there is no rebound or guarding. She has no palpable abdominal masses and there is no abdominal distention; a urine pregnancy test is negative.

Imaging Considerations

Prior to imaging, a pregnancy test must be obtained, since this can assist the clinician in considering an appropriate imaging modality selection to evaluate nongynecologic and gynecologic causes of abdominal pain and to avoid fetal exposure to ionizing radiation. The American College of Radiology (ACR) has Appropriateness Criteria® (AC) useful for selecting among various imaging modalities for the evaluation of female acute pelvic pain in the reproductive age group, based on gynecologic and nongynecologic suspected etiologies and whether the patient is pregnant or not. As the patient had a negative serum pregnancy test, Variant 2 of the AC for "gynecological etiology suspected, serum β-hCG negative" applies (Table 23.1).[1] The ACR Appropriateness Criteria® content is updated regularly and users should go to the website (https://www.acr.org/Clinical-Resources/ACR-Appropriateness-Criteria®) to access the most current and complete version of the AC.

PLAIN RADIOGRAPHY

While plain radiography of the abdomen may be utilized in cases of abdominal pain, it is not indicated as a first-line imaging study in patients who have suspected ovarian pathology as a source of their pain.

ULTRASOUND (US)

Readily available and without ionizing radiation exposure, US is an excellent means by which to visualize the ovary and surrounding structures. This is the first-line imaging modality for cases of suspected ovarian torsion or other gynecologic pathology where imaging is indicated.[2]

A mid- to high-frequency curvilinear transducer is used and the bladder is used as a sonographic window and therefore must be full to obtain meaningful results.[3-5] In pediatric patients, a transabdominal approach is usually employed, although in select patients such as sexually active adolescents, a transvaginal technique may be utilized.[5] The clinician should be aware of local statutes regarding informed consent for performing a transvaginal US, which vary among jurisdictions. The decision to perform transvaginal US should be based on sexual and clinical history, and age of the patient. The preference of the patient, parent/guardian, and physician are factors in the decision to utilize a transvaginal approach and informed consent for the procedure should be obtained.[5] The patient should also be made aware that the study can be stopped at any time, if the patient wishes.[5] Clinicians may utilize institutional protocols if they are available.

Suggested transabdominal technique includes the following[5]:

- A scout scan of the entire pelvis in two planes, making sure the bladder is full.
- Low-frequency color Doppler use to ensure proper penetration.
- Imaging the uterus in two planes, with uterine volume.
- Measuring the anteroposterior thickness of the endometrium in the midsagittal plane and color Doppler assessment of the endometrium, looking for endometrial lesions.
- Measurement of the ovaries in three orthogonal planes with calculation of the ovarian volume.
- Other organ assessment (appendix, kidneys, bowel wall) as clinically indicated.

Doppler sonography has been the traditional imaging method to evaluate for the presence of ovarian torsion, since both venous and arterial flow can be compromised during this process. A lack of normal blood flow is suspicious for ovarian torsion. Abnormal blood flow has modest accuracy for identifying ovarian torsion and while abnormal arterial blood flow is often a concern, abnormal venous blood flow is seen earlier in ovarian torsion.[1,6-12] The presence of arterial blood flow to the ovary does not exclude ovarian torsion, due to secondary ovarian vascular supply, and does not rule out intermittent, or even partial torsion. Other findings should be considered, such as the size and

Table 23.1   American College of Radiology (ACR) Appropriateness Criteria®.

CLINICAL CONDITION: ACUTE PELVIC PAIN IN THE REPRODUCTIVE AGE GROUP
VARIANT 2: GYNECOLOGICAL ETIOLOGY SUSPECTED, SERUM β-hCG NEGATIVE.

Radiologic Procedure	Rating	Comments	RRL*
US pelvis transvaginal	9	Both transvaginal and transabdominal US should be performed if possible	O
US pelvis transabdominal	9	Both transvaginal and transabdominal US should be performed if possible	O
US duplex Doppler pelvis	8		O
MRI pelvis without and with IV contrast	6	This procedure can be performed if US is inconclusive or nondiagnostic. See the Summary of Literature Review and ACR Manual on Contrast Media for the use of contrast media.	O
MRI abdomen and pelvis without and with IV contrast	6	This procedure can be performed if US is inconclusive or nondiagnostic. See the Summary of Literature Review and ACR Manual on Contrast Media for the use of contrast media.	O
MRI pelvis without IV contrast	4	This procedure can be performed if US is inconclusive or nondiagnostic. See the Summary of Literature Review and ACR Manual on Contrast Media for the use of contrast media.	O
MRI abdomen and pelvis without IV contrast	4	This procedure can be performed if US is inconclusive or nondiagnostic. See the Summary of Literature Review and ACR Manual on Contrast Media for the use of contrast media.	O
CT abdomen and pelvis with IV contrast	4	This procedure can be performed if US is inconclusive or nondiagnostic and MRI is not available. See the Summary of Literature Review for the use of contrast media.	☢☢☢
CT pelvis with IV contrast	4	This procedure can be performed if US is inconclusive or nondiagnostic and MRI is not available. In young women undergoing repeat imaging, the cumulative radiation dose should be considered. See the Summary of Literature Review for the use of contrast media.	☢☢☢
CT pelvis without IV contrast	2	This procedure can be performed if US is inconclusive or nondiagnostic and MRI is not available. In young women undergoing repeat imaging, the cumulative radiation dose should be considered.	☢☢☢
CT pelvis without and with IV contrast	2		☢☢☢☢
CT abdomen and pelvis without IV contrast	2		☢☢☢
CT abdomen and pelvis without and with IV contrast	2		☢☢☢☢
Rating Scale: 1, 2, 3 Usually not appropriate; 4, 5, 6 May be appropriate; 7, 8, 9 Usually appropriate			*Relative Radiation Level

CT, Computed tomography; *hCG*, human chorionic gonadotropin; *IV*, intravenous; *MRI*, magnetic resonance imaging; *US*, ultrasound.
From https://acsearch.acr.org/docs/69503/Narrative/. The ACR Appropriateness Criteria® content is updated regularly and users should go to the website (https://www.acr.org/Clinical-Resources/ACR-Appropriateness-Criteria®) to access the most current and complete version of the AC.

morphology of the affected ovary (compared to the unaffected ovary), venous blood flow, the presence of free fluid, or ovarian masses. Ovarian enlargement is particularly concerning for torsion, and lack of venous blood flow is a frequent finding with ovarian torsion.[10,11] A number of studies confirm cases of proven ovarian torsion where patients have either an enlarged ovary or lack of venous blood flow despite having arterial blood flow by Doppler sonography.[6,7,10,11,13,14] Combining abnormal findings, particularly ovarian enlargement and the presence of free fluid, increases the sensitivity of sonography to detect ovarian torsion.[6,7,10,13,15] Detection of the twisting of the vascular pedicle—the "Whirlpool Sign"—demonstrated as a round hyperechoic structure with concentric hypoechoic stripes or as a tubular structure with internal heterogeneous echoes,[11] suggests ovarian torsion. Sensitivities and specificities for various US findings for ovarian torsion have been reported[1,16]:

ULTRASOUND FINDING	SENSITIVITY[a]	SPECIFICITY[a]
Tissue edema	21%	100%
Absence of intraovarian vascularity	52%	91%
Absence of arterial flow	76%	99%
Absence or abnormal venous flow	100%	97%

[a]These values represent upper estimates and may be lower based on the skill of the providers performing and interpreting the test.

US can also detect other gynecologic entities that may mimic symptoms of ovarian torsion, including ovarian (simple, complex, and hemorrhagic) cysts, tubo-ovarian abscesses, and ovarian masses, as well as nongynecologic etiologies, such as appendicitis.[3,17]

US is the diagnostic imaging modality of choice for all patients when ovarian torsion is suspected, but the presence of arterial flow by Doppler alone cannot be solely and exclusively relied upon to exclude this condition in patients whose symptoms and exam are consistent with ovarian torsion. The clinician should also consider the history, clinical exam, and other ovarian US findings when interpreting sonography results.

COMPUTED TOMOGRAPHY (CT)

Computed tomography is utilized frequently during the evaluation of abdominal pain. With pediatric patients, ALARA (as low as reasonably achievable) principles should be practiced.

There are no well-defined CT criteria for ovarian torsion, but there are findings that suggest this process. Ovarian enlargement, pelvic free fluid, a twisted vascular pedicle, inflammatory fat stranding, and deviation of the uterus to the side of the torsion have been reported CT findings in patients with proven ovarian torsion.[7,10,13,18] Some studies have proposed that a well-visualized, normal-appearing ovary on CT can exclude torsion; in these studies, patients with proven ovarian torsion had abnormalities on imaging, including an enlarged ovary, free pelvic fluid, abnormal ovarian enhancement, uterine deviation, and a twisted pedicle.[10,19–21] Notably, there are findings on CT that can mimic ovarian torsion, including ectopic pregnancy, endometriosis, hemorrhagic functional cyst, or tumors.[18]

While CT is not a first-line imaging modality to investigate ovarian torsion and should not be solely relied upon to exclude this diagnosis, a normal CT scan appears to make torsion less likely. This modality may be useful if US findings are equivocal or indeterminant, but suspicious, for torsion or if nongynecologic pathology such as appendicitis is suspected.[4,7,10,19,20] However, if available, magnetic resonance imaging (MRI) with intravenous (IV) contrast is preferred over CT as the second-line imaging modality for gynecologic pathology including ovarian torsion, if sonography is nondiagnostic. This is promulgated by the ACR Appropriateness Criteria®—Variant 2.[1]

MAGNETIC RESONANCE IMAGING

While also not a first-line imaging modality for ovarian torsion, MRI is excellent at visualizing Mullerian structures and the ovaries.[6,7] Findings on MRI suggestive of torsion are similar to those seen with CT: ovarian enlargement, masses (well visualized on T2 weighted images), twisted pedicles, and free fluid (to which MRI is very sensitive).[4,7,10] Although used infrequently for ovarian torsion, MRI is the study of choice for gynecologic pathology, including ovarian torsion, after an inconclusive pelvic sonogram. MRI is especially useful if the diagnosis of ovarian torsion is suspected in a pediatric patient, a pregnant patient, patients with renal failure, or patients with severe IV contrast allergies when a secondary imaging test is needed to clarify US results.

Imaging Findings

While IV access was established, pediatric surgical consultation was obtained. The patient appeared improved on examination, although still with pain. A request was made for a transabdominal pelvic US. The need for a full urinary bladder was discussed at length with the patient and her parents; they did not consent to the placement of a urinary catheter. Rather, several normal saline boluses were given, and the patient, after the second bolus, stated she felt a strong urge to urinate, at which time the US was obtained. Selected images from that study are presented here. The right ovary is enlarged, and ovarian parenchyma is diffusely heterogeneous with a prominent cyst or follicle and a few peripherally arranged small follicles. The right ovary appears to be shifted toward the midline of the pelvis and Doppler evaluation showed no convincing arterial or venous flow in the right ovary; comparison is made to the left ovary (Figs. 23.1–23.4).

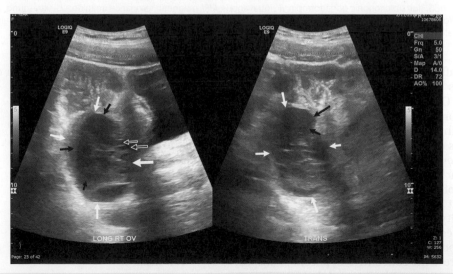

Fig. 23.1 Longitudinal and transverse ultrasound images demonstrating an enlarged right ovary *(white arrows)* with a subtle hypoechoic lesion *(black arrows)* corresponding to a hemorrhagic cyst at surgery. Also, note is made of small peripherally arranged follicles *(open white arrows).*

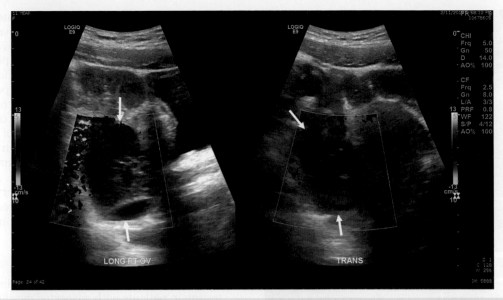

Fig. 23.2 Longitudinal and transverse color Doppler ultrasound images of the right ovary *(white arrows)*. Color Doppler and spectral Doppler interrogation of the right ovary showed no discernible arterial or venous blood flow in the enlarged right ovary. The only color seen over the ovary on these images was due to artifactual "noise," rather than evidence of blood flow.

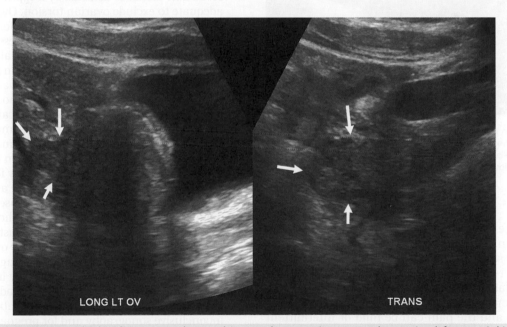

Fig. 23.3 Longitudinal and transverse ultrasound images demonstrating a normal-appearing left ovary *(white arrows)*.

Case Conclusion

With these imaging findings, the patient was taken to the operating suite by Pediatric Surgery to undergo laparoscopic exploration. This procedure revealed a partially torsed ovary, which was somewhat dusky in appearance, accompanied by a large hemorrhagic ovarian cyst. The ovary was detorsed and an oophoropexy was performed. The hemorrhagic cyst was excised. Prior to the end of the

procedure, the left ovary was evaluated and was found to be normal. The patient recovered uneventfully.

Ovarian torsion (while this is the commonly used term, "adnexal torsion" is more accurate, since both the ovary and the fallopian tube are involved[11]) has significant implications if prompt diagnosis and treatment are not instituted. This process commonly occurs in women of reproductive age, but pediatric torsion does occur, including during infancy and childhood (including in utero); the

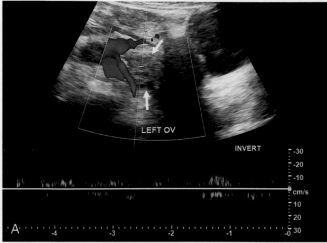

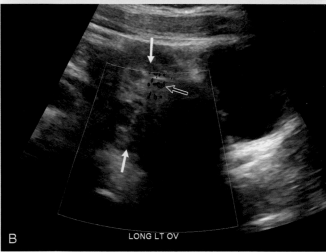

Fig. 23.4 Doppler ultrasound images demonstrating arterial and venous flow in the left ovary *(white arrows)*. (A) Spectral Doppler tracings of blood flow in the left ovary and (B) color Doppler imaging showed pulsatile flow in the left ovary *(open white arrow)*.

Treatment for ovarian torsion is immediate operative intervention to restore blood flow and prevent ovarian loss. Studies have supported untwisting the ovary rather than frank oophorectomy in an attempt to preserve ovarian function, with close monitoring of the affected ovary, and follow-up surgery if indicated.[10] In the pediatric population, the laparoscopic approach is preferred.[6] While ischemia can begin within hours of symptom onset, there is no specific time that determines the limit of ovarian viability.[13,25] One study that induced torsion in rat models showed no histological difference in ovaries that underwent 4 hours and 24 hours of torsion, but irreversible damage occurred after 36 hours.[13] Nevertheless, current treatment recommendations support operative intervention as quickly as possible and consultation with a gynecological specialist or qualified surgeon.[13]

IMAGING PEARLS

1. Pelvic US with Doppler imaging is the first-line imaging testing in patients with suspected ovarian torsion. The availability, lack of ionizing radiation, and excellent ability to visualize the ovary make this an ideal modality.
2. US sensitivity for ovarian torsion varies (up to 85%) and is operator dependent. Evaluation of arterial blood flow alone, as detected by Doppler, is not always adequate to exclude ovarian torsion. Ovarian morphology, venous blood flow, and free fluid, for example, are important imaging findings when assessing for ovarian torsion. The clinician should consider all findings from a US study when determining if torsion is present.
3. CT may show findings suggestive of ovarian torsion, but CT is more useful as an imaging modality to evaluate for suspected nongynecological pathology, such as appendicitis. An enlarged/asymmetric ovary, free fluid, a twisted pedicle, and abnormal ovarian enhancement are suggestive of ovarian torsion. However, CT is not a first-line modality for ovarian torsion and involves ionizing exposure as well as IV contrast use. CT alone should not be used to exclude or diagnose ovarian torsion and results should be interpreted in the context of clinical history and exam.
4. MRI may be used in the evaluation for ovarian torsion, and is the preferred second-line imaging test, after sonography, for gynecologic pathology including ovarian torsion. The lack of ionizing radiation makes this modality attractive for pediatric patients with inconclusive sonography and for pregnant patients. However, possible lack of availability, the time needed to obtain imaging, and expense make this a second-line imaging modality.

exact prevalence is not known.[13,15,22] One study found pediatric ovarian torsion to be 2.7% of abdominal pain cases.[6] Another study found the incidence of ovarian torsion in females 1–20 years of age to be 4.9 per 100,000 patients.[23] A classic presentation of ovarian torsion is acute onset of severe lower abdominal pain, but this is not always the case and the pain can be mild or intermittent and can be difficult to appreciate on physical examination; radiation of pain to the back, nausea, and emesis are also symptoms.[6,7,13,22] Ultimately, although imaging can suggest torsion, the diagnosis is clinical[8] and confirmed during operative exploration and repair. Attempts to develop a diagnostic algorithm for ovarian torsion through systemic and literature reviews have not been successful.[22]

Studies have examined what, if any, risk factors exist for ovarian torsion. Predisposing factors include ovarian cysts (found to be three times more common in ovarian torsion cohorts), ovarian masses, pregnancy ovarian hyperstimulation, and previous abdominal surgery (other than hysterectomy); however, younger patients may not have such predisposing factors.[4,6,7,10,24]

References

1. American College of Radiology appropriateness criteria for acute pelvic pain in the reproductive age group. https://acsearch.acr.org/docs/69503/Narrative/. Published 2008. Updated 2015. Accessed July 1, 2020.
2. Rialon KL, Wolf S, Routh JC, et al. Diagnostic evaluation of ovarian torsion: An analysis of pediatric patients using the Nationwide Emergency Department Sample. *Am J Surg.* 2017; 213(4):637-639.

3. Sintim-Damoa A, Majmudar AS, Cohen HL, et al. Pediatric ovarian torsion: spectrum of imaging findings. *Radiographics.* 2017;37(6):1892-1908.

4. Rha SE, Byun JY, Jung SE, et al. CT and MR imaging features of adnexal torsion. *Radiographics.* 2002;22(2):2832-2894.

5. Deslandes A, Pannucio C, Parasivam S, et al. How to perform a gynaecological ultrasound in the paediatric or adolescent patient. *AJUM.* 2020;23(1):10-21.

6. Childress KJ, Dietrich JE. Pediatric ovarian torsion. *Surg Clin North Am.* 2017;97(1):209-221.

7. Lourenco AP, Swenson D, Tubbs RJ, et al. Ovarian and tubal torsion: imaging findings on US, CT, and MRI. *Emerg Radiol.* 2014;21(2):179-187.

8. Grunau GL, Harris A, Buckley J, et al. Diagnosis of ovarian torsion: is it time to forget about Doppler? *J Obstet Gynaecol Can.* 2018;40(7):871-875.

9. Oltmann SC, Fischer A, Barber R, et al. Cannot exclude torsion—a 15-year review. *J Pediatr Surg.* 2009;44(6):1212-1216.

10. Chang HC, Bhatt S, Dogra VS. Pearls and pitfalls in diagnosis of ovarian torsion. *Radiographics.* 2008;28(5):1355-1368.

11. Wilkinson C, Sanderson A. Adnexal torsion—a multimodality imaging review. *Clin Radiol.* 2012;67(5):476-483.

12. Mashiach R, Melamed N, Gilad N, et al. Sonographic diagnosis of ovarian torsion accuracy and predictive factors. *J Ultrasound Med.* 2011;30(9):1205-1210.

13. Robertson JJ, Long B, Koyfman A. Myths in the evaluation and management of ovarian torsion. *J Emerg Med.* 2017;52(4):449-456.

14. Shadinger LL, Andreotti RF, Kurian RL, et al. Pre-operative sonographic and clinical characteristics as predictors of ovarian torsion. *J Ultrasound Med.* 2008;27(1):7-13.

15. Sheth R, Hoelzer D, Scattergood E, et al. In utero fetal ovarian torsion with imaging findings on ultrasound and MRI. *Case Rep Radiol.* 2012;2012:151020.

16. Nizar K, Deutsch M, Filmer S, et al. Doppler studies of the ovarian venous blood flow in the diagnosis of adnexal torsion. *J Clin Ultrasound.* 2009;37(8):436-439.

17. Schmahmann S, Haller JO. Neonatal ovarian cysts: pathogenesis, diagnosis and management. *Pediatr Radiol.* 1997;27(2):101-105.

18. Dhanda S, Quek ST, Ting MY, et al. CT features in surgically proven cases of ovarian torsion-a pictorial review. *Br J Radiol.* 2017;90(1078):20170052.

19. Moore C, Meyers AB, Capotasto J, et al. Prevalence of abnormal CT findings in patients with proven ovarian torsion and a proposed triage schema. *Emerg Radiol.* 2009;16(2):115-120.

20. Lam A, Nayyar M, Helmy M, et al. Assessing the clinical utility of color Doppler ultrasound for ovarian torsion in the setting of a negative contrast-enhanced CT scan of the abdomen and pelvis. *Abdom Imaging.* 2015;40(8):3206-3213.

21. Swenson DW, Lourenco AP, Beaudoin FL, et al. Ovarian torsion: case-control study comparing the sensitivity and specificity of ultrasonography and computed tomography for diagnosis in the emergency department. *Eur J Radiol.* 2014;83(4):733-738.

22. Rey-Bellet Gasser C, Gehri M, Joseph JM, et al. Is it ovarian torsion? A systematic literature review and evaluation of prediction signs. *Pediatr Emerg Care.* 2016;32(4):256-261.

23. Guthie B, Adler MD, Powell EC. Incidence and trends of pediatric ovarian torsion hospitalizations in the United States, 2000–2006. *Pediatrics.* 2010;125(3):532-538.

24. Asfour V, Varma R, Menon P. Clinical risk factors for ovarian torsion. *J Obstet Gynaecol.* 2015;35(7):721-725.

25. Ghandehari H, Kahn D, Tomlinson G, et al. Ovarian Torsion: Time Limiting Factors for Ovarian Salvage. *Emergency Medicine: Open Access (Los Angel).* 2015;5(5).

24 All Pain and No Gain: Renal Stones

ROBERT VEZZETTI, MD, FAAP, FACEP

Case Presentation

An 11-year-old male presents with acute onset of left-sided lower abdominal pain and left-sided flank pain, which began 1–2 hours prior to presentation. The patient was not engaged in any particular activity; he states that he was "just relaxing" when the pain began. He denies trauma. There has been no fever, back pain, dysuria, hematuria, testicular pain/swelling, or other abdominal pain. While he has not had vomiting, he does report nausea.

The patient appears uncomfortable on physical examination but is not toxic. His vital signs show a temperature of 98 degrees Fahrenheit, a heart rate of 100 beats per minute, a respiratory rate of 22 breaths per minute, a blood pressure of 108/58 mm Hg, and a room air oxygen reading of 100%. His physical examination is unremarkable. He has no abdominal tenderness, rebound, or guarding; there is no costovertebral angle tenderness. The thoracic and lumbar spine exams are normal. His genital examination reveals Tanner stage II; there is no scrotal edema, erythema, or tenderness. He is circumcised. The inguinal area has no obvious masses and there is no tenderness.

Imaging Considerations

Imaging is useful to determine not only the presence of nephrolithiasis but also associated complications, such as ureteral obstruction and hydronephrosis. The primary imaging modalities utilized during the evaluation of a pediatric patient with suspected nephrolithiasis are generally available, including ultrasound and computed tomography (CT).

PLAIN RADIOGRAPHY

Plain radiography can detect radiopaque stones but has low sensitivity and specificity (62% and 67%, respectively).[1] One study found plain radiography (a kidney-ureter-bladder image, or KUB) to be of limited value as a sole imaging modality for small renal stones, stones detected by KUB were mostly detected by ultrasound (US), and adding KUB to US did not improve the detection rate.[2] Guidelines exist suggesting the use of a combination of US and plain radiography for following diagnosed renal stones,[3,4] but this remains somewhat controversial and is best left to the discretion of a consulting pediatric urologist. As a rule, plain radiography has little use in the acute detection and management of renal stones and is not typically utilized.

ULTRASOUND

US is the imaging modality of choice in pediatric patients with suspected nephrolithiasis, and the technology has improved over the past 10 years.[5,6] The lack of ionizing radiation and the general availability of this technique are attractive attributes. US is not as sensitive or specific for nephrolithiasis when compared to CT,[6–9] with previous studies demonstrating a sensitivity of approximately 30%–50% compared to noncontrast CT.[10,11] Recent studies have found US to have a sensitivity and specificity of 70% and 100%, respectively, with the ability to detect clinically significant stones.[6,7,9] Another study demonstrated a sensitivity of 67% with a high specificity (97%) compared with noncontrast CT,[12] which is consistent with previously recently published literature. Notably, US has been shown to have a high detection rate (90%) for renal stones but a low rate (38%) for ureteral stones.[1,8]

COMPUTED TOMOGRAPHY

CT is considered the gold standard for the detection of nephrolithiasis, with near 100% sensitivity and specificity.[1,3,5–7] While this study is generally rapid and intravenous (IV) contrast is not needed, exposure of the pediatric patient to ionizing radiation is a concern. One study of nearly 8000 children found that, on average, pediatric patients received two CT scans for a single nephrolithiasis episode.[13] In another study, CT use was noted to have increased and linked to various patient demographic factors (age, race, and insurance status), as well as strongly linked to the treating hospital, which was the single strongest factor.[13] Due to improvement in US technology and techniques, CT can be used as a second-line study in patients with a high clinical and historical suspicion for nephrolithiasis but in whom US is nondiagnostic.[3,4,6,7]

In an effort to reduce ionizing radiation exposure, professional societies have developed imaging recommendations: the American Urological Association (2012) and the European Association of Urology (2013) have both recommended ultrasonography as the first-line imaging modality in pediatric patients, with CT reserved for patients with equivocal US findings or negative US findings in the setting of a strong clinical suspicion for a renal stone.[3,4,6,7,14] These recommendations are in keeping with the Society for Pediatric Radiology, the American College of Radiology, and the American Society of Radiologic Technologists Image Gently campaign to reduce ionizing exposure for pediatric patients.[14]

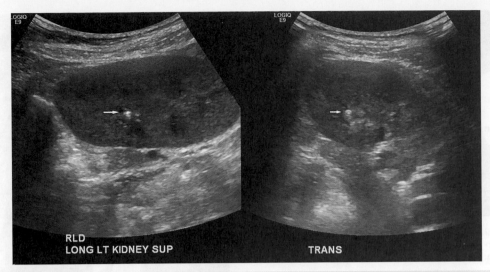

Fig. 24.1 Longitudinal and transverse ultrasound images of the left kidney demonstrate echogenic renal calculi *(arrows)*.

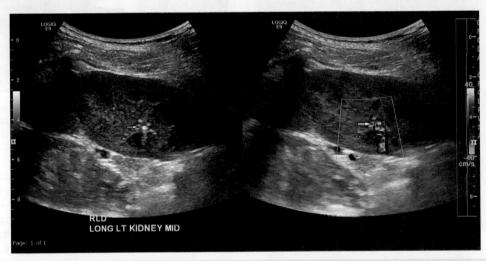

Fig. 24.2 Longitudinal images of the left kidney demonstrating an echogenic renal calculus and an associated "twinkle" sign on color Doppler imaging *(arrows)*. A "twinkle" sign, a focus of alternating colors at rough acoustic interfaces, can increase the conspicuity of calculi on sonography but is not a specific sign for calculus.

Imaging Findings

This patient underwent renal US. The right kidney is normal in size and echotexture, with normal corticomedullary differentiation, normal renal cortical thickness; the left kidney is normal in size and echotexture, with normal corticomedullary differentiation, normal renal cortical thickness (Figs. 24.1–24.3). There is a 3-mm stone located in the upper pole of the left kidney and a 4-mm stone in the midportion of the kidney.

For comparison, another case is presented here. This child presented with right flank pain radiating to the right upper quadrant along with nonbilious, nonbloody emesis and nausea. An initial US did not demonstrate a renal stone, and due to clinical suspicion, a noncontrast CT scan was obtained. CT revealed a 2-mm stone in the distal right ureter, adjacent to the right ureterovesicle junction. The right ureter is mildly dilated with mild right hydronephrosis (Figs. 24.4–24.6).

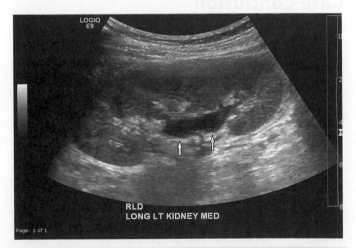

Fig. 24.3 Longitudinal ultrasound image shows normal size, echotexture, and cortical thickness of the left kidney, with mild dilatation of the left renal pelvis *(arrows)*.

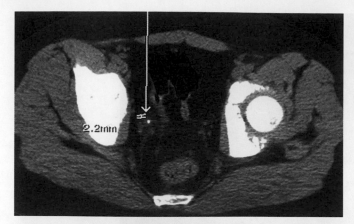

Fig. 24.4 Axial unenhanced computed tomography image of the pelvis shows a two-mm stone in the distal right ureter, adjacent to the right ureterovesicular junction.

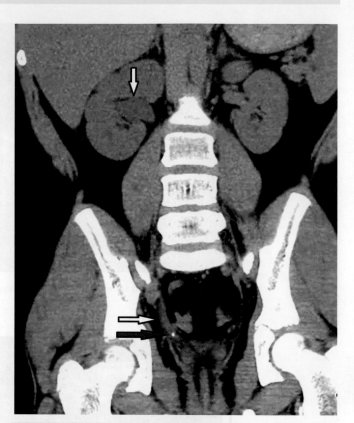

Fig. 24.6 Coronal computed tomography image demonstrates the distal right ureteral stone *(red arrow)* and dilatation of the right renal pelvis and distal right ureter *(arrows)*.

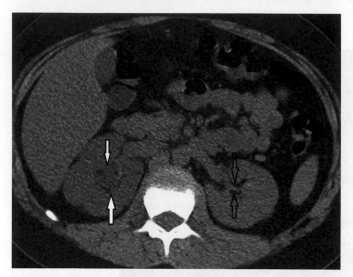

Fig. 24.5 Axial unenhanced computed tomography image demonstrating mild dilatation of the right renal pelvis *(arrows)*. Note comparison to the normal, nondilated left renal pelvis *(open arrows)*.

Case Conclusion

The child was given IV fluids, IV odansetron, and pain control with IV ketorolac. This resulted in resolution of the child's pain. A urinalysis showed large blood with 11–20 red blood cells per high-powered field but was otherwise normal. Pediatric Urology was consulted and they recommended continued hydration and pain control. Since the child responded well to initial therapy and was tolerating oral fluids, he was discharged with close observation and follow-up.

Pediatric nephrolithiasis has been increasing over the past years, 6%–10% annually[1,5,6,15] with an incidence of 50 per 100,000 adolescents.[5] The majority of calculi are composed of calcium oxalate.[6,7,16] Several associations have been made with increased nephrolithiasis, including sex, socioeconomic status, race, geographic factors, and diet/fluid intake.[1,5,6,15] One study has proposed that obesity may be a risk factor for stone development, since there is an association with lower urine pH, increased urinary oxalate, uric acid, and sodium and phosphate excretion,[5,17] although

this theory has not been universally accepted.[5,18] The presentation of nephrolithiasis in children varies among age groups. Older children and adolescents often complain of abdominal or flank pain, whereas younger children often have more nonspecific symptoms, including vague abdominal pain, vomiting, and nausea. Notably, hematuria is not common.[5] Infants are more likely to present with irritability and vomiting.[5,19]

Medical management is predicated on the likelihood that a stone will pass on its own. While it does appear that the size and location of the stone are factors associated with spontaneous passage, there has been little investigation into which factors are most likely to allow a stone to spontaneously pass, including stone size. For example, studies have stated that stones smaller than 10 mm and located in the distal ureter are thought likely to pass,[7,20] whereas other studies have asserted a size less than 4 mm as a reasonable size to allow passage without intervention.[1,21] However, studies have demonstrated that the overall likelihood of stone passage is quite good.[5,20,22] There have been few pediatric studies on the use of medical therapy for nephrolithiasis management, but there have been several studies evaluating the effectiveness of tamsulosin for medical management, demonstrating that tamusulosin had some effectiveness in promoting stone passage.[19,23] Medical therapy is most likely to be effective in stones that are smaller or distally located.[3,24,25] Younger children are more likely to present with renal stones, whereas older children had more ureteral stones; younger children are more likely to pass stones and have successful medical management.[26]

Stones that are unlikely to pass with observation or medical therapy or stones that cause obstruction and are unlikely to pass warrant surgical intervention. Surgical options include urinary decompression, uteroscopy, and extracorporeal shock-wave lithrotripsy (ESWL). ESWL is particularly attractive, given the noninvasiveness of this technique and high stone free rate (between 70% and 100%,[3,5,27] with other studies quoting a lower rate of 59% to 80%[1,28]), and has become the procedure of choice for pediatric patients. Children with a previous urologic history have a lower ESWL success rate of around 15%.[1,29] Another advantage of ESWL is the ability to perform this procedure on a variety of stone types. There are associated complications, including hematuria and even renal scarring, but these are self-limiting.[1,5,27]

Stone recurrence is less common in pediatric patients than in the adult population. Reported recurrence is approximately 16%,[7,24] with some studies reporting rates as high as 50%.[1,30] Hypercalciuria is a known risk factor for stone recurrence.[31]

IMAGING PEARLS

1. Plain radiography is of limited use in the acute evaluation of pediatric patients with suspected renal stones. There may be a role for plain radiography combined with ultrasonography in continued evaluation of children with known renal stones.
2. Renal ultrasonography is the diagnostic imaging modality of choice in pediatric patients with suspected renal stones.
3. Noncontrast CT should be reserved for patients with a high clinical suspicion for renal stones but in whom US is nondiagnostic.

References

1. Schissel BL, Johnson BK. Renal stones: evolving epidemiology and management. *Pediatr Emerg Care.* 2011;27(7):676-681.
2. Kanno T, Kubota M, Funada S, et al. The utility of the kidneys-ureters-bladder radiograph as the sole imaging modality and its combination with ultrasonography for the detection of renal stones. *Urology.* 2017;104:40-44.
3. Fulgham PF, Assimos DG, Pearle MS, et al. Clinical effectiveness protocols for imaging in the management of ureteral calculous disease: AUA technology assessment. *J Urol.* 2012;189:1203.
4. Grivas N, Thomas K, Drake T, et al. Imaging modalities and treatment of paediatric upper tract urolithiasis: A systematic review and update on behalf of the EAU urolithiasis guidelines panel. *J Pediatr Urol.* 2020;4:S1477-5131.
5. Miah T, Kamat D. Pediatric nephrolithiasis: a review. *Pediatr Ann.* 2017;46(6):e242-e244.
6. Morrison JC, Kawal T, Van Batavia JP, et al. Use of ultrasound in pediatric renal stone diagnosis and surgery. *Curr Urol Rep.* 2017;18(3):22.
7. Tasian GE, Copelovitch L. Evaluation and medical management of kidney stones in children. *J Urol.* 2014;192(5):1329-1336.
8. Palmer JS, Donaher ER, O'Riordan MA, et al. Diagnosis of pediatric urolithiasis: role of ultrasound and computerized tomography. *J Urol.* 2005;174(4 pt 1):1413-1416.
9. Passerotti C, Chow JS, Silva A, et al. Ultrasound versus computerized tomography for evaluating urolithiasis. *J Urol.* 2009;182(suppl 4):1829-1834.
10. Fowler KA, Locken JA, Duchesne JH, et al. US for detecting renal calculi with nonenhanced CT as a reference standard. *Radiology.* 2002;222(1):109-113.
11. Ulusan S, Koc Z, Tokmak N. Accuracy of sonography for detecting renal stone: comparison with CT. *J Clin Ultrasound.* 2007;35(5):256-261.
12. Roberson NP, Dillman JR, O'Hara SM, et al. Comparison of ultrasound versus computed tomography for the detection of kidney stones in the pediatric population: a clinical effectiveness study. *Pediatr Radiol.* 2018;48(7):962-972.
13. Routh JC, Graham DA, Nelson CP. Trends in imaging and surgical management of pediatric urolithiasis at American pediatric hospitals. *J Urol.* 2010;184 (suppl 4):1816.
14. Goske MJ, Applegate KE, Boylan J, et al. The Image Gently campaign: working together to change practice. *AJR Am J Roentgenol.* 2008;190(2):273-264.
15. Tasian GE, Ross ME, Song L, et al. Annual incidence of nephrolithiasis among children and adults in South Carolina from 1997 to 2012. *Clin. J Am Soc Nephrol.* 2016;11(3):488-496.
16. Sternberg K, Greenfield SP, Williot P, et al. Pediatric stone disease: an evolving experience. *J Urol.* 2005;174:1711-1714.
17. Kovesdy CP, Furth SL, Zoccali C; World Kidney Day Steering Committee. Obesity and kidney disease: hidden consequences of the epidemic. *Kidney Int.* 2017;91(2):260-262.
18. Van Dervoort K, Wiesen J, Frank R, et al. Urolithiasis in pediatric patients: a single center study of incidence, clinical presentation and outcome. *J Urol.* 2007;177(6):2300-2305.
19. Tasian GE, Cost NG, Granberg CF, et al. Tamsulosin and the spontaneous passage of ureteral stones in children: a multi-institutional cohort study. *J Urol.* 2014;192(2):506-511.
20. Mokhless I, Zahran AR, Youssif M, et al. Factors that predict the spontaneous passage of ureteric stones in children. *Arab J Urol.* 2012;10(4):402-407.
21. Van Savage JG, Palanca LG, Andersen RD, et al. Treatment of distal ureteral stones in children: similarities to the American Urological Association guidelines in adults. *J Urol.* 2000;164 (3 pt 2):1089-1093.
22. van Batavia JP, Tasian GE. Clinical effectiveness in the diagnosis and acute management of pediatric nephrolithiasis. *Int J Surg.* 2016;36(Pt D):698-704.
23. Mokhless I, Zahran AR, Youssif M, et al. Tamsulosin for the management of distal ureteral stones in children: a prospective randomized study. *J Pediatr Urol.* 2012;8(5):544-548.
24. Pietrow PK, Pope JC IV, Adams MC, et al. Clinical outcome of pediatric stone disease. *J Urol.* 2002;167(2 pt 1):670-673.
25. Velazquez N, Zapata D, Wang HH, et al. Medical expulsive therapy for pediatric urolithiasis: systemic review and meta-analysis. *J Pediatr Urol.* 2015;11(6):321-327.
26. Kalorin CM, Zabinski A, Okpareke I, et al. Pediatric urinary stone disease—does age matter? *J Urol.* 2009;181(5):2267-2271.
27. Yucel S, Akin Y, Danisman A, et al. Complications and associated factors of pediatric extracorporeal shock wave lithotripsy. *J Urol.* 2012;187(5):1812-1816.
28. D'Addessi A, Bongiovanni L, Sasso F, et al. Extracorporeal shockwave lithotripsy in pediatrics. *J Endourol.* 2008;22(1):1-12.
29. Mandeville JA, Nelson CP. Pediatric urolithiasis. *Curr Opin Urol.* 2009;19(4):419-423.
30. Tasian GE, Kabarriti AE, Kalmus A, et al. Kidney stone recurrence among children and adolescents. *J Urol.* 2017;197(1):246-252.
31. Srivastava T, Alon US. Urolithiasis in adolescent children. *Adolesc Med Clin.* 2005;16(1):87-109.

25 *Belly Getting Bigger? Wilms Tumor*

ROBERT VEZZETTI, MD, FAAP, FACEP

Case Presentation

A 14-month-old female is referred from her primary care pediatrician for increasing abdominal girth and an abdominal mass. For the past month, the child's abdomen has been increasing in size, as noted by her parents. There has been no associated fever, vomiting, diarrhea, trauma, back pain, urinary complaints, difficulty breathing, or cough. She is otherwise behaving at her baseline.

Physical examination reveals a well-appearing child in no distress. Her vital signs are unremarkable and appropriate for her age. She has a remarkable abdominal examination: There is obvious abdominal distention and a palpable right flank mass. There is no tenderness, guarding, or rebound.

Imaging Considerations

ULTRASOUND (US)

This imaging modality is a first-line imaging choice in pediatric patients suspected of having an intraabdominal mass.[1,2] The study is generally readily available and requires no sedation to complete. Additionally, there is no exposure to ionizing radiation and US can differentiate between abdominal masses and other causes of mass effect such as hydronephrosis, distended bowel, or a distended urinary bladder. These attributes make ultrasonography an excellent screening modality. Wilms tumor usually appears as a well-defined mass arising from the kidney; however, when the mass is very large, the site of origin can be difficult to determine. Doppler flow studies should also be obtained at the time of imaging, since Wilms tumor can invade the renal vein, the inferior vena cava, or, rarely, the right atrium (termed intracardiac Wilms tumor).[1]

PLAIN RADIOGRAPHY

Plain radiography may initially be used in patients with abdominal distention. Findings may be nonspecific and masses may or may not be visualized. As a general rule, plain radiography of the abdomen is not useful for abdominal mass detection per se but will provide a view of the bowel gas pattern, may detect calcifications, and may demonstrate mass effect if an intraabdominal tumor is present, prompting additional imaging with US or computed tomography (CT).

If an abdominal mass suspicious for Wilms tumor is found on imaging, chest x-ray may be utilized as the lungs are a primary site of metastasis for this tumor.[1-4]

COMPUTED TOMOGRAPHY

CT is an excellent imaging modality used to evaluate intraabdominal pathology. While readily available and rapid, the patient is exposed to ionizing radiation. Intravenous contrast should be utilized. CT of the abdomen and pelvis should be obtained if ultrasonography demonstrates a renal mass; if Wilms tumor is suspected, additional CT of the chest may be obtained, since the lung is a common site of metastases for this lesion, with up to 15% of patients having lung involvement at the time of diagnosis.[1-4] CT of the chest may also be utilized if plain chest radiography is abnormal.[1,2,4] Wilms tumor is visualized as a solid mass arising from the kidney, with renal parenchyma splayed around the border with the mass (the "claw sign"); calcifications within the tumor are possible, but not commonly seen. Once treatment is completed, CT is used to monitor for recurrence.[5]

The decision to utilize plain radiography or CT for chest imaging may be determined after consultation with Pediatric Oncology and/or Pediatric Surgery.

MAGNETIC RESONANCE IMAGING (MRI)

This imaging modality, like CT, is utilized as a secondary test when US is abnormal. Like CT, MRI provides visualization of the contralateral kidney and intraabdominal contents. However, availability may be a barrier and sedation is generally required to complete a meaningful study. MRI is often utilized as a surveillance imaging modality.

Imaging Findings

The CT study (with intravenous contrast) obtained by the primary care provider was reviewed. Selected images are provided here. There is a large renal mass, which is solid in appearance; the remaining intraabdominal organs appear normal (Figs. 25.1–25.3).

Case Conclusion

The patient was admitted to the hospital; Pediatric Surgery and Pediatric Oncology were consulted. CT of the chest was obtained, which demonstrated no pulmonary involvement. The child underwent right nephrectomy and tumor removal. Pathology confirmed Wilms tumor with favorable histology, and intraabdominal lymph node biopsies were negative for disease. The patient completed a course of chemotherapy appropriate for the disease

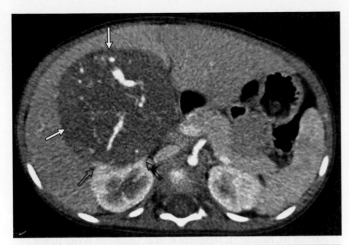

Fig. 25.1 Axial intravenous contrast-enhanced computed tomography image demonstrating a large right-sided abdominal mass *(white arrows)*. Enhancing right renal parenchyma is splayed around the posterior edge of the mass (the "claw sign," denoted by *open arrows*), confirming renal origin of the mass.

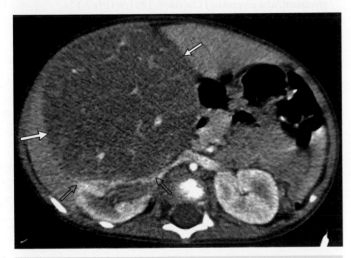

Fig. 25.2 Axial intravenous contrast-enhanced computed tomography image demonstrates a large right sided abdominal mass *(white arrows)*. Enhancing right renal parenchyma is splayed around the posterior edge of the mass (the "claw sign," denoted by *open arrows*), confirming renal origin of the mass.

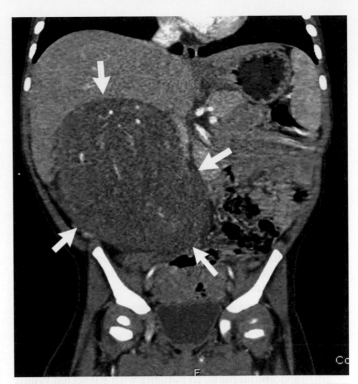

Fig. 25.3 Coronal intravenous contrast-enhanced computed tomography image demonstrates a large right-sided abdominal mass *(white arrows)* consistent with a Wilms tumor.

extent and histology. Subsequent surveillance revealed no recurrence of disease.

Pediatric nephroblastoma is also known by its more common name, Wilms tumor. This lesion is named for Max Wilms (1867–1918), a pathologist and surgeon who extensively studied this tumor.[1]

Wilms tumor represents 5% of pediatric neoplasms, with an equal distribution between males and females and a mean age at presentation of between 2 and 3 years of age.[1,6] While most cases are spontaneous, there is a familial variety, which usually presents at a younger age and is due to an inherited genomic mutation.[1] The most common presentation of Wilms tumor is that of an asymptomatic abdominal mass, although hematuria or hypertension may be present.[1,4,6] Wilms tumor can be associated with genetic syndromes and conditions, including WAGR (Wilms tumor, aniridia, genitourinary anomalies, and developmental retardation); the genitourinary anomalies seen include hypospadias and cryptorchidism.[1,4,6] Aniridia, which is not common in the general population, may be seen.[1] Aniridia in a pediatric patient should prompt the clinician to recommend sonographic screening for Wilms tumor, which should be obtained until 9 years of age, since Wilms tumor is commonly not encountered after this age.[1] Wilms tumor may also be seen in patients with Beckwith-Wiedemann syndrome and hemihypertrophy of the extremities. Patients with these conditions should undergo routine screening for Wilms tumor.

Wilms tumor may spread to the abdominal lymph nodes; lung and liver metastases are also common sites.[1] Wilms tumor typically involves one kidney. However, 5% of patients will have bilateral disease or will develop another lesion in the contralateral kidney at some point in time; 7% may present with more than one primary kidney tumor; this is usually seen in patients with the familial variety of the disease.[1]

Management of Wilms tumor requires a multidisciplinary approach. Consultation with Pediatric Surgery and/or Pediatric Urology, as well as Pediatric Oncology is required. Unilateral Wilms tumor is managed with resection; depending on the size of the tumor, chemotherapy may be initiated prior to resection, but this is not routinely recommended in the United States, since pretreatment with chemotherapy may alter histologic studies and potentially impact staging as well as prognosis.[1,6] The decision to use chemotherapy prior to surgery is made on an individual basis.[1,4] Biopsies of regional lymph nodes, suspicious hepatic nodules, and pulmonary nodules that do not look typical for Wilms tumor are usually performed.[1]

Staging of Wilms tumor is based on radiographic and surgical findings[1,4]:

Stage I (37% of tumors)—limited to the kidney

Stage II (20% of tumors)—extend beyond the renal capsule or into the renal sinus

Stage III (20% of tumors)—residual abdominal disease following resection

Stage IV (23% of tumors)—pulmonary or hepatic metastasis

Stage V (7%-13% of tumors)—bilateral tumors

Chemotherapy is based on histological grade as well as tumor metastasis, with a variety of treatment protocols available.[1,4] Abdominal radiotherapy tends to be avoided out of concerns for the long-term effects that this may have on the remaining kidney's function and is usually reserved for patients with unresectable disease.[5] Factors that suggest a good prognosis include initial tumor stage I or II, treatment with vincristine and dactinomycin only, no prior radiotherapy, and favorable histology.[4,7]

IMAGING PEARLS

1. Plain radiography may be initially used in patients with abdominal distention to evaluate the bowel gas pattern and may demonstrate signs suspicious for an intraabdominal mass. In patients with suspected Wilms tumor, chest radiography may be obtained but often is deferred in favor of CT.

2. Ultrasonography is a first-line imaging modality in patients with suspected intraabdominal masses.

3. Intravenous contrast-enhanced CT of the abdomen is the imaging modality of choice to follow up abnormal abdominal US findings. If Wilms tumor is suspected, CT of the chest is often employed, since the lungs are a primary site of metastasis for this tumor.

4. MRI may be employed as a second-line imaging modality in patients with abnormal abdominal US.

References

1. Friedman AD. Wilms tumor. *Pediatr Rev*. 2013;34(7):328-330.
2. Aldrink JH, Heaton TE, Dasgupta R, et al. Update on Wilms tumor. *J Pediatr Surg*. 2019;54(3):390-397.
3. Ehrlich PF. Wilms tumor: progress to date and future considerations. *Expert Rev Anticancer Ther*. 2001;1(4):555-564.
4. Sonn G, Shortliffe LM. Management of Wilms tumor: current standard of care. *Nat Clin Pract Urol*. 2008;5(10):551-560.
5. Coppes MJ, Wilson PC, Weitzman S. Extrarenal Wilms' tumor: staging, treatment, and prognosis. *J Clin Oncol*. 1991;9(1):167-174.
6. Aune GJ. Wilms tumor. *Pediatr Rev*. 2008;29(4):142-143.
7. Kalapurakal JA, Dome JS, Perlman EJ, et al. Management of Wilms' tumour: current practice and future goals. *Lancet Oncol*. 2004; 5(1):37-46.

26 TOA (Tubo-ovarian Abscess): Three Letters You Don't Want to Hear

ROBERT VEZZETTI, MD, FAAP, FACEP

Case Presentation

An 11-year-old female presents with severe right-sided abdominal pain that began 5 days ago. The patient reports that she was in her usual state of good health until she experienced the pain, which initially seemed generalized, intermittent, and achy but has become more constant, sharp, and now is located primarily in the right lower quadrant. She developed a fever to 102 degrees Fahrenheit 2 days ago. She reports nausea but no emesis, diarrhea, hematuria, or trauma; she endorses dysuria. She also states that she had right flank pain several days ago, which has now resolved. She is generally healthy but does have a history of frequent urinary tract infections and at the age of 2 years had ureteral reimplant surgery on the right side for vesicoureteral reflux. She began her menses several months ago, but this has been somewhat irregular and occasionally associated with bilateral lower quadrant pain.

Examination reveals a visibly uncomfortable child who complains of right lower quadrant pain. She is afebrile, has a heart rate of 118 beats per minute, a respiratory rate of 20 breaths per minute, and a blood pressure of 120/80 mm Hg. She has focal right lower quadrant pain to palpation, with moderate guarding and rebound. There is no costovertebral tenderness. There are no signs of trauma.

Laboratory values demonstrate a total peripheral white blood cell (WBC) count of 11,000 cc/mm, a C-reactive protein level of 2.4 mg/dL, and a urinalysis with + nitrite, 1+ leukocyte esterase, few WBCs, and few bacteria.

Imaging Considerations

Since the diagnosis of tubo-ovarian abscess (TOA) requires the presence of an inflammatory mass,[1] imaging is usually employed.

PLAIN RADIOGRAPHY

Plain radiography may be employed as an imaging modality during the evaluation of abdominal pain but is not helpful in identifying TOA.

ULTRASOUND (US)

US is often employed as a first-line imaging modality in adolescent patients with abdominal pain.[2,3] The general availability, rapidity of the study, and lack of ionizing radiation make this an attractive means to evaluate reproductive organs. US is useful in detecting ovarian pathology (torsion, cysts, masses) and pregnancy, both intrauterine and ectopic.

Transvaginal US is the imaging modality of choice when a TOA is suspected (or transabdominal US with a full bladder).[3] In one study, 89% of patients with suspected ovarian pathology had imaging studies performed, and of these, 97% were pelvic US.[3] A TOA appears as a complex multilocular cystic mass with thick irregular walls, partitions, and internal echoes.[1,4–6] The sensitivity of transvaginal and transabdominal US for the diagnosis of TOA has been reported to be 75% and 83%, respectively.[7]

COMPUTED TOMOGRAPHY (CT)

This modality is often employed when there is suspicion for complex disease or an alternative diagnosis is under consideration, such as appendicitis or an inflammatory bowel process. CT may have an advantage over US in the visualization of a TOA. Compared to US, CT may have increased sensitivity to detect a TOA (78% to 100% vs. 75% to 82%, respectively) and improved specificity (100% to 91%).[1,8] Frequent findings of a TOA on CT include unilateral location (73%), multilocularity (89%), and thick, uniform, enhancing walls; less common findings included bowel thickening (59%), uterosacral ligament thickening (64%), and pyosalpinx (50%).[1,9,10] A TOA appears on CT imaging as a multilocular, septate, cystic mass surrounded by a thick enhancing wall.[11] CT, though, requires the use of intravenous (IV) contrast material and exposes the patient to ionizing radiation.

MAGNETIC RESONANCE IMAGING (MRI)

MRI can detect TOA. The abscess appears as a uni- or multilocular adnexal mass with thick and intensely enhancing walls, with low signal intensity on T1-weighted images and heterogeneous high signal intensity on T2-weighted images, although this may vary depending on the protein content of the abscess.[10–12] Thick walls, multiple internal septa, and lymphadenopathy may also be seen.[13] This modality is typically not employed as a first-line imaging modality in patients with suspected TOA but may be utilized if there is concern for a more complex infection or underlying genitourinary anatomic abnormalities.

Imaging Findings

Initially, a limited abdominal US of the right lower quadrant was obtained to look for appendicitis. The appendix was identified and was normal. Because the patient has started her menstrual cycles and due to the previous report of right lower quadrant pain associated with these cycles, a pelvic US was obtained (transabdominal with a full bladder); there are several images presented here. The right ovarian borders are difficult to visualize, but there is a complex 7.1 × 6.3 × 6.0-cm mass-like structure in the right adnexa, containing the ovary, with a peripherally positioned dilated fluid-filled tubular structure. The left ovary measures 3.9 × 2.4 × 2.5 cm. Color-flow with spectral Doppler analysis shows normal arterial and venous blood flow to both ovaries (Figs. 26.1–26.3). Although the findings are not specific, the right ovary does not appear normal and differential considerations include an ovarian torsion (arterial flow on Doppler examination of an ovary does not exclude ovarian torsion) or an infectious process.

Case Conclusion

Pediatric Surgery was consulted to evaluate the patient in the emergency department. The decision was made to obtain an IV contrast-enhanced CT scan, since the history, physical examination, and US results were not specific and better visualization of the ovary and surrounding structures was desired. Select images from this study are presented here. These images demonstrate that the right ovary is large, with ill-defined borders, with a large dilated tubular structure around the right ovary, and surrounding edema is also seen (Fig. 26.4 and 26.5).

The patient was taken to the operating suite, where a right TOA was identified and drained. Cultures from this abscess

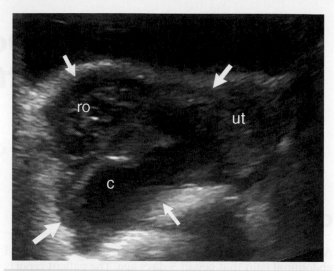

Fig. 26.2 Transverse ultrasound image shows a large complex cystic and solid mass in the right adnexa *(white arrows)*, containing the right ovary *(ro)*. The posterior cystic structure *(c)* is seen to be an elongated, tubular, fluid-filled structure along the periphery, consistent with a dilated fallopian tube. The uterus is seen *(ut)*.

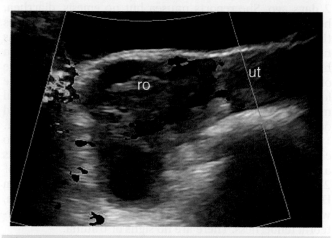

Fig. 26.3 Transverse color Doppler imaging shows color flow in the ovarian structure in the right adnexa. *ro*, Right ovary; *ut*, uterus.

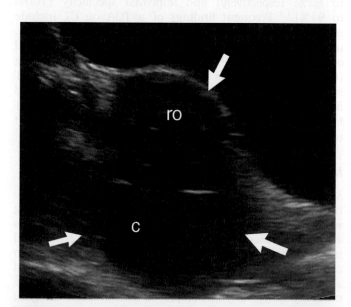

Fig. 26.1 Longitudinal transabdominal ultrasound image shows a large complex cystic and solid mass *(white arrows)* in the right adnexa, containing the right ovary *(ro)*, but ovarian borders cannot be defined and there is a cystic focus posteriorly *(c)*.

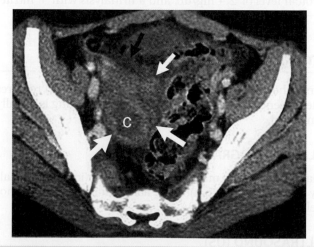

Fig. 26.4 Axial contrast-enhanced computed tomography image demonstrates the complex cystic and solid mass of the right adnexa *(white arrows)* and low-density fluid seen adjacent to the mass *(black arrow)*. *c*, cystic fluid collection.

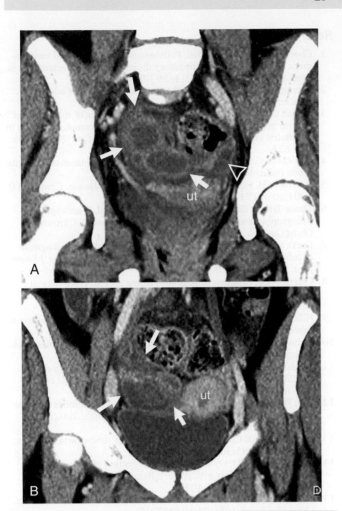

Fig. 26.5 Coronal contrast-enhanced computed tomography images show the complex cystic and solid mass of the right adnexa *(white arrows)* (A, B) and the normal left ovary is seen *(arrowhead,* A). The uterus *(ut)* is seen as well.

A TOA is the result of infection of the upper genital tract and may result in irreversible damage to the fallopian tubes and ovaries and may lead to infertility.[1,15] Sexually active patients present the highest risk group for PID and TOA development.[14] PID is any combination of endometritis, salpingitis, TOA, and pelvic peritonitis.[1,16,17] While *N. gonorrhoeae* and *C. trachomatis* are commonly implicated in PID, these organisms may not be as common as previously thought, with less than 50% of patients diagnosed with PID testing positive for these organisms. A wide variety of other microorganisms (*Escherichia coli, Bacteriodes fragilis, Bacteriodes* species, *Peptostreptococcus, Peptococcus,* and aerobic streptococcus) are now implicated both in PID and TOA.[1,16–18]

TOA is often considered the end result of PID, but the literature has reported that only up to one-half of patients with TOA have had PID.[14] Nevertheless, PID is a risk factor for the development of a TOA, and up to one-third of patients with PID develop an abscess.[1,4,15,19,20] The rate of TOA in the context of adolescent patients with PID has been decreasing, possibly due to better adherence to and implementation of the Centers for Disease Control and Prevention diagnostic and treatment guidelines for PID, which in 2002 were broadened.[3] An abscess will form due to an untreated infection, producing an inflammatory process that extends from the fallopian tube to the ovary.[1,4,15] Perfusion to the inner portion of the abscess is compromised, creating an environment for both aerobic and anaerobic organisms to grow. The microbiology associated with PID and TOA is often polymicrobial.[1,21]

There are literature reports of TOA in non–sexually active adolescent patients, highlighting an important point that TOAs are not exclusive to sexually active patients. The literature investigating this population has found that the majority of non–sexually active patients with TOA have associated comorbidities, such as ascending infection secondary to urinary tract infection, bacterial translocation from the gastrointestinal tract (e.g., due to Crohn disease or appendicitis), previous pelvic surgery, congenital genitourinary anomalies, or bloodborne infections.[19,22,23] TOA has also mimicked ovarian masses that were initially thought to be tumors.[20]

PID caused by *N. gonorrhea* and *C. trachomatis* is associated with heavy or irregular vaginal bleeding.[14] However, patients with PID may have subtle or nonspecific symptoms and may go unrecognized.[1,16] There is no single historical or physical examination finding that is specific for PID, and the clinical diagnosis for PID has a positive predictive value of 65%–90%.[16,24,25] Diagnostic criteria for PID can include:[1,16,21]

Cervical motion tenderness OR uterine tenderness OR adnexal tenderness.

If one of these is present, presumptive treatment for PID should be initiated.[16] Additionally, one or more of these criteria enhance the likelihood that PID is present:[1,16]

Oral temperature >101°F (>38.3°C); abnormal cervical mucopurulent discharge or cervical friability; presence of abundant numbers of WBC on saline microscopy of vaginal fluid; elevated erythrocyte sedimentation rate; elevated C-reactive protein; and laboratory documentation of cervical infection with N. gonorrhoeae or C. trachomatis.

grew multiple organisms but not *Neisseria gonorrhoeae* or *Chlamydia trachomatis.* The urine culture grew multiple species as well. The patient did well and was discharged on postoperative day 2 with doxycycline and metronidazole treatment. Follow-up was arranged with Pediatric Surgery and Adolescent Medicine. There was no report of, or concern for, sexual abuse in this patient after extensive evaluation by Social Services and the treatment team.

The differential diagnosis for patients presenting with lower abdominal pain and an adnexal mass found on imaging is extensive. Common etiologies include ectopic pregnancy, TOA, ovarian cysts, ovarian tumors, and ovarian torsion, and symptoms of these conditions can overlap.[2] One study examining clinical variables and the ability to recognize TOA in adolescent patients with pelvic inflammatory disease (PID) found that patients with TOA present later in the menstrual cycle and may appear less ill, having a lower heart rate, temperature, WBC count, and erythrocyte sedimentation rate compared to PID.[14] Adolescents with TOA were also more likely to have had PID before, suggesting that previous infection and inflammation are associated with the development of a TOA, but clinical signs and symptoms may be less acute than in patients without a TOA.[14]

Abdominal or pelvic pain and fever are common presenting symptoms of TOA.[1,2] Fever, pelvic pain, vaginal discharge/bleeding, and nausea may also be seen.[1] Patients may have significant pain and a physical examination may be difficult due to discomfort.[4] While leukocytosis is often seen, patients may have normal total WBC counts.[1,2]

Management of TOA can be complicated by the delay in seeking care that adolescent patients may exhibit.[14] All patients diagnosed with PID and/or TOA should be tested for human immunodeficiency virus (HIV), gonorrhea, and chlamydia.[16] There are multiple treatment regimens for PID that are promulgated by the Centers for Disease Control and Prevention that utilize both oral and parenteral routes and both outpatient and inpatient management.[16] No one particular regimen has been proven to be superior to the other; coverage should include *N. gonorrhoeae*, *C. trachomatis*, and *Mycoplasma genitalium*, but also streptococcus, Gram-negative enteric bacteria (*E. coli*, *Klebsiella* spp., and *Proteus* spp.), and bacteria vaginosis-associated anaerobic organisms.[1,16] If there is any doubt about patient compliance, then hospitalization should be strongly considered. Patients with a TOA should be admitted to the hospital for management, which consists of medical and, in some cases, surgical means; other clinical situations that warrant consideration for hospitalization include pregnancy, other possible surgical conditions, poor response to therapy if being treated as an outpatient for PID, or toxic appearance.[16] There are no data to suggest routine hospitalization for adolescents with PID; however, these criteria should be applied to this population when considering management decisions.[16] All sexual partners should be evaluated and treated.

Special consideration for either sexual abuse or sex trafficking should be given to any pediatric patient with PID or TOA. Documented infection with gonorrhea and/or chlamydia outside the neonatal age range is *generally* considered suspicious for sexual abuse[1,26] and a thorough social history should be obtained by the clinician. Social Work or Law Enforcement should be involved if there is suspicion of either scenario and every state in the United States has mandatory reporting laws. Additionally, HIV prophylaxis should be offered and discussed, along with evaluation and treatment for bacterial vaginosis and trichomonas infection if indicated.

IMAGING PEARLS

1. Plain radiography may be used to investigate abdominal pain but has no role in the diagnosis of a TOA.
2. US is the preferred initial imaging modality when there are concerns for an ovarian process, such as torsion or a TOA.
3. CT can detect a TOA, but is not a first-line imaging test. It is typically used when US is equivocal, there is suspicion for complex disease, or alternative diagnoses (e.g., appendicitis, inflammatory bowel disease) are considered.
4. MRI can detect a TOA but is not used as a first-line imaging modality. Indications for use are similar to CT, but MRI has the advantage of avoiding ionizing radiation and is thus useful in pediatric and pregnant patients. MRI also provides multiplanar imaging, and additional genitourinary tract detail that may be useful, especially if genitourinary tract anomalies are suspected.

References

1. Chappell CA, Wiesenfeld HC. Pathogenesis, diagnosis, and management of severe pelvic inflammatory disease and tuboovarian abscess. *Clin Obstet Gynecol.* 2012;55(4):893-903.
2. Huang A, Jay MS, Uhler M. Tuboovarian abscess in the adolescent. *J Pediatr Adolesc Gynecol.* 1997;10(2):73-77.
3. Mollen CJ, Pletcher JR, Bellah RD, et al. Prevalence of tubo-ovarian abscess in adolescents diagnosed with pelvic inflammatory disease in a pediatric emergency department. *Pediatr Emerg Care.* 2006;22(9): 621-625.
4. Banikarim C, Chacko MR. Pelvic inflammatory disease in adolescents. *Semin Pediatr Infect Dis.* 2005;16(3):175-180.
5. Horrow MM. Ultrasound of pelvic inflammatory disease. *Ultrasound Q.* 2004;20(4):171-179.
6. Timor-Tritsch IE, Lerner JP, Monteagudo A, et al. Transvaginal sonographic markers of tubal inflammatory disease. *Ultrasound Obstet Gynecol.* 1998;12(1):56-66.
7. Lee D, Swaminathan A. Sensitivity of ultrasound for the diagnosis of tubo-ovarian abscess: a case report and literature review. *J Emerg Med.* 2011;40(2):170-175.
8. Cacciatore B, Leminen A, Ingman-Friberg S, et al. Transvaginal sonographic findings in ambulatory patients with suspected pelvic inflammatory disease. *Obstet Gynecol.* 1992;80(6):912-916.
9. Hiller N, Sella T, Lev-Sagi A, et al. Computed tomographic features of tuboovarian abscess. *J Reprod Med.* 2005;50(2):203-208.
10. Iraha Y, Okada M, Iraha R, et al. CT and MR imaging of gynecologic emergencies. *Radiographics.* 2017;37(5):1569-1586.
11. Revzin MV, Mathur M, Dave HB, et al. Pelvic inflammatory disease: multimodality imaging approach with clinical-pathologic correlation. *Radiographics.* 2016;36(5):1579-1596.
12. Sam JW, Jacobs JE, Birnbaum BA. Spectrum of CT findings in acute pyogenic pelvic inflammatory disease. *Radiographics.* 2002;22(6): 1327-1334.
13. Ha HK, Lim GY, Cha ES, et al. MR imaging of tubo-ovarian abscess. *Acta Radiol.* 1995;36(5):510-514.
14. Slap GB, Forke CM, Cnaan A, et al. Recognition of tubo-ovarian abscess in adolescents with pelvic inflammatory disease. *J Adolesc Health.* 1996;18(6):397-403.
15. Osborne NG. Tubo-ovarian abscess: pathogenesis and management. *J Natl Med Assoc.* 1986;78(10):937-951.
16. Workowski KA, Bolan GA; Centers for Disease Control and Prevention. Sexually transmitted diseases treatment guidelines, 2015. *MMWR Recomm Rep.* 2015;64(RR-03):1-137.
17. Wiesenfeld HC, Sweet RL, Ness RB, et al. Comparison of acute and subclinical pelvic inflammatory disease. *Sex Transm Dis.* 2005;32(7): 400-405.
18. Burnett AM, Anderson CP, Zwank MD. Laboratory-confirmed gonorrhea and/or chlamydia rates in clinically diagnosed pelvic inflammatory disease and cervicitis. *Am J Emerg Med.* 2012;30(7): 1114-1117.
19. Hakim J, Childress KJ, Hernandez AM, et al. Tubo-ovarian abscesses in nonsexually active adolescent females: a large case series. *J Adolesc Health.* 2019;65(2):303-305.
20. Dogan E, Altunyurt S, Altındag T, et al. Tubo-ovarian abscess mimicking ovarian tumor in a sexually inactive girl. *J Pediatr Adolesc Gynecol.* 2004;17(5):351-352.
21. Saito JM. Beyond appendicitis: evaluation and surgical treatment of pediatric acute abdominal pain. *Curr Opin Pediatr.* 2012;24(3): 357-634.
22. Hartmann KA, Lerand SJ, Jay MS. Tubo-ovarian abscess in virginal adolescents: exposure of the underlying etiology. *J Pediatr Adolesc Gynecol.* 2009;22(3):e13-e16.
23. Arda IS, Ergeneli M, Coskun M, et al. Tubo-ovarian abscess in a sexually inactive adolescent patient. *Eur J Pediatr Surg.* 2004;14(1): 70-72.
24. Gaitan H, Angel E, Diaz R, et al. Accuracy of five different diagnostic techniques in mild-to-moderate pelvic inflammatory disease. *Infect Dis Obstet Gynecol.* 2002;10(4):171-180.
25. Peipert JF, Ness RB, Blume J, et al. Clinical predictors of endometritis in women with symptoms and signs of pelvic inflammatory disease. *Am J Obstet Gynecol.* 2001;184(5):856-863.
26. Jenny C, Crawford-Jakubiak JE, Committee on Child Abuse and Neglect, American Academy of Pediatrics. The evaluation of children in the primary care setting when sexual abuse is suspected. *Pediatrics.* 2013;132(2):e558-e567.

Neurologic

27 Don't Lose Your Head: Ventriculoperitoneal (VP) Shunt Issues

ROBERT VEZZETTI, MD, FAAP, FACEP

Case Presentation

An 83-day-old female, with a history of congenital hydrocephalus and chronic subdural fluid collections, presents with a 1-week history of increasing fussiness and decreasing oral intake. She has a ventriculoperitoneal (VP) shunt that was placed soon after birth; there has been no revision of the shunt since placement. The mother reports to you that there has been no fever, vomiting, diarrhea, or rash, and there has been good urine output. She tells you that the child was seen by her primary care provider several days ago and was noted to have an increased head circumference compared to previous measurements, but she cannot elaborate further except to say she was told to make a follow-up appointment with the child's pediatric neurosurgeon.

The child's physical exam reveals an irritable, yet nontoxic, child. She is afebrile. Her respiratory rate is 40 breaths per minute with a heat rate of 180 beats per minute. A blood pressure is not documented. She has a small anterior fontanelle that seems full although the mother is unable to tell you how the fontanelle usually feels. She has palpable shunt tubing on the right parietal portion of her scalp; you are unable to feel a reservoir. The rest of her examination is unremarkable.

Imaging Considerations

PLAIN RADIOGRAPHY

A series of plain radiographs, more commonly known as a shunt series, is often the first step in the evaluation of a possible shunt malfunction. The purpose of these images is to examine the shunt tubing for cracks, kinking, or disconnections. A full series will evaluate the entire length of the shunt. The tubing is often coiled in the peritoneal cavity; this is to allow a patient to "grow" into their shunt and reduce the number of revisions necessary to compensate for a child's growth. Recently, however, the utility of obtaining a traditional shunt series has come into question.[1,2] Some experts have proposed proceeding directly to neuroimaging in children when shunt malfunction is suspected, given the low sensitivity of plain radiography in detecting shunt malfunction.[1,2]

The programmable valve settings on a shunt may be seen with a "valve view."[3] This view can be used to confirm shunt settings.

ULTRASOUND

Ultrasound has been used to evaluate optic nerve sheath diameter as a measurement of intracranial pressure and has begun to be explored as a possible imaging test to evaluate a patient for shunt malfunction.[4–6] In some studies, when combined with plain radiography shunt series imaging, ultrasound has been shown to be helpful in detecting shunt malfunction in patients with low pretest probability of shunt malfunction.[4] However, another study using ocular ultrasound as a single imaging modality to screen for shunt malfunction demonstrated low sensitivity and specificity.[5] Further research is needed to understand the potential role of ultrasound in patients with suspected shunt malfunction.

NEUROIMAGING

Computed Tomography (CT)

Usually readily available, and performed without intravenous (IV) contrast for this indication, CT offers rapid assessment of the size of a child's ventricles, assisting the clinician in ascertaining if a shunt malfunction exists. Sedation is rarely, if ever, required. CT exposes the patient to ionizing radiation. These children often have had multiple studies, and the potential of sequelae from exposure to ionizing radiation is cumulative. Minimizing the duration and amount of radiation exposure by practicing ALARA (as low as reasonably achievable) principles helps mitigate this risk. Limited-use CT protocols have been proposed; one center initiated a pilot study using a four-slice protocol (third ventricle, fourth ventricle, lateral ventricle, and basal ganglia levels) to evaluate ventricular size.[7] Another institution created a clinical pathway that used a full coverage (i.e., complete brain visualization) but reduced-dose cranial CT and eliminated routine radiographic shunt series, with directed plain films obtained only for specific indications. Results showed this clinical pathway to reduce CT effective radiation dose by approximately 50% and to decrease effective dose from radiographs by 64%, with no adverse effect on patient care.[8] CT may be the only option available (even in tertiary care pediatric facilities), and the risk of complications by either not identifying shunt malfunction or delaying treatment can be significant.

Magnetic Resonance Imaging (MRI)

MRI has seen increasing use in VP shunt evaluation.[9] There is no exposure to ionizing radiation and IV contrast is not required. Fast acquisition MRI has become an alternative to conventional brain MRI, allowing good visualization of ventricular size with a short scanning time. Diagnostic accuracy is comparable to CT, and sedation needs have diminished with rapid acquisition protocols.[4,10]

Several issues complicate the use of MRI. MRI is often not readily available on demand, even in pediatric facilities. The time required to complete an adequate study sometimes necessitates the use of sedation, particularly in patients who may be agitated, although fast acquisition MRI has made this need less common.

Most programmable VP shunt valves are MRI-compatible. However, some programmable shunt valves are programmed using magnets, and an MRI evaluation can reset the current shunt settings. It is important to ascertain if the child has a programmable shunt and if the shunt valve setting requires evaluation after scanning. One can still obtain the study, but a post-MRI "valve view" (a one-view plain radiograph) to confirm that the settings have not changed should be performed.[3,10]

Regardless of the neuroimaging method used, there are two important aspects to consider. First, expertise in the interpretation of pediatric neuroimaging is important in determining if shunt malfunction exists. Second, prior neuroimaging studies are critical. A comparison should be made between the current neuroimaging study results and past study results. Ideally, similar modalities should be compared, but comparison of current CT to prior MRI and vice versa are acceptable.

Imaging Findings

This child had a radiographic shunt series (Figs. 27.1–27.4) and a fast acquisition MRI (Figs. 27.5–27.7). Selected views are included.

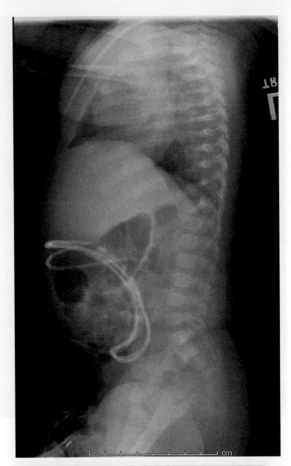

Fig. 27.2 Lateral view of the intact shunt tubing.

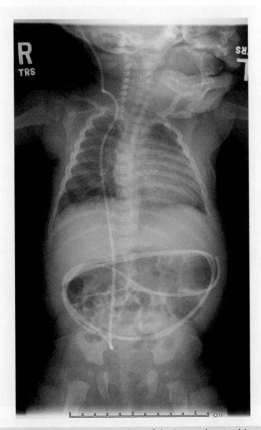

Fig. 27.1 Anteroposterior view of the intact shunt tubing.

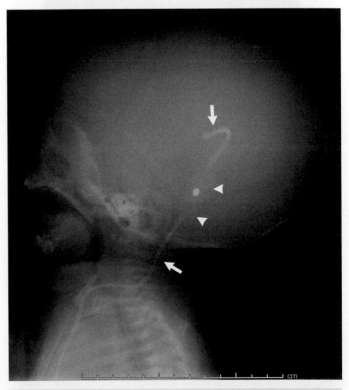

Fig. 27.3 Lateral view of the intact shunt tubing *(arrows)*. A normal area of radiolucency is seen in areas of connections around the shunt valve *(arrowheads)*.

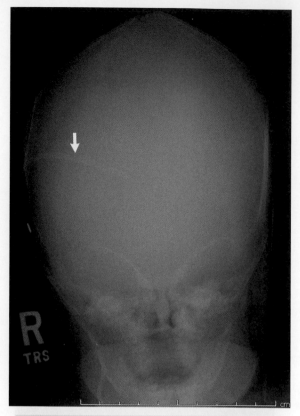

Fig. 27.4 Anteroposterior view of the shunt tubing (arrow).

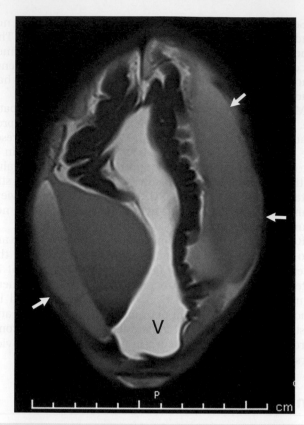

Fig. 27.6 Axial MRI image shows bilateral chronic subdural collections (arrows) and enlargement of a dysmorphic ventricle (V).

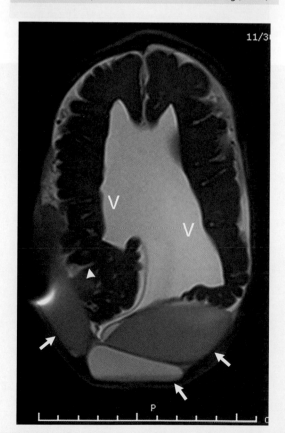

Fig. 27.5 Axial MRI image shows enlargement of dysmorphic appearing lateral ventricles (V) and chronic subdural fluid collections (arrows). The tip of the shunt is seen (arrowhead) but no shunt is seen in the lateral ventricles.

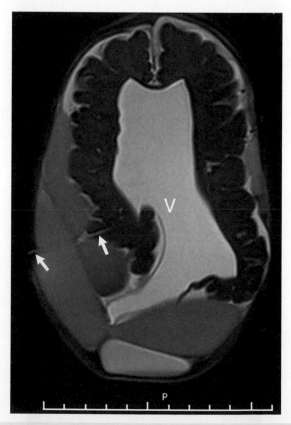

Fig. 27.7 Axial MRI shows more of the shunt tubing (arrows) than in Fig.27.5, but still does not show the shunt to extend into the ventricles (V).

The shunt series identified the VP shunt. There is no obvious disconnection or breakage of the tubing.

The fast acquisition MRI scan is quite revealing. When compared to previous imaging, the shunt tip is now positioned in the right parietal cortical mantle and is not communicating with the ventricular system. There is an interval increase in the size of the chronic subdural fluid collections and lateral ventricular size. These findings are consistent with shunt failure.

Case Conclusion

Congenital hydrocephalus has multiple etiologies. Treatment is often relief of the increased intracranial pressure by placing a shunt, which may be VP or at other sites, such as lumbar-peritoneal or ventriculoatrial. VP shunting is more commonly encountered in pediatric patients. Shunt infection is most often seen in the acute period following shunt placement (the first 1 to 2 months postsurgery).[4] A more common shunt complication is shunt failure, producing either overshunting or undershunting of cerebral spinal fluid, leading to a variety of symptoms. These symptoms can be nonspecific and sometimes subtle; they include vomiting, fussiness, decreased mental status, and headache. Asking the child's caregiver if the child has had an acute change in their usual behavior is helpful when evaluating these patients.

Neuroimaging is commonly employed to determine if a child is experiencing shunt malfunction. The extent to which repeated imaging of these children is useful has been called into question, particularly given the exposure to ionizing radiation involved when CT is utilized.[11] Utilization of MRI, especially fast acquisition MRI, can mitigate such exposure and the potential complications associated with it.

Given the apparent change of ventricular size and the location of the shunt versus previous neuroimaging, a pediatric neurosurgical consultation was obtained. The child was taken to the operating room for shunt revision.

IMAGING PEARLS

1. Children with VP shunts may present with a variety of symptoms that may indicate shunt malfunction. Imaging should be used in these patients if there is any suspicion of shunt malfunction.
2. A shunt series, consisting of several plain radiographic views, is helpful in determining disconnection, breakage, or kinking of the shunt. The entire shunt should be visualized on these images. There is debate by some experts about the utility of a traditional shunt series to detect shunt malfunction, except in cases of broken shunt tubing.
3. Non—contrast-enhanced CT is a rapid imaging modality that can identify findings of potential shunt malfunction.

While generally readily available, exposure to radiation should be considered. Consideration can be given to performing lower-dose cranial CT.

4. Fast acquisition MRI is an excellent study to utilize for the evaluation of shunt malfunction. Limitations include availability and the occasional need for sedation.
5. Prior neuroimaging studies are important. Comparison of current to previous ventricular size, the degree of hydrocephalus (if present), and the overall picture of the brain and associated structures can help determine if shunt malfunction is present.
6. Do not delay neurosurgical consultation or transfer (if indicated) to a pediatric facility in order to obtain neuroimaging in patients who have clinical findings concerning for or consistent with shunt failure, especially in critically ill children. Obtaining a neuroimaging study prior to neurosurgical consultation is ideal but should not delay treatment.

References

1. Desai KR, Babb JS, Amodio JB. The utility of the plain radiograph "shunt series" in the evaluation of suspected ventriculoperitoneal shunt failure in pediatric patients. *Pediatr Radiol.* 2007;37(5): 452-456.
2. Lehnert BE, Rahbar H, Relyea-Chew S, et al. Detection of ventricular shunt malfunction in the ED: relative utility of radiography, CT, and nuclear imaging. *Emerg Radiol.* 2011;18(4):299-305.
3. Lollis SS, Mamourian AC, Vaccaro TJ, et al. Programmable CSF shunt valves: radiographic identification and interpretation. *AJNR Am J Neuroradiol.* 2010;31(7):1343-1346.
4. Pershad J, Taylor A, Hall MK, et al. Imaging strategies for suspected acute cranial shunt failure: a cost-effectiveness analysis. *Pediatrics.* 2017;140(2):2016-4263. Erratum in: *Pediatrics.* 2017;140(5).
5. Hall MK, Spiro DM, Sabbaj A, et al. Bedside optic nerve sheath diameter ultrasound for the evaluation of suspected pediatric ventriculoperitoneal shunt failure in the emergency department. *Childs Nerv Syst.* 2013;29(12):2275-2280.
6. Komut E, Kozaci N, Sönmez BM, et al. Bedside sonographic measurement of optic nerve sheath diameter as a predictor of intracranial pressure in ED. *Am J Emerg Med.* 2016;34(6):963-967.
7. Koral K, Blackburn T, Bailey AA, et al. Strengthening the argument for rapid brain MR imaging: estimation of reduction of lifetime attributable risk of developing fatal cancer in children with shunted hydrocephalus by instituting a rapid brain MR imaging protocol in lieu of head CT. *AJNR Am J Neuroradiol.* 2012;33(10):1851-1854.
8. Marchese RF, Schwartz ES, Heuer GG, et al. Reduced radiation in children presenting to the ED with suspected ventricular shunt complication. *Pediatrics.* 2017;139(5):2016-2431.
9. Trost MJ, Robison N, Coffey D, et al. Changing trends in brain imaging technique for pediatric patients with ventriculoperitoneal shunts. *Pediatr Neurosurg.* 2018;53(2):116-120.
10. Captiano JF, Venier A, Mazzeo LA, et al. Prospective study to evaluate rate and frequency of perturbations of implanted programmable Hakim Codman valve after 1.5-Tesla magnetic resonance imaging. *World Neurosurg.* 2016;88:297-293.
11. Antonucci MC, Zuckerbraun NS, Tyler-Kabara EC, et al. The burden of ionizing radiation studies in children with ventricular shunts. *J Pediatr.* 2017;182:210-216.

28 *More Than a Migraine: Intracranial Mass - Medulloblastoma*

ROBERT VEZZETTI, MD, FAAP, FACEP

Case Presentation

A 6-year-old male with no significant medical history presents with headaches for the past 2 weeks. The headache is described as diffuse and, while occurring throughout the day, seems to be worse at night, at times waking him from sleep. He has also had daily first morning nonbilious, nonbloody emesis for the past week. There is no complaint of abdominal pain and there has been no fever or diarrhea. He does not appear to have vision changes and the parents report no difficulty ambulating or problems with balance. There is a strong family history of migraines in both his mother and older sisters. The child was seen by his primary care provider a few days after the headaches began and probable migraines were diagnosed. Oral magnesium was prescribed and his mother was asked to keep a headache diary and to give ibuprofen if acetaminophen was not helping. The mother has complied with these instructions. The ibuprofen and acetaminophen initially provided some relief but now do not seem to be helping. There is no recent travel and no other family members the child lives with have concurrent headaches.

The child's physical examination reveals no fever, a heart rate of 83 beats per minute, respiratory rate of 24 breaths per minute, and blood pressure of 103/69 mm Hg. He does not appear ill but does complain of headache. He is normocephalic and there are no signs of trauma. His pupils are equal and reactive; there is no photophobia and no nystagmus. He ambulates without difficulty and has equal tone and strength throughout. There are no rashes or skin lesions.

Imaging Considerations

In an acute setting, the common causes of pediatric headache include viral illness and migraine.[1] The decision to obtain imaging in the pediatric patient with headache is based on history and physical examination findings. Most headaches in the pediatric population are not due to intracranial pathology. Over 90% of children who have an intracranial mass will have other historic or physical examination findings.[2] Historic "red flags" include progressively worsening headache, waking in the middle of the night with a headache, complaints of morning headache upon awakening, morning emesis upon waking, duration of symptoms less than 6 months, and lack of a family history of migraine. Physical examination "red flags" include focal neurologic findings, worsening headache with Valsalva maneuver, and gait/balance disturbances.[1] Children with these findings should be considered for neuroimaging.

PLAIN RADIOGRAPHY

Plain radiography does not have a role in the evaluation of the pediatric patient with headache.

COMPUTED TOMOGRAPHY (CT)

CT is often used as a first-line imaging modality to detect intracranial pathology.[3] This modality is readily available in most urgent and emergent settings. If an intracranial mass is suspected, a non—contrast study can be utilized.

MAGNETIC RESONANCE IMAGING (MRI)

This imaging modality is the preferred method to visualize intracranial pathology, including brain tumors, and is often obtained following the detection of a brain mass on CT. Conventional MRI techniques can provide anatomic information regarding the dimensions and location of a brain tumor; advanced MRI imaging techniques, such as diffusion weighted imaging, functional MRI, and diffusion tensor imaging, can be utilized to provide physiologic information regarding hemodynamics and cellularity.[4] Barriers to MRI use include the time necessary to complete a study and lack of immediate availability in many cases. In young children, sedation is often required to complete the study.

Imaging Findings

The child had non—contrast-enhanced CT of his brain. There is a large, relatively homogeneous hyperdense mass centered in the fourth ventricle measuring 3.4 × 3.9 × 3.5 cm without significant internal calcifications. The mass is completely obstructing the fourth ventricle, with moderate to severe dilatation of the lateral and third ventricles (hydrocephalus) (Figs. 28.1–28.3).

Case Conclusion

Given the imaging findings, Pediatric Neurosurgery was consulted. Therapy with intravenous dexamethasone

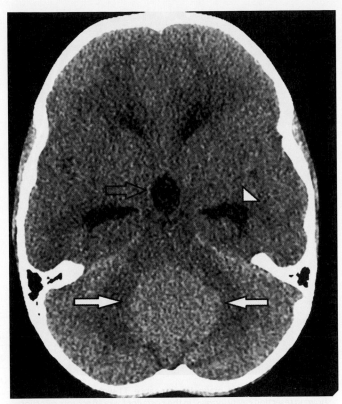

Fig. 28.1 Computed tomography axial image demonstrates a large homogenous hyperdense posterior fossa mass *(arrows)* filling and obstructing the fourth ventricle. The third ventricle *(open arrow)* and temporal horns of the lateral ventricles *(arrowhead)* are dilated.

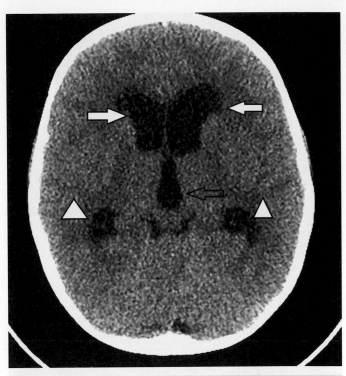

Fig. 28.3 Computed tomography axial image demonstrates enlargement of bilateral frontal *(arrows)* and temporal *(arrowheads)* horns of the lateral ventricles, and third ventricular dilatation *(open arrow)*, consistent with obstructive hydrocephalus.

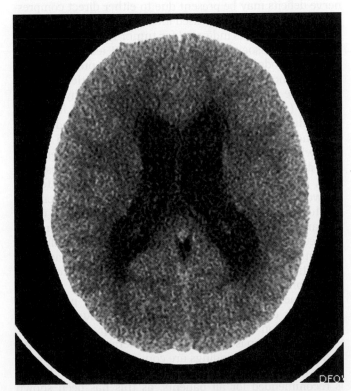

Fig. 28.2 Computed tomography axial image demonstrates bilateral lateral ventricular enlargement consistent with obstructive hydrocephalus.

(0.6 mg/kg/dose every 6 hours) was initiated and the child was admitted to the pediatric intensive care unit. The next day, the child underwent MRI of his brain and entire spine. The mass was again visualized (Fig. 28.4). The spine images revealed leptomeningeal spread (Fig. 28.5). Several days later, the child underwent suboccipital craniotomy for resection of the fourth ventricular tumor with microscopic dissection and insertion of an external ventricular drain. A selected image of the postoperative MRI is provided (Fig. 28.6). The patient tolerated the procedure well. Pediatric Oncology was consulted and an appropriate chemotherapy and radiation therapy regimen was instituted.

Brain tumors are the second most common malignancy and the most common solid tumor in pediatric patients.[5–7] Medulloblastoma occurs in the posterior fossa, represents 10%–15% of pediatric brain tumors, and has a potential for leptomeningeal spread.[3,8] These tumors are more common in the first decade if life, with a bimodal peak incidence at 3–4 years and 8–10 years of age.[8] This tumor has been described as the most common pediatric brain neoplasm,[5] and overall 5-year survival rates have improved from 30% in the 1960s to greater than 80% over the past few decades,[9,10] depending on age and tumor characteristics.

The symptoms caused by medulloblastoma typically evolve quickly due to the rapid growth rate typical of these tumors. Symptoms are due to increased intracranial pressure and cerebellar dysfunction. Irritability, decreased mentation, vomiting, headaches (especially in the morning), and behavioral changes are common signs of increased intracranial pressure. Symptoms due to cerebellar dysfunction depend on the tumor location. Midline tumors of the

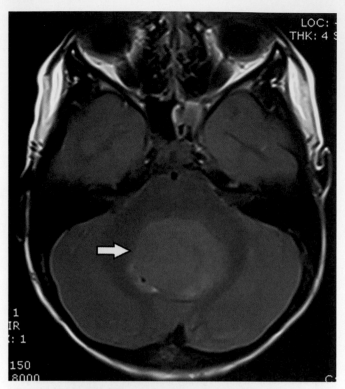

Fig. 28.4 Magnetic resonance axial image demonstrating the mass (*arrow*) filling and distending the fourth ventricle.

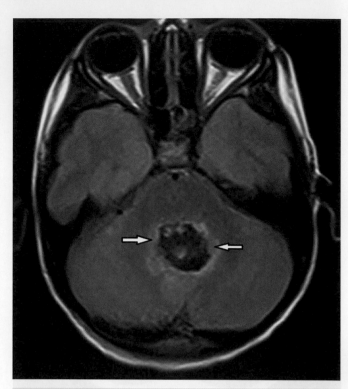

Fig. 28.6 Postoperative magnetic resonance T1-weighted axial image showing resection cavity (*arrows*) in the posterior fossa after gross resection of the mass.

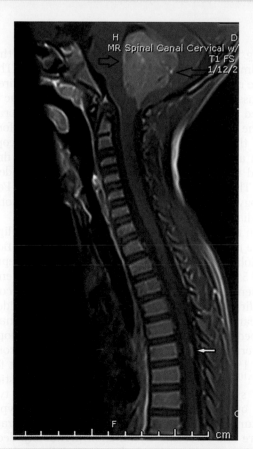

Fig. 28.5 Contrast-enhanced sagittal T1-weighted MRI image demonstrates leptomeningeal spread with an enhancing lesion along the posterior surface of the thoracic spinal cord (*arrow*). The primary mass is again seen in the posterior fossa (*open arrows*).

cerebellum tend to produce truncal ataxia; those of the hemispheres manifest as appendicular ataxia.[8] Cranial nerve deficits may be present due to either direct compression or the effects of increased intracranial pressure.

Neuroimaging is indicated for tumor location and identification of associated complications. CT and MRI are the imaging modalities most utilized for this purpose. Both imaging modalities demonstrate characteristics that are suggestive of medulloblastoma. CT reveals hyperdense tumors (some with calcifications) that arise from the cerebellum (the vermis is a common location) and extend into the fourth ventricle. Hydrocephalus is often identified, with effacement and dilation of the fourth ventricle and dilatation of the lateral and third ventricles.[8] On MRI, these tumors are hypointense to gray matter on T1-weighted imaging with heterogeneous enhancement, iso- to hyperintense to gray matter on T2-weighted imaging, and hyperintense on fluid-attenuated inversion recovery sequences and show restricted diffusion on diffusion-weighted imaging.[3,8] It is appropriate to obtain imaging of the entire spine since medulloblastoma has a propensity for leptomeningeal spread.[3,8]

Treatment for medulloblastoma is based on patient age and tumor classification. A combination of surgical resection, radiation therapy, and chemotherapy is employed. Surgical resection is a cornerstone of therapy for all patients, and if radiographic findings are consistent with a diagnosis of medulloblastoma, biopsy is not indicated.[8] Chemotherapy is recommended for all patients, as this has been shown to improve outcomes.[8,11] Radiation therapy is effective and recommended when possible.[9]

Patients greater than 3 years old are stratified based on the measurement of postoperative residual tumor and the presence or absence of metastases into standard-risk and high-risk categories:

Standard Risk (less than 1.5 cm^2 of postoperative residual disease)—These patients are treated with postoperative radiation therapy and adjunct chemotherapy. Overall 5-year survival rate is 85%.[8,12]

High risk (greater than 1.5 cm^2 of postoperative residual disease)—These patients are treated with postoperative radiation therapy and adjunct chemotherapy. Overall 5-year survival rate is 70%.[8,13]

Infants or children less than 3 years of age with medulloblastoma represent a unique category of patient. Overall outcomes are poor in these patients, compared to older children. Radiation therapy negatively impacts neurodevelopmental outcomes in young children; therefore, this arm of the typical medulloblastoma treatment regimen is omitted in these children, who can be treated with surgical resection and chemotherapy only.[8,9] Several studies have reported 5-year progression-free rates and overall survival rates of 38%–50% and 43%–80%, respectively, using this treatment approach.[8,14–16]

Patients with relapsed medulloblastoma have an overall poor prognosis; reported 5-year survival rates are approximately 25%.[8,17] Treatment options include repeat surgical resection, reirradiation, high-dose chemotherapy, and stem cell therapy.[8,18,19] For young children who were initially not candidates for radiation therapy, studies have shown that, in some cases, initiation of radiation therapy in this age group has been an effective treatment.[20]

IMAGING PEARLS

1. History and physical examination findings will help identify which children with headache require neuroimaging. Those with "red flag" findings should strongly be considered for neuroimaging.
2. Non—contrast CT is most commonly the initial imaging modality utilized in pediatric patients with suspected intracranial tumors in the acute care setting, as this modality is rapid and readily available.
3. MRI is the gold standard for intracranial imaging in pediatric patients with suspected intracranial tumor. However, MRI may not be readily available in the acute setting and sedation is often required in young children. When MRI is unavailable or not feasible in the acute setting, unenhanced CT may be performed and MRI performed as a secondary test when indicated.
4. Advanced MRI techniques, such as diffusion-weighted imaging, can be used to provide information regarding tumor cellularity, hemodynamics, and other physiologic characteristics, helpful for tumor management.
5. Often, the imaging characteristics and location of a tumor will provide clues to the likely diagnosis in pediatric patients.

References

1. Blume HK. Childhood headache: a brief review. *Pediatr Ann.* 2017; 46(4):e155-e165.
2. Lanphear J, Sarnaik S. Presenting symptoms of pediatric brain tumors diagnosed in the emergency department. *Pediatr Emerg Care.* 2014;30(2):77-80.
3. Massimino M, Biassoni V, Gandola L, et al. Childhood medulloblastoma. *Crit Rev Oncol Hematol.* 2016;105:35-51.
4. Lequin M, Hendrikse J. Advanced MR imaging in pediatric brain tumors, clinical applications. *Neuroimaging Clin N Am.* 2017; 27(1):167-190.
5. Udaka YT, Packer RJ. Pediatric brain tumors. *Neurol Clin.* 2018; 36(3):533-556.
6. Segal D, Karajannis MA. Pediatric brain tumors: an update. *Curr Probl Pediatr Adolesc Health Care.* 2016;46(7):242-250.
7. Glod J, Rahme GJ, Kaur H, et al. Pediatric brain tumors: current knowledge and therapeutic opportunities. *J Pediatr Hematol Oncol.* 2016;38(4):249-260.
8. Millard NE, De Braganca KC. Medulloblastoma. *J Child Neurol.* 2016;31(12):1341-1353.
9. Dressler EV, Dolecek TA, Liu M, et al. Demographics, patterns of care, and survival in pediatric medulloblastoma. *J Neurooncol.* 2017;132(3):497-506.
10. Chintagumpala M, Gajjar A. Brain tumors. *Pediatr Clin North Am.* 2015;62(1):167-178.
11. Tait DM, Thornton-Jones H, Bloom HJ, et al. Adjuvant chemotherapy for medulloblastoma: the first multi-centre control trial of the International Society of Paediatric Oncology (SIOP I). *Eur J Cancer.* 1990;26(4):46446-46449.
12. Packer RJ, Gajjar A, Vezina G, et al. Phase III study of craniospinal radiation therapy followed by adjuvant chemotherapy for newly diagnosed average-risk medulloblastoma. *J Clin Oncol.* 2006;24(25):4202-4208.
13. Gajjar A, Chintagumpala M, Ashley D, et al. Risk-adapted craniospinal radiotherapy followed by high-dose chemotherapy and stem-cell rescue in children with newly diagnosed medulloblastoma (St Jude Medulloblastoma-96): long-term results from a prospective, multicentre trial. *Lancet Oncol.* 2006;7(10):813-820.
14. Geyer JR, Sposto R, Jennings M, et al. Multiagent chemotherapy and deferred radiotherapy in infants with malignant brain tumors: a report from the Children's Cancer Group. *J Clin Oncol.* 2005;23(30): 7621-7631.
15. Rutkowski S, Gerber NU, von Hoff K, et al. Treatment of early childhood medulloblastoma by postoperative chemotherapy and deferred radiotherapy. *Neuro Oncol.* 2009;11(2):201-210.
16. von Bueren AO, von Hoff K, Pietsch T, et al. Treatment of young children with localized medulloblastoma by chemotherapy alone: results of the prospective, multicenter trial HIT 2000 confirming the prognostic impact of histology. *Neuro Oncol.* 2011;13(6):669-679.
17. Bowers DC, Gargan L, Weprin BE, et al. Impact of site of tumor recurrence upon survival for children with recurrent or progressive medulloblastoma. *J Neurosurg.* 2007;107(suppl 1):5-10.
18. Dunkel IJ, Gardner SL, Garvin Jr JH, et al. High-dose carboplatin, thiotepa, and etoposide with autologous stem cell rescue for patients with previously irradiated recurrent medulloblastoma. *Neuro Oncol.* 2010;12(3):297-303.
19. Bakst RL1, Dunkel IJ, Gilheeney S, et al. Reirradiation for recurrent medulloblastoma. *Cancer.* 2011;117(21):4977-4982.
20. Gururangan S, Krauser J, Watral MA, et al. Efficacy of high-dose chemotherapy or standard salvage therapy in patients with recurrent medulloblastoma. *Neuro Oncol.* 2008;10(5):745-751.

29 *Diffuse Intrinsic Pontine Glioma: DIPG*

ROBERT VEZZETTI, MD, FAAP, FACEP

Case Presentation

A 4-year-old female presents with the parents noting that the child has been "not walking right" and "wobbly" for the past 3 weeks. She sustained a head injury 1 month prior to her current presentation but there was no reported loss of consciousness at that time and the fall was off a chair, onto a hardwood floor, less than 2 feet. At the time, she did not appear injured and had been at her baseline until the onset of current symptoms. There has been no reported fever, recent illness, emesis, neck pain, back pain, or incontinence. The family has noted that her "eyes look funny" and she appears to "have trouble focusing her vision." She also has been drooling (new for this child) and seems to have difficulty speaking, which is also new for the child as she has been developmentally appropriate.

Physical examination reveals age-appropriate vital signs and the child is in no overall distress. She is normocephalic and there are no signs of trauma. Pupils are round and equally reactive to light and there is no photophobia. The child has bilateral ptosis and she appears to have difficulty focusing her vision on objects. She has equal tone and strength throughout, but when she ambulates, she is ataxic and has dysmetria. She is drooling and is difficult to understand when she speaks.

Imaging Considerations

Imaging is often employed in patients with general neurologic complaints, such as severe headache, and focal neurologic findings (such as ataxia or abnormal neurologic examination), or if there are symptoms that raise suspicion for an intracranial process, such as emesis, vision changes, or concerning historical findings (such as awakening in the middle of the night with headache, first morning emesis, or persistent/worsening headache).[1] Imaging options include computed tomography (CT) and magnetic resonance imaging (MRI); which modality is employed depends largely on history, physical examination, and institutional resources.

While the use of neuroimaging has become commonplace for the evaluation of a variety of symptoms in pediatric patient populations, including concussion,[2,3] first-time seizures,[2,4] headache,[2,5] and dizziness,[2,6] neuroimaging may not be indicated in all patients. Several studies looking at acute and subacute ataxia in pediatric patients found conditions that required intervention in approximately 13% of patients imaged.[2,7] Of note, the clinical features most predictive of imaging abnormalities were the age of the child (older children had more significant intracranial pathology), the duration of symptoms (more than 3 days was significant), and the presence of additional neurological signs on examination, such as cranial nerve deficits or hemiparesis.[2,7] Cranial nerve deficits are associated with a variety of intracranial pathologies, including demyelinating disease and tumors; more than 80% of children with space-occupying tumors will have signs of increased intracranial pressure, in addition to ataxia.[2,8] Therefore it is a constellation of symptoms and examination findings that leads the clinician to suspect an intracranial process, rather than individual symptoms alone.

PLAIN RADIOGRAPHY

This modality has no role in the evaluation of pediatric patients with focal neurologic findings.

COMPUTED TOMOGRAPHY

CT is often used as a first-line imaging modality to detect intracranial pathology. This modality is readily available in most urgent and emergent settings and sedation is not required. If an intracranial mass is suspected, a non—contrast study can be utilized.

MAGNETIC RESONANCE IMAGING

MRI is the preferred method to visualize intracranial pathology, including brain tumors, and is often obtained following the detection of a brain mass on CT. In cases with a high index of suspicion, MRI is appropriate as an initial imaging test or after a CT with unrevealing or nonspecific findings. Conventional MRI techniques can provide anatomic information regarding dimensions and location of a brain tumor; advanced MRI imaging techniques, such as diffusion-weighted imaging, functional MRI, and diffusion tensor imaging, can be utilized to provide physiologic information regarding hemodynamics and cellularity.[9] Barriers to MRI use include the time necessary to complete a study and lack of immediate availability in many cases. In young children, sedation is often required to complete the study.

Imaging Findings

The child's history and physical examination were concerning for an intracranial process, especially a space-occupying lesion. A non—contrast CT scan was obtained and selected images are provided. There is diffuse enlargement and low

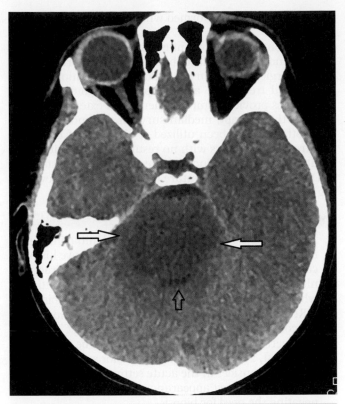

Fig. 29.1 Computed tomography axial image demonstrates a large low-density pontine mass that expands the brainstem (*arrows*) and compresses/effaces the fourth ventricle (*open arrow*).

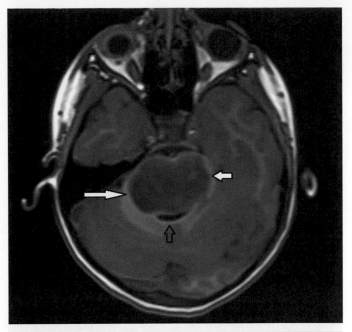

Fig. 29.2 T1-weighted magnetic resonance axial image demonstrates low signal mass expanding the brainstem (*arrows*) and compressing the fourth ventricle (*open arrow*).

attenuation throughout the brainstem, but particularly in the pontine region, and there is compression and effacement of the fourth ventricle but no hydrocephalus; these findings are concerning for a brainstem glioma (Fig. 29.1).

In light of these imaging findings, the child underwent MRI of the brain and spine with and without intravenous (IV) contrast. Selected images are provided. Sedation was required to complete the study. This study demonstrated a large T2 hyperintense pontine mass without enhancement or hemorrhage, with some exophytic extension around the basilar artery, and compression of the fourth ventricle without hydrocephalus (Figs. 29.2 and 29.3). There is no cerebrospinal fluid dissemination of the tumor.

Case Conclusion

Based on imaging findings, the child was diagnosed with diffuse intrinsic pontine glioma (DIPG). Pediatric Neurosurgery and Pediatric Oncology were consulted and the child was admitted for planned radiation therapy. In this case, the family requested a biopsy, but after extensive discussions, they opted not to have the procedure done. The child was begun on radiation therapy. For comparison, a follow-up MRI is provided, demonstrating slightly diminished size of the tumor with central necrosis, likely secondary to radiotherapy response (Fig. 29.4).

DIPG is a leading cause of pediatric brain tumor deaths, with a median survival of 9 months; 90% of children will die within 2 years of initial diagnosis, with a survival rate

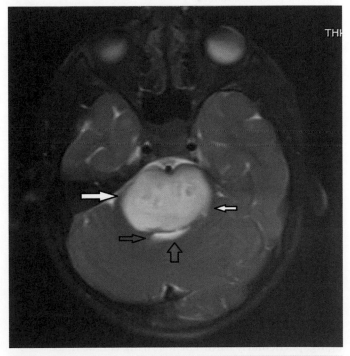

Fig. 29.3 T2-weighted axial magnetic resonance image demonstrates high T2 signal mass expanding the brainstem (*arrows*) and compressing the fourth ventricle (*open arrows*).

of less than 1% at 5 years.[10–12] Interestingly, patients with predominately exophytic tumor, tumors in patients with neurofibromatosis, or tumors that originate near the cerebellar peduncles or cervicomedullary junction have a slightly more favorable course.[12] The tumor arises in the ventral pons and is the most common pediatric brainstem

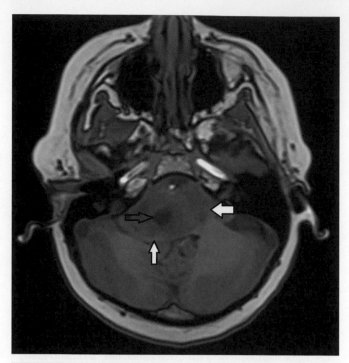

Fig. 29.4 Magnetic resonance imaging postradiation therapy. T1-weighted magnetic resonance axial image following radiation therapy shows mild decrease in tumor size *(arrows)* with a focus of necrosis within the lesion *(open arrow)*.

glioma (80% of all brainstem tumors), affecting some 300–400 children a year.[12–14] Dissemination to the midbrain and cerebellum, leptomeningeal dissemination, and supratentorial extension have all been described.[15,16] This tumor is aggressive and carries a very poor prognosis.

Symptoms are rapidly progressive and clinical manifestations are the result of compression of the nerve structures surrounding the ventral pons. Most patients diagnosed with this tumor present with symptoms for less than 1–2 months.[10,12] An initial sign and poor prognostic indicator is the presence of cranial nerve six palsy (abducens palsy), resulting in dysconjugate gaze and diplopia; extremity and facial weakness have been reported; weakness and gait disturbances may also be seen.[10,12] The so-called classic triad of DIPG (ataxia, dysmetria, and dysarthria) is seen in only one-half of patients with this tumor.[10,12]

The diagnosis of DIPG is based on physical examination and radiographic findings. Due to the infiltrative nature of the tumor, characteristic findings can be noted on neuroimaging, particularly MRI. The following can be noted[10–12]:

1. Poorly demarcated tumor margins.
2. Engulfs the basilar artery.
3. Involves greater than 50% of the pontine axial diameter.
4. Does not enhance with IV gadolinium contrast.

Traditionally, surgical biopsy has not been recommended or offered. This has been based on imaging pattern that is used to diagnose DIPG, the perceived associated risks with the biopsy procedure, and the fact that biopsy does not guide therapy.[10,12] However, the recommendation not to biopsy has started to be questioned, and in some

countries, biopsy is performed when radiographic imaging is unclear.[10]

Treatment options are limited. Because of the infiltrative nature and invasion into brainstem structures of this tumor, surgical resection is not possible. Radiation therapy is standard treatment, as it helps to mitigate symptoms (sometimes providing improvement) and extends survival; without this therapy, median survival is 5 months.[10,12,17] Chemotherapy has been utilized at all stages of the radiation treatment process with no resulting survival improvement.[18–21] Recent advances in the genomic understanding of DIPG may help devise future treatments of this devastating tumor.[10,21,22]

IMAGING PEARLS

1. Non—contrast CT is a commonly used initial imaging modality for patients with headache who have historical or physical examination concerns for an intracranial mass or pathology, especially in the acute setting when MRI may not be readily available or feasible.
2. MRI is utilized as an initial test for this indication, or as a secondary study once initial imaging with CT has been performed. While this modality can be used as an initial test, availability and the need for sedation are factors to consider in the acute setting.
3. DIPG has a distinct appearance on neuroimaging, often negating the need for biopsy.

References

1. Lanphear J, Sarnaik S. Presenting symptoms of pediatric brain tumors diagnosed in the emergency department. *Pediatr Emerg Care.* 2014;30(2):77-80.
2. Luetje M, Kannikeswaran N, Arora R, et al. Utility of neuroimaging in children presenting to a pediatric emergency department with ataxia. *Pediatr Emerg Care.* 2019;35(5):335-340.
3. Zonfrillo MR, Kim KH, Arbogast KB. Emergency department visits and head computed tomography utilization for concussion patients from 2006 to 2011. *Acad Emerg Med.* 2015;22:872-878.
4. Maytel J, Krauss JM, Novak G, et al. The role of brain computed tomography in evaluating children with new onset of seizures in the emergency department. *Epilepsia.* 2000;41:950-954.
5. Sheridan DC, Meckler GD, Spiro DM, et al. Diagnostic testing and treatment of pediatric headache in the emergency department. *J Pediatr.* 2013;163:1634-1637.
6. Raucci U, Vanacore N, Paolino MC, et al. Vertigo/dizziness in pediatric emergency department: five years' experience. *Cephalalgia.* 2015; 36:593-598.
7. Rudloe T, Prabhu SP, Gorman MP, et al. The yield of neuroimaging in children presenting to the emergency department with acute ataxia in the post-varicella vaccine era. *J Child Neurol.* 2015;30: 1333-1339.
8. Wilne S, Collier J, Kennedy C, et al. Presentation of childhood CNS tumours: a systematic review and meta-analysis. *Lancet Oncol.* 2007;8:685-695.
9. Lequin M, Hendrikse J. Advanced MR Imaging in Pediatric Brain Tumors, Clinical Applications. *Neuroimaging Clin N Am.* 2017; 27(1): 167-190.
10. Johung TB, Monje M. Diffuse intrinsic pontine glioma: new pathophysiological insights and emerging therapeutic targets. *Curr Neuropharmacol.* 2017;15(1):88-97.
11. Donaldson SS, Laningham F, Fisher PG. Advances toward an understanding of brainstem gliomas. *J Clin Oncol.* 2006;24:1266-1272.
12. Cohen KJ, Broniscer A, Glod J. Pediatric glial tumors. *Curr Treat Options Oncol.* 2001;2(6):529-536.
13. Freeman CR, Farmer JP. Pediatric brain stem gliomas: a review. *Int J Radiat Oncol Biol Phys.* 1998;40(2):265-271.
14. CBTRUS Statistical report: Primary brain and other central nervous system tumors diagnosed in the United States in 2012-2016. *Neuro Oncol.* 2019;21(Suppl 5):v1-v100.

15. Gururangan S, McLaughlin CA, Brashears, et al. Incidence and patterns of neuraxis metastases in children with diffuse pontine glioma. *J Neurooncol.* 2006;77(2):207-212.

16. Caretti V, Bugiani M, Freret M, et al. Subventricular spread of diffuse intrinsic pontine glioma. *Acta Neuropathol.* 2014;128(4):605-607.

17. Langmoen IA, Lundar T, Storm-Mathisen I, et al. Management of pediatric pontine gliomas. *Childs Nerv Syst.* 1991;7(1):13-15.

18. Jennings MT, Sposto R, Boyett JM, et al. Preradiation chemotherapy in primary high-risk brainstem tumors: phase II study CCG-9941 of the Childrens Cancer Group. *J Clin Oncol.* 2002;20(16):3431-3437.

19. Bouffet E, Raquin M, Doz F, et al. Radiotherapy followed by high dose busulfan and thiotepa: a prospective assessment of high dose chemotherapy in children with diffuse pontine gliomas. *Cancer.* 2000;88(3):685-692.

20. Jalali R, Raut N, Arora B, et al. Prospective evaluation of radiotherapy with concurrent and adjuvant temozolomide in children with newly diagnosed diffuse intrinsic pontine glioma. *Int J Radiat Oncol Biol Phys.* 2010;77(1):113-118.

21. Cohen KJ, Jabado N, Grill J. Diffuse intrinsic pontine gliomas-current management and new biologic insights. Is there a glimmer of hope? *Neuro Oncol.* 2017;19(8):1025-1034.

22. Schroeder KM, Hoeman CM, Becher OJ. Children are not just little adults: recent advances in understanding of diffuse intrinsic pontine glioma biology. *Pediatr Res.* 2014;75(1):205-209.

30 Not Actin' Right: Lacunar Infarct and Pediatric Stroke

ROBERT VEZZETTI, MD, FAAP, FACEP and BHAIRAV PATEL, MD

Case Presentation

A 17-year-old male presents with right-sided facial numbness and extremity weakness that has been intermittent for the past 1 month. Several hours ago, the patient noted he had difficulty ambulating when rising out of bed due to the weakness, causing him to fall. He was able to prevent injury by steadying himself on a chair. He went back to lie down and then called his mother, who noted that he had slurred speech. He was taken to an outside facility after being transported by emergency medical services. There, he was told he was "fine" and was discharged home. His mother then brought him for evaluation to your department after he felt weak and was having slurred speech again; he also was noted to have a right facial droop. He denies visual changes, ataxic episodes, altered consciousness, recent illness, and recent trauma. He has no significant medical or familial history.

Physical examination reveals a well-appearing patient in no distress. He has age-appropriate vital signs including his blood pressure. His physical examination is remarkable for right facial droop, tongue deviation to the right, and right upper extremity weakness. He has no other neurologic deficits.

Imaging Considerations

Pediatric patients presenting with symptoms concerning for a stroke or who have previously had a stroke and there is concern for recurrence should undergo imaging as soon as possible.[1] There are several options available to the clinician.

COMPUTED TOMOGRAPHY (CT)/CT ANGIOGRAPHY (CTA)/CT VENOGRAPHY (CTV)

This imaging modality is rapid and available but does involve exposure to ionizing radiation. Unenhanced CT is useful in detecting hemorrhage and changes of ischemic stroke within 6 hours after the onset of the ischemic process, although prior to this, the study may be unremarkable.[1,2] The sensitivity and specificity of CT for pediatric stroke have not been validated in studies, but expert opinion for its use has been based on extrapolation and application from existing adult data.[1] Non—contrast CT is the initial imaging modality in patients with a history and examination concerning for hemorrhagic and, in some cases, ischemic stroke.

CTA and perfusion studies may also be performed in children with suspected ischemic events and are often utilized in patients in whom magnetic resonance imaging (MRI) might be contraindicated, such as those with cochlear implants or other medical devices that are not MRI compatible.[1] CTV is very useful in detecting cavernous sinus thrombosis.[3,4]

MRI/MRI-ANGIOGRAM (MRA)–VENOGRAM (MRV)

MRI is an excellent modality for imaging patients with concerns for an ischemic event. A typical standard stroke protocol includes fluid attenuated inversion recovery (FLAIR), diffusion-weighted imaging, and susceptibility-weighted imaging (SWI) and T1 sequences.[2] Certain sequences of MRI are highly sensitive in the detection of parenchymal hemorrhage, subarachnoid hemorrhage (FLAIR and SWI sequences particularly), and, using perfusion techniques, cerebral blood flow, cerebral blood volume, and transit times.[1,2,5] MRA and MRV can be used to evaluate cerebral blood vessel patency and evaluate vascular anatomy, and vascular imaging should be obtained when the cause of stroke is suspected to be ischemic or hemorrhagic.[1–3] MRI is more sensitive than CT for acute ischemia and is better at evaluating the posterior fossa and can be useful in diagnosing stroke mimics.[3]

The International Pediatric Stroke Study Neuroimaging Consortium recommends MRI as a first-line imaging study.[3,4] Due to the time required to perform the study, sedation, especially in younger patients, may be required. There are fast-acquisition protocols that some institutions have implemented, but this is still a 20-minute study, and sedation, even when these protocols are utilized, may still be required.[3]

ULTRASOUND (US)

This modality is useful in neonates or infants with open fontanelles, allowing for imaging of the cerebral parenchyma, although visualization of the posterior fossa may be limited.[1] Ischemic injury of the parenchyma may be seen as areas of increased echogenicity with mass effect.[1] However, US has been shown to be less sensitive compared to CT and MRI in detecting ischemic lesions.[1,6] While this limits the usefulness of cranial US in detecting ischemia, the availability, lack of ionizing radiation, and portability of this modality make it useful in neonates to evaluate parenchymal hemorrhage, intraventricular hemorrhage, and gross anatomic evaluation of the cerebrum in neonates.

CATHETER ANGIOGRAPHY

Cerebral angiography is useful in evaluating vascular malformations and is an accurate modality to evaluate the cerebral vasculature, providing great detail about blood vessels, including smaller vessels and branches, although the likelihood of identifying a vascular abnormality in patients with a normal MRI scan is low.[1,7] Angiography can also be therapeutic if neurointerventional radiology specialists are available. However, there are several limitations to the utilization of this test. Catheter angiography is often available only at specialty pediatric centers and sedation may be required in young children since the risk of arterial injury during the procedure is higher in uncooperative children.[1]

Imaging Findings

With the history and physical examination, the decision was made to obtain imaging. An MRI study of the brain, with and without intravenous contrast, was obtained. Selected images from that study are provided here. These images demonstrate a focal area of restricted diffusion involving the left corpus striatum and left corona radiata without evidence of acute hemorrhage and a suspected chronic lacunar infarct within the left thalamocapsular region (Figs. 30.1 and 30.2).

Case Conclusion

Pediatric Neurology was consulted. The patient also underwent CTA of the head and neck, which were normal. The

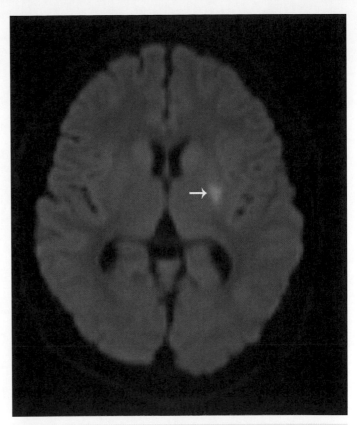

Fig. 30.2 Magnetic resonance imaging (axial diffusion-weighted image) demonstrating an area of restricted diffusion involving the left corpus striatum/left corona radiata without acute hemorrhage (white arrow).

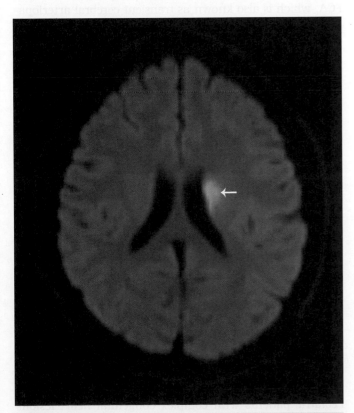

Fig. 30.1 Magnetic resonance imaging (axial diffusion-weighted image) demonstrating an area of restricted diffusion involving the left corpus striatum/left corona radiata without acute hemorrhage (white arrow).

patient was initially started on unfractionated heparin and Pediatric Hematology was also consulted. After extensive discussion between the family and the consultants, the patient was transitioned to aspirin. His symptoms resolved within 48 hours. He was carefully monitored by Pediatric Neurology and Pediatric Hematology and had no further symptoms. Follow-up imaging (selected images provided here) demonstrates encephalomacia and gliosis in the location of previous acute infarction (Figs. 30.3 and 30.4).

Stroke is a cerebrovascular event that may be ischemic or hemorrhagic. While approximately 80% of adult strokes are ischemic, only approximately 55% of pediatric strokes are ischemic.[1,7–9] The incidence of pediatric stroke has been reported to be 2–3/100,000 children per year in the United States.[10,11] Over one-half of pediatric patients who have suffered a stroke will have cognitive and motor disabilities and up to one-third will have recurrent stroke.[9] Lacunar infarctions are not commonly seen in the pediatric population. Lacunar strokes involve a branch of a cerebral artery that, when occluded, produces a small noncortical infarction. These branches originate from the Circle of Willis, middle cerebral artery, or the basilar artery.

There are comorbidities that are associated with ischemic and hemorrhagic stroke in pediatric patients. These include sickle cell disease, vascular anomalies, hypertension, congenital heart disease, head and neck trauma, coagulation disorders, and infection.[1,6,10,12–15] Vascular wall injuries are also a risk factor for ischemic stroke in this population.[11] About one-half of pediatric patients have a

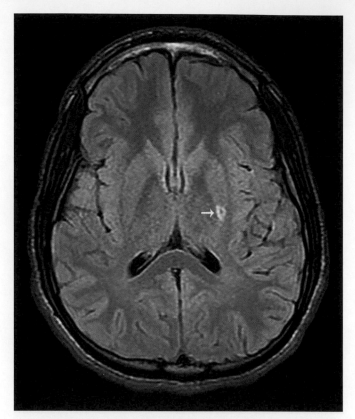

Fig. 30.3 Follow-up magnetic resonance imaging (axial fluid attenuated inversion recovery sequence) demonstrating encephalomacia and gliosis in the location of previous acute infarction *(white arrow)*.

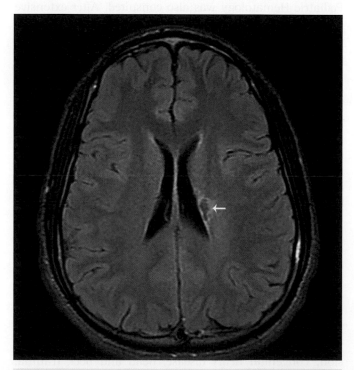

Fig. 30.4 Follow-up magnetic resonance imaging (axial fluid attenuated inversion recovery sequence) demonstrating encephalomacia and gliosis in the location of previous acute infarction *(white arrow)*.

previously identified risk factor for stroke at the time of infarction, and after a complete evaluation, up to two-thirds have more than one identifiable risk factor; however, up to one-third of pediatric patients with stroke do not have an apparent underling etiology.[1,9,13]

SICKLE CELL DISEASE

Patients with sickle cell disease carry a higher risk of stroke compared to the general population. In sickle cell patients with stroke, 60% to 90% will have abnormalities of the cerebral vasculature on angiography or MRA, including stenosis and occlusion.[10,16,17]

VASCULAR ANOMALIES/ANEURYSMS

Symptomatic aneurysms are not common in pediatric patients.[1] Cerebral aneurysms can be associated with genetic conditions, such as Ehlers-Danlos syndrome, coarctation of the aorta, and autosomal dominant polycystic kidney disease. Pediatric patients may present with subarachnoid, intraventricular, or intracerebral hemorrhage, and vascular anomalies are present in a wide age range, including newborns.[1] One study demonstrated that 70% of children with vascular anomalies had recurrent stroke, whereas children without vascular anomalies had none.[8]

FOCAL CEREBRAL ARTERIOPATHY

One of the most common causes of stroke in a previously healthy child is focal cerebral arteriopathy of childhood, or FCA, which is also known as transient cerebral arteriopathy. The exact pathophysiology is not well understood. This is an acute, monophasic disease causing unilateral stenosis of the intracranial cerebral arteries, mainly involving the anterior circulation and places the child at high risk for recurrent stroke (up to 25% within 1 year).[18–20] Herpes viruses, especially varicella and herpes virus simplex 1, have been identified as a possible trigger of FCA, secondary to inflammation of the walls of affected arterial segments.[19,20–22] Pediatric patients with FCA can have rapid progression over days to weeks, and rapid progression is associated with a risk of recurrent ischemia.[19,21,23] Patients with enhancing arteriopathies on vessel wall imaging have been shown to have a higher risk of arteriopathy progression than those without enhancement.[19,21,23]

HYPERTENSION

Hypertension is a known risk factor for stroke in the adult population and may be a risk factor for stroke in pediatric patients.[8,9,12,13] One case series of pediatric patients demonstrated a significant association between blood pressure greater than the 90th percentile and cerebral arterial abnormalities.[13]

CARDIAC DISEASE

Pediatric patients with complex congenital heart lesions with right-to-left shunting and cyanosis are prone to stroke, but stroke can be associated with any heart lesion.[1] Stroke is more common among patients with uncorrected heart disease.[1,24] Stroke may also be seen in patients with valvular heart disease as a result of infection (e.g., rheumatic fever), those with prosthetic heart valves, and as a complication of cardiac catheterization procedures.

TRAUMA

Carotid artery or vertebral artery dissection as a result of a traumatic injury is a recognized risk factor for stroke.[10]

HEMATOCRIT ABNORMALITIES/COAGULOPATHIES

Abnormal hematocrit is a risk factor for the development of stroke. Patients with low hematocrit (commonly seen in pediatric patients with iron deficiency) are at high risk for arterial stroke, while those with an elevated hematocrit are at risk for central venous thrombosis.[1] Coagulation disorders and thrombocytopenia are risk factors for pediatric hemorrhagic stroke, and the degree of severity of the underlying disorder correlates with risk of hemorrhage.[1,25] In a review of the association between stroke and iron deficiency anemia, previously healthy children with stroke were significantly more likely to have iron-deficiency anemia and children with iron deficiency anemia accounted for more than half of stroke cases in the study population (children 12 to 389 months of age).[26] A case control study found previously healthy children with stroke were 10 times more likely to have iron-deficiency anemia than healthy children without stroke and children with iron-deficiency anemia accounted for more than half of all stroke cases in children without an underlying medical illness.[26]

INFECTION

In the pediatric population, stroke has been associated with infection. Recent varicella infection has been shown to be associated with stroke involving the middle cerebral artery.[10,13] Patients with prior immunodeficiency or leukocytosis are at risk for stroke as well.[10,27] In patients with otitis media and meningitis, dural sinus venous thrombosis may be a complication, although this entity is not exclusive to infectious processes and may be a result of other underlying conditions, including autoimmune diseases, anemias, prothrombotic disorders, and metabolic conditions. Intracranial complications from infection may present with subdural effusion or hematoma, subarachnoid hemorrhage, or intracerebral hemorrhage; often, clinical signs are nonspecific, such as seizure and headache.[1,28-30]

The NIH Pediatric Stroke Scale (PedNIHSS) is an adaptation of the adult NIH Stroke Scale (NIHSS) and designed for use in children 2 years and older with concerns for ischemic stroke (hemorrhagic stroke has not been validated). The NIHSS has been used to quantitate stroke severity and outcomes at 7 and 90 days.[31,32] The PedNIHSS closely resembles the NIHSS. A multicenter cohort study found that the PedNIHSS demonstrated excellent interrater reliability and may be predictive of future disability.[32,33] An online tool is available to calculate this score at https://www.mdcalc.com/pediatric-nih-stroke-scale-nihss.

The management of pediatric stroke depends on the underlying etiology. It is important to note that there are no standardized treatment protocols for the treatment of acute pediatric stroke. A notable exception to this is the management of sickle cell disease patients. Stroke in these patients is managed with hydration, correction of underlying metabolic derangements (such as hypoxemia), and exchange transfusion.[1,10,33] In general, acute management of pediatric stroke may include the use of antiinflammatory medications (such as aspirin or steroids) and antithrombotic therapies (such as low-molecular-weight heparin or warfarin).[1,10] Treatment strategies are based on limited pediatric studies, expert opinion, anecdotal evidence, and adult studies; they are designed to treat the immediate stroke but also to prevent recurrence, which occurs in up to 25% of patients.[1] Regardless of the etiology of the ischemic event, management includes providing oxygen for hypoxemic patients, maintaining normothermia, addressing electrolyte abnormalities, providing rehydration, treating anemia, and treating seizures, although there is no strong evidence that routine administration of antiepileptic medications for seizure prophylaxis in the absence of seizures is beneficial.[1] Hypothermic measures are not recommended.[1] Studies have indicated that having an established pediatric stroke protocol benefits patients with rapid diagnosis, including decreased time to imaging and decreased time to treatment.[34,35]

Thrombolytic therapy is a particularly interesting area of pediatric ischemic stroke treatment. Low-molecular-weight heparin is preferred over unfractionated heparin because it is easier to administer and monitor but has the disadvantage of being more difficult to reverse rapidly.[1,36] Both of these medications are used for short-term anticoagulation; long-term anticoagulation can be achieved with low-molecular-weight heparin or warfarin.[1,37] Aspirin may be another option in patients without sickle cell disease who do not have a hypercoagulable disorder.[1] Tissue plasminogen activator (tPA) has not been well studied in pediatric patients. There have been case reports of its use in pediatric patients.[38-40] It may be reasonable to consider use of tPA if certain criteria are met, such as persistent disabling neurologic deficits or radiographically confirmed cerebral large artery occlusion.[33] Until more definitive data are available, routine use of tPA is not recommended and consultation with a pediatric neurologist is reasonable. Endovascular thrombectomy has also been explored as an acute thrombolytic therapy and may be useful in the pediatric population, given concerns about introducing catheters into small groin and cerebral arteries, size-based limitations on contrast dye, and radiation exposure.[41] Since safety and efficacy data are lacking and there are no definitive guidelines regarding thrombectomy in pediatric patients, consultation with an expert in the care of pediatric stroke is reasonable if this therapy is being considered. Aneurysms in pediatric patients are treated much in the same manner as in adults. Microsurgical and endovascular techniques are utilized.[1,42,43] Consultation with Pediatric Neurosurgery can be helpful in the management of these patients.

Corticosteroids are used with increasing frequency in children with FCA, although the evidence for this is not abundant.[18,44] One study in particular demonstrated improvement in children with FCA treated with a combination of steroid and antithrombotic therapy versus antithrombotic therapy alone, finding lower levels of neurologic impairment in the combination therapy group.[45] However, one must balance the possible benefits of the use of corticosteroid therapy with the potential worsening of an existing infectious process.

Management of hemorrhagic stroke is extrapolated from adult studies. Generally, management or blood pressure to prevent hypotension, strategies to prevent increased intracranial pressure, and hyperosmotic agents (hypertonic saline) are utilized.[3] Prevention of further bleeding can be done with transfusion of platelets, clotting factors, fresh frozen plasma, or vitamin K, depending on the etiology of the bleeding.[3] Reversal of antithrombotic therapy may be indicated and there are a variety of agents available for this purpose. If clinically indicated, surgical craniectomy can be performed when there is a need for decompression (brainstem compression, bleeds >3 cm, hydrocephalus).[3,46]

IMAGING PEARLS

1. Initial imaging in patients with suspected stroke may be with CT or MRI:
   • CT (non—contrast) brain + CTA head ± neck (in cases of suspected carotid dissection).
   • MRI brain + MRA head ± neck.
2. CT is rapid and readily available. This modality can detect hemorrhage as well as changes of acute ischemic events.
3. CTA can be utilized to evaluate vascular anatomy and relative cerebral blood flow.
4. MRI is an excellent imaging modality to evaluate cerebral ischemic events. Using different sequences, MRI can evaluate cerebral blood flow, the presence of hemorrhage, and cerebral vasculature.
5. Catheter angiography can be used to evaluate the cerebral vasculature and for interventional procedures but often requires sedation and carries a risk of vascular injury during the procedure.

References

1. Roach ES, Golomb MR, Adams R, et al. Management of stroke in infants and children. *Stroke.* 2008;39(1):2644-2691.
2. Heit JJ, Iv M, Wintermark M. Imaging of intracranial hemorrhage. *J Stroke.* 2017;19(1):11-27.
3. Buckwoski A, Rose E. Pediatric stroke: diagnosis and management in the emergency department. *Pediatr Emerg Med Pract.* 2019;16(11):1-20.
4. Mirsky DM, Beslow LA, Amlie-Leford, et al. Pathways for neuroimaging of childhood stroke. *Pediatr Neurol.* 2017;69:11-23.
5. Mitchell P, Wilkinson ID, Hoggard N, et al. Detection of subarachnoid haemorrhage with magnetic resonance imaging. *J Neurol Neurosurg Psychiatry.* 2001;70:205-211.
6. Golomb MR, Dick PT, MacGregor DL, et al. Cranial ultrasonography has a low sensitivity for detecting arterial ischemic stroke in term neonates. *J Child Neurol.* 2003;18(2):98-103.
7. Husson B, Rodesch G, Lasjaunias P, et al. Magnetic resonance angiography in childhood arterial brain infarcts: a comparative study with contrast angiography. *Stroke.* 2002;33(5):1280-1285.
8. Kupferman JC, Singh A, Pavlakis SG. Lacunar stroke and masked hypertension in an adolescent male. *Pediatr Neurol.* 2007;36(2):125-127.
9. Lynch JK, Hirtz DG, Deveber G, et al. Report of the National Institute of Neurological Disorders and Stroke Workshop on perinatal and childhood stroke. *Pediatrics.* 2002;109(1):116-123.
10. Seidman C, Kirkham F, Pavlakis S. Pediatric stroke: current developments. *Curr Opin Pediatr.* 2007;19(6):657-662.
11. Laugesaar R, Kolk A, Tomberg T, et al. Acutely and retrospectively diagnosed perinatal stroke: a population-based study. *Stroke.* 2007;38(8):2234-2238.
12. Nowak-Gottl U, Gunther G, Kurnik K, et al. Arterial ischemic stroke in neonates, infants and children: an overview of underlying conditions, imaging methods and treatment modalities. *Semin Thromb Hemost.* 2003;29(4):405-414.
13. Ganesan V, Prengler M, McShane MA, et al. Investigation of risk factors in children with arterial ischemic stroke. *Ann Neurol.* 2003;53(2):167-173.
14. Lynch JK, Han CJ. Pediatric stroke: What do we know and what do we need to know? *Semin Neurol.* 2005;25(4):410-423.
15. Kirkham F, Sebire G, Strater R. Arterial ischaemic stroke in children: review of the literature and strategies for future stroke studies. *Thromb Haemost.* 2004;92(4):697-706.
16. Kirkham FJ, Calamante F, Bynevelt M, et al. Perfusion magnetic resonance abnormalities in patients with sickle cell disease. *Ann Neurol.* 2001;49(4):477-485.
17. Kirkham FJ. Therapy insight: stroke risk and its management in patients with sickle cell disease. *Nat Clin Pract Neurol.* 2007;3(5):264-278.
18. Fullerton HJ, Wu YW, Sidney S, et al. Risk of recurrent childhood arterial ischemic stroke in a population-based cohort: the importance of cerebrovascular imaging. *Pediatrics.* 2007;119(3):495-501.
19. Fullerton HJ, Stence N, Hills NK, et al. Focal cerebral arteriopathy of childhood: novel severity score and natural history. *Stroke.* 2018;49(11):2590-2596.
20. Fullerton HJ, Wintermark M, Hills NK, et al. Risk of recurrent arterial ischemic stroke in childhood: a prospective international study. *Stroke.* 2016;47(1):53-59.
21. Stence NV, Pabst LL, Hollatz AL, et al. Predicting progression of intracranial arteriopathies in childhood stroke with vessel wall imaging. *Stroke.* 2017;48(8):2274-2277.
22. Elkind MS, Hills NK, Glaser CA, et al. Herpesvirus infections and childhood arterial ischemic stroke: results of the VIPS study. *Circulation.* 2016;133(8):732-741.
23. Braun KP, Bulder MM, Chabrier S, et al. The course and outcome of unilateral intracranial arteriopathy in 79 children with ischaemic stroke. *Brain.* 2009;132(Pt 2):544-557.
24. Kumar K. Neurological complications of congenital heart disease. *Indian J Pediatr.* 2000;67(4):287-291.
25. Ghosh K, Nair AP, Jijina F, et al. Intracranial haemorrhage in severe haemophilia: prevalence and outcome in a developing country. *Haemophilia.* 2005;11(5):459-462.
26. Maguire JL, deVeber G, Parkin PC. Association between iron-deficiency anemia and stroke in young children. *Pediatrics.* 2007;120(5):1053-1057.
27. Ganesan V, Prengler M, Wade A, et al. Clinical and radiological recurrence after childhood arterial ischemic stroke. *Circulation.* 2006;114(20):2170-2177.
28. Biousse V, Ameri A, Bousser MG. Isolated intracranial hypertension as the only sign of cerebral venous thrombosis. *Neurology.* 1999;53(7):1537-1542.
29. Cumurciuc R, Crassard I, Sarov M, et al. Headache as the only neurological sign of cerebral venous thrombosis: a series of 17 cases. *J Neurol Neurosurg Psychiatry.* 2005;76(8):1084-1087.
30. Marquardt G, Weidauer S, Lanfermann H, et al. Cerebral venous sinus thrombosis manifesting as bilateral subdural effusion. *Acta Neurol Scand.* 2004;109(6):425-428.
31. Adams Jr HP, Davis PH, Leira EC, et al. Baseline NIH Stroke Scale score strongly predicts outcome after stroke: a report of the Trial of Org 10172 in Acute Stroke Treatment (TOAST). *Neurology.* 1999;53(1):126-131.
32. Beslow LA, Kasner SE, Smith SE, et al. Concurrent validity and reliability of retrospective scoring of the Pediatric National Institutes of Health Stroke Scale. *Stroke.* 2012;43(2):341-345.
33. Ichord RN, Bastian R, Abraham L, et al. Interrater reliability of the Pediatric National Institutes of Health Stroke Scale (PedNIHSS) in a multicenter study. *Stroke.* 2011;42(3):613-617.
34. Shack M, Andrade A, Shah-Basak PP, et al. A pediatric institutional acute stroke protocol improves timely access to stroke treatment. *Dev Med Child Neurol.* 2017;59(1):31-37.
35. DeLaroche AM, Siviswamy L, Farooqi A, et al. A pediatric stroke clinical pathway improves the time to diagnosis in an emergency department. *Pediatr Neurol.* 2016;65:39-44.
36. Massicotte P, Adams M, Marzinotto V, et al. Low-molecular-weight heparin in pediatric patients with thrombotic disease: a dose finding study. *J Pediatr.* 1996;128(3):313-318.

37. Monagle P, Chan A, Massicotte P, et al. Antithrombotic therapy in children: the Seventh ACCP Conference on Antithrombotic and Thrombolytic Therapy. *Chest.* 2004;126(suppl 3):645S-687S.

38. Carlson MD, Leber S, Deveikis J, et al. Successful use of rt-PA in pediatric stroke. *Neurology.* 2001;57(1):157-158.

39. Thirumalai SS, Shubin RA. Successful treatment for stroke in a child using recombinant tissue plasminogen activator. *J Child Neurol.* 2000;15(8):558.

40. Medley TL, Miteff C, Andrews I, et al. Australian clinical consensus guideline: the diagnosis and acute management of childhood stroke. *Int J Stroke.* 2019;14(1):94-106.

41. Ferriero DM, Fullerton HJ, Bernard TJ, et al. Management of stroke in neonates and children: a scientific statement from the American Heart Association/American Stroke Association. *Stroke.* 2019; 50(3):e51-e96.

42. Sanai N, Quinones-Hinojosa A, Gupta NM, et al. Pediatric intracranial aneurysms: durability of treatment following microsurgical and endovascular management. *J Neurosurg.* 2006;104(suppl 2): 82-89.

43. Buis DR, van Ouwerkerk WJ, Takahata H, et al. Intracranial aneurysms in children under 1 year of age: a systematic review of the literature. *Childs Nerv Syst.* 2006;22(11):1395-1409.

44. Steinlin M, Bigi S, Stojanovski B, et al, and the Swiss NeuroPediatric Stroke Registry. Focal cerebral arteriopathy: do steroids improve outcome? *Stroke.* 2017;48(9):2375-2382.

45. Fearn ND, Mackay MT. Focal cerebral arteriopathy and childhood stroke. *Curr Opin Neurol.* 2020;33(1):37-46.

46. Lo WD. Childhood hemorrhagic stroke: an important but understudied problem. *J Child Neurol.* 2011;26(9):1174-1185.

31 *Hard to Wake Up: Cerebritis*

ROBERT VEZZETTI, MD, FAAP, FACEP

Case Presentation

A 20-month-old patient presents with decreased activity, including eating and drinking, over the past 2 days. He is currently completing a second course of oral antibiotics for acute otitis media and 1 week ago completed a 10-day course of cefdinir. He was especially sleepy today, per the parents, who decided to bring him to his primary care physician for evaluation. He was also found to have a temperature of 101 degrees Fahrenheit in the office. While en route to the office, the patient was noted to be staring ahead without interacting with his parents; he then developed right hand and arm twitching, which lasted for several minutes, then resolved. After the event, he has remained difficult to arouse. The parents state that he is an otherwise healthy child who has all of his recommended immunizations. They deny any possibility of ingestion or trauma.

His physical examination in the emergency department reveals an afebrile child who is in no acute distress but is quite sleepy and difficult to awaken. He has a heart rate of 130 beats per minute, a respiratory rate of 25 breaths per minute, and a blood pressure of 90/60 mm Hg; his oxygen saturation is 95% on room air. He has no signs of obvious trauma. His pupils are 3 mm, equal and reactive; he appears to have photophobia. His tympanic membranes and oropharynx are all clear. His cardiovascular and abdominal examinations are unremarkable. It is difficult to conduct a neurologic examination due to the child's sleepiness, but he is moving all of his extremities, and grossly, the tone and strength appear to be equal. There are no skin lesions or rashes.

Imaging Considerations

Patients with suspected intracranial pathology often undergo neuroimaging as part of a medical evaluation.

COMPUTED TOMOGRAPHY (CT)

Non–contrast-enhanced CT is an imaging test often utilized in patients with concerns for intracranial pathology. In its initial stages, cerebritis appears as an area of low attenuation; edema may be present.[1] If intravenous contrast is used, CT may show patchy enhancement.[1] CT is widely available and has the advantage of rapidity, usually obviating the need for sedation. However, CT does expose the patient to ionizing radiation.

Initially, CT in patients with cerebritis may appear normal. As the process progresses, a poorly defined area of cortical or subcortical hypodensity may be noted, accompanied by edema and mass effect of varying degrees.[1-3] As the

disease progresses, a better defined area of hypodensity with some ring enhancement may be seen.[1-3]

MAGNETIC RESONANCE IMAGING (MRI)

MRI is more sensitive than CT in the detection of early changes seen in cerebritis.[1-3] In early cerebritis, MRI will demonstrate iso- or hypointense signals on T1-weighted imaging; T2-weighted signal imaging or fluid attenuated inversion recovery (FLAIR) sequences will demonstrate increased signal intensity and vasogenic edema.[1-3] Late-stage cerebritis on MRI is demonstrated by progressive enhancement without obvious abscess.[1-3]

Diffusion-weighted imaging can prove useful in the detection of cerebritis and subsequent brain abscess.[4] On diffusion-weighted imaging, areas of cerebritis demonstrate restricted diffusion. Low diffusion coefficient values strongly suggest the presence of infection, including pus and abscess.

Imaging Findings

The patient underwent non–contrast-enhanced cranial CT. A selected image from this study is provided. There is low attenuation in the left frontal lobe without evidence of hemorrhage (Fig. 31.1).

Case Conclusion

The results of the CT prompted MRI of the brain, with and without intravenous contrast. An MR arteriogram (MRA) and magnetic resonance venogram (MRV) were also obtained, since the CT findings can be attributed to an infectious or vascular process. Selected images are provided. The MRA/MRV studies were normal. The MRI demonstrated restricted diffusion, abnormal enhancement, and abnormal T2-weighted signal within the left frontal cortex, suggesting cerebritis (Figs. 31.2 and 31.3).

The patient was admitted to the pediatric intensive care unit. Intravenous antibiotics were initiated and a lumbar puncture was performed, since there was no sign of abscess or increased intracranial pressure. MRI 10 days later revealed interval development of a small left frontal subdural fluid collection and a decrease in previously noted signal abnormality in the left frontal lobe (Fig. 31.4). The child gradually improved and was discharged with anticonvulsant therapy and three additional weeks of intravenous antibiotics provided through a peripherally inserted central catheter line. Spinal fluid cultures revealed *Streptococcus pneumoniae*, which was pan-sensitive to antibiotics. The child underwent an immunology evaluation, which was

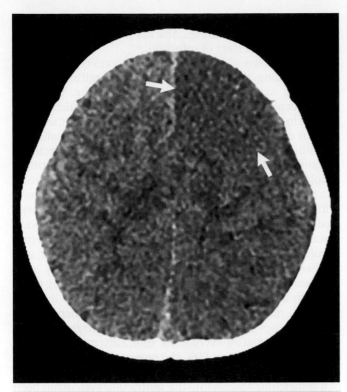

Fig. 31.1 Non–contrast-enhanced axial computed tomography image demonstrating low attenuation in the left frontal lobe *(arrows)* consistent with cerebritis.

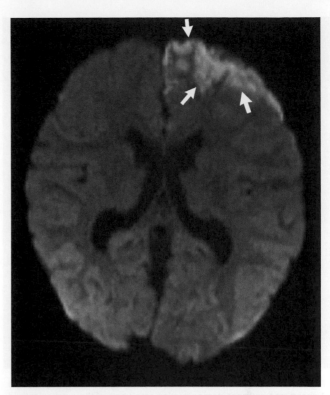

Fig. 31.3 Axial magnetic resonance imaging (diffusion-weighted sequence) demonstrating increased signal of restricted diffusion within the left frontal cortex *(arrows)*.

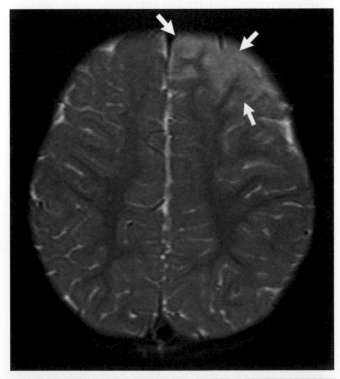

Fig. 31.2 Axial magnetic resonance imaging (T2-weighted image) demonstrating abnormal increased signal within the left frontal lobe *(arrows)*.

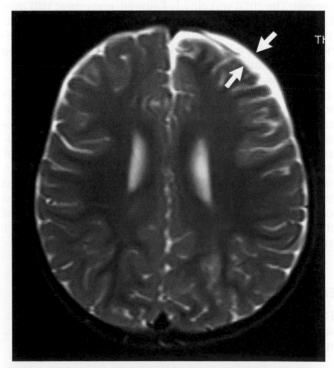

Fig. 31.4 Magnetic resonance imaging (axial T2-weighted image) demonstrating interval development of a small subdural fluid collection *(arrows)* over the left frontal lobe. Previously noted abnormal signal and swelling in the left frontal lobe is no longer seen.

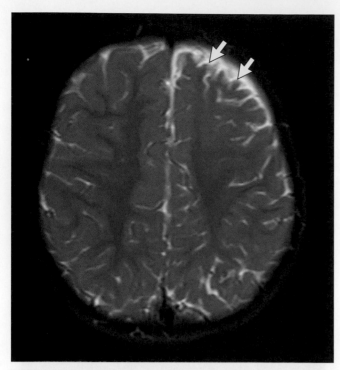

Fig. 31.5 Axial magnetic resonance imaging (T2-weighted image) 1 year post treatment demonstrating resolution of the extra-axial fluid collection and volume loss/encephalomalacia *(arrows)* in the anterior left frontal lobe, at the prior site of cerebritis.

of the involved tissue. From this stage, progression to a cerebral abscess is possible. Abscess formation may occur 2 weeks from the start of infection.

The symptoms of cerebritis mimic a variety of pathologies, including viral syndrome and meningitis. Common presenting symptoms include fever, headache, vomiting, focal neurologic findings, and seizures; many patients present late in the disease course.[1,5,7,8] The location of the development of a brain abscess is dependent on the location of the initial cerebritis.[7] Management of cerebritis is directed at the suspected underlying cause. Antimicrobial treatment should be directed at the most likely pathologic organism. Since meningitis can present with symptoms similar to cerebritis, performance of a lumbar puncture may be considered. In patients with focal neurologic findings or if a brain abscess is a diagnostic consideration, lumbar puncture should be delayed due to the potential risk of herniation and the likelihood of recovery of a pathogen is generally low.[7] Admission to the hospital for monitoring and ongoing treatment, in addition to subspecialty consultation, is a sound plan of care. If a brain abscess has developed, then antimicrobial therapy and prompt pediatric neurosurgical consultation is mandatory.[7] While the mortality rate of a brain abscess is around 5% to 10%, the presence of hydrocephalus due to compression from a posterior fossa abscess or rupture of a ventricular abscess into the ventricular system has been associated with a mortality rate of up to 85%.[7]

IMAGING PEARLS

1. Neuroimaging is indicated in patients with acute mental status changes in whom an intracranial process is suspected. CT and MRI are available options.
2. Non–contrast-enhanced CT is a reasonable first-line imaging choice in patients with concern for an intracranial process.
3. MRI is often used as a follow-up study in patients with abnormal CT findings or if there is a strong clinical concern for an intracranial process and initial imaging is unremarkable.

normal. The child was closely followed, and repeat MRI over 1 year post treatment demonstrates resolution of the extra-axial fluid collection, with encephalomalacia in the anterior left frontal lobe (Fig. 31.5). The child was able to be weaned off anticonvulsant therapy and did well.

Cerebritis is an area of poorly defined inflammation in the brain with increased vascular permeability.[1,2,5] This process is often due to hematogenous or localized spread of infection and is composed of vascular congestion, infiltration of inflammatory cells, and edema.[1,5,6] These components comprise the early stages of cerebritis; later stages of the disease include liquefaction and cavitary formation processes.[1] Untreated cerebritis may progress to localized brain abscess.[5,7] Up to 25% of cases of cerebritis are found in patients less than 25 years of age.[5] While a bacterial etiology is commonly found, up to 30% of cases are of undetermined etiology.[5]

Cerebritis can be divided into two main stages[1,2,7]:

EARLY CEREBRITIS

This stage is characterized by edema, vascular congestion, and coagulative necrosis. It is usually short in duration, approximately 2–3 days.

LATE CEREBRITIS

This stage usually occurs 1 week after the onset of illness. It is a progressive infection leading to the liquefaction necrosis

References

1. Rath TJ, Hughes M, Arabi M, et al. Imaging of cerebritis, encephalitis, and brain abscess. *Neuroimaging Clin N Am*. 2012;22(4):585-607.
2. Hygino de la Cruz LC. Intracranial infection. In: Atlas S, ed. *Magnetic Resonance Imaging of the Brain and Spine*, 5th ed. Philadelphia: Wolters Kluwer; 2017.
3. Smirniotopoulos JG, Murphy FM, Rushing EJ, et al. Patterns of contrast enhancement in the brain and meninges. *Radiographics*. 2007;27(2):525-551.
4. Stadnik TW, Demaerel P, Luypaert RP, et al. Imaging tutorial: differential diagnosis of bright lesions on diffusion-weighted MR images. *Radiographics*. 2003 Jan;23(1):e7.
5. Nguyen I, Urbanczyk K, Mtui E, et al. Intracranial CNS infections: a literature review and radiology case studies. *Semin Ultrasound CT MR*. 2020;41(1):106-120.
6. Lee KS, Lee BL. Cerebritis arising from acute sinusitis evolving into a large brain abscess. *Pediatr Neurol*. 2013;48(6):475-476.
7. Weinberg GA. Brain abscess. *Pediatr Rev*. 2018;39(5):270-272.
8. Shih RY, Koeller KK. Bacterial, fungal, and parasitic infections of the central nervous system: radiologic-pathologic correlation and historical perspectives: from the radiologic pathology archives. *Radiographics*. 2015;35(4):1141-1169.

32 Nothing Cute About It: Acute Flaccid Myelitis

ROBERT VEZZETTI, MD, FAAP, FACEP

Case Presentation

A 2-year-old child presents with difficulty ambulating for the past 24 hours. His parents state that the child has had fever, cough, and congestion for the past 5 days. He was seen twice by his primary care provider and diagnosed with a viral upper respiratory infection. A chest x-ray 1 day ago was interpreted as consistent with a viral process. The parents tell you that the child had had no bowel movement for the past 2 days, and today, in addition to his difficulty ambulating, he has not urinated. They also tell you that the child began to indicate soreness or discomfort in his arms and his legs.

Physical examination is remarkable for a quiet child, who, while not toxic, does not want to ambulate. He does not appear to be in obvious distress. He has a temperature of 102 degrees Fahrenheit and a heart rate of 130 beats per minute. His neurologic examination is significant for diminished strength throughout, although he is able to sit up. He appears to have equal tone. Reflexes are diminished bilaterally. Sensation is grossly intact. There are no rashes.

Imaging Considerations

COMPUTED TOMOGRAPHY (CT)

CT of the brain may be helpful in patients who present with acute mental status changes or neurologic findings. This modality is useful at detecting intracranial masses and acute hemorrhage, is widely available, and does not require sedation in the majority of instances. However, the utility of CT is limited in the evaluation of neurologic symptoms where the etiology is suspected to be infectious, such as cerebritis or encephalitis, or inflammatory, such as demyelinating disorders. If a demyelinating disorder is suspected, CT is not the imaging study of choice.

MAGNETIC RESONANCE IMAGING (MRI)

MRI is the modality of choice in patients whose neurologic symptoms are suspected to be due to an infectious etiology or a demyelinating disorder. MRI provides optimal imaging of brain and spinal cord anatomy, including gray and white matter as well as nerve roots. While the lack of ionizing radiation is advantageous, barriers to MRI use include the time necessary to complete a study and lack of immediate availability in many cases. In young children, sedation is often required to complete the study.

Imaging Findings

The child was admitted and MRI of the brain and spinal cord was obtained. Selected imaging is provided. Figs. 32.1 and 32.2 demonstrate abnormal T2 hyperintense signal of the central gray matter of essentially the entire spinal cord, most severe in the cervical spine.

Case Conclusion

The child was admitted to the hospital with a diagnosis of acute flaccid myelitis (AFM). A lumbar puncture revealed mild pleocytosis and a negative Gram stain. On admission, consultation with Pediatric Neurology and Pediatric Infectious Disease was obtained and intravenous immunoglobulin (IVIG) and intravenous steroids were begun once the MRI and cerebrospinal fluid results were known. He was initially placed in a floor bed, but his weakness rapidly progressed and there was concern about his respiratory drive and he was transferred to the pediatric intensive care unit. Gradual improvement was noted. A repeat MRI on hospital day 9 showed significant improvement in previous abnormal cord signal with minimal residual T2 hyperintense signal, remaining most prominent in the upper cervical cord (Figs. 32.3 and 32.4). At the time of discharge, the patient had improved motor strength but still had deficits. Follow-up with subspecialty services was arranged, including aggressive physical therapy with Pediatric Rehabilitation Medicine. He made a full recovery after 1 year of therapy.

AFM came to prominence after cohorts of children with clinically similar symptoms of sudden and unexplained paralysis emerged. These clusters of cases were initially reported in California (2012), then Colorado (2014), and then Utah (2014). By late 2014, 120 children from 34 states met the Centers for Disease Control and Prevention (CDC) criteria, which were acute onset of flaccid limb weakness with spinal cord or brainstem gray matter lesions.[1–3] Early on during the reporting and investigation of this entity, terms such as "poliomyelitis" or "polio-like syndrome" were coined. The term "acute flaccid myelitis" was devised to avoid confusion with symptoms caused by poliovirus.

AFM is a disorder affecting the gray matter of the brainstem and spinal cord. While there has been a wide age range of children who are affected, older children seem to be predominantly affected, with an average age of 4 to 7 years.[1,4] Most affected children appear to have been previously healthy.[1,5] There appears to be a seasonality to infection,

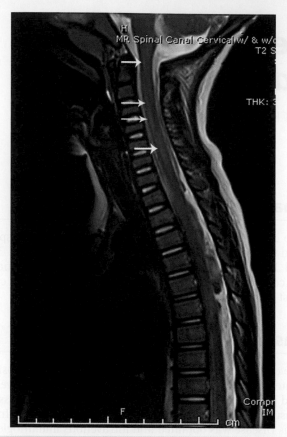

Fig. 32.1 Pretreatment magnetic resonance imaging. Sagittal T2-weighted magnetic resonance image shows T2 hyperintense signal of the central gray matter of essentially the entire spinal cord, most severe in the cervical spine (arrows).

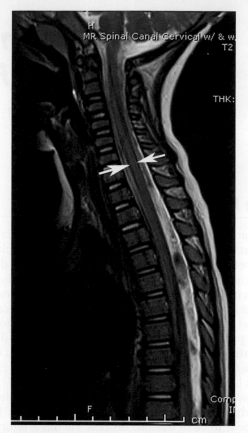

Fig. 32.2 Pretreatment magnetic resonance imaging. Sagittal T2-weighted magnetic resonance image shows T2 hyperintense signal of the central gray matter of essentially the entire spinal cord, most severe in the cervical spine (arrows).

with infections more commonly seen in later summer and fall.[6] The disorder usually starts as a febrile illness, often with symptoms of upper respiratory infection (such as rhinorrhea and cough); gastrointestinal symptoms (such as vomiting or diarrhea) are not uncommon; this is followed by limb myalgias, which occur around the time weakness develops.[1,2,6,7] There is rapid progression of limb weakness, over hours to days, which is often asymmetric, can involve any of the limbs (although there is a propensity for upper limb involvement), and ranges from mild to complete paralysis.[1–3,5–8] Other reported symptoms from the original cohort groups have been variable, including accompanying numbness,[1,7] cranial nerve dysfunction (hypotonia, dysarthria, and dysphagia),[1,2,7] constipation or other bowel dysfunction and bladder dysfunction, and altered mental status.[1,2,5,7]

The exact cause of AFM remains unknown; however, a possible association with various viruses, including rhinovirus, respiratory syncytial virus, parainfluenza virus, and adenovirus, which have all been isolated from patients diagnosed with AFM, is currently being explored.[1,2,5,7] There is an intriguing possibility of infection with enterovirus D68 and the development of AFM, since this virus was isolated from many patients with AFM and in several cases was the only virus found.[1–3,5–8] Increased circulation of this virus occurred during the time of increased identification

of AFM, during late summer and fall. Conversely, in 2015, when enterovirus D68 was not in high circulation, there were no cases in the United States and only 21 cases of AFM were diagnosed worldwide. In 2016, there were 122 cases identified in the United States, coinciding with increased enterovirus D68 activity.[9,10] Notably, not all patients test positive for enterovirus D68, although this may be due to late specimen collection; more investigation is needed to establish this link.[1,3,4]

There are standard diagnostic criteria that have been promulgated by the CDC, based on historical and clinical examination, including cerebrospinal fluid and MRI findings. Clinical criteria consistent with the diagnosis of AFM are[1–3,5–7]:

1. Acute onset of flaccid limb paralysis.
2. Spinal cord lesion on MRI largely restricted to gray matter and spanning one or more spinal segments.

The clinical criteria for the diagnosis of a probable AFM include:

1. Acute onset of flaccid limb paralysis.
2. Cerebral spinal fluid pleocytosis.

Patients with AFM have characteristic MRI findings. Lesions noted on MRI do not enhance with gadolinium and are seen optimally on a T2 series; poorly defined signal

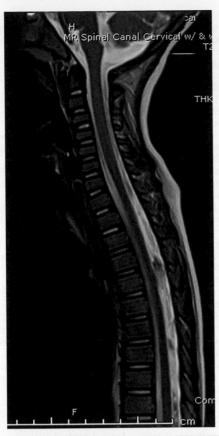

Fig. 32.3 Posttreatment magnetic resonance imaging. Sagittal T2-weighted magnetic resonance images 9 days later show significant improvement in previous abnormal cord signal with only minimal residual T2 hyperintense signal, remaining most prominent in the cervical spine.

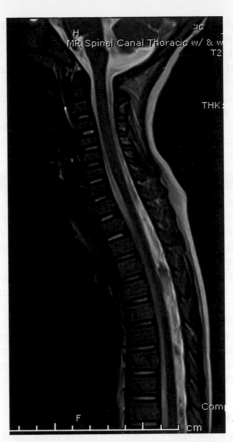

Fig. 32.4 Posttreatment magnetic resonance imaging. Sagittal T2-weighted magnetic resonance images 9 days later show significant improvement in previous abnormal cord signal with only minimal residual T2 hyperintense signal, remaining most prominent in the cervical spine

abnormalities are seen in the gray matter of the spinal cord in most cases, which, with disease progression, become better defined in the anterior horn cell area.[1,3,4,8,11] These lesions involve multiple segments of the spinal cord in the majority of patients. The cervical region is commonly involved, although affected areas can extend throughout the entire length of the cord.[1,2,4,5,7] Lesions of the brainstem may be present if there are cranial nerve findings. The pons is most commonly involved.[11] With illness resolution, these MRI findings typically resolve as well.[1,4,8]

Treatment for AFM is controversial, and no one standard regimen exists at this time. Supportive care is universally recommended.[1–3,5,7] Management options that have been advocated include the use of IVIG, steroids, plasmapheresis, and antiviral medication.[1–3,5,7,12] Antivirals have not been shown to be effective against enterovirus D68 and should not be utilized unless a different viral etiology, such as herpesvirus, is suspected. One small case series has shown fluoxetine to have activity against enterovirus D68 and is well tolerated but did not improve neurologic outcomes.[3,13] The CDC published guidelines for the management of AFM[14]:

1. There is no specific therapy or intervention that is preferred or should be avoided.
2. Consultation with neurology and infectious disease is recommended as quickly as possible.

3. Corticosteroids have no clear efficacy in controlled trials, and use is neither recommended nor discouraged. Consideration should be given to the potential immunosuppressive effects of corticosteroid use.
4. IVIG use has not been shown to be beneficial in controlled trials, and use is neither recommended nor discouraged. Use of IVIG does not appear to be harmful.
5. Plasmapheresis has not been shown to be beneficial in controlled trials, and use is neither recommended nor discouraged. Use of plasmaphresis is not likely to be harmful.
6. Fluoxetine has not been shown to be efficacious in controlled trials and should not be routinely used.
7. Antiviral agents (e.g., acyclovir) should not be routinely used, unless there is suspected herpesvirus infection. In this case it is recommended that appropriate antiviral medications be initiated until herpesvirus infection has been excluded.
8. Interferon should not be used, as there is no indication of efficacy and it may potentially be harmful.
9. Biologic agents should not be used as there is no proven efficacy and potential for harm exists.

Outcomes following AFM are variable. Many patients do have improvement, but most have some residual functional deficits.[1,3,4,8,12,15] Upper extremity motor deficits are more severe and have been shown to be more persistent compared to lower extremity deficits. Cranial nerve deficits, while mostly recovering, were mildly persistent at 1 year after diagnosis.[15] In one study, MRI findings were not consistent with clinical findings in the months after diagnosis and did not correlate with clinical outcomes,[15] although these results have not been consistently replicated.[16] Children who have comprehensive rehabilitation intervention have been shown to have improvement in neurologic and functional outcomes.[17] Ultimately, the long-term prognosis of patients with AFM is not known.

IMAGING PEARLS

1. CT can be helpful in the evaluation of children with acute onset of weakness, mental status changes, or other focal neurologic findings, but the utility of CT for infectious or inflammatory etiologies of such symptoms is limited.

2. MRI is the modality of choice when AFM is suspected. Imaging of the brain and entire spine is recommended.

3. AFM has characteristic findings on MRI, including gray matter involvement and T2 signal abnormalities. AFM can affect the brain, most commonly the pons, and the entire spinal cord, although the cervical cord is most commonly involved, followed by the upper thoracic cord.

References

1. Messacar K, Schreiner TL, Van Haren K, et al. Acute flaccid myelitis: a clinical review of US cases 2012–2015. *Ann Neurol.* 2016;80(3): 326-338.
2. Van Haren, K, Ayscue P, Waubant E, et al. Acute flaccid myelitis of unknown etiology in California, 2012–2015. *JAMA.* 2015;314(4):2663-2671.
3. Fatemi Y, Chakraborty R. Acute flaccid myelitis: a clinical overview for 2019. *Mayo Clin Proc.* 2019;94(5):875-881.
4. Christy A, Messacar K. Acute flaccid myelitis associated with enterovirus D68: A review. *J Child Neurol.* 2019;34(9):511-516.
5. Nelson GR, Bonkowsky JL, Doll E, et al. Recognition and management of acute flaccid myelitis in children. *Pediatr Neurol.* 2016;55:17-21.
6. Helfferich J, Knoester M, Van Leer-Buter CC, et al. Acute flaccid myelitis and enterovirus D68: lessons from the past and present. *Eur J Pediatr.* 2019;178(9):1305-1315.
7. Sejvar JJ, Lopez AS, Cortese MM, et al. Acute flaccid myelitis in the United States—August–December 2014: results of nation-wide surveillance. *Clin Infect Dis.* 2016;63(6):737-745.
8. Esposito S, Chidini G, Cinnante C, et al. Acute flaccid myelitis associated with enterovirus-D68 infection in an otherwise healthy child. *Virol J.* 2017;14(1):4.
9. Massacar K, Asturias EJ, Hixon AM, et al. Enterovirus D68 and acute flaccid myelitis-evaluating the evidence for causality. *Lancet Infect Dis.* 2018;18(8):e239-e247.
10. Centers for Disease Control and Prevention. *Acute flaccid myelitis surveillance.* 2017. www.cdc.gov/acute-flaccid-myelitis. Accessed October 19, 2019.
11. Maloney JA, Mirsky DM, Messacar K, et al. MRI findings in children with acute flaccid paralysis and cranial nerve dysfunction occurring during the 2014 enterovirus D68 outbreak. *AJNR Am J Neuroradiol.* 2015;36(2):245-250.
12. Andersen EW, Kornberg AJ, Freeman JL, et al. Acute flaccid myelitis in childhood: a retrospective cohort study. *Eur J Neurol.* 2017;24(8):1077-1083.
13. Massacar K, Sillau S, Hopkins SE, et al. Safety, tolerability, and efficacy of fluoxetine as an antiviral for acute flaccid myelitis. *Neurology.* 2019;92(18):e2118-e2126.
14. CDC Acute flaccid myelitis (AFM): Clinical guidance for the acute medical treatment of AFM. www.cdc.gov/acute-flaccid-myelitis/hcp/clinical-management.html. Accessed October 19, 2019.
15. Martin JA, Messacar K, Yang ML, et al. Outcomes of Colorado children with acute flaccid myelitis at 1 year. *Neurology.* 2017; 89(2):129-137.
16. McCoy DB, Talbot JF, Wilson M, et al. MRI atlas-based measurement of spinal cord injury predicts outcome in acute flaccid myelitis. *Am J Neuroradiol.* 2017;38(2):410-417.
17. Melicosta ME, Dean J, Hagen K, et al. Acute flaccid myelitis: rehabilitation challenges and outcomes in a pediatric cohort. *J Pediatr Rehabil Med.* 2019;12(3):245-253.

33 What Headache? Pediatric Arteriovenous Malformation

ROBERT VEZZETTI, MD, FAAP, FACEP, and BHAIRAV PATEL, MD

Case Presentation

A 13-year-old male presents with acute onset of mental status changes. He was found in his room, lying facedown. Emergency medical services was called. On their arrival, the patient was conversing but appeared sleepy; he was responsive to questions but confused. He was attempting to speak but was able to manage only a few words.

Once in the Emergency Department, the patient was able to speak more easily and seemed to be more at his baseline. He reports having a left frontal headache prior to "passing out." He denies illegal substance use. He has no history of prior episodes of "passing out" and is otherwise healthy. There is no family history of sudden cardiac death but there is a cousin with epilepsy.

He continues to complain of a left frontal headache. He does remember standing up and then "the lights went out." His vital signs reveal no fever, a heart rate of 90 beats per minute, a respiratory rate of 18 breaths per minute, and a blood pressure of 112/63 mm Hg. He has a normal physical examination other than a large frontal hematoma with tenderness to palpation.

The patient states that he has been having left frontal headaches for the past 2 weeks, which he describes as "severe sometimes." He has had some morning nausea and did have nonbilious/nonbloody morning emesis 2 days ago.

Imaging Considerations

There are several imaging options available to the clinician when a pediatric patient presents with acute mental status changes. The initial imaging modality of choice may be dependent on the suspected diagnosis and institutional resources.

COMPUTED TOMOGRAPHY (CT)

Acute mental status changes in pediatric patients have a broad differential diagnosis; when an intracranial etiology is suspected, such as masses or hemorrhage, CT is an excellent first-line imaging modality. Widely available and rapid, this modality does not require sedation. In addition to hemorrhage and intracranial mass, CT can detect calcifications. If a neurovascular cause is suspected, CT angiography can provide important information about the size, location, and drainage of an arteriovenous malformation.[1] If emergent surgical intervention is required, this modality can provide needed information for surgical planning more rapidly than other modalities.

MAGNETIC RESONANCE IMAGING (MRI)

MRI (with and without contrast) and magnetic resonance angiography (MRA) are important imaging modalities that can be utilized when a neurovascular cause of a patient's presenting symptoms is suspected clinically or by CT. MRI is valuable when evaluating arteriovenous malformations for several reasons: the localization of the malformation; comparison of contrast, non—contrast, and gradient echo sequences helps to rule out other hemorrhagic lesions; MRA helps delineate the vascular anatomy of the lesion; and it can be used intraoperatively to guide surgical procedures.[1] The main obstacle to more immediate utilization of this modality is the time needed to complete the study and the common need for sedation in pediatric patients.

CEREBRAL ANGIOGRAPHY

Conventional cerebral angiography is the gold standard for diagnosing arteriovenous malformations, providing characteristics of the malformation, including location, size, associated vascular lesions, draining veins, and other vital information.[1,2] Conventional angiography also has the advantage of detecting small malformations that may not be seen on MRI or MRA.[1]

There are instances of malformations being radiographically occult; usually, these are located in the region of the middle cerebral artery.[1] Pediatric patients who present with a spontaneous intraparenchymal hemorrhage and have negative imaging studies may indeed have an arteriovenous malformation, as the resulting hematoma can compress the malformation; in this instance, delayed imaging is indicated, which can reveal the malformation as the clot resolves.[1]

Imaging Findings

The patient was observed in the Emergency Department while blood work and an electrocardiogram were obtained. With the history of recent headaches and nausea, as well as the apparent, sudden onset of the patient's collapse, the decision was made to obtain non—contrast CT of the brain. A selected image from that study is provided here. There is a subtle, ill-defined, increased attenuation in the anterior left frontal lobe deep white matter and evidence of prominent vascular structures around the periphery of the anterior left frontal lobe; there is no calcification or acute hemorrhage in the region and the bones are normal (Fig. 33.1).

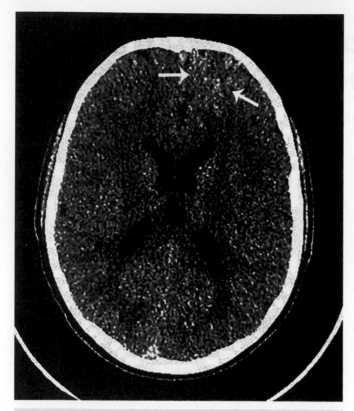

Fig. 33.1 Axial non—contrast computed tomography demonstrates ill-defined high attenuation in the inferior left frontal lobe *(arrows)*.

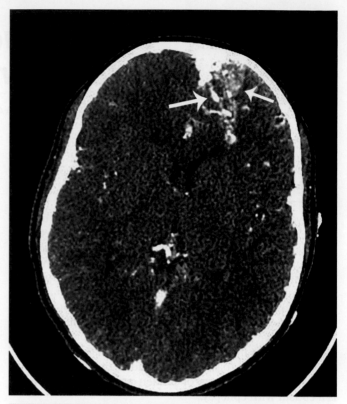

Fig. 33.2 Axial computed tomography (CT) angiography demonstrates multiple enhancing vessels in the inferior left frontal lobe in the area of high attenuation on non—contrast CT *(arrows)*.

Case Conclusion

The patient was admitted with Pediatric Neurosurgical consultation. CT angiography was obtained, and a selected image from that study is provided here. This study demonstrated an ill-defined area of high attenuation in the left frontal lobe (Fig. 33.2). MRI was also obtained, demonstrating multiple tightly packed vessels with surrounding enlarged feeding arteries (Fig. 33.3A, B) and a vascular nidus with enlarged left anterior and middle cerebral feeding arteries and multiple enlarged draining cortical veins (Fig. 33.4). These findings are consistent with a vascular malformation. The patient had endovascular embolization followed by surgical resection and did well.

Arteriovenous malformations are the most common cause of spontaneous intraparenchymal hemorrhage in pediatric patients, and the annual hemorrhage rate has been reported to be between 2% and 10%.[1-4] Mortality rate for each rupture event is 25%, and the risk is higher in the first 5 years after diagnosis.[1,2,4-6] There is debate regarding the size of an arteriovenous malformation and the risk for rupture.[2,7] Reported risk factors for arteriovenous malformation rupture include increasing age, hemorrhagic presentation, deep brain location, deep venous drainage, diffuse morphology, and female sex.[1,2,7,8] Patients with diffuse arteriovenous malformations have a high risk for hemorrhagic presentation.[8] Pediatric patients appear to have a higher risk for rebleeding compared to their adult counterparts, although this is debated in the literature.[1,4,9]

Pediatric arteriovenous malformations carry a higher rate of rupture compared to adult counterparts, with 80%–85% of pediatric patients presenting initially with hemorrhage, compared to 50%–65% of adult cases.[1,2,5,9] Previous studies have reported the mean age of diagnosis of an arteriovenous malformation to be 31 years; the overall yearly risk for hemorrhage from an arteriovenous malformation across all age groups is between 2% and 4%,[2,10,11] and pediatric patients are thought to represent 3% of all arteriovenous malformations.[2,5] Adult patients with rupture of an arteriovenous malformation often present with neurologic symptoms, such as headache, dizziness, scizures, and progressive neurologic abnormalities (suggesting ischemia) and epilepsy compared to pediatric patients who typically present with altered mental status and headache.[1,12] Interestingly, children tend to have a higher percentage of malformations in the basal ganglia and thalamus, which are more prone to bleeding, compared to adults.[1,9,13] The exact reason why arteriovenous malformations occur is unknown. Two proposed mechanisms for formation are the persistence of embryonal arteriovenous connections (which form primarily during the third week of embryogenesis) or the development of new connections after closure of the embryonal one.[2]

Treatment for arteriovenous malformations includes vascular resection surgical procedures, radiosurgery, and endovascular embolization. The goal of treatment is complete angiographic obliteration of the malformation. How this is accomplished depends on several factors, including

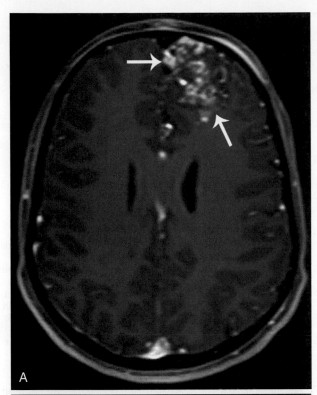

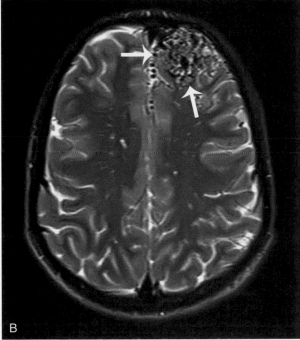

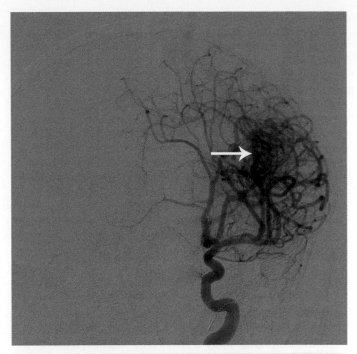

Fig. 33.4 Anterior-posterior projection of left ICA (internal carotid artery) injection of catheter angiography demonstrates a vascular nidus with enlarged left ACA (anterior cerebral artery) and MCA (middle cerebral artery) feeding arteries and multiple enlarged draining cortical veins *(white arrow)*.

Fig. 33.3 Axial T1 postcontrast (A) and T2 (B) images demonstrate multiple tightly packed vessels with surrounding enlarged feeding arteries in the left frontal lobe *(arrows)*. Vessels appear bright due to contrast enhancement (A) and dark due to flow voids (B).

the properties of the malformation, the condition of the patient, and which treatment modality is selected.[2] Previously, conservative management was advocated in pediatric patients with arteriovenous malformation, but that approach has become less used, except in cases where therapy

might prove more harmful than beneficial or is deemed ineffective.[1,2]

Surgical resection is the standard in pediatric patients.[1,2] This allows for removal of the malformation and the hematoma. Therapy focuses on the complete surgical resection, if possible. Arteriovenous malformations are classified according to the Spetzler-Martin Grading System,[14,15] which assigns a grade based on size, location, and venous draining system; this scoring system is used to assess a patient's risk for neurologic sequelae after open surgical resection, but caution must be exercised when applying this to pediatric patients, as there is little evidence in its application in this population.

Radiosurgery has been employed in the pediatric population but does involve exposure to radiation, making this treatment modality less attractive. This treatment option is exercised for malformations in locations that make surgical resection difficult and there is risk of significant complications.[1,2,16–20] Radiotherapy is efficacious in pediatric patients, but long-term complications, such as malignancy development, are not well studied.[1,18,19] Endovascular embolization is used as an adjunct to other treatments, with staged embolization particularly used for large malformations, followed by surgical resection.[1,2,9,20] Smaller malformations are more amenable to complete obliteration than larger ones.[6,21] This procedure is tolerated and efficacious in the pediatric population.[22–24]

The natural course of pediatric arteriovenous malformations is not well described in the literature, but one study reported the risk for hemorrhage after treatment relative to treatment modalities used: microsurgical resection with or without embolization had no subsequent hemorrhages (0.0%), 0.8% with radiosurgery with or without embolization,

0.8% with conservative management (observation), 2.8% with embolization only, and 3.5% with incomplete resection (surgery with radiotherapy, with or without embolization).[4] Patients who presented with hemorrhage had a higher risk of posttreatment hemorrhage as well.[4] In this study, seizure presentation, frontal lobe location, nonheadache presentation, and treatment modality (e.g., surgery with radiotherapy with or without embolization) were all associated with poor functional outcomes.[4] Previous studies have reported that 86% of patients with arteriovascular malformations (grade I–III) had good functional outcomes after surgical resection and multimodal therapy was associated with good functional outcomes as well.[20] A more recent study reported that patients treated with microvascular surgical resection had good functional outcomes but there was a persistent neurologic deficit rate of 38%, which was associated with preoperative neurologic deficits, malformation size >3 cm, and eloquent cortex location.[25]

IMAGING PEARLS

1. Non—contrast CT is an excellent first-line imaging modality when an intracranial etiology for a patient's acute mental status change is suspected. Consider catheter angiography if there is strong suspicion for a vascular problem.
2. MRI and MRA are useful to localize arteriovenous malformations, delineate malformation anatomy, rule out other causes of hemorrhage, and guide intraoperative procedures.
3. Cerebral angiography is the gold standard for the diagnosis of arteriovenous malformations.
4. There are instances of radiographically occult vascular malformations. In these instances, delayed imaging may be helpful as the clot resolves.

References

1. Niazi TN, Klimo Jr P, Anderson RC, et al. Diagnosis and management of arteriovenous malformations in children. *Neurosurg Clin N Am.* 2010;21(3):443-456.
2. El-Ghanem M, Kass-Hout T, Kass-Hout O, et al. Arteriovenous malformations in the pediatric population: review of the existing literature. *Interv Neurol.* 2016;5(3-4):218-225.
3. Darsaut TE, Guzman R, Marcellus ML, et al. Management of pediatric intracranial arteriovenous malformations: experience with multimodality therapy. *Neurosurgery.* 2011;69(3):540-556.
4. Yang W, Anderson-Keightly H, Westbroek EM, et al. Long-term hemorrhagic risk in pediatric patients with arteriovenous malformations. *J Neurosurg Pediatr.* 2016;18(3):329-338.
5. Di Rocco C, Tamburrini G, Rollo M. Cerebral arteriovenous malformations in children. *Acta Neurochir (Wien).* 2000;142(2):145-156.
6. Kondziolka D, Kano H, Yang HC, et al. Radiosurgical management of pediatric arteriovenous malformations. *Childs Nerv Syst.* 2010; 26(10):1359-1366.
7. Stapf C, Mast H, Sciacca RR, et al. Predictors of hemorrhage in patients with untreated brain arteriovenous malformation. *Neurology.* 2006;66(9):1350-1355.
8. Ai X, Ye Z, Xu J, et al. The factors associated with hemorrhagic presentation in children with untreated brain arteriovenous malformation: a meta-analysis. *J Neurosurg Pediatr.* 2018;23(3):343-354.
9. Hoh BL, Ogilvy CS, Butler WE, et al. Multimodality treatment of nongalenic arteriovenous malformations in pediatric patients. *Neurosurgery.* 2000;47(2):346-357.
10. Hofmeister C, Stapf C, Hartmann A, et al. Demographic, morphological, and clinical characteristics of 1289 patients with brain arteriovenous malformation. *Stroke.* 2000;31(6):1307-1310.
11. Smyth MD, Sneed PK, Ciricillo SF, et al. Stereotactic radiosurgery for pediatric intracranial arteriovenous malformations: the University of California at San Francisco experience. *J Neurosurg.* 2002;97(1):48-55.
12. Kondziolka D, Humphreys RP, Hoffman HJ, et al. Arteriovenous malformations of the brain in children: a forty year experience. *Can J Neurol Sci.* 1992;19(1):40-45.
13. Kiriş T, Sencer A, Sahinbas M, et al. Surgical results in pediatric Spetzler-Martin grades I–III intracranial arteriovenous malformations. *Childs Nerv Syst.* 2005;21(1):69-74.
14. Spetzler RF, Martin NA. A proposed grading system for arteriovenous malformations. *J Neurosurg.* 1986;65(4):476-483.
15. Kim H, Abla AA, Nelson J, et al. Validation of the supplemented Spetzler-Martin grading system for brain arteriovenous malformations in a multicenter cohort of 1009 surgical patients. *Neurosurgery.* 2015; 76(1):25-31.
16. Blamek S, Larysz D, Miszczyk L. Stereotactic linac radiosurgery and hypofractionated stereotactic radiotherapy for pediatric arteriovenous malformations of the brain: experiences of a single institution. *Childs Nerv Syst.* 2013;29(4):651-656.
17. Yamamoto M, Akabane A, Matsumaru Y, et al. Long-term follow-up results of intentional 2-stage Gamma Knife surgery with an interval of at least 3 years for arteriovenous malformations larger than 10 cm³. *J Neurosurg.* 2012;117 Suppl:126-134.
18. Kano H, Kondziolka D, Flickinger JC, et al. Stereotactic radiosurgery for arteriovenous malformations, part 2: management of pediatric patients. *J Neurosurg Pediatr.* 2012;9(1):1-10.
19. Yen CP, Monteith SJ, Nguyen JH, et al. Gamma Knife surgery for arteriovenous malformations in children. *J Neurosurg Pediatr.* 2010; 6(5):426-434.
20. Darsaut TE, Guzman R, Marcellus ML, et al. Management of pediatric intracranial arteriovenous malformations: experience with multimodality therapy. *Neurosurgery.* 2011;69(3):540-556.
21. Bristol RE, Albuquerque FC, Spetzler RF, et al. Surgical management of arteriovenous malformations in children. *J Neurosurg.* 2006; 105(suppl 2):88-93.
22. Soltanolkotabi M, Schoeneman SE, Alden TD, et al. Onyx embolization of intracranial arteriovenous malformations in pediatric patients. *J Neurosurg Pediatr.* 2013;11(4):431-437.
23. Zheng T, Wang QJ, Liu YQ, et al. Clinical features and endovascular treatment of intracranial arteriovenous malformations in pediatric patients. *Childs Nerv Syst.* 2014;30(4):647-653.
24. Berenstein A, Ortiz R, Niimi Y, et al. Endovascular management of arteriovenous malformations and other intracranial arteriovenous shunts in neonates, infants, and children. *Childs Nerv Syst.* 2010; 26(10):1345-1358.
25. Ravindra VM, Bollo RJ, Eli IM, et al. A study of pediatric cerebral arteriovenous malformations: clinical presentation, radiological features, and long-term functional and educational outcomes with predictors of sustained neurological deficits. *J Neurosurg Pediatr.* 2019;24(1):1-8.

34 Can You See It? Orbital Cellulitis

ROBERT VEZZETTI, MD, FAAP, FACEP

Case Presentation

A 10-year-old male presents with left eye edema and pain for the past 2–3 days. The child reports mild congestion for the past week but there has been no fever, vomiting, cough, vision changes, eye discharge, or trauma. He states that it is difficult for him to completely open the eye because of the swelling. When he does, he complains of generalized eye pain. He has not had fever, although during your evaluation, you note that the child has a temperature of 100.9 degrees Fahrenheit, with a heart rate of 105 beats per minute, a respiratory rate of 18 breaths per minute, and a blood pressure of 100/75 mm Hg. The physical examination is unremarkable except for obvious left upper and lower eyelid edema with erythema and warmth. There is mild induration and no palpable fluctuance. The patient is able to open his eye, and you note there is no scleral edema or erythema; there is no obvious proptosis; there is no hyphema; his pupil is briskly reactive and equal with his other pupil. He has mild photophobia. When testing his extraocular muscles, the child complains of pain looking primarily medially and laterally. He has a nonfocal neurologic examination.

Imaging Considerations

Imaging is often utilized to assist in distinguishing periorbital from orbital or intracranial complications and identifying patients who would benefit from surgical intervention. There have been studies that employed clinical findings, particularly proptosis and limited or painful ocular motion, to risk stratify patients who require imaging.[1,2] Not all patients have classic findings for orbital or intracranial involvement[1,2] and the decision to obtain imaging depends upon the patient's presenting history, examination findings, and provider experience and index of suspicion.

PLAIN RADIOGRAPHY

Orbital radiography may be of some use in a trauma setting, but this modality is not useful in children with suspected orbital infection.

COMPUTED TOMOGRAPHY (CT)

Intravenous (IV) contrast–enhanced CT is the imaging modality of choice to evaluate orbital infections and associated complications.[3] Patients with signs of orbital infection (fever, severe eyelid edema, proptosis, pain with movement

of the eye) or for whom physical examination is unreliable or unable to be properly performed (e.g., very young or uncooperative patients) are candidates for orbital imaging. A patient with no improvement (worsening clinical condition or persistent symptoms after 24–48 hours of appropriate antibiotics) or with neurologic findings on clinical examination should also undergo imaging.[3] An abscess will first appear as a soft tissue density, evolving into a fluid-filled ring enhancing mass. CT is useful in identifying infection extent and the presence of an abscess but may not identify an abscess in its very early stages.[3] Sedation is rarely required to obtain this study and this modality is readily available in most institutions. Although a disadvantage is exposure to ionizing radiation, which can be limited through the application of ALARA (as low as reasonably achievable) principles, the morbidity and potential mortality of not adequately identifying and treating an orbital infection and any associated complications are high.

MAGNETIC RESONANCE IMAGING (MRI)

This modality provides superior resolution of orbital soft tissues compared to CT and is especially useful in the identification of subperiosteal or orbital abscesses.[3,4] MRI is also useful in detecting intracranial complications of orbital cellulitis. In cases where a diagnosis is unclear, MRI may provide delineation of infectious and other inflammatory processes. Gadolinium administration is typically used, but diffusion-weighted imaging has proven useful in abscess detection and may be considered in children with renal compromise.[3,4] However, MRI is not readily available in many centers and often requires sedation to obtain an adequate study.

ULTRASOUND

Orbital ultrasonography does not have a role in the identification of orbital cellulitis. It can detect orbital abscesses but lacks sensitivity compared to other imaging modalities, such as CT and MRI,[1] and cannot image the posterior one-third of the orbit and sinuses.[5]

Imaging Findings

The child underwent IV contrast–enhanced orbital CT. Selected images are seen. There is a 3 mm × 18 mm × 7 mm left medial subperiosteal orbital abscess with slight lateral displacement of the medial rectus muscle. There is preseptal soft tissue edema and left ethmoid sinus opacification (Figs. 34.1–34.3).

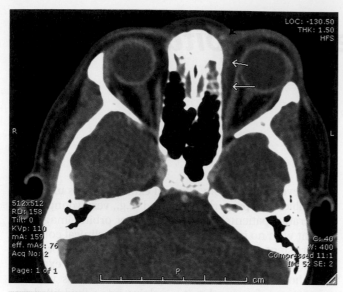

Fig. 34.1 Axial contrast-enhanced orbital CT image shows a medial subperiosteal orbital abscess *(white arrows)* with preseptal soft tissue edema *(red arrow)*.

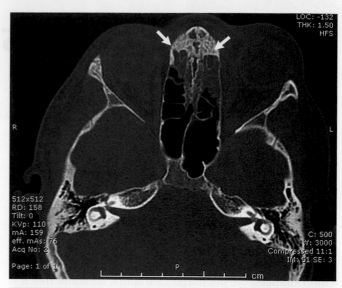

Fig. 34.3 Axial CT bone window image demonstrating left greater than right ethmoid sinus opacification *(arrows)*.

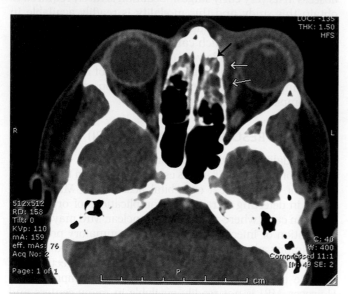

Fig. 34.2 Axial contrast-enhanced CT image shows the abscess *(white arrows)* with ethmoid opacification *(red arrow)*.

Case Conclusion

The child was admitted to the inpatient service and begun on IV antibiotics. Pediatric Ophthalmology was consulted. The imaging was reviewed and it was decided that the abscess was not amenable to drainage. Antibiotics and careful monitoring were continued. After clinical improvement, the child was discharged on oral antibiotics with follow-up arranged with his primary care provider and Pediatric Ophthalmology. He did not require surgical intervention.

Orbital cellulitis is not commonly encountered in the general population, but pediatric patients are a commonly involved age group.[3,5] There are several scenarios that predispose patients to orbital cellulitis with or without

subperiosteal abscess: spread from an existing sinus infection (estimated between 1% and 5% with less than 1% developing an abscess), spread from an upper respiratory infection, trauma or foreign bodies, and spread from dental infections. *Staphylococcus aureus* and *Streptococcus* species are typical etiologic organisms.[6,7] There are several classification systems for identifying orbital complications from sinusitis.

Presenting symptoms include erythema and edema of the orbital area (usually the first symptoms) and progressive pain, especially with eye movements. Fever may be present, but the lack of fever does not exclude an orbital infection. Proptosis and vision changes are later findings, resulting from infection progression, which can be rapid. Complications of orbital infections include meningitis, development of a cerebral abscess, and loss of vision.

Treatment includes medical and surgical management.[3,5,8–10] Medical management involves appropriate IV antibiotics, with coverage aimed at the most common organisms, including coverage for anaerobic organisms. In locations where methicillin-resistant *Staphylococcus aureus* (MRSA) is problematic or if the patient has a history of MRSA, antibiotic choice should also include coverage of this organism. There are multiple antibiotic regimens that have been proposed.[1,2] If there are questions regarding antibiotic regimen choice, discussion with qualified subspecialists, such as pediatric infectious disease or pediatric ophthalmology, is appropriate.

Surgical management is somewhat controversial and may be indicated in select patients; however, any sign of vision compromise or medical treatment failure are indications for surgical management.[5,8–10] Interestingly, medial and inferior abscesses are more likely to respond to medical management. Intracranial complications should prompt consultation with pediatric neurosurgery. Retained foreign bodies should be removed surgically. Many patients require additional surgical intervention for concurrent severe sinus infection; consultation with Pediatric Otolaryngology is appropriate when managing these patients.

IMAGING PEARLS

1. Imaging is indicated in patients with severe orbital edema, severe pain, or pain with ocular movements, proptosis, or a worsening clinical course despite appropriate antibiotic therapy.
2. IV contrast–enhanced CT is the imaging modality of choice in children with suspected orbital cellulitis and associated complications.
3. CT may not identify an abscess if the study is obtained early in the course of illness. If a strong clinical suspicion exists, then an MRI may be helpful in determining the presence of an abscess.
4. MRI should be considered in patients with suspected intracranial complications, such as cerebral abscess. The need for sedation and availability can be barriers to obtaining this study at some facilities.

References

1. Rudloe TF, Harper MB, Prabhu SP, et al. Acute periorbital infections: who needs emergent imaging? *Pediatrics*. 2010;125(4):e719-e726.
2. Jabarin B, Eviatar E, Israel O, et al. Indicators for imaging in periorbital cellulitis secondary to rhinosinusitis. *Eur Arch Otorhinolaryngol*. 2018;275(4):943-948.
3. Tsirouki T, Dastiridou AI, Ibáñez Flores N, et al. Orbital cellulitis. *Surv Ophthalmol*. 2018;63(4):534-553.
4. Sepahdari AR, Aakalu VK, Kapur R, et al. MRI of orbital cellulitis and orbital abscess: the role of diffusion-weighted imaging. *AJR Am J Roentgenol*. 2009;193(3):W244–W250.
5. Jain A, Rubin PA. Orbital cellulitis in children. *Int Ophthalmol Clin*. 2001;41:71-86.
6. Givner LB. Periorbital versus orbital cellulitis. *Pediatr Infect Dis J*. 2002;21(12):1157-1158.
7. Wald ER. Periorbital and orbital infections. *Pediatr Rev*. 2004;25(9): 312-320.
8. Brown CL, Graham SM, Griffin MC, et al. Pediatric medial subperiosteal orbital abscess: medical management where possible. *Am J Rhinol*. 2004;18(5):321-327.
9. Wong SJ, Levi J. Management of pediatric orbital cellulitis: a systemic review. *Int J Pediatr Otorhinolaryngol*. 2018;110:123-129.
10. Bedwell J, Bauman NM. Management of pediatric orbital cellulitis and abscess. *Curr Opin Otolaryngol Head Neck Surg*. 2011;19(6): 467-473.

35 *Something in Your Eye: Periorbital Cellulitis*

ROBERT VEZZETTI, MD, FAAP, FACEP

Case Presentation

A 7-month-old baby presents with left infraorbital swelling and erythema for the past 2 days, which has progressed rapidly. There has been a fever of 101.5 degrees Fahrenheit for the past 24 hours. He has not had cough, congestion, vomiting, or diarrhea. Four days ago, the child was playing with his older sibling, who, during the course of play, threw a small toy car at the child, striking him in the left side of the face (under the eye) and causing a small abrasion. The wound did not appear large and the mother has been keeping the area clean with soap and water. He has been eating and drinking well and is otherwise at his baseline.

Physical examination reveals a child in no distress. His temperature is 100.1 degrees Fahrenheit, his heart rate is 137 beats per minute, and his respiratory rate is 30 breaths per minute. He has obvious erythema and swelling to the left periorbital area, particularly the infraorbital area, which is warm and is painful when palpated. There is no fluctuance, but there is induration. The child is unable to open the eye (which you find very difficult to open due to the swelling) and consequently the pupil, conjunctiva, and sclera are not visible. There is no proptosis. There is moderate yellow eye discharge and eyelash mattering.

Imaging Considerations

PLAIN RADIOGRAPHY

Plain radiography is not a first-line imaging modality in patients with suspected periorbital infection and associated complications. While indications suggestive of sinus disease can be visualized, signs of sinus mucosal thickening may be nonspecific in pediatric patients, and neither cellulitis nor an abscess will be visualized with this imaging test.

COMPUTED TOMOGRAPHY (CT)

This modality is the imaging modality of choice to evaluate periorbital and orbital infections.[1–3] Examination of the child with periorbital cellulitis can be difficult, since pediatric patients are often anxious and uncooperative, and there may be significant swelling and/or pain. CT has been increasingly used to determine the extent of infection and evaluate patients for possible orbital involvement.[4] One study reported the use of CT in almost 94% of patients.[1] In patients with a clinical examination that is consistent with an uncomplicated periorbital infection, it is reasonable to withhold CT imaging and initiate antibiotic therapy with

close observation. If there is no improvement in 48 hours, worsening clinical examination, or signs of complications (neurologic symptoms or increasing pain), then obtaining imaging is reasonable.[5] CT is appropriate when there is concern for orbital infection, abscess, or intracranial complication and when clinical examination is difficult.[1–3,6,7] Periorbital cellulitis will appear as diffuse soft-tissue thickening and areas of enhancement anterior to the orbital septum on CT.[8] Intravenous contrast should be utilized. As contemporary scanners are rapid, sedation is usually not required. The use of pediatric protocols to lower ionizing radiation exposure time is recommended per American College of Radiology guidelines.

MAGNETIC RESONANCE IMAGING (MRI)

This modality is excellent at detecting infectious and inflammatory processes but is not a first-line imaging test. A study with and without contrast can be obtained to complement CT findings if further detail of an identified pathologic process is necessary.[9] If intracranial extension is a concern, MRI is recommended, as MRI is better at soft tissue detail than CT.[9,10]

ULTRASOUND (US)

Orbital US is an emerging imaging modality but currently is not used routinely in the evaluation of periorbital infection.[10,11]

Imaging Findings

The physical examination findings were suggestive of a periorbital infection; however, the swelling was significant, hindering the ability to complete a thorough physical examination. After much discussion with the family, the decision was made to obtain an intravenous contrast–enhanced orbital CT. Selected images from this study are presented here. There is diffuse left preseptal periorbital soft tissue swelling with no sign of abscess, intraorbital, or intracranial involvement (Figs. 35.1–35.3).

Case Conclusion

The child was admitted to the inpatient service, and ceftriaxone with clindamycin, per hospital protocol, was initiated. Pediatric Ophthalmology was consulted, and an eye examination was able to be performed using retractors; there was

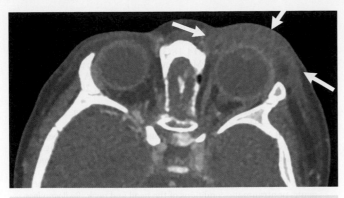

Fig. 35.1 Axial contrast-enhanced computed tomography soft tissue window image demonstrates left periorbital soft tissue swelling *(arrows)* with no sign of abscess or postseptal, intraorbital involvement.

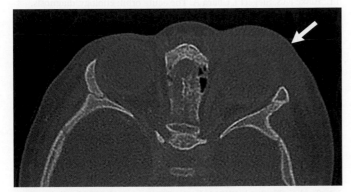

Fig. 35.2 Axial computed tomography bone window image of the orbits demonstrates periorbital soft tissue swelling *(arrow)*, but no evidence of fracture or bone destruction.

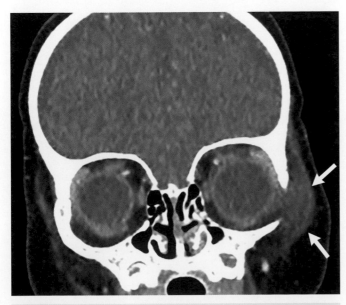

Fig. 35.3 Coronal computed tomography soft tissue window image demonstrates left periorbital soft tissue swelling laterally *(arrows)*, with no sign of abscess. No evidence of intraorbital involvement.

more discharge noted and conjunctival erythema, but the exam was otherwise normal. Cultures of the eye discharge were obtained and ultimately grew methicillin-resistant *Staphylococcus aureus* (MRSA). The patient improved dramatically on intravenous antibiotics and was able to be transitioned to oral antibiotics based on sensitivities from the culture. On hospital day 3, the patient was discharged and completed his antibiotic course at home.

Periorbital cellulitis (or preseptal cellulitis) does not involve the orbital septum and generally does not have serious complications, although there are literature reports of lacrimal gland abscess, vision loss from ischemic retinopathy and optic neuropathy, restricted ocular movements, and spread of infection locally and centrally leading to cavernous sinus thrombosis, meningitis, and cerebral abscess.[8,10,12,13] Periorbital cellulitis is more common than orbital cellulitis.[14] This disease process can affect any age of patient, but is more common in pediatric patients. The mean age of patients is around 3 years, but all pediatric age groups are affected.[1,3,12] Predisposing factors to the development of periorbital cellulitis include sinusitis, upper respiratory infection, insect bites, trauma, conjunctivitis, and dental abscess.[1–3,6,15] Hematogenous spread occurs in children under the age of 3 years.[3] Common symptoms of periorbital cellulitis include localized erythema, swelling, warmth, and tenderness, with unilateral involvement more common, although bilateral involvement has been reported.[1,3] Ophthalmoplegia and proptosis are usually seen in orbital infection rather than periorbital cellulitis.[1]

Evaluation of periorbital cellulitis often consists of laboratory testing, including complete blood count, C-reactive protein, and blood cultures. Complete blood count and C-reactive protein are commonly elevated in periorbital infections and blood cultures are typically sterile, although infants under 3 months of age have a higher positive culture rate.[1,2,6,14] In the absence of systemic symptoms, blood cultures are not recommended.[3,16] However, ocular discharge, if present, should be cultured since this has a high yield rate.[3] Laboratory results should not be used exclusively to diagnose periorbital infections.[3]

Management for periorbital cellulitis involves both inpatient management with intravenous antibiotics[1,3,6,17] and outpatient management with oral antibiotics.[3,15] One study found that the majority of patients with periorbital cellulitis were treated as outpatients, but 46% ultimately were admitted for intravenous antimicrobial therapy secondary to failure to respond to oral antimicrobial therapy. Patients with fevers greater than 39 degrees Celsius (102.2 degrees Fahrenheit) had a higher admission rate.[15] In hospitalized patients, various intravenous antibiotic regimens are available and have been used. A third-generation cephalosporin (ceftriaxone) is a typical first-line therapeutic agent[1,6,15,17] Once clinical improvement is demonstrated, antibiotics are transitioned to oral administration for 10–14 days in uncomplicated cases.[1,3] Antimicrobial agents should have coverage against *Staphylococcus aureus* and *Streptococcus pyogenes*.[2,3,7,14,15] MRSA has been increasingly prevalent in patients with periorbital infections. One study documented that over 70% of patients had this organism as a cause of their infection.[3,18,16] Adjunct therapies, such as antihistamines, nasal steroids, and decongestants, are not recommended.[3,19] Hospital protocols for the management of periorbital cellulitis, including use of CT, antimicrobial agent choice, recommendations for admission, and guidelines for subspecialty consultation, are helpful for proper management of these patients.[2,7,15] The commonly reported reasons for admission for patients with periorbital cellulitis include cellulitis with systemic illness, inability to examine the eye properly, neurologic symptoms, diplopia, and failure to respond to oral antibiotic therapy.[1,2,15]

IMAGING PEARLS

1. The diagnostic imaging modality of choice in patients with periorbital cellulitis is intravenous contrast–enhanced CT.

2. It is reasonable to forego imaging studies in patients who do not have systemic signs of illness, have no signs of orbital involvement, and do not have neurologic symptoms (i.e., diplopia, other vision changes, or severe headache).

3. If there are worsening clinical findings, no improvement after 48 hours of appropriate antibiotic therapy, neurologic symptoms, or there is suspicion of an abscess or orbital involvement, then intravenous contrast–enhanced CT should be obtained.

4. MRI is not a first-line imaging modality in patients with periorbital cellulitis. If greater anatomic detail is desired or there is suspicion of intracranial complications, either clinically or on CT, then MRI should be considered.

References

1. Gonçalves R, Menezes C, Machado R, et al. Periorbital cellulitis in children: analysis of outcome of intravenous antibiotic therapy. *Orbit.* 2016;35(4):175-180.
2. Howe L, Jones NS. Guidelines for the management of periorbital cellulitis/abscess. *Clin Otolaryngol Allied Sci.* 2004;29(6):725-728.
3. Hauser A, Fogarasi S. Periorbital and orbital cellulitis. *Pediatr Rev.* 2010;31(6):242-249.
4. Le TD, Liu ES, Adatia FA, et al. The effect of adding orbital computed tomography findings to the Chandler criteria for classifying pediatric orbital cellulitis in predicting which patients will require surgical intervention. *J AAPOS.* 2014;18(3):271-277.
5. Botting AM, McIntosh D, Mahadevan M. Paediatric pre- and post-septal peri-orbital infections are different diseases. A retrospective review of 262 cases. *Int J Pediatr Otorhinolaryngol.* 2008;72(3):377-383.
6. Malinow I, Powell KR. Periorbital cellulitis. *Pediatr Ann.* 1993;22(4):241-246.
7. Crosbie RA, Nairn J, Kubba H. Management of paediatric periorbital cellulitis: our experience of 243 children managed according to a standardised protocol 2012-2015. *Int J Pediatr Otorhinolaryngol.* 2016;87:134-138.
8. Capps EF, Kinsella JJ, Gupta M, et al. Emergency imaging assessment of acute, nontraumatic conditions of the head and neck. *Radiographics.* 2010;30(5):1335-1352.
9. Expert Panel on Neurologic Imaging, Kennedy TA, Corey AS, Policeni B, et al. ACR Appropriateness Criteria ® orbits vision and visual loss. *J Am Coll Radiol.* 2018;15(5S):S116-S131.
10. Eustis HS, Mafee MF, Walton C, Mondonca J. MR imaging and CT of orbital infections and complications in acute rhinosinusitis. *Radiol Clin North Am.* 1998;36(6):1165-1183.
11. Blake FAS, Siegert J, Gbara A. The acute orbit: etiology, diagnosis, and therapy. *J Oral Maxillofac Surg.* 2006;64:87-93.
12. Parvizni N, Choudhury N, Singh A. Complicated periorbital cellulitis: case report and literature review. *J Laryngol Otol.* 2012;126(1):94-96.
13. Herrmann BW, Forsen JW. Simultaneous intracranial and orbital complications of acute rhinosinusitis in children. *Int J Pediatr Otorhinolaryngol.* 2004;68(5):619-625.
14. Georgakopoulos CD, Eliopoulou MI, Stasinos S, et al. Periorbital and orbital cellulitis: a 10-year review of hospitalized children. *Eur J Ophthalmol.* 2010;20(6):1066-1072.
15. James V, Mohamad Ikbal MF, Min NC, et al. Periorbital cellulitis in paediatric emergency medicine department patients. *Ann Acad Med Singapore.* 2018;47(10):420-423.
16. McKinley SH, Yen MT, Miller AM, et al. Microbiology of pediatric orbital cellulitis. *Am J Ophthalmol.* 2007;144(4):497-501.
17. Starkey CR, Steele RW. Medical management of orbital cellulitis. *Pediatr Infect Dis J.* 2001;20(10):1002-1005.
18. Blomquist PH. Methicillin-resistant *Staphylococcus aureus* infections of the eye and orbit. *Trans Am Ophthalmol Soc.* 2006;104:322-345.
19. Wald ER, Applegate KE, Bordly C, et al. Clinical practice guideline for the diagnosis and management of acute bacterial sinusitis in children aged 1 to 18 years. *Pediatrics.* 2013;132(1):e262-e280.

36 Somethin' Growin': Pediatric Arachnoid Cysts

ROBERT VEZZETTI, MD, FAAP, FACEP

Case Presentation

A 16-year-old female presents with a history of severe headaches, nausea, and vomiting for the past 3 weeks. She was seen at an urgent care facility where she was diagnosed with sinusitis and was given prescriptions for odansetron, prednisone, and amoxicillin. After several days of these medications, she did not experience any relief, so she was seen by her primary care provider. She was given an injection of ceftriaxone, her oral antibiotics were changed to cefdinir, and the steroid dose was lowered. The child's headaches, nausea, and vomiting were persistent, so she was brought to the emergency department for evaluation.

The headaches have become daily and occur throughout the day. She does have nighttime headache, which started 1 week ago. She states that the headaches cause nausea, which leads to emesis. There has been no fever, neck pain, back pain, vision changes, incontinence, or weakness; she has noted intermittent numbness to the fingertips of both her hands. There has been no report of trauma. She has been taking nonsteroidal antiinflammatory medications, which have become less effective over the past week.

Her examination is unremarkable, other than complaint of mild headache, which is primarily left frontal in location. She is afebrile; her heart rate is 84 beats per minute, respiratory rate is 18 breaths per minute, and blood pressure is 120/80 mm Hg. She is awake, alert, and age appropriate. Her pupils are equal, round, and reactive to light. There is no evidence of papilledema and her extraocular movements are intact. She has no visual field cuts and cranial nerves II–XII are grossly intact. Deep tendon reflexes are 2+ and symmetric. She moves her extremities symmetrically with no apparent weakness, spasticity, or hypotonia. Her gait is steady and there are no cerebellar findings. Her sensation appears intact.

Imaging Considerations

Imaging is often employed in patients with general neurologic complaints, such as severe headache, focal neurologic findings including ataxia, or if there are symptoms that raise suspicion for an intracranial process, such as emesis or vision changes, or concerning historical findings (such as wakening in the middle of the night with headache, first morning emesis, or persistent/worsening headache).[1] The choice of imaging modality may be influenced by the resources available at a particular facility.

COMPUTED TOMOGRAPHY (CT)

This imaging modality is an excellent first-line choice when there is concern for an intracranial hemorrhage, mass, or lesion. CT is widely available, sedation is generally not required, and intravenous contrast is not generally indicated.

MAGNETIC RESONANCE IMAGING (MRI)

This imaging modality can provide details of the intracranial structures and anatomy. Often, this test is obtained to further delineate findings initially identified on CT. Cost, availability, and the potential need for sedation are barriers to MRI use as a first-line imaging modality.

Imaging Findings

The patient underwent noncontrast CT imaging of the brain. A selected image from that study is included. These images demonstrate an approximately 8 × 7 × 6-cm arachnoid cyst in the region of the left Sylvian fissure, extending from the mid-left frontal extra-axial space to the floor of the left middle cranial fossa. There is mild mass effect and bilateral extra-axial fluid collections, most consistent with hygromas (Fig. 36.1).

Case Conclusion

Pediatric Neurosurgery was consulted. The patient was admitted to the hospital for observation and remained stable. After discussion with the family, the decision was made to perform an arachnoid fenestration. The next day, she had an MRI study, prior to surgery to assess for any other structural anomalies. This study again demonstrated the left frontotemporal arachnoid cyst causing distortion of the left frontal and temporal lobe contours and mild effacement of the left lateral ventricle from mass effect. There are 6-mm-thick bilateral frontoparietal subdural hygromas. There is mild flattening of the lateral hemispheric parenchymal contour from mass effect (Figs. 36.2 and 36.3). The child was electively taken to the operating room for arachnoid cyst fenestration, which was performed successfully. She recovered uneventfully.

The etiology of arachnoid cysts is not known. They are thought to be secondary to malformation of the embryonal arachnoid membrane, by splitting or duplication, leading to an accumulation of fluid.[2–5] Arachnoid cysts are commonly found incidentally in pediatric patients.[4–8] The increased use

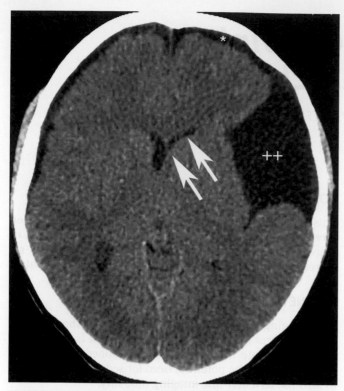

Fig. 36.1 Axial CT image demonstrating the large cyst *(crosses)* with mass effect *(arrows)* and bilateral subdural hygromas *(asterisk)*.

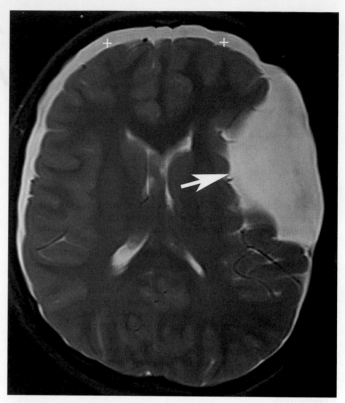

Fig. 36.3 Axial T2 MRI image demonstrating the cyst *(arrow)* and bilateral subdural hygromas *(crosses)*.

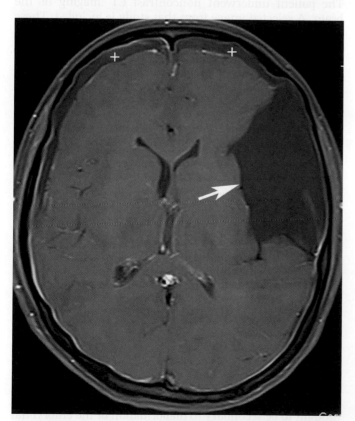

Fig. 36.2 Axial contrast-enhanced T1 weighted MRI image demonstrating the unenhancing cyst *(arrow)* and bilateral subdural hygromas *(crosses)*.

of neuroimaging, including CT and MRI, has led to increasing detection of arachnoid cysts.[6,9,10] Cysts have also been found on prenatal ultrasonography.[6,11] In a study of nearly 12,000 pediatric patients who underwent neuroimaging (MRI) over an 11-year study period, a prevalence rate of 2.6% was found; males were more commonly found to have arachnoid cysts, with prevalence peaking at 1 and 5 years of age.[6] Interestingly, multiple arachnoid cysts were found in several patients in this study.[6] The most common reasons listed for obtaining a neuroimaging study included headaches, acute mental status changes, and seizure.[6] Arachnoid cysts can be found in a variety of locations: Sylvian fissure/middle cranial fossa is the most common location, but arachnoid cysts can occur suprasellar, intrasellar, or uncommonly in the posterior fossa.[5]

Neuroimaging easily demonstrates arachnoid cysts. On CT, these cysts appear extraaxial, are the same density as cerebrospinal fluid, and do not enhance.[5] On MRI, arachnoid cysts have similar signal intensity as cerebrospinal fluid on T1- and T2-weighted images and do not enhance with gadolinium.[5] Diffusion-weighted MRI can be used to distinguish between arachnoid cysts and epidermoid tumors.[5,12]

Consultation with Neurosurgery is appropriate. Arachnoid cysts are generally thought not to be symptomatic and treatment is not routinely indicated.[5–7] These cysts have been reported to expand, and while there are numerous theories speculating why this can happen, the exact mechanism that causes this expansion is not clear.[5] Asymptomatic cysts can likely be followed without surgery and some authors propose serial MRI studies to monitor cyst progression, which is not common, especially in older patients.[6] These lesions, however, can be associated with increasing head size, hydrocephalus, headache, cognitive symptoms, vision problems, aphasia, and cranial neuropathy, although it can be difficult to ascribe headache to the presence of an arachnoid cyst itself.[4–6,13,14] These cysts can cause pain secondary to expansion or hemorrhage.[4] If a patient is experiencing symptoms due to an arachnoid cyst, or if there is radiologic worsening of the cyst, surgical treatment is often recommended.[2,6,13] Hydrocephalus and intracranial hypertension are absolute indications for surgery.[5] A study examining surgical intervention in pediatric patients found that surgical intervention was more often performed if the cyst was large, caused hydrocephalus, or had ruptured/hemorrhaged.[15] Spontaneous resolution, although rare, has been reported.[4,16]

There are several surgical options available: open craniotomy for cyst excision and fenestration, endoscopic fenestration, and cystoperitoneal shunting are commonly employed, with craniotomy and cyst fenestration the preferred procedure for many cases depending on specialist opinion and cyst location.[2,17]

IMAGING PEARLS

1. Noncontrast CT is the initial imaging modality of choice in patients in whom an intracranial abnormality is suspected.
2. MRI is often utilized as a second-line imaging modality in patients who have abnormal findings on initial CT.
3. Consider neuroimaging in patients who present with persistent/worsening headache, headache that wakes the patient from sleep, persistent, or first morning emesis, changes in previous symptoms, or focal neurologic findings on physical examination.

References

1. Lanphear J, Sarnaik S. Presenting symptoms of pediatric brain tumors diagnosed in the emergency department. *Pediatr Emerg Care*. 2014; 30(2):77-80.
2. Cincu R, Agrawal A, Eiras J. Intracranial arachnoid cysts: current concepts and treatment alternatives. *Clin Neurol Neurosurg*. 2007; 109(10):837-843.
3. Ali ZS, Lang SS, Bakar D, et al. Pediatric intracranial arachnoid cysts: comparative effectiveness of surgical treatment options. *Childs Nerv Syst*. 2014;30(3):461-469.
4. Eidlitz-Markus T, Zeharia A, Cohen YH, et al. Characteristics and management of arachnoid cyst in the pediatric headache clinic setting. *Headache*. 2014;54(10):1583-1590.
5. Gosalakkal JA. Intracranial arachnoid cysts in children: a review of pathogenesis, clinical features, and management. *Pediatr Neurol*. 2002;26(2):93-98.
6. Al-Holou WN, Yew AY, Boomsaad ZE, et al. Prevalence and natural history of arachnoid cysts in children. *J Neurosurg Pediatr*. 2010;5(6):578-785.
7. Marin-Sanabria EA, Yamamoto H, NagashimaT, et al. Evaluation of the management of arachnoid cyst of the posterior fossa in pediatric population: experience over 27 years. *Childs Nerv Syst*. 2007;23(5):535-442.
8. Pradilla G, Jallo G. Arachnoid cysts: case series and review of the literature. *Neurosurg Focus*. 2007;22(2):E7.
9. Kim BS, Illes J, Kaplan R, et al. Incidental findings on pediatric MR images of the brain. *AJNR Am J Neuroradiol*. 2002;23(10): 1674-1677.
10. Weber F, Knopf H. Incidental findings in magnetic resonance imaging of the brains of healthy young men. *J Neurol Sci*. 2006; 240(1-2):81-84.
11. Haino K, Serikawa T, Kikuchi A, et al. Prenatal diagnosis of fetal arachnoid cyst of the quadrigeminal cistern in ultrasonography and MRI. *Prenat Diagn*. 2009;29(11):1078-1080.
12. Tsuruda JS, Chew WM, Moseley ME, et al. Diffusion weighted MR imaging of the brain: value of differentiating between extraaxial cysts and epidermoid tumors. *AJR Am J Roentgenol*. 1990;155(5):1059-1065.
13. Kang JK, Lee KS, Lee IW, et al. Shunt-independent surgical treatment of middle cranial fossa arachnoid cysts in children. *Childs Nerv Syst*. 2000;16(2):111-116.
14. Ashker L, Weinstein JM, Dias M, et al. Arachnoid cyst causing third cranial nerve palsy manifesting as isolated internal ophthalmoplegia and iris cholinergic supersensitivity. *J Neuroophthalmol*. 2008;28(3):192-197.
15. Ali M, Bennardo M, Almenawer SA, et al. Exploring predictors of surgery and comparing operative treatment approaches for pediatric intracranial arachnoid cysts: a case series of 83 patients. *J Neurosurg Pediatr*. 2015;16(3):275-282.
16. Adilay U, Guclu B, Tiryaki M, et al. Spontaneous resolution of a Sylvian arachnoid cyst in a child: a case report. *Pediatr Neurosurg*. 2017;52(5):343-345.
17. Tamburrini G, Dal Fabbro M, Di Rocco C. Sylvian fissure arachnoid cysts: a survey on their diagnostic workout and practical management. *Childs Nerv Syst*. 2008;24(5):593-604.

Pulmonary

37 Rattlin' in the Chest: Community-Acquired Pneumonia

COBURN ALLEN, MD and CHRISTOPHER MICHAEL WRIGHT, MD

Case Presentation

A 7-year-old male with a medical history of asthma presents with 7 days of cough and "not feeling well." Four days ago, the patient developed fever to 103 degrees Fahrenheit. He was seen at his primary care provider 2 days ago and started on azithromycin, but he has not been eating or drinking well for the past several days and has had decreased urine output. He has complained of difficulty breathing today despite albuterol use, prompting the evaluation in the Emergency Department. He has not had emesis, diarrhea, or abdominal pain. Physical examination reveals a temperature of 103 degrees Fahrenheit, heart rate of 120 beats per minute, respiratory rate of 25 breaths per minute, blood pressure of 100/60 mm Hg, and an oxygen saturation of 94% on room air. He has mildly dry mucous membranes. His pulmonary examination reveals crackles and diminished breath sounds in the right upper lobe.

Imaging Considerations

Imaging is frequently utilized in the evaluation of children with respiratory symptoms. The initial differential diagnosis is broad, with history and physical examination serving to narrow the differential diagnosis and assist the clinician in choice of imaging, if clinically indicated.

PLAIN RADIOGRAPHY

Pediatric patients with suspected viral etiology or uncomplicated bacterial pneumonia do not require routine imaging, since the diagnosis of pneumonia may be made clinically.[1,2] Studies of pre-guideline management and post-guideline adherence have shown a notable decrease in the frequency of radiographs being obtained without significant increase in clinically diagnosed pneumonia.[3-5] Plain radiography is the first-line imaging choice for confirmation/exclusion of disease, for those who are not following an expected clinical course, if there are concerns for complications, if the child is severely ill, or for alternative diagnoses under consideration, such as foreign body ingestion.[1,2] Two views of the chest allow for proper and complete visualization of chest anatomy, including areas obscured by the heart and mediastinal structures.[1,2] This imaging modality provides low exposure to ionizing radiation and is readily available.

However, this imaging modality is not without limitations; findings of community-acquired pneumonia can vary, as can interoperator description and diagnosis of these findings.[6] One multisite, international study looked at observer agreement for radiographic findings of pneumonia utilizing World Health Organization standardized interpretation guidelines. The study showed good agreement for the finding of consolidation but poor agreement for other types of infiltrates on plain films, as has been reported elsewhere.[6,7] Imaging alone is incapable of distinguishing viral from bacterial etiology.[2,8] Still, radiography is often used to confirm a suspected bacterial etiology and has been shown to correlate well with that diagnosis in children who have *Pneumococcus* species as a cause of their pneumonia; negative radiographs have been found to have a high negative predictive value for bacterial source in those diagnosed with pneumonia clinically.[9,10]

COMPUTED TOMOGRAPHY (CT)

CT is generally not a first-line imaging modality. Use of this technology may be indicated in children with complex illness such as effusion or empyema requiring invasive interventions (i.e., imaging-guided thoracentesis and drainage catheter placement, video-assisted thoracoscopic surgery [VATS]) or when a diagnosis is uncertain.[17]

ULTRASOUND (US)

Interest in ultrasonography to diagnose pneumonia continues to increase due to its lack of ionizing radiation and relatively low cost compared to other imaging modalities. Ultrasound has proven adept at locating effusions and is more sensitive than CT.[13] Consolidations can be detected, but distinguishing between atelectasis and true pneumonia can be difficult, affecting accuracy. Studies have reported equivalent sensitivity for US and plain radiography at detecting pneumonia, although plain radiography has been shown to have a higher specificity.[12] Several studies have shown US to be effective at diagnosing community-acquired pneumonia in selected patients,[12,14,15] and the use of chest sonography may result in shorter length of stay and lower costs compared to chest radiography.[16] In cases of complicated pneumonia, US is useful to evaluate for an effusion or abscess, as it can be more sensitive than CT for small-volume effusions.[13]

The usage of transthoracic US to aid in diagnosing pediatric pneumonia continues to evolve. This modality may be useful, either as a first-line test or as an adjunct to better define abnormal plain radiography findings. US has the advantage of a lack of exposure to ionizing radiation and the study is rapid to perform. However, this modality requires specific training to perform appropriately and may not be generalizable to providers without skill in thoracic US.[17]

MAGNETIC RESONANCE IMAGING (MRI)

MRI is not a first-line imaging modality for CAP. Technical challenges previously limited the use of this modality, but recent studies have shown MRI to be sensitive for complications of pneumonia, although it is less sensitive than CT at detecting bronchiectasis, and may be considered a viable alternative to CT.[16,18,19] MRI is accurate at detecting pulmonary consolidation, pulmonary necrosis/abscess, and pleural effusion.[12]

The lack of ionizing radiation is advantageous. The availability of MRI may be a limiting factor in the further spread of use for this modality, as well as the likely need for sedation in younger children.

Imaging Findings

While the patient's history and physical examination findings are suggestive of pneumonia, there has been a worsening clinical course despite antimicrobial treatment. The decision was made to obtain two-view plain chest radiography. These images are provided here. There is a lung opacity in the right upper lobe without associated effusion or pneumothorax (Figs. 37.1 and 37.2).

Case Conclusion

The patient was given antipyretics and intravenous (IV) fluids with improvement of his temperature and vital signs. He was then able to tolerate oral fluids well in the emergency department. Strict return precautions were given, and he was placed on a 10-day course of oral amoxicillin and discharged home.

Community-acquired pneumonia is a leading cause of morbidity and mortality worldwide and a leading cause for hospitalization in the United States.[20,21] It is defined as an acute infection of the lung parenchyma and its etiology varies with age. Presenting symptoms may be nonspecific—especially in infants—but fever, cough, and respiratory complaints are often present.

Community-acquired pneumonia has a variety of etiologies, with over 90% attributed to a viral source with age-dependent variance.[20] In those less than 2 years of age, viral sources predominate.[20–22] As children age, viruses become less common; bacterial (especially atypical bacterial) causes increase in frequency.[22,23] Among bacterial etiologies, *Streptococcus pneumoniae*, *Staphylococcus aureus*, *Moraxella catarrhalis*, and *Haemophilus influenzae* are the most common agents.[22,23]

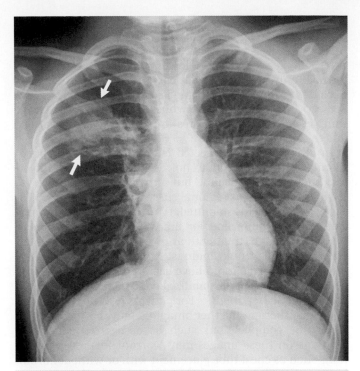

Fig. 37.1 Posterior-anterior chest radiograph demonstrating lung opacity in the right upper lobe *(arrows)*, which appears rounded on the frontal view, without associated effusion.

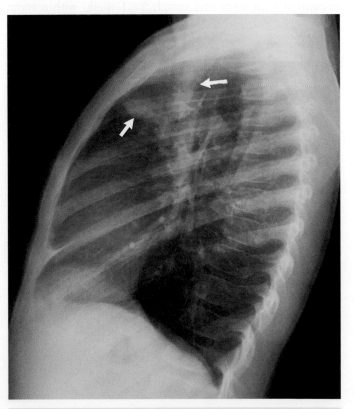

Fig. 37.2 Lateral chest radiograph demonstrating lung opacity in the right upper lobe *(arrows)*, without associated effusion.

Diagnostic testing for bacterial etiologies of CAP is often low yield, and no gold standard exists.[9,20] Polymerase chain reaction (PCR) is commonly employed to assess respiratory tract samples for viral etiologies. Blood cultures are performed only when needed per the Infectious Diseases Society of America (IDSA) and Pediatric Infectious Diseases Society (PIDS) guidelines, while bronchoalveolar lavage samples and needle aspirates are not typically performed due to their invasive nature.[1,20,21]

In children with suspected community-acquired pneumonia, first-line antibiotic choices are beta lactam antibiotics, such as amoxicillin, but providers should refer to local antibiogram as regional susceptibility exists.[1,22,23] For those patients being admitted, IV antibiotics are commonly utilized (e.g., ampicillin for amoxicillin). The decision of whether or not to treat with antibiotics is not greatly influenced by radiographic findings.[24] Adjunct laboratory studies such as procalcitonin have been reported as a potential delineator for which hospitalized patients may be safe without antibiotic treatment.[25] For patients who do not respond to initial therapy, further imaging may be indicated to assess for complications such as abscess or effusion.[1,6] Findings on these images may warrant further interventions such as chest tube placement with or without fibrinolytics or VATS procedure.[1] If atypical causes of pneumonia are suspected, such as *Mycoplasma* pneumoniae, macrolide antibiotics are recommended. Given the frequency of a viral source, recent studies have questioned the rate of antibiotic prescribing.[26]

For comparison, several cases are presented here:

This 35-month-old patient in Figs. 37.3 and 37.4 presented with fever and cough for 1 week, with a room

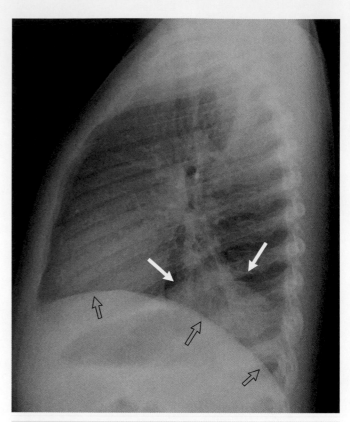

Fig. 37.4 Lateral chest radiograph demonstrates a left lower lobe consolidation *(white arrows)* that obscures visualization of the left hemidiaphragm, such that only the right hemidiaphragm *(open black arrows)* is visualized on the lateral view.

air pulse oximetry reading of 91% and mild tachypnea. A two-view chest radiography demonstrates a left lower lobe consolidation without effusion. While the consolidation is seen on both views in this patient, if a lower lobe consolidation is only in the retrocardiac region, it may be possible to overlook on the frontal view and more easily be seen on the lateral view. This highlights the importance of obtaining two-view chest radiographs in the pediatric population.

This 11-month-old child presented with fever and difficulty breathing and was quite ill-appearing (Figs. 37.5–37.8). Plain radiographs of the chest demonstrated opacification of the left chest, with mass effect, as the mediastinum was shifted to the right, away from the opacified hemithorax. In a child presenting clinically with pneumonia, these findings are most suggestive of pneumonia with pleural effusion, but the chest radiographic findings are not specific. Transthoracic ultrasonography of the chest was obtained, revealing a large left pleural effusion with multiple septations and loculations (Fig. 37.7). Pediatric Surgery was consulted and the child was taken for a VATS procedure with drainage of an empyema and chest tube placement (Fig. 37.8). Methicillin-resistant *Staphylococcus* grew from the effusion culture.

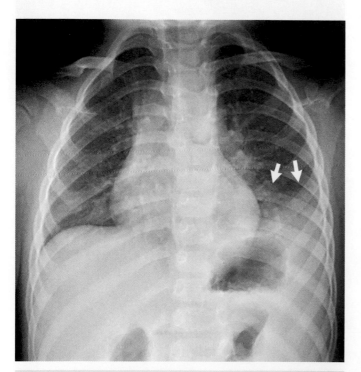

Fig. 37.3 Anterior-posterior chest radiograph demonstrates a left lower lobe consolidation *(white arrows)* that obscures visualization of the left hemidiaphragm.

IMAGING PEARLS

1. Children with a diagnosis of clinical, community-acquired pneumonia do not require routine chest imaging.

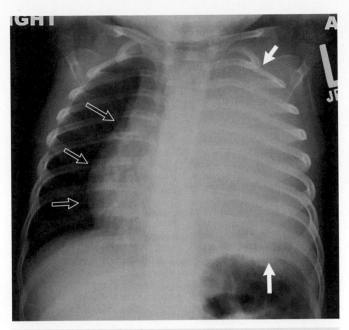

Fig. 37.5 Anterior-posterior chest radiography demonstrates complete opacification of the left hemithorax *(white arrows)* on the frontal view with increased volume and mass effect, as the mediastinum is shifted to the right *(open arrows)*.

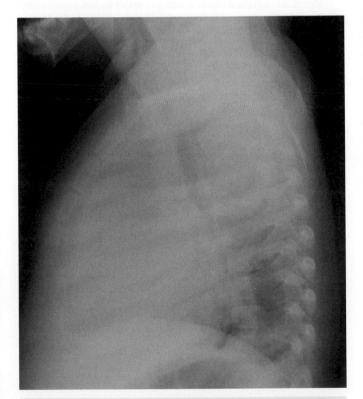

Fig. 37.6 Lateral chest radiography demonstrates complete opacification of the left hemithorax. The lateral view is limited in utility compared with Fig. 37.5, but only the right hemidiaphragm is seen; the left is obscured by the left chest opacification. In a child presenting clinically with pneumonia, these findings are most suggestive of left-sided pneumonia with pleural effusion or empyema, but the findings are not diagnostic by plain radiography.

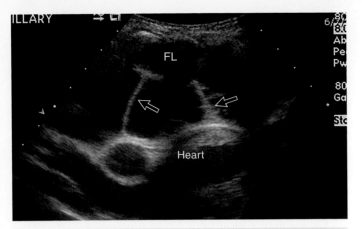

Fig. 37.7 Transthoracic longitudinal ultrasound image of the left chest, demonstrating left pleural fluid *(FL)*, with loculations and septations *(arrows)*, most consistent with empyema with this clinical presentation. The heart is also seen and labeled on this image.

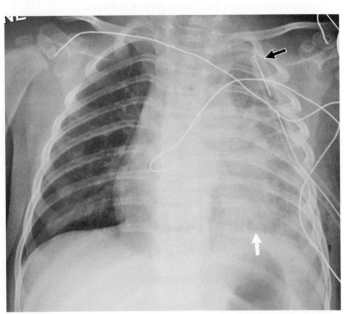

Fig. 37.8 Following a video-assisted thoracoscopic surgery procedure with drainage of left pleural empyema, an anterior-posterior chest radiograph shows decreased opacification of the left hemithorax with re-expansion of the left lung *(white arrow)*. A left chest tube is present *(black arrow)*.

2. Plain chest radiography (two views) is the modality of choice in children with suspected pneumonia in whom imaging is indicated or would be helpful (i.e., hospital admission, atypical course, complication concerns, suspected alternative diagnoses).
3. Transthoracic lung ultrasonography is a useful imaging modality in children with community-acquired pneumonia for the identification of pleural effusions and fluid collections.
4. CT and MRI are not first-line imaging tests but may be indicated for complex disease or when an alternate diagnosis is suspected.

References

1. Bradley JS, Byington CL, Shah SS, et al. Executive summary: the management of community-acquired pneumonia in infants and children older than 3 months of age: clinical practice guidelines by the pediatric infectious diseases society and the Infectious Diseases Society of America. *Clin Infect Dis.* 2011;53(7):617-630.
2. Harris M, Clark J, Coote N, et al. British Thoracic Society guidelines for the management of community acquired pneumonia in children: update 2011. *Thorax.* 2011;66(suppl 2):ii1-ii23.
3. McLaren SH, Mistry RD, Neuman MI, et al. Guideline adherence in diagnostic testing and treatment of community-acquired pneumonia in children. *Pediatr Emerg Care.* 2019 Feb 14. doi: 10.1097/PEC.0000000000001745. Epub ahead of print.
4. Geanacopoulos AT, Porter JJ, Monuteaux MC, et al. Trends in chest radiographs for pneumonia in emergency departments. *Pediatrics.* 2020;145(3):e20192816.
5. Neuman MI, Shah SS, Shapiro DJ, et al. Emergency department management of childhood pneumonia in the United States prior to publication of national guidelines. *Acad Emerg Med.* 2013;20(3):240-246.
6. Fancourt N, Deloria Knoll M, Barger-Kamate B, et al. Standardized interpretation of chest radiographs in cases of pediatric pneumonia from the PERCH Study. *Clin Infect Dis.* 2017;64(suppl 3):S253-S261.
7. Fancourt N, Deloria Knoll M, Bagget HC, et al. Chest radiograph findings in childhood pneumonia cases from the multisite PERCH study. *Clin Infect Dis.* 2017;64(suppl 3):S262-S270.
8. Andronikou S. Imaging community-acquired pneumonia in children. *Pediatr Radiol.* 2017;47(11):1390-1391.
9. Nascimento-Carvalho CM, Araújo-Neto CA, Ruuskanen O. Association between bacterial infection and radiologically confirmed pneumonia among children. *Pediatr Infect Dis J.* 2015;34(5):490-493.
10. Lipsett SC, Monuteaux MC, Bachur RG, et al. Negative chest radiography and risk of pneumonia. *Pediatrics.* 2018;142(3):e20180236.
11. Andronikou S, Goussard P, Sorantin E. Computed tomography in children with community-acquired pneumonia. *Pediatr Radiol.* 2017;47(11): 1431-1440.
12. Boursiani C, Tsolia M, Koumanidou C, et al. Lung ultrasound as first-line examination for the diagnosis of community-acquired pneumonia in children. *Pediatr Emerg Care.* 2017;33(1):62-66.
13. Principi N, Esposito A, Giannitto C, et al. Lung ultrasonography to diagnose community-acquired pneumonia in children. *BMC Pulm Med.* 2017;17(1):212.
14. Stadler JAM, Andronikou S, Zar HJ. Lung ultrasound for the diagnosis of community-acquired pneumonia in children. *Pediatr Radiol.* 2017;47(11):1412-1419.
15. Yilmaz HL, Özkaya AK, Sarı Gökay S, et al. Point-of-care lung ultrasound in children with community acquired pneumonia. *Am J Emerg Med.* 2017;35(7):964-969.
16. Harel-Sterling M, Diallo M, Santhirakumaran S, et al. Emergency department resource use in pediatric pneumonia: point-of-care lung ultrasonography versus chest radiography. *J Ultrasound Med.* 2019;38(2):407-414.
17. Ambroggio L, Sucharew H, Rattan MS, et al. Lung ultrasonography: a viable alternative to chest radiography in children with suspected pneumonia? *J Pediatr.* 2016;176:93-98.e7.
18. Liszewski MC, Görkem S, Sodhi KS, et al. Lung magnetic resonance imaging for pneumonia in children. *Pediatr Radiol.* 2017;47(11): 1420-1430.
19. Wagner WL, Schenk JP, Alrajab A, et al. The value of chest magnetic resonance imaging compared to chest radiographs with and without additional lung ultrasound in children with complicated pneumonia. *PLoS One.* 2020;15(3):e0230252.
20. Jain S, Williams DJ, Arnold SR, et al. Community acquired pneumonia requiring hospitalization among US children. *N Engl J Med.* 2015;372(9):835-845.
21. Tramper-Stranders GA. Childhood community-acquired pneumonia: a review of etiology- and antimicrobial treatment studies. *Paediatr Respir Rev.* 2018;26:41-48.
22. Gereige RS, Laufer PM. Pneumonia. *Pediatr Rev.* 2013;34(10): 438-456.
23. Messinger AI, Kupfer O, Hurst A, Parker S. Management of pediatric community-acquired bacterial pneumonia. *Pediatr Rev.* 2017;38(9): 394-409.
24. Nelson KA, Morrow C, Wingerter SL, et al. Impact of chest radiography on antibiotic treatment for children with suspected pneumonia. *Pediatr Emerg Care.* 2016;32(8):514-519.
25. Stockman C, Ampofo K, Killpack J, et al. Procalcitonin accurately identifies hospitalized children with low risk of bacterial community-acquired pneumonia. *J Pediatric Infect Dis Soc.* 2018;7(1):46-53.
26. Lipshaw MJ, Eckerle M, Florin TA, et al. Antibiotic use and outcomes in children in the emergency department with suspected pneumonia. *Pediatrics.* 2020;145(4):e20193138.

38   Is That Pneumonia? Atelectasis

ROBERT VEZZETTI, MD, FAAP, FACEP

Case Presentation

A 22-month-old female presents with cough and congestion for the past 5 days. She was noted to have persistent fever to 102 degrees Fahrenheit. She has been taking oral fluids well, but this has decreased over the past few days, although she still has good urine output. There has been no vomiting, diarrhea, or concern for foreign body ingestion/choking episodes. Her physical examination reveals a febrile child (101.5 degrees Fahrenheit) with a respiratory rate of 25 breaths per minute, a heat rate of 140 beats per minute, and a pulse oximetry reading of 85% on room air. She is alert and vigorous but with mild respiratory distress. There are scattered crackles and wheezing throughout her lung fields, but especially at the left lower lobe. She has moderate intercostal retractions without stridor or grunting. The remainder of her examination is unremarkable.

Imaging Considerations

PLAIN RADIOGRAPHY

This is often the first-line imaging modality in patients with concern for a pulmonary process, usually pneumonia. Atelectasis on plain radiography may be difficult to distinguish from a lobar consolidation that may be seen with other processes, such as pneumonia. There are radiographic features that can assist with the differentiation of atelectasis and consolidation. Compared to pneumonia, atelectasis is a process of volume loss and is associated with signs of volume loss such as a shift in the normal position of fissures or pulmonary vessels, a mediastinal shift toward the side of the atelectasis, or unilateral diaphragmatic elevation.[1] While atelectasis can involve any lobe of the lungs, the right and left lower lobes and the right middle lobe are frequent sites of atelectasis, especially in patients with asthma.[1] Plain radiography does not expose the patient to significant amounts of ionizing radiation compared to other ionizing modalities (e.g., computed tomography [CT]). Two views of the chest are recommended.[1]

ULTRASOUND (US)

US is an emerging imaging modality in many pediatric imaging applications. There are some reports using US to detect atelectasis, particularly in the neonatal population, which have shown promise, but US is not typically a first-line imaging modality.[2,3]

COMPUTED TOMOGRAPHY

CT can detect atelectasis but is not employed as a first-line imaging modality in general.

Imaging Findings

Plain radiography of the chest was obtained. Here, a two-view (posterior-anterior and lateral) study is provided (Figs. 38.1 and 38.2). The examination demonstrates increased parahilar interstitial markings and peribronchial thickening bilaterally. There is consolidation in the retrocardiac left lower lobe, with angular borders, that has a bandlike appearance on the lateral view, an appearance consistent with atelectasis. There is no effusion or pneumothorax. In light of the history, radiographic appearance, and clinical exam, these findings are consistent with atelectasis due to airway disease rather than pneumonia.

Case Conclusion

The child was placed on high-flow nasal cannula oxygen with improvement of her symptoms. She had vigorous nasal suctioning performed. Due to her hypoxia and respiratory distress, she was admitted to the hospital for monitoring and supportive care. After several days, she improved and was able to be discharged with close monitoring and follow-up.

Pediatric atelectasis has various etiologies. These can be categorized as:[1,4]

1. Airway obstruction—either from exogenous causes (such as an airway foreign body or recurrent aspiration) or endogenous causes (mucous plugs in cystic fibrosis or infectious processes, such as pneumonia, bronchiolitis, or ciliary mobility syndromes).
2. Compression of lung parenchyma—due to chest masses (either primary or due to metastasis), cardiomegaly, pneumothorax, pleural effusion, hemothorax, or neuromuscular diseases (such as spinal muscular atrophy).
3. Surfactant deficiency—as can be seen in pulmonary edema, submersion injuries, and acute respiratory distress syndrome.

A common cause of atelectasis in the pediatric population is mucous plugging associated with an infectious process.[1] The clinical presentation of atelectasis can be nonspecific but often is dependent on the underlying process. For example, in bronchiolitis, fever, wheezing, rhonchi, and crackles are usually present in some degree. Although none of these findings are specific for atelectasis, the presence of focal wheezing or diminished breath sounds can be found and can be suggestive of atelectasis.[1] A thorough history and physical examination can assist the clinician in determining the most probable etiology of atelectasis.

Special mention should be made of right middle lobe syndrome, originally described by Graham to describe atelectasis from compression of the right middle lobe bronchus

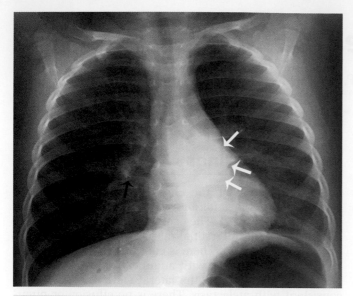

Fig. 38.1 Posterior-anterior view of the chest demonstrates parahilar bronchial wall thickening, a representative thick-walled bronchus seen clearly on the right *(black arrow)*. There is focal consolidation in the retrocardiac left lower lobe *(white arrows)*, with angular borders, especially in the left parahilar region, that has a collapsed, bandlike appearance on the lateral view (Fig 38.2). This appearance is consistent with atelectasis rather than pneumonia.

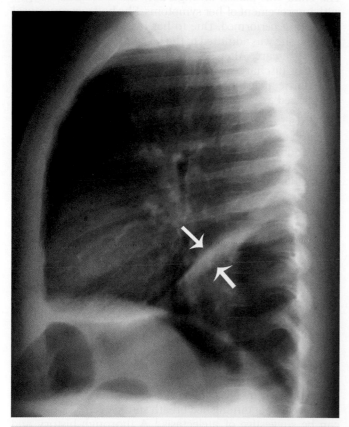

Fig. 38.2 Lateral view of the chest demonstrates parahilar bronchial wall thickening. There is focal consolidation in the retrocardiac left lower lobe (Fig. 38.1), with angular borders, especially in the left parahilar region, that has a collapsed, bandlike appearance on the lateral view *(white arrows)*. This appearance is consistent with atelectasis rather than pneumonia.

due to peribronchial lymphadenopathy.[4,5] Findings similar to right middle lobe syndrome have been reported in other sections of the lung as well.[4,6] The precise prevalence is unknown, but this entity is more commonly found in the preschool-age population.[4] Right middle lobe syndrome should be suspected when patients present with chronic or persistent cough, wheezing, or recurrent/persistent "pneumonia" in the right middle lobe.[4] Interestingly, this entity is frequently overlooked by physicians, and patients often have been treated with multiple courses of antibiotics prior to diagnosis.[4] Right middle lobe syndrome, commonly seen in pediatric asthma patients, is most commonly due to bronchial wall inflammation and plugging in the right middle lobe with persistent atelectasis.[1,4] Radiographic findings are often misinterpreted as pneumonia and treated as such, although antibiotics are not indicated.[4] Chest radiography is the first-line imaging modality for investigating middle lobe syndrome; CT can be utilized as a secondary imaging study to investigate the patency of the bronchial apparatus, evaluate for bronchiectasis, as well as assess for any causes of extrinsic compression, such as adenopathy or masses, or endobronchial lesion such as mass or foreign body.[4] While the role of US in the investigation of middle lobe syndrome remains to be defined, magnetic resonance imaging has emerged as an imaging option.[4] Management is dependent on the underling etiology of the middle lobe syndrome and often involves subspecialty consultation, particularly with pediatric pulmonology. The outcomes of patients with middle lobe syndromes are overall favorable, although long-term outcome data are lacking.[4,7] There are reports of up to one-third of patients having residual respiratory symptoms, including mild obstructive airway disease.[4,7,8]

Treatment of atelectasis is dependent on the underlying disease process. Patients with asthma, cystic fibrosis, and underlying chronic illnesses are managed with appropriate medications and treatments appropriate to the underlying disease process. Chest physiotherapy is another method that has been employed, especially in the inpatient setting, to help relieve atelectasis and improve pulmonary mucous clearance.[1,9] There are few published studies evaluating the management of pediatric atelectasis, although various modalities, such as nebulized medications and intrapulmonary percussive therapy, in addition to chest physiotherapy, have been investigated.[9–11] Patients with persistent atelectasis should have a pediatric pulmonology consultation and flexible bronchoscopy should be considered.[4,12] There are entities (e.g., endobronchial tumors) that can present with persistent atelectasis that require further investigation beyond plain radiography.[13,14]

For comparison, several cases are presented here:

A 6-year-old girl with a history of asthma presented with two separate episodes of fever, cough, and wheezing, 5 months apart. At her first presentation, opacity and volume loss were noted in the right lower lobe on chest radiograph, consistent with right lower lobe atelectasis. When she was again symptomatic 5 months later, chest radiograph shows the right lower lobe to be re-expanded and normal, but there is opacity and volume loss in the left lower lobe, consistent with left lower lobe atelectasis. Note the similar appearance of atelectasis in either lower lobe, as both lower lobes characteristically collapse inferiorly and medially (Figs. 38.3 and 38.4).

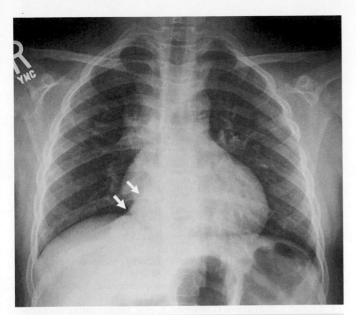

Fig. 38.3 Posterior-anterior view of the chest in the same patient as Fig. 38.4, 5 months apart. Here, there is asymmetric increased opacity in the retrocardiac right lower lobe, due to right lower lobe atelectasis *(arrows)*. Note the angular, sharply defined right superolateral border of this opacity, which is the depressed major fissure *(arrows)*.

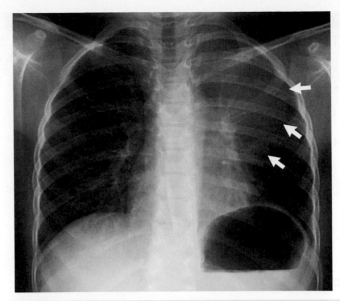

Fig. 38.5 Posterior-anterior (PA) view of left upper lobe atelectasis. This figure demonstrates a hazy increased opacity of the left mid to upper lung *(arrows)* which is associated with prominence and poor definition of the left hilar structures and poor definition of the left upper cardiac border.

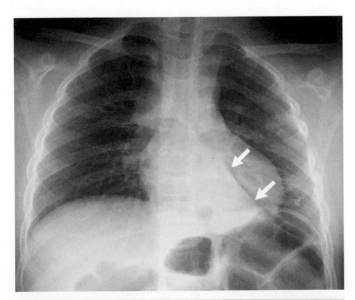

Fig. 38.4 Posterior-anterior view of the chest in the same patient, 5 months later. Here, the right lower lobe opacity has resolved, but there is interval development of opacity and volume loss consistent with atelectasis in the left lower lobe *(arrows)*. Note depression of the major fissure on the left *(arrows)* consistent with lower lobe volume loss.

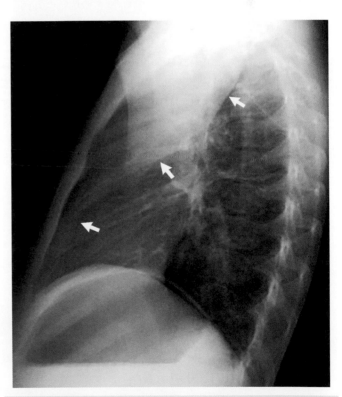

Fig. 38.6 Lateral view of left upper lobe atelectasis. This figure demonstrates the opacity is anterior *(arrows)*, as the left upper lobe collapses anteriorly.

An 8-year-old patient presents with cough and wheezing. A two-view chest series demonstrates opacity of the left mid to upper lung on the frontal view, obscuring the left hilar structures and the upper left cardiac border. On the lateral view, the opacity is anterior. This is the characteristic appearance of atelectasis of the left upper lobe and does not represent pneumonia or a mass. Although the right upper lobe is well known to collapse superiorly and medially, the left upper lobe instead collapses anteriorly, creating the characteristic appearance seen in this child. It is important to recognize this as left upper lobe atelectasis and to avoid the misconception that there is pneumonia or a hilar mass (Figs. 38.5 and 38.6).

IMAGING PEARLS

1. Plain chest radiography is the first-line imaging modality in patients with suspected pulmonary disease. A two-view study is preferable.
2. CT can detect atelectasis but should not be the primary imaging modality in the majority of cases.
3. The role of US in detecting atelectasis in pediatric patients is evolving, but shows promise.
4. Radiographically distinguishing atelectasis from other pulmonary processes, such as infiltrate or effusion, can be difficult. In general, atelectasis is associated with volume loss and most often will involve the right middle or lower lobes, but it can involve any lobe. Certain disease processes, such as uncomplicated bronchiolitis or asthma, are commonly associated with atelectasis and not bacterial pneumonia.

References

1. Peroni DG, Boner AL. Atelectasis: mechanisms, diagnosis and management. *Paediatr Respir Rev.* 2000;1(3):274-278.
2. Liu J, Chen SW, Liu F, et al. The diagnosis of neonatal pulmonary atelectasis using lung ultrasonography. *Chest.* 2015;147(4):1013-1019.
3. Caiulo VA, Gargani L, Caiulo S, et al. Usefulness of lung ultrasound in a newborn with pulmonary atelectasis. *Pediatr Med Chir.* 2011;33 (5-6):253-255.
4. Romagnoli V, Priftis KN, de Benedictis FM. Middle lobe syndrome in children today. *Paediatr Respir Rev.* 2014;15(2):188-193.
5. Graham EA, Burford TH, Mayer JH. Middle lobe syndrome. *Postgrad Med.* 1948;4(1):29-34.
6. Hamad AM, Elmistekawy E, Elatafy E. Chronic atelectasis of the left lower lobe: a clinicopathological condition equivalent to middle lobe syndrome. *Interact Cardiovasc Thorac Surg.* 2012;15(4):618-621.
7. Priftis KN, Mermiri D, Papadopoulou A, et al. The role of timely intervention in middle lobe syndrome in children. *Chest.* 2005; 128(4):2504-2510.
8. De Boeck K, Willems T, Van Gysel D, et al. Outcome after right middle lobe syndrome. *Chest.* 1995;108(1):150-152.
9. Schindler MB. Treatment of atelectasis: where is the evidence? *Crit Care.* 2005;9(4):341-342.
10. Yen Ha TK, Bui TD, Tran AT, et al. Atelectatic children treated with intrapulmonary percussive ventilation via a face mask: clinical trial and literature overview. *Pediatr Int.* 2007;49(4):502-507.
11. Soyer O, Ozen C, Cavkaytar O, et al. Right middle lobe atelectasis in children with asthma and prognostic factors. *Allergol Int.* 2016; 65(3):253-258.
12. Midulla F, de Blic J, Barbato A, et al. Flexible endoscopy of pediatric airways. *Eur Respir J.* 2003;22(4):698-708.
13. Ruttan T, Vezzetti R, Scalo J. Persistent pneumonia: time to take a closer look. *Pediatr Emerg Care.* 2017;33(1):31-33.
14. Dhouib A, Barrazzone C, Reverdin A, et al. Inflammatory myofibroblastic tumor of the lung: a rare cause of atelectasis in children. *Pediatr Radiol.* 2013;43(3):381-384.

39 Will the Cough Ever Stop? Atypical Pneumonia

ROBERT VEZZETTI, MD, FAAP, FACEP

Case Presentation

A 12-year-old male with a history of autism presents with cough for the past 3 weeks. There was initially fever to 102 degrees Fahrenheit, but this lasted for 2–3 days, then resolved. He was seen by his primary care provider 2 weeks ago and was diagnosed with a viral upper respiratory infection. He has not had congestion, vomiting, diarrhea, or abdominal pain. There is no report of choking or concern for foreign body ingestion. He has been eating and drinking well. Examination reveals a temperature of 99 degrees Fahrenheit, a heart rate of 90 beats per minute, a respiratory rate of 20 breaths per minute, a blood pressure of 110/75 mm Hg, and an oxygen saturation of 93% on room air. He appears comfortable and in no respiratory distress. He has no stigmata of allergies. His pulmonary examination reveals scattered rhonchi without crackles; there is slight bibasilar wheezing. He has no rash.

Imaging Considerations

Imaging is often employed in the evaluation of children with respiratory complaints. The differential diagnosis can be broad, and the imaging modality that a clinician may employ is dependent on history and physical examination.

PLAIN RADIOGRAPHY

Pediatric patients with suspected viral etiology or uncomplicated bacterial pneumonia do not generally require imaging. Plain radiography is an excellent first-line imaging choice in patients who are not following an expected clinical course, if there are concerns for complications from a previously diagnosed pulmonary infection, the child is severely ill, or if there is an alternative diagnosis under consideration, such as foreign body ingestion. Two views of the chest are needed to allow for proper and complete visualization of chest anatomy, including areas obscured by the heart and mediastinal structures.[1] Plain radiography does have limitations, including variability with image interpretation and image technique, which may make it difficult to obtain meaningful studies in select patients.

Viral infection is the most common cause of pneumonia in the pediatric population. While controversial, radiography is often used to confirm a suspected bacterial etiology and has been shown to correlate well with that diagnosis in children who have *Pneumococcus* species as a cause of their pneumonia; children with a normal radiograph who have been diagnosed with clinical bacterial pneumonia are not prone to have pneumococcal infection.[2] In one study, the majority of children hospitalized with severe community-acquired pneumonia had radiographs demonstrating alveolar infiltrates, and those with upper lobe infiltrates along with effusions were found to have more serious disease.[3] (For a complete discussion of bacterial pneumonia and radiography, please see Chapter 37: Community-Acquired Pneumonia).

ULTRASOUND

Interest in sonography to aid in the diagnosis of pneumonia has increased. Ultrasound has the advantage of a lack of ionizing radiation and is fairly inexpensive compared to other imaging modalities. Ultrasound has proven adept at locating effusions and is more sensitive than computed tomography.[1,4] Consolidation can be detected, seen as a hypoechogenic area with poor border definition, but distinguishing between atelectasis and true pneumonia can be difficult, affecting accuracy.[1,5] Other studies have shown ultrasound to be effective at diagnosing community-acquired pneumonia in selected patients[4–7] and may result in shorter length of stay and lower costs compared to chest radiography.[8] Standardized usage for transthoracic ultrasound to aid diagnosing pediatric pneumonia is a developing practice. Studies thus far have shown this modality may be useful, either as a first-line test or as an adjunct to better define abnormal plain radiography findings, although this modality requires specific training to perform appropriately and the noted accuracy may not be generalizable to providers without skill in thoracic ultrasound.

COMPUTED TOMOGRAPHY

Computed tomography is generally not a first-line imaging modality. Use of this technology may be indicated in children with complex illness or when a diagnosis is uncertain.

Imaging Findings

The patient had two-view radiography of the chest. The images demonstrate interstitial opacities in the lungs, with a hazy more focal parenchymal opacity in the right lower lung, best seen on the AP view. There are no signs of pleural effusion/fluid. The cardiac silhouette is normal with a left-sided aorta (Figs. 39.1 and 39.2).

Case Conclusion

The child's clinical history, examination, and chest radiography were suggestive of infection with *Mycoplasma*

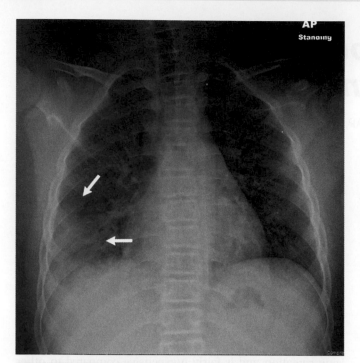

Fig. 39.1 Anterior-posterior view: multiple areas of interstitial opacities with more focal confluent opacity *(arrows)* in the right lower lobe, partially obscuring the lateral right hemidiaphragm.

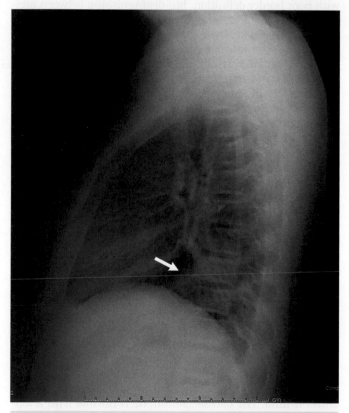

Fig. 39.2 The right lower lobe opacity is seen more subtly on the lateral view, as opacity extending posterior to the major fissure *(arrow)*, causing loss of visualization of the posterior right hemidiaphragm.

pneumoniae. The patient was discharged from the pediatric emergency department with close monitoring, treatment with azithromycin for 5 days, and follow-up with his primary care provider. Serologic testing was not performed.

The term "walking pneumonia" has been used to describe infections with *Mycoplasma* pneumonia. Current convention uses the term "atypical pneumonia" to describe infections attributed to *Mycoplasma* and *Chlamydial* species. *Mycoplasma pneumoniae* has been recognized as a significant, common etiology of respiratory tract infections among school-aged children.[9] A positive polymerase chain reaction (PCR) test or positive serology for this organism has been reported in up to one-third of children hospitalized with community-acquired pneumonia.[9–11] Most infections with *Mycoplasma* are mild and self-limited. Common symptoms include signs of respiratory infection, including low-grade fever and cough, including asthma-like symptoms.[9,12,13] Severe infection is possible and extrapulmonary complications have been reported, including dermatologic (nonspecific exanthems and erythema multiformae) and neurologic conditions (encephalitis and Guillain-Barré syndrome), although all body systems can be affected.[9,10,12–14]

Chest radiography typically demonstrates bilateral, diffuse interstitial infiltrates but may also show effusions.[10,13] Some studies have reported peripheral infiltration in older children and hilar adenopathy in younger children.[13] Volume loss and multilobar involvement are also common.[15,16] However, plain radiography findings are variable and these findings are not specific for *Mycoplasma* infection. A combination of historical and clinical findings, in combination with radiography, can help make the diagnosis of *Mycoplasma* infection. Advanced imaging, in general, is not indicated for patients with clinically suspected uncomplicated *Mycoplasma* infections.

There are several diagnostic testing options that may be utilized to confirm *Mycoplasma* infection. PCR is considered the "gold standard" due to excellent sensitivity and rapid time to results. Serology for IgM and IgG and rapid antigen tests are less sensitive than PCR, and agglutination assays have been replaced by PCR and serology testing. Culture is not used, due to special medium requirements and the length of time needed to obtain a result.[10,12,17] No single testing method, however, can reliably confirm *Mycoplasma* infection in children.

Treatment for this infection is dependent on clinical suspicion and radiographic findings. In children with suspected community-acquired pneumonia, first-line antibiotic choices are beta-lactam antibiotics, such as amoxicillin.[10,18] However, due to the lack of a cell wall, beta-lactam antibiotics are not effective against *Mycoplasma*. As such, macrolide antibiotics, such as azithromycin, are recommended for the treatment of *Mycoplasma* infections, although the evidence supporting their use is limited and resistance has been increasing.[9,10,11,18–20] The clinician should also consider treatment for *Mycoplasma* in children who are being treated for community-acquired pneumonia with appropriate first-line antibiotics and are not improving or not responding as expected.[10,11]

IMAGING PEARLS

1. Children with a diagnosis of clinical, uncomplicated pneumonia do not require routine chest imaging.
2. Most pneumonia in children is viral in etiology. If antibiotics are considered, treatment choice is based on historical and clinical findings.
3. Plain chest radiography (ideally two views) is the modality of choice in children with suspected pneumonia in whom imaging is indicated or would be helpful. Children with an atypical course of a suspected viral infection, concerns for complications, or in whom an alternative diagnosis is suspected are appropriate candidates for imaging.
4. Transthoracic ultrasonography has emerged as a potentially useful imaging test in children with community-acquired pneumonia. This modality is very useful for the identification of pleural effusions and fluid collections. Ultrasound has mixed efficacy in distinguishing between atelectasis and infiltrate in the pediatric population; more study is needed.
5. Computed tomography is not a first-line imaging test in the vast majority of children in whom pneumonia is suspected. In children with complex disease or where an alternative diagnosis is suspected, this modality may be useful.

References

1. Principi N, Esposito A, Giannitto C, et al. Lung ultrasonography to diagnose community-acquired pneumonia in children. *BMC Pulm Med.* 2017;17(1):212.
2. Nascimento-Carvalho CM, Araújo-Neto CA, Ruuskanen O. Association between bacterial infection and radiologically confirmed pneumonia among children. *Pediatr Infect Dis J.* 2015;34(5):490-493.
3. Ferrero F, Nascimento-Carvalho CM, Cardoso MR, et al. Radiographic findings among children hospitalized with severe community-acquired pneumonia. *Pediatr Pulmonol.* 2010;45(10):1009-1013.
4. Iuri D, De Candia A, Bazzocchi M. Evaluation of the lung in children with suspected pneumonia: usefulness of ultrasonography. *Radiol Med.* 2009;114(2):321-330.
5. Boursiani C, Tsolia M, Koumanidou C, et al. Lung ultrasound as first-line examination for the diagnosis of community-acquired pneumonia in children. *Pediatr Emerg Care.* 2017;33(1):62-66.
6. Yilmaz HL, Özkaya AK, Sarı Gökay S, et al. Point-of-care lung ultrasound in children with community acquired pneumonia. *Am J Emerg Med.* 2017;35(7):964-969.
7. Claes AS, Clapuyt P, Menten R, et al. Performance of chest ultrasound in pediatric pneumonia. *Eur J Radiol.* 2017;88:82-87.
8. Harel-Sterling M, Diallo M, Santhirakumaran S, et al. Emergency department resource use in pediatric pneumonia: point-of-care lung ultrasonography versus chest radiography. *J Ultrasound Med.* 2019;38(2):407-414.
9. Meyer Sauteur PM, Unger WW, Nadal D, et al. Infection with and carriage of *Mycoplasma pneumoniae* in children. *Front Microbiol.* 2016;7:329.
10. Meyer Sauteur PM, Unger WWJ, van Rossum AMC, et al. The art and science of diagnosing *Mycoplasma pneumoniae* infection. *Pediatr Infect Dis J.* 2018;37(11):1192-1195.
11. Harris M, Clark J, Coote N, et al. British Thoracic Society guidelines for the management of community acquired pneumonia in children: update 2011. *Thorax.* 2011;66(suppl 2):ii1-ii23.
12. Parrott GL, Kinjo T, Fujita J. A compendium for *Mycoplasma pneumoniae. Front Microbiol.* 2016;7:513.
13. Søndergaard MJ, Friis MB, Hansen DS, et al. Clinical manifestations in infants and children with *Mycoplasma pneumoniae* infection. *PLoS One.* 2018;13(4):e0195288.
14. Narita M. Classification of extrapulmonary manifestations due to *Mycoplasma pneumoniae* infection on the basis of possible pathogenesis. *Front Microbiol.* 2016;7:23.
15. Tomoo K. Community-acquired pneumonia caused by *Mycoplasma pneumoniae*: how physical and radiological examination contribute to successful diagnosis. *Front Med (Lausanne).* 2016;3:28.
16. Guo WL, Wang J, Zhu LY, et al. Differentiation between mycoplasma and viral community-acquired pneumonia in children with lobe or multi foci infiltration: a retrospective case study. *BMJ Open.* 2015;5(1):1-6.
17. Meyer Sauteur PM, van Rossum AM, Vink C. *Mycoplasma pneumoniae* in children: carriage, pathogenesis, and antibiotic resistance. *Curr Opin Infect Dis.* 2014;27(3):220-227.
18. Pereyre S, Goret J, Bébéar C. *Mycoplasma pneumoniae*: current knowledge on macrolide resistance and treatment. *Front Microbiol.* 2016;7:974.
19. Spuesens EB, Meyer Sauteur PM, Vink C, et al. *Mycoplasma pneumoniae* infections—does treatment help? *J Infect.* 2014;69(suppl 1):S42-S46.
20. Gardiner SJ, Gavranich JB, Chang AB. Antibiotics for community-acquired lower respiratory tract infections secondary to *Mycoplasma pneumoniae* in children. *Cochrane Database Syst Rev.* 2015;1:CD004875.

40 *Of Course You Have Asthma: Persistent Wheezing*

TIM RUTTAN, MD

Case Presentation

An 8-year-old boy presents with 3 days of cough, fever, and headache. He had been seen the previous day by his primary care physician and he was told to come to the Emergency Department after a chest x-ray performed as an outpatient demonstrated findings concerning for pneumonia. Six weeks ago, he was diagnosed with a right lower lobe pneumonia and treated with oral amoxicillin but failed to clinically improve and was admitted to the hospital for further management. He improved clinically and was discharged to complete a course of oral antibiotics.

Medical history is notable for a diagnosis of reactive airway disease at 3 years of age, which mostly responded to treatment with bronchodilators. His mother observed that he seemed to have more breathing problems over the last 3 years, and he was diagnosed as an outpatient multiple times over this time period with clinical pneumonia and "bronchitis."

Physical examination reveals a nontoxic child whose only complaint is right-sided chest pain with deep inspiration. His vital signs demonstrate a temperature of 102 degrees Fahrenheit, a heart rate of 130 beats per minute, a respiratory rate of 24 breaths per minute, a blood pressure of 127/68 mm Hg, and a pulse oximetry reading of 95% on room air. He has an unremarkable examination other than his pulmonary exam, which has decreased breath sounds on the right without crackles or rhonchi, but there is mild inspiratory and expiratory wheezing; he has no retractions or grunting.

Imaging Considerations

PLAIN RADIOGRAPHY

While the vast majority of pediatric patients with wheezing will have a viral etiology, the clinician should broaden the differential diagnosis in patients with persistence of respiratory symptoms. This can be divided into two major categories: structural causes and functional causes. Structural causes include vascular rings and slings, tracheomalacia, tracheal stenosis, tracheal webs, and masses. Functional causes include asthma/reactive airway disease, gastroesophageal reflux disease (especially in infants), vocal cord dysfunction (especially in adolescent patients), persistent or recurrent infection, and foreign bodies. Plain radiography is the initial imaging modality of choice for patients with persistent wheezing or other respiratory symptoms (such as tachypnea or hypoxia).

A two-view study (posterior-anterior or anterior-posterior and lateral) should be obtained when possible.

COMPUTED TOMOGRAPHY (CT)

CT is a second-line imaging modality for evaluating complicated lung disease, particularly lesions affecting the bronchus or if there is a concern for a bronchial foreign body. CT provides greater definition of the underlying pathology than plain film. In addition, given the typically broad differential, CT can help to give guidance on the next steps in diagnosis and treatment, and can localize pathology, to help direct bronchoscopy or surgery. If CT is being obtained for acute foreign body aspiration, intravenous (IV) contrast is not necessary. However, for more subacute processes or processes that may be infectious or related to a malignancy, IV contrast should be used to define the vasculature, differentiate vasculature from adenopathy or other mass, and to help characterize a mass, pneumonia, or abscess.

ULTRASOUND (US)

Unlike in the evaluation of more typical pneumonias and effusions, lung US does not provide sufficient detail for evaluation of processes involving the bronchial tree.

MAGNETIC RESONANCE IMAGING (MRI)

This modality is not used for first-line imaging and may be employed in patients who require further clarification of plain radiographic or CT findings.

Imaging Findings

The patient underwent plain chest radiography. A selected image from this study is provided here. This examination was compared to chest radiograph from 6 weeks prior (not shown) and revealed persistent right lower lobe consolidation and volume loss with no significant interval change (Fig. 40.1).

Case Conclusion

The child was admitted to the hospital for further evaluation and diagnostic management. An IV contrast–enhanced CT of the chest was obtained. Selected images from the CT are provided here, demonstrating complete opacification of the right lower lobe with a filling defect of the right lower lobe bronchus, suggesting an endobronchial lesion such as foreign body, mass, or granuloma (Figs. 40.2 and 40.3). Pediatric Pulmonology was consulted and flexible bronchoscopy was performed, which led to a tissue diagnosis of

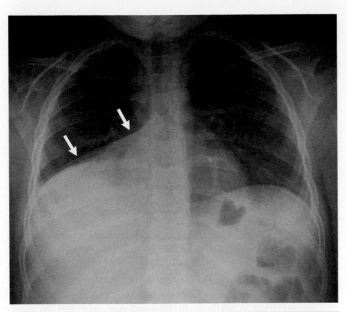

Fig. 40.1 Frontal chest radiograph demonstrates consolidation and volume loss in the right lower lobe *(arrows)*, with appearance unchanged since a prior chest radiograph 6 weeks earlier.

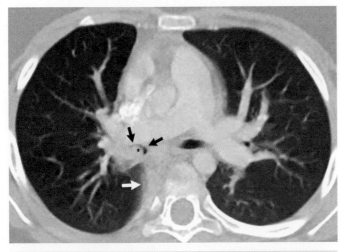

Fig. 40.2 Axial computed tomography lung window image demonstrates an endobronchial mass on the right *(*)*, with a crescent of air partially surrounding the mass in the involved right bronchus *(black arrows)*. The right lower lobe is collapsed and consolidated *(white arrow)*.

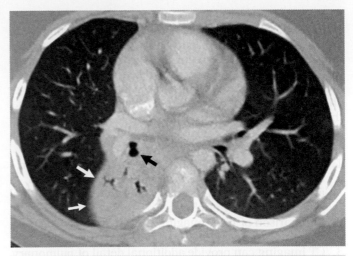

Fig. 40.3 Axial computed tomography lung window image inferior to Fig. 40.2 shows air in the more peripheral right lower lobe bronchi *(black arrow)* but dense atelectasis and consolidation in the basilar right lower lobe *(white arrows)*.

an endobronchial mucoepidermoid carcinoma. The patient was treated with laser photoablation and ultimately did well with improvement in lung function.

Most medical trainees can recite the dogma that "all that wheezes is not asthma," but in the setting of a busy clinical environment, it can be challenging to think beyond common etiologies. Diagnoses that may mimic asthma or pneumonia include congenital malformations (vascular rings and slings, tracheomalacia and bronchomalacia, congenital pulmonary airway malformations, and pulmonary sequestrations), foreign bodies, tuberculosis, myocarditis, mucous plugs, and pulmonary hemosiderosis.[1–3]

Wheezing and reactive airway disease are common in the pediatric population, and considerable interest exists in limiting chest x-rays in patients with suspected asthma.[4] While it is clear that imaging tests can be overused, certain factors should prompt the clinician to pursue imaging. Unusual age of onset, severity of disease, atypical response to treatment, and recurrent symptoms all may indicate the need for imaging. Moreover, a careful history could help to identify pathology such as a retained foreign body. For example, a child with recurrent pneumonias after an initial choking episode should have further investigation to evaluate for a foreign body. In addition, review of previous imaging (if available) can help to evaluate for change as well as indicate patterns of airway compromise.

Several case reports in the literature have illustrated the ability of malignancies to mimic pneumonia and asthma.[1,5,6] Clinicians should maintain a high index of suspicion for atypical presentations of common disease to make an earlier diagnosis for the patient.

Mucoepidermoid carcinoma was described in 1952 by Hubbell and Liebow.[7] These lesions are malignant tumors that arise from the epithelial mucous-secreting cells and affect a large age range.[8] Patients with lower histological grades and earlier-stage lesions at diagnosis have better outcomes and survival.[8]

The presentation of these tumors in children can be subtle. Several signs and symptoms, however, are commonly reported, including recurrent pneumonia, recurrent and frequent wheezing (often unresponsive to standard treatment for reactive airways disease), chronic cough, and occasionally hemoptysis.

Radiographic findings in mucoepidermoid carcinoma usually include an area of persistent lobar collapse or consolidation that persists despite appropriate treatment. Bronchoscopy is essential for airway evaluation in cases of chronic consolidation or atypical wheezing to determine etiology, and sometimes treatment.[9–11] Further imaging with CT or MRI can be helpful but is not universally used.[1,9–11] The choice of imaging studies is often physician and institution dependent.

The primary treatment modality for endobronchial tumors is surgical resection and can sometimes be accomplished during bronchoscopy. In some cases, lobar or lung resection may be necessary. The recurrence rate of these tumors is low once complete resection has been accomplished.[9,12] If complete resection cannot be achieved, then radiotherapy or chemotherapy can be used; how effective this additional therapy is has not been determined.[1,9,11]

IMAGING PEARLS

1. Consider obtaining chest imaging in a patient with an atypical history or response to treatment for asthma and pneumonia. Plain radiography should be the initial imaging modality of choice.
2. Comparison of prior imaging studies, if available, to current imaging studies is recommended.
3. CT imaging can provide additional detail of pulmonary pathologies when an abnormality has been identified on chest x-ray and can help to guide treatment.

References

1. Ruttan T, Vezzetti R, Scalo J. Persistent pneumonia: time to take a closer look. *Pediatr Emerg Care*. 2017;33(1):31-33.
2. Park DB, Dobson JV, Losek JD. All that wheezes is not asthma: cognitive bias in pediatric emergency medical decision making. *Pediatr Emerg Care*. 2014;30(2):104-107.
3. Gokdemir Y, Cakir E, Kut A, et al. Bronchoscopic evaluation of unexplained recurrent and persistent pneumonia in children. *J Paediatr Child Health*. 2013;49(3):E204-E207.
4. Cohen E, Rodean J, Diong C, et al. Low-value diagnostic imaging use in the pediatric emergency department in the United States and Canada. *JAMA Pediatr*. 2019;178(8):e191439.
5. Lin CH, Chao YH, Wu KH, et al. Primary mucoepidermoid carcinoma at the carina of trachea presenting with wheezing in an asthmatic child mimicking an attack of asthma: a case report. *Medicine (Baltimore)*. 2016;95(44):e5292.
6. Firinci F, Ates O, Karaman O, et al. A 7-year-old girl with cough, fever, pneumonia. Diagnosis: mucoepidermoid carcinoma (MEC). *Pediatr Ann*. 2011;40(3):124-127.
7. Hubbell DS, Liebow AA. Thymic tumors characterized by lymphangioendothelial structure. *Am J Pathol*. 1952;28:321-345.
8. Chin CH, Huang CC, Lin MC, et al. Prognostic factors of tracheobronchial mucoepidermoid carcinoma—15 years experience. *Respirology*. 2008;13(2):275-280.
9. Hause DW, Harvey JC. Endobronchial carcinoid and mucoepidermoid carcinoma in children. *J Surg Oncol*. 1991;46(4):270-272.
10. Roby BB, Drehner D, Sidman JD. Pediatric tracheal and endobronchial tumors: an institutional experience. *Arch Otolaryngol Head Neck Surg*. 2011;137(9):925-929.
11. Smiddy PF, Abdul Manaf ZM, Roberts IF, et al. Endobronchial mucoepidermoid carcinoma in childhood: case report and literature review. *Clin Radiol*. 2000;55(8):647-649.
12. Al-Qahtani AR, Di Lorenzo M, Yazbeck S. Endobronchial tumors in children: institutional experience and literature review. *J Pediatr Surg*. 2003;38(5):733-736.

Trauma

41 Buckle Up: Abdominal Trauma

ROBERT VEZZETTI, MD, FAAP, FACEP

Case Presentation

A 4-year-old male arrives via air ambulance after being involved in an all-terrain vehicle (ATV) accident. The child was riding with his older sister (he was in the front, riding on his sister's lap) when the ATV turned over at a high rate of speed, causing the vehicle to flip onto the child. The ATV was pushed over by his father and several other witnesses to the accident and emergency medical services were called. The child was complaining of severe abdominal pain and had a Glasgow Coma Scale score (GCS) of 12. The accident occurred 1 to 2 hours by car from the nearest pediatric trauma center, so the decision was made to transport the child by air.

On arrival, he is alert and crying but consoles and tells you he has "tummy pain." His vital signs are significant for a heart rate of 114 beats per minute, respiratory rate of 22 breaths per minute, and blood pressure of 95/65 mm Hg. He has diffuse abdominal tenderness with guarding and there is mild bruising to the right upper quadrant. His liver function tests are elevated: AST (aspartate aminotransferase) of 1721 U/L and ALT (alanine transaminase) of 1083 U/L.

Imaging Considerations

Imaging is routinely employed in the evaluation of blunt abdominal trauma and its use is fairly routine in adult trauma victims. The role of imaging during the evaluation of abdominal trauma in the pediatric population, however, is somewhat controversial. Indeed, not all pediatric patients who sustain abdominal trauma require imaging. Several clinical decision tools have been devised to assist the clinician in determining which patients might have an intraabdominal injury[1,2] and benefit from imaging and which patients can forego computed tomography (CT) imaging safely, employing historical, clinical examination, and laboratory findings to render an imaging decision.[3-7] Such decision rules do appear to reduce imaging use (specifically CT), reduce cost of care, and potentially reduce the risk of future cancer cases.[6,8] An example of one such decision rule is given below, devised by Streck et al.,[3] which takes into account five variables in patients with blunt abdominal trauma:

1. AST >200 U/L.
2. Abdominal wall trauma, tenderness, or distention.
3. Abnormal chest x-ray.
4. Complaint of abdominal pain.
5. Abnormal pancreatic enzymes.

This study included almost 2200 children with a mean age of 8 years. Patients who were negative for all five variables had a 0.6% risk of intraabdominal injury and 0.0% risk of intraabdominal injury requiring intervention. Thus, this clinical prediction model had a negative predictive value of 99.4% for intraabdominal injury and 100.0% for intraabdominal injury requiring acute intervention in patients with none of the prediction rule variables present.[3]

PLAIN RADIOGRAPHY

This modality can be used to detect free abdominal air and associated pelvic fractures. However, plain radiography is not useful to visualize intraabdominal solid organ injury.

ULTRASOUND (US)

The use of US in the Focused Assessment with Sonography for Trauma (FAST) technique for routine adult abdominal trauma evaluation has been well documented and well supported, proving to be efficacious in detecting abdominal organ injury and useful in guiding management, including further imaging and operative repair. The advantages of sonography for the pediatric patient include a rapid examination time, general availability, and eliminating ionizing radiation exposure.

However, studies have shown FAST US to be less reliable in pediatric patients. A large meta-analysis of approximately 4000 patients that included both prospective and retrospective studies found a sensitivity of 66% and a specificity of 95% for FAST in the detection of intraabdominal solid organ injury in adult patients.[9,10] Other studies have found similar results.[11,12] In a recent multicenter study of children 16 years of age and less, FAST was shown to have a sensitivity for intraabdominal injury of 27% and a specificity of 91%; CT utilization rate among FAST and non-FAST groups was approximately the same; centers that performed FAST at a higher frequency did not have improved accuracy; and all patients who required intervention had abnormal physical examinations, including 15 children with negative FAST examinations.[13] In another study, in hemodynamically stable children, the routine use of FAST compared to standard trauma care was not supported, as the rate of abdominal CT scans, time in the Emergency Department, hospital charges, or missed intraabdominal injuries was not improved in patients randomized to FAST versus those randomized to standard trauma care.[14] Studies have sought to improve the low sensitivity associated with pediatric FAST examinations by utilizing liver function tests along with FAST. One study of approximately 3000 patients found that FAST alone produced low sensitivity (50%), but when combined with liver function testing, sensitivity improved to 88%.[10,15]

An intriguing development is the use of intravenous contrast–enhanced US (IV CEUS). The use of IV CEUS greatly improves sensitivity in detecting intraabdominal solid organ injury, as compared to standard sonography.[16–18] IV CEUS is operator dependent and not yet available in most centers in the United States. Currently, application appears most promising for hemodynamically stable children, with suspicion for solid organ injury from low-energy blunt abdominal trauma, or for follow-up imaging of known injuries. More investigation is needed with this imaging technique before this technique gains a wider application, but preliminary investigations seem promising.

The place of US in the evaluation of pediatric trauma is evolving. Notably, the American Academy of Pediatrics has released a guideline supporting the use of US as a diagnostic and procedural adjunct, promulgating effective training programs/curricula, credentialing, and quality control measures.[3,10,19] For many pediatric emergency medicine fellowships, point of care US has become part of the training curricula, although implementation does vary.[19,20] Currently, though, use of abdominal ultrasonography as a sole imaging modality to reliably exclude intraabdominal injury is not supported.

COMPUTED TOMOGRAPHY

The American College of Surgery Advanced Trauma Life Support manual states that CT should be used in hemodynamically stable children only when necessary, but there is a lack of specific guidelines in this regard.[21] CT exposes children to ionizing radiation that has the potential to cause adverse effects later on in life. This modality is excellent at identifying intraabdominal injury. The clinician should keep the following in mind:

1. Utilize CT only when necessary (i.e., study results will impact management decisions).
2. Practice gentle imaging (i.e., As Low As Reasonably Achievable [ALARA] principles).
3. Avoid "pan-scanning" in pediatric patients. While this technique is utilized frequently in adult trauma patients, it exposes pediatric patients to unnecessary radiation with little impact on clinical management or outcomes.[22–24]

A significant percentage of pediatric patients have required repeat imaging of the same body part at a pediatric trauma center after initial imaging at a referring hospital, increasing radiation dose to the patient.[25] If CT is utilized prior to transfer to a pediatric trauma center, the study should be done with intravenous (IV) contrast and using proper technique to avoid the need to repeat a poor study.

MAGNETIC RESONANCE IMAGING (MRI)

This modality is currently not considered a first-line test for pediatric abdominal trauma. There is scant literature describing the role of MRI in pediatric patients with blunt abdominal trauma. There are case reports of MRI use in adult patients with abdominal trauma.[26,27] An initial study demonstrated that noncontrast MRI offered no advantage to contrast-enhanced CT imaging in the diagnosis of solid organ injury,[28] and another study reported IV contrast–enhanced MRI was comparable to CT for evaluating blunt abdominal trauma.[29]

However, there are instances where MRI may prove useful. Patients with a previously documented severe reaction to iodinated IV contrast, patients with decreased renal function, pregnant patients,[30] or patients in whom CT or other imaging modality results are indeterminant may be candidates for MRI.[31] What role MRI can or will play in the evaluation of blunt pediatric trauma remains undetermined at this time.

Imaging Findings

Given the history and physical examination, IV contrast–enhanced CT of the abdomen and pelvis was performed. Thoracic and lumbar spine image reconstructions were also obtained. CT demonstrates a hepatic laceration extending from the anterolateral liver margin to the liver hilum, with perihepatic hemorrhage (Fig. 41.1). The degree of injury is consistent with a grade IV liver laceration. On the early phase images, there is a 2-cm lobulated high attenuation area at the site of injury, which increases in size on delayed phase imaging, consistent with active contrast extravasation due to active bleeding (Figs. 41.2 and 41.3).

Selected imaging of a different patient with a spleen laceration is provided (Fig. 41.4). The patient in this case fell off a horse, landing on her left side. There is perisplenic hemorrhage, with a full-thickness splenic laceration extending to the splenic hilum, and devascularization in the middle to lower third of the spleen, without active arterial extravasation. These findings are consistent with a grade IV splenic laceration.

The patient in Fig. 41.5 was involved in a motor vehicle crash and CT demonstrates a grade III laceration of the left kidney with approximately 2.7-cm hematoma, which

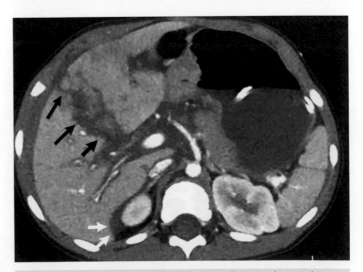

Fig. 41.1 Axial contrast-enhanced CT image depicting hepatic laceration *(black arrows)*, extending from the anterolateral liver capsule to the liver hilum. Hemoperitoneum is present, seen in perihepatic spaces, including the hepatorenal fossa *(white arrows)*.

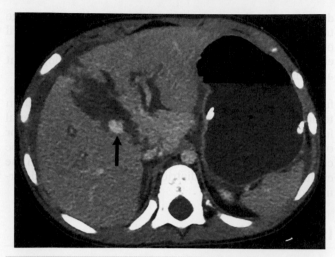

Fig. 41.2 Axial contrast-enhanced CT image demonstrating an area of high attenuation within the liver laceration *(arrow)*.

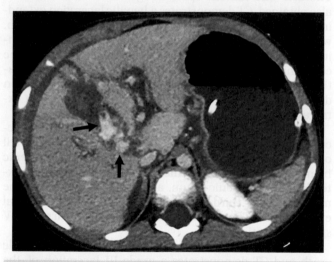

Fig. 41.3 Delayed phase axial computed tomography demonstrating increased size of high-attenuation focus *(arrows)* within the liver laceration, consistent with vascular contrast extravasation due to active hemorrhage.

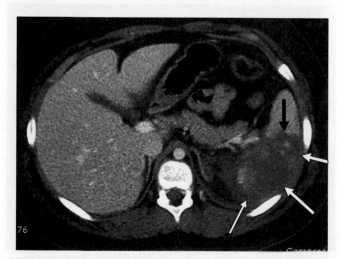

Fig. 41.4 Axial contrast-enhanced CT image demonstrating splenic laceration extending to the splenic hilum *(black arrow)*, with lack of contrast enhancement of the posterior two-thirds of the spleen *(white arrows)* consistent with devascularization.

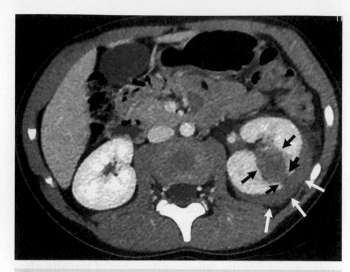

Fig. 41.5 Contrast-enhanced axial CT image shows a grade III laceration with hematoma *(black arrows)* of the left kidney, which extends to the renal hilum. A left perirenal hematoma is also present *(white arrows)*.

extends to the renal hilum, and a perinephric hematoma. There was no collecting system contrast extravasation on delayed imaging (not shown).

Case Conclusion

The Pediatric Trauma Service was consulted. Due to the concern for ongoing hemorrhage, abdominal embolization by Interventional Radiology was thought to be appropriate. The child underwent embolization of the right hepatic artery without incident. His postinjury course was complicated by the development of a biloma, which became infected, and the child developed sepsis. He also had a large right intrahepatic bile duct leak which was treated with endoscopic retrograde cholangiopancreatography. The patient tolerated this procedure and recovered from his sepsis after appropriate antibiotic administration.

Blunt abdominal trauma is a leading cause of abdominal injury in children, accounting for up to 90% of injuries in this population; motor vehicle crashes and falls are leading causes; nonaccidental trauma should also be considered in the differential diagnosis.[1-3,7,32] The spleen and liver are the most commonly affected organs, followed by the kidneys. Pancreatic, bladder, and urethral injuries are not as common. Bowel injuries are rare and can be difficult to detect radiographically, and their presentation can be delayed. Use of validated clinical decision tools to assist in the detection of intraabdominal injury can be helpful.[1,3,5,7]

The majority of pediatric intraabdominal injuries are managed nonoperatively.[32,33] The American Association for the Surgery of Trauma has a validated scoring system, used to identify the degree of injury for solid abdominal organs and which can assist in the management of specific injuries,[34] although more recently, hemodynamic status has become the important factor in guiding care.[35,36] Consultation with a pediatric surgeon or a qualified trauma surgeon is helpful when managing these patients. Strict return precautions should be provided to any discharged child who has sustained blunt abdominal trauma.

In adult populations, transcatheter arterial embolization is commonly utilized as a means to control hemorrhage in a rapid manner, but large pediatric studies are lacking. However, previous studies have demonstrated that pediatric abdominal and pelvic embolization procedures can be successful with a low complication rate[37–39] and complications from such a procedure tend to resolve in time.[37] What role embolization procedures have in the routine management of pediatric blunt abdominal trauma remains to be seen.

IMAGING PEARLS

1. Apply ALARA principles when imaging the child with blunt abdominal trauma.
2. Plain radiography is useful in detecting significant abdominal free air and pelvic fractures but otherwise has limited use in pediatric blunt trauma.
3. Although CT remains the gold standard for imaging children with significant abdominal trauma, routine, reflexive use of CT in pediatric blunt abdominal trauma patients should be discouraged. Validated clinical decision tools exist to assist the clinician in determining which children might benefit from imaging with CT and involve history, physical examination, and laboratory investigation.
4. If CT is used, avoid "pan-scanning." This method has not proven beneficial and does not impact clinical management or improve outcomes in the pediatric population.
5. Interpretation of imaging results from abdominal US in the pediatric trauma setting should be done with caution, given the low sensitivity of the study at this time. History, physical examination, and laboratory values should be taken into consideration in addition to US findings when making management decisions in these patients.
6. A combination of history, physical examination, and abnormal laboratory results (elevated liver function tests, for example) may improve the sensitivity of US in blunt pediatric trauma.
7. Contrast-enhanced US appears to improve sensitivity when used to evaluate children with blunt abdominal trauma. However, more study is needed.
8. MRI is not a first-line imaging test in the evaluation of pediatric abdominal trauma but may be an option instead of CT in patients with documented severe CT-contrast allergies, pregnant patients, and in those with renal failure who have sustained blunt abdominal trauma and would benefit from imaging.

References

1. Holmes JF, Sokolove PE, Brant WE, et al. Identification of children with intra-abdominal injuries after blunt trauma. *Ann Emerg Med.* 2002;39(5):500-509.
2. Holmes JF, Lillis K, Monroe D, et al. Identifying children at very low risk of clinically important blunt abdominal injuries. *Ann Emerg Med.* 2013;62:107-116.
3. Streck CJ, Vogel AM, Zhang J, et al. Identifying children at very low risk for blunt intra-abdominal injury in whom CT of the abdomen can be avoided safely. *J Am Coll Surg.* 2017;224(4):449-458.
4. Holmes JF, Mao A, Awasthi S, et al. Validation of a prediction rule for the identification of children with intra-abdominal injuries after blunt torso trauma. *Ann Emerg Med.* 2009;54(4):528-533.
5. Nishijima DK, Yang Z, Clark JA, et al. A cost-effectiveness analysis comparing a clinical decision rule versus usual care to risk stratify children for intraabdominal injury after blunt torso trauma. *Acad Emerg Med.* 2013;20(11):1131-1138.
6. Bregstein JS, Lubell TR, Ruscica AM, et al. Nuking the radiation: minimizing radiation exposure in the evaluation of pediatric blunt trauma. *Curr Opin Pediatr.* 2014;26(3):272-278.
7. Hynick NH, Brennan M, Schmit P, et al. Identification of blunt abdominal injuries in children. *J Trauma Acute Care Surg.* 2014;76(1): 95-100.
8. Nishijima DK, Yang Z, Clark JA, et al. A cost-effectiveness analysis comparing a clinical decision rule versus usual care to risk stratify children for intraabdominal injury after blunt torso trauma. *Acad Emerg Med.* 2013;20(11):1131-1138.
9. Holmes JF, Gladman A, Chang CH. Performance of abdominal ultrasonography in pediatric blunt trauma patients: a meta-analysis. *J Pediatr Surg.* 2007;42(9):1588-1594.
10. Guttman J, Nelson BP. Diagnostic point-of-care ultrasound: assessment techniques for the pediatric trauma patient. *Pediatr Emerg Med Pract.* 2019;16(suppl 7):1-50.
11. Fox JC, Boysen M, Gharahbaghian L, et al. Test characteristics of focused assessment of sonography for trauma for clinically significant abdominal free fluid in pediatric blunt abdominal trauma. *Acad Emerg Med.* 2011;18(5):477-482.
12. Coley BD, Mutabagani KH, Martin LC, et al. Focused abdominal sonography for trauma (FAST) in children with blunt abdominal trauma. *J Trauma.* 2000;48(5):902-906.
13. Calder BW, Vogel AM, Zhang J, et al. Focused Assessment with Sonography for Trauma in children after blunt abdominal trauma: A multi-institutional analysis. *J Trauma Acute Care Surg.* 2017;83(2): 218-224.
14. Holmes JF, Kelley KM, Wootton-Gorges SL, et al. Effect of abdominal ultrasound on clinical care, outcomes, and resource use among children with blunt torso trauma: a randomized clinical trial. *JAMA.* 2017;317(22):2290-2296.
15. Sola JE, Cheung MC, Yang R, et al. Pediatric FAST and elevated liver transaminases: An effective screening tool in blunt abdominal trauma. *J Surg Res.* 2009;157(1):103-107.
16. Armstrong LB, Mooney DP, Paltiel H, et al. Contrast enhanced ultrasound for the evaluation of blunt pediatric abdominal trauma. *J Pediatr Surg.* 2018;53(3):548-552.
17. Trinci M, Piccolo CL, Ferrari R, et al. Contrast-enhanced ultrasound (CEUS) in pediatric blunt abdominal trauma. *J Ultrasound.* 2019;22(1): 27-40.
18. Valentino M, Serra C, Pavlica P, et al. Blunt abdominal trauma: diagnostic performance of contrast-enhanced US in children—initial experience. *Radiology.* 2009;24(3): 903-909.
19. Marin JR, Lewiss RE, American Academy of Pediatrics, Committee on Pediatric Emergency Medicine, Society for Academic Emergency Medicine, Academy of Emergency Ultrasound, American College of Emergency Physicians, Pediatric Emergency Medicine Committee; World Interactive Network Focused on Critical Ultrasound. Point-of-care ultrasonography by pediatric emergency medicine physicians. *Pediatrics.* 2015;135(4):e1113-e1122.
20. Hoeffe J, Desjardins MP, Fischer J, et al. Emergency point-of-care ultrasound in Canadian pediatric emergency fellowship programs: current integration and future directions. *CJEM.* 2016;18(6):469-474.
21. Blumgart LH, DeMatteo RP. American College of Surgeons Committee on Trauma. Pediatric trauma. In: *Advanced Trauma Life Support for Doctors.* 9th ed. Chicago, IL: American College of Surgeons; 2012:261.
22. Belabbas D, Auger M, Lederlin M, et al. Whole-body CT after motor vehicle crash: no benefit after high-energy impact and with normal physical examination. *Radiology.* 2019;292(1):94.
23. Pandit V, Michailidou M, Rhee P, et al. The use of whole body computed tomography scans in pediatric trauma patients: are there differences among adults and pediatric centers? *J Pediatr Surg.* 2016;51(4):649.
24. Abe T, Aoki M, Deshpande G, et al. Is whole-body CT associated with reduced in-hospital mortality in children with trauma? A nationwide study. *Pediatr Crit Care Med.* 2019;20(6):e245.
25. Chwals WJ, Robinson AV, Sivit CJ, et al. Computed tomography before transfer to a level I pediatric trauma center risks duplication

with associated increased radiation exposure. *J Pediatr Surg.* 2008; 43(12):2268-2272.

26. Hedrick TL, Sawyer RG, Young JS. MRI for the diagnosis of blunt abdominal trauma: a case report. *Emerg Radiol.* 2005;11(5):309-311.
27. Barbiera F, Nicastro N, Finazzo M et al. The role of MRI in traumatic rupture of the diaphragm: our experience in three cases and review of the literature. *Radiol Med.* 2003;105(3):188-194.
28. McGehee M, Kier R, Cohn SM, et al. Comparison of MRI with post-contrast CT for the evaluation of acute abdominal trauma. *J Comput Assist Tomogr.* 1993;17(3):410-413.
29. Weishaupt K, Hetzer FH, Ruehm SG, et al. Three-dimensional contrast-enhanced MRI using an intravascular contrast agent for detection of traumatic intra-abdominal hemorrhage and abdominal parenchymal injuries: an experimental study. *Eur Radiol.* 2000;10(12):1958-1964.
30. Raptis CA, Mellnick VM, Raptis DA, et al. Imaging of trauma in the pregnant patient. *Radiographics.* 2014;34(3):748-763.
31. Gordic S, Alkadhi H, Simmen HP, et al. Characterization of indeterminate spleen lesions in primary CT after blunt abdominal trauma: potential role of MR imaging. *Emerg Radiol.* 2014;21(5):491-498.
32. Miele V, Piccolo CL, Trinci M, et al. Diagnostic imaging of blunt abdominal trauma in pediatric patients. *Radiol Med.* 2016;121(5):409-430.

33. Vane D, Keller M, Sartorelli K, et al. Pediatric trauma: current concepts and treatments. *J Intensive Care Med.* 2002;17(5):230-249.
34. Tinkoff G, Esposito TJ, Reed J, et al. American Association for the Surgery of Trauma Organ Injury Scale I: spleen, liver, and kidney, validation based on the National Trauma Data Bank. *J Am Coll Surg.* 2008;207(5):646-655.
35. Notrica DM. Pediatric blunt abdominal trauma: current management. *Curr Opin Crit Care.* 2015;21(6):531-537.
36. St Peter SD, Aguayo P, Juang D, et al. Follow up of prospective validation of an abbreviated bedrest protocol in the management of blunt spleen and liver injury in children. *J Pediatr Surg.* 2013;48: 2437-2441.
37. Vo NJ, Althoen M, Hippe DS, et al. Pediatric abdominal and pelvic trauma: safety and efficacy of arterial embolization. *J Vasc Interv Radiol.* 2014;25(2):215-220.
38. Kiankhooy A, Sartorelli KH, Vane DW, et al. Angiographic embolization is safe and effective therapy for blunt abdominal solid organ injury in children. *J Trauma.* 2010;68(3):526-531.
39. Ohtsuka Y, Iwasaki K, Yoshida H, et al. Management of blunt hepatic injury in children: usefulness of emergency transcatheter arterial embolization. *Pediatr Surg Int.* 2003;19(1-2):29-34.

42 *Where's the Air? Pneumothorax*

ROBERT VEZZETTI, MD, FAAP, FACEP

Case Presentation

A 16-year-old male presents with left-sided chest pain for the past week. He states that the pain began during band practice. He plays the trombone and states that he "must have pulled a chest muscle" because he was "playing really loud." He immediately felt the pain but continued playing. He reports no shortness of breath, but the pain is worse with deep inspiration and he feels like he is breathing faster than usual after marching. He denies recent illness and abdominal or back pain. He was seen by his primary care provider 2 days ago and had an electrocardiogram that was normal. He was told to take ibuprofen which has helped some.

Physical examination reveals a tall, thin, pleasant adolescent in no obvious distress. He is afebrile; his heart rate is 85 beats per minute, respiratory rate is 18 breaths per minute, and blood pressure is 118/70 mm Hg, and he has a pulse oxygenation reading of 93% on room air. He converses easily but does complain of chest pain to the left side. He has slightly diminished breath sounds to the left without crackles or rhonchi. He has no retractions. The remainder of his physical examination is unremarkable.

Imaging Considerations

Patients with suspected pneumothorax may have imaging to confirm the diagnosis. In patients with concern for tension pneumothorax or decompensating clinical status, imaging should not delay immediate treatment and stabilization.

PLAIN RADIOGRAPHY

This imaging modality is the initial test of choice for patients when a pneumothorax is a clinical consideration. It is readily available and inexpensive relative to other modalities. The presence of a pleural line and the absence of vascular markings beyond this line are the hallmarks of pneumothorax identification on chest radiography.[1] The deep sulcus sign, which is an area of hyperluncency in a depressed costophrenic angle, is pathognomonic for pneumothorax and seen on nonerect radiographs.[1] Pleural air may also be seen in the subpulmonic and anteromedial areas and laterally.[1,2] In an adult meta-analysis, the pooled sensitivity and specificity of chest radiography for pneumothorax were 52% and 100%, respectively.[1,3]

The optimal position of the pediatric patient undergoing radiography for suspected pneumothorax has not been well studied. Traditionally upright inspiratory chest radiographs have been utilized,[1] but this may not be feasible in the pediatric population, since cooperation may be an issue, or in the trauma patient, who may be immobilized. While upright inspiratory films are preferred, supine or lateral decubitus views may be obtained.[1] A chest radiograph should visualize the entire chest and lungs.

COMPUTED TOMOGRAPHY (CT)

CT is often used as a follow-up study in patients with recurrent pneumothorax or if there is a clinical concern for pleural bullae/blebs.[4] It is generally not a first-line imaging modality; however, in cases of penetrating thoracic trauma or concern for vascular injury, CT may be utilized.

For patients with chest radiography that reveals large pulmonary bullae or if there is concern for structural anomalies of the lung, CT may be indicated and is often utilized if operative management is being considered.[1,5,6] CT for first-time spontaneous pneumothorax is not recommended by the American College of Chest Physicians guidelines.[1,7] However, there are authors that recommend obtaining CT on all patients with first time primary spontaneous pneumothorax to evaluate for pulmonary abnormalities and to assist in a management plan but this is not universally recommended.[1] In one series of patients, Tsou et al. did not find differences in length of stay, length of operation, or rate of complications in patients who underwent CT prior to thoracoscopic surgical procedures.[1,8]

ULTRASOUND (US)

The use of ultrasound to identify pneumothorax has gained interest. The advantages are the lack of ionizing radiation, lower expense relative to other advanced modalities, and general availability. There are several findings suggestive of pneumothorax on sonography. The absence of lung sliding and so-called comet tails (grayscale artifacts that are present in normal lung parenchyma) has been shown to have a sensitivity and specificity of 100% and 96.5% for pneumothorax[9]; the absence of comet tails was found to be present in 100% of patients with pneumothorax.[10]

MAGNETIC RESONANCE IMAGING (MRI)

This modality is not indicated for the evaluation of patients with suspected pneumothorax.

Imaging Findings

Chest radiography was obtained. This two-view study demonstrates a left-sided pneumothorax, and a very small left

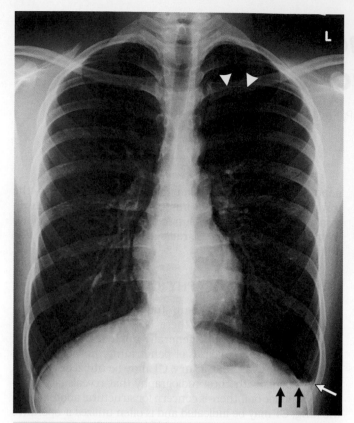

Fig. 42.1 Posterior-anterior upright chest radiograph demonstrates a left-sided pneumothorax. The white visceral pleural line of the apical left lung is seen *(white arrowheads)*, separated from the chest apex. A small left pleural effusion is also seen, blunting the left lateral costophrenic angle *(white arrow)*. Pleural effusion is also seen as a straight line, indicating an air fluid level of hydropneumothorax, in the left lung base *(black arrows)*.

pleural effusion, without tension or other obvious pulmonary abnormalities (Fig. 42.1).

Case Conclusion

The Pediatric Surgery team evaluated the patient in the emergency department. Oxygen by face mask delivery was initiated and the decision was made to admit the patient to the hospital for monitoring and serial chest radiography. Later during the admission day, it was revealed that the patient had two prior episodes of chest pain and similar symptoms which resolved on their own after several days. This prompted concern for recurrent episodes of pneumothorax. Chest CT was obtained to evaluate for the presence of underlying blebs or bullae. CT showed the pneumothorax, but no other findings. A pigtail catheter chest tube was placed for decompression of the pneumothorax, which was successful (Fig. 42.2). The patient was observed in the hospital for several days with serial radiography documenting pneumothorax resolution. The chest tube was removed and follow-up radiography demonstrated no residual pneumothorax. He was discharged with follow-up and did well.

Pneumothorax is defined as the presence of air between the visceral and parietal pleura and, due to pressure differences between the lung and the pleura space, leads to lung collapse.

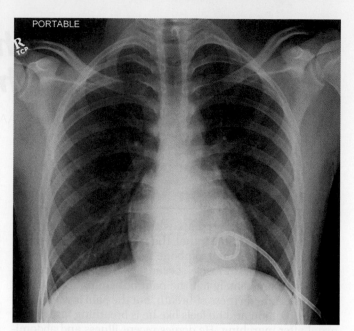

Fig. 42.2 Portable chest radiograph after pigtail catheter placement shows no significant pneumothorax or pleural effusion.

Pneumothorax can be spontaneous or traumatic.[4] Typical presenting symptoms of pneumothorax include ipsilateral chest pain, which may radiate to the ipsilateral shoulder, and dyspnea. Symptom severity is related to the size of the pneumothorax.[4]

There are several manifestations of pneumothorax.[1,4]

PRIMARY SPONTANEOUS PNEUMOTHORAX

This form of pneumothorax is not associated with radiographically identified lung disease.[1,4] Primary spontaneous pneumothorax occurs more commonly in adolescent males who are thin and tall; most cases occur while at rest.[1,4] Smoking is a known risk factor.[1,4] Although patients with primary spontaneous pneumothorax do not have clinically apparent lung disease on chest radiography, the majority are found to have subpleural bullae when undergoing video-assisted thoracoscopic surgery (VATS).[4]

SECONDARY SPONTANEOUS PNEUMOTHORAX

Patients with asthma, cystic fibrosis, Marfan syndrome/ Marfanoid habitus, and connective tissue disorders are prone to the development of secondary spontaneous pneumothorax.[1,4] Patients may develop a pneumothorax as a sequelae from severe coughing or pneumonia.[1] These patients tend to have a more severe clinical presentation and have higher recurrence rates.[4]

TRAUMATIC PNEUMOTHORAX

Traumatic pneumothorax may be due to iatrogenic causes (such as when a patient is on ventilatory support, after undergoing transthoracic needle biopsy, which is a leading cause of iatrogenic pneumothorax, and after central line placement)[4] or due to blunt or penetrating thoracic trauma. In the latter case, there may be significant associated injury.

OPEN PNEUMOTHORAX

This variety or pneumothorax is often associated with other injuries resulting from thoracic trauma.

TENSION PNEUMOTHORAX

Tension pneumothorax is due to the entry of air into the pleural space that cannot exit, leading to ipsilateral lung collapse with a mediastinal shift toward the contralateral side. This can impede venous return, reduce cardiac output, and compromise normal cardiovascular status and hemodynamic stability. Clinical symptoms suggestive of tension pneumothorax include hypotension, tracheal deviation, tachycardia, and cyanosis, in addition to chest pain and dyspnea.[1,4]

There are no consensus guidelines for the management of pediatric pneumothorax, but in general, management depends on many factors, including the type, size, and location of pneumothorax. The patient's history, including existing medical conditions and previous episodes, also is taken into consideration. The size of the pneumothorax is a critical factor in determining a treatment plan.[1,4] There are, however, no universally accepted normal lung volume values in pediatric patients.[1] The American College of Chest Physicians classifies pneumothorax size by using the distance between the lung apex and the ipsilateral dome of the thoracic cavity; a small pneumothorax is less than 3 cm and a pneumothorax is considered large when this distance is greater than 3 cm.[1,4,11] Other classification systems include the British Thoracic Society system, which utilizes a greater than 2-cm gap between the pleural edge and the chest wall as a large pneumothorax.[1,12]

Management

SMALL PRIMARY SPONTANEOUS PNEUMOTHORAX

Small pneumothoraces are generally treated with observation only and generally reabsorb at a rate of 1% to 2% per day.[1,13] Some authors recommend oxygen therapy, which, due to "nitrogen washout" (a process that increases nitrogen absorption, increasing the rate of pneumothorax reabsorption), has been shown in some studies to increase the rate of pneumothorax reabsorption to 5% per day.[1,4,14] Other studies have demonstrated no acceleration in pneumothorax reabsorption with oxygen administration.[15] A follow-up chest radiograph, which may be obtained based on ongoing clinical examination, should reveal a stable, if not smaller, pneumothorax; if this is the case, no further treatment is indicated; treatment is indicated if there is worsening of the pneumothorax.[1,4] Patients with a small, minimally symptomatic, clinically stable pneumothorax who have follow-up can be managed as outpatients after a period of observation with repeat imaging in the emergency department.[1,4,11] If adequate outpatient observation and follow-up cannot be assured, the patient should be admitted to the hospital.[1,11] A conservative management option would also be admission for supplemental oxygen, serial radiography, and subspecialty consultation.[1]

LARGE PRIMARY OR SMALL SYMPTOMATIC PRIMARY PNEUMOTHORAX

Patients with a large pneumothorax generally are admitted to the hospital and are treated with placement of either a chest tube or a small-bore ("pigtail") catheter.[1,4,11] There are few studies comparing the use of pigtail catheters versus traditional chest tubes in the pediatric population, but one study demonstrated similar efficacy, similar lengths of stay, and less need for analgesic medications in patients who had pigtail catheter placement.[1,16] The use of a modified Seldinger technique has been shown to be an effective and less invasive method for managing pneumothoraces.[1,17,18] The British Thoracic Society guidelines suggest attempting needle aspiration of the pneumothorax followed by careful observation in the emergency department for several hours; hospital admission is recommended for pneumothorax that recurs, if there is inadequate pain control, or if outpatient follow-up cannot be assured.[1,12] The American College of Chest Physicians does not recommend drainage of pneumothorax by needle aspiration.[1,11]

SECONDARY PNEUMOTHORAX

Patients with secondary pneumothorax often are managed by subspecialists due to underlying chronic medical conditions. Management of these patients should be done in consultation with the subspecialist who is caring for the patient.[1]

TENSION PNEUMOTHORAX

Since tension pneumothorax is a life-threatening condition, immediate recognition and management are warranted. If a tension pneumothorax is suspected, do not delay treatment for confirmatory imaging. Needle decompression is the first intervention, followed by chest tube thoracostomy.[1] Management should also address coexisting injuries.

OPEN PNEUMOTHORAX

Initial management consists of the application of a "flutter valve" dressing (a dressing secured on three sides with the fourth side open) and placement of a chest tube.[1] Patients require surgical intervention for definitive management.

There are other management options available for pediatric patients with pneumothorax, although when to utilize these techniques is a matter of debate. Surgical management involves the resection of blebs or bullae, or apical resection.[6] VATS has been proven to be effective and well tolerated.[19–21] The use of sclerosing agents may also be considered. The instillation of these agents causes irritation between the parietal and visceral pleural layers, causing scarring and closing this space, with the goal of preventing recurrence.[4,6] Indications for surgical management include second ipsilateral pneumothorax, first contralateral pneumothorax, bilateral pneumothorax, and persistent air leak.[6,11,12]

The recurrence rate for a primary spontaneous pneumothorax has been reported to be 30% to 50%, with the majority recurring within the first 2 years after diagnosis.[1,4] Risk factors for recurrence include young age, thin body habitus, evidence of pulmonary fibrosis, and smoking.[4]

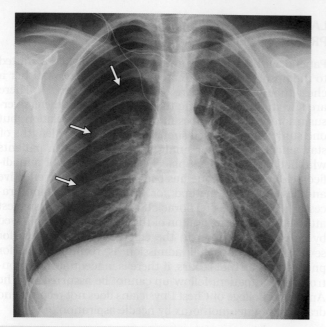

Fig. 42.3 Posterior-anterior upright chest radiograph demonstrates a large right-sided pneumothorax *(white arrows)*, without tension.

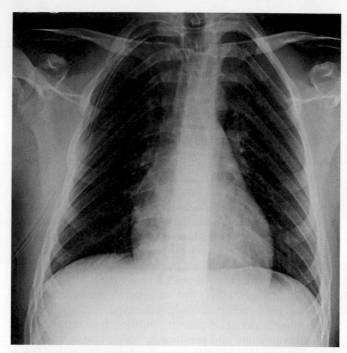

Fig. 42.5 This figure shows resolution or near-complete resolution of right pneumothorax following right chest tube placement.

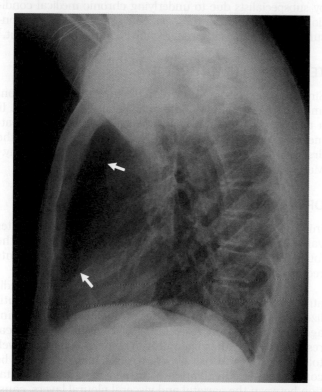

Fig. 42.4 Lateral upright chest radiograph demonstrates a large right-sided pneumothorax *(white arrows)*, without tension.

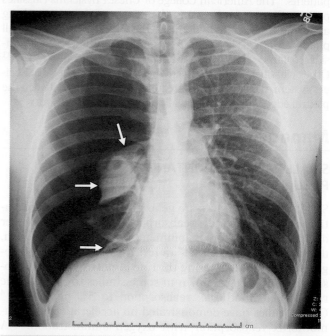

Fig. 42.6 Chest radiography prior to video-assisted thoracoscopic surgery. This figure demonstrates a large right pneumothorax, filling most of the right thorax, with collapse of the right lung *(white arrows denote collapsed right lung)*. There is subtle, minimal shift of the heart to the left, consistent with very minimal mass effect/tension, but the mediastinum is otherwise in usual position.

The patient in Figs. 42.3–42.5, a 16-year-old male, developed acute onset of right-sided chest pain while taking an examination at school. He presented with mild tachypnea and a room air oxygenation of 92%. Chest radiography revealed a large right-sided pneumothorax. He had a chest tube placed with subsequent resolution of the pneumothorax. He presented several months later with a recurrence of the pneumothorax, had CT imaging revealing several blebs, and underwent a VATS with apical blebectomy, pleurodesis, and chest tube placement.

The adolescent patient in Figs. 42.6 and 42.7 presented with acute onset of right-sided chest pain, hypoxia, and

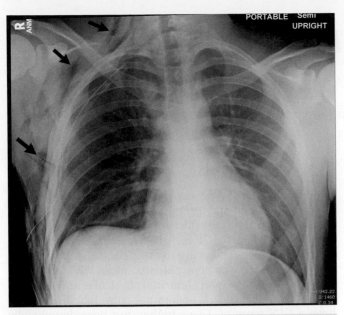

Fig. 42.7 Chest radiography following video-assisted thoracoscopic surgery (VATS). The figure shows right lung reexpansion after VATS with right chest tube placement. There is postoperative right chest wall and cervical emphysema *(black arrows).*

difficulty breathing. Chest radiography revealed a large right pneumothorax with near complete collapse of the right lung with minimal mass effect and shift of the heart toward the left. Pediatric Surgery was consulted and discussed the options of primary chest tube placement versus proceeding to VATS with the patient's family. At VATS, several pulmonary blebs were found; the patient was treated with chest tube placement and pleurodesis.

IMAGING PEARLS

1. Plain radiography is the initial imaging modality of choice in patients with suspected pneumothorax.
2. CT is not generally a first-line imaging modality for patients with suspected pneumothorax. CT may be obtained following plain radiography if there is concern for anatomic anomalies, such as blebs or bullae or in patients with repeated episodes of pneumothorax. If a patient is a victim of trauma and there is concern for vascular injury, CT is appropriate.
3. Ultrasonography is becoming another imaging modality to use for the diagnosis of pneumothorax and may be an alternative to traditionally used modalities. Expertise in the technique and interpretation of chest sonography is required.

References

1. Harris M, Rocker J. Pneumothorax in pediatric patients: management strategies to improve patient outcomes. *Pediatr Emerg Med Pract.* 2017;14(3):1-28.
2. Tocino IM, Miller MH, Fairfax WR. Distribution or pneumothorax in the supine and semirecumbant critically ill adult. *AJR Am J Roentgenol.* 1985;144(5):901-905.
3. Ding W, Shen Y, Yang J, et al. Diagnosis of pneumothorax by radiography and ultrasonography: a meta-analysis. *Chest.* 2011;140(4):859-866.
4. Posner K, Needleman JP. Pneumothorax. *Pediatr Rev.* 2008;29(2):69-70.
5. Warner BW, Bailey WW, Shipley RT. Value of computed tomography of the lung in the management of primary spontaneous pneumothorax. *Am J Surg.* 1991;162(1):39-42.
6. Robinson PD, Cooper P, Ranganathan SC. Evidence-based management of paediatric primary spontaneous pneumothorax. *Paediatr Respir Rev.* 2009;10(3):110-117.
7. Ayed Ak, Chandrasekaran C, Sukumar M. Aspiration versus tube drainage in primary spontaneous pneumothorax: a randomized study. *Eur Respir J.* 2006;27(3):477-482.
8. Tsou KC, Huang PM, Hsu HH, et al. Role of computed tomography scanning prior to thoracoscopic surgery for primary spontaneous pneumothorax. *J Formos Med Assoc.* 2014;113(9):606-611.
9. Wilkerson RG, Stone MB. Sensitivity of bedside ultrasound and supine anteriorposterior chest radiographs for the identification of pneumothorax after blunt trauma. *Acad Emerg Med.* 2010;17(1):11-17.
10. Lichtenstein D, Meziere G, Biderman P, et al. The comet-tail artifact: an ultrasound sign ruling out pneumothorax. *Intensive Care Med.* 1999;25(4):383-388.
11. Baumann MH, Stange C, Heffner JE, et al. Management of spontaneous pneumothorax: an American College of Chest Physicians Delphi consensus statement. *Chest.* 2001;119(2):590-602.
12. Henry M, Arnold T, Harvey J. BTS guidelines for the management of spontaneous pneumothorax. *Thorax.* 2003;5(suppl 2):ii39-ii52.
13. Kelly AM. Treatment of primary spontaneous pneumothorax. *Curr Opin Pulm Med.* 2009;15(4):376-379.
14. Zierold D, Lee SL, Subramania S, et al. Supplemental oxygen improves resolution of injury-induced pneumothorax. *J Pediatr Surg.* 2000;35(6):998-1001.
15. Clark SD, Saker F, Schneeberger MT, et al. Administration of 100% oxygen does not hasten resolution of symptomatic spontaneous pneumothorax in neonates. *J Perinatol.* 2014;34(7):528-531.
16. Dull KE, Fleischer GR. Pigtail catheters versus large-bore chest tubes for pneumothoraces in children treated in the emergency department. *Pediatr Emerg Care.* 2002;18(4):265-267.
17. Horsley A, Jones L, White J, et al. Efficacy and complications of small bore, wire-guided chest drains. *Chest.* 2006;130(6):1857-1863.
18. Tsai Wk, Chen W, Lee JC, et al. Pigtail catheters vs large-bore chest tubes for management of secondary spontaneous pneumothoraces in adults. *Am J Emerg Med.* 2006;24(7):795-800.
19. Ozcan C, McGahren ED, Rodgers BM. Thoracoscopic treatment of spontaneous pneumothorax in children. *J Pediatr Surg.* 2003;38(10):1459-1464.
20. Butterworth SA, Blair GK, LeBlanc JG, et al. An open and shut case for early VATS treatment of primary spontaneous pneumothorax in children. *Can J Surg.* 2007;50(3):171-174.
21. Zganjer M, Kljenak A. Video-assisted thoracoscopic surgery for spontaneous pneumothorax in children-our experience. *Bratisl Lek Listy.* 2007;108(4-5):200-202.

43 Can't Pee: Pediatric Bladder Trauma

ROBERT VEZZETTI, MD, FAAP, FACEP

Case Presentation

An 8-year-old female is brought into the Emergency Department by private vehicle after being run over by a car. The child was in her driveway when her father, who was backing the family van out of the garage, struck and ran over her. She is accompanied by both of her parents. The mother corroborates the father's history. There is no reported loss of consciousness and the parents are sure that the child did not strike her head. There is no complaint of neck pain, chest pain, or difficulty breathing. She does complain of abdominal and lower back pain, but this has improved since the accident. Due to the history and her symptoms, the child is brought immediately to the trauma resuscitation bay.

Her physical examination reveals an afebrile child with a heart rate of 170 beats per minute, respiratory rate of 32 breaths per minute, a blood pressure of 87/56 mm Hg, and a room air oxygen saturation of 97%. Her Glasgow Coma Scale (GCS) score is 15. She is complaining of diffuse hip pain and bilateral lower leg pain. There are no signs of head, neck, chest, or abdominal trauma. A cervical collar is placed, given her other injuries. Her abdominal examination shows diffuse tenderness and bilateral lower quadrant guarding. She has multiple abrasions to the suprapubic area, bilateral lower abdominal quadrants, and the bilateral upper thighs. There is blood at the meatus. The vaginal area shows no other signs of trauma.

Imaging Considerations

Imaging is indicated if there is suspicion, either by history or physical examination, of an intraabdominal injury (including bladder injury), significant microscopic hematuria, or gross hematuria. The amount of microscopic hematuria that is considered significant, prompting a clinician to obtain imaging, is a matter of debate and there is no universally accepted standard. Some authors have suggested that imaging is not indicated in patients with microscopic hematuria of less than 25 red blood cells per high-powered field.[1]

PLAIN RADIOGRAPHY

This imaging modality is readily available and is utilized as a first-line modality for suspected pediatric pelvic injuries. The standard view is anteroposterior (AP). Plain radiography can be used to diagnose pelvic fractures but may not demonstrate certain fractures well, such as those of the posterior pelvic ring,[2,3] and is less sensitive than computed tomography (CT).[4] The detection of pelvic fractures on plain radiography may prompt the clinician to investigate for the presence of a bladder injury. Some authors recommend proceeding to CT if pelvic fractures are present.[5] Other recommendations are to avoid routine pelvic radiography in low-risk pediatric patients: those who lack lower extremity injury, lack an abnormal physical examination of the pelvis and hip, lack abdominal pain, lack hematuria, have a GCS score of 13 or higher, are hemodynamically stable and have no need for abdominal/pelvis CT.[6,7] If a patient is to undergo CT of the abdomen/pelvis, plain radiography of the pelvis can be deferred.[4]

Traditionally, plain radiographic or fluoroscopic cystography has been used to evaluate for the presence of a bladder injury. This study is performed by instilling iodinated contrast into the bladder and obtaining imaging to assess for contrast extravasation; postvoid imaging is important to avoid missing bladder injury and extravasation not evident on initial imaging.[8] However, the density of contrast utilized for conventional (plain film or fluoroscopic) cystography will preclude performance of a CT of the abdomen and pelvis after the cystogram.

COMPUTED TOMOGRAPHY

CT is the imaging modality of choice for blunt or penetrating abdominal or genitourinary trauma. Standard CT imaging, though, is not adequate to diagnose bladder rupture. CT cystography, with retrograde filling of the bladder with very dilute iodinated contrast, is indicated for this purpose and is the preferred method over conventional cystography in patients undergoing CT imaging of the abdomen and pelvis for other injuries.[9]

Authors have recommended CT cystography if certain injuries or findings are present: gross hematuria, pelvic free fluid on intravenous (IV) contrast–enhanced abdominal/pelvic CT, specific pelvic fractures (pubic symphysis diastasis, sacroiliac diastasis, and sacral, iliac, pubic rami fractures), and microscopic hematuria with pelvic fractures.[1,5,9]

Whichever method is utilized to perform cystography, the bladder should be fully distended. Instructions on how to perform a CT cystogram, and suggested bladder volumes for a cystogram, are presented later.

MAGNETIC RESONANCE IMAGING (MRI)

MRI is not generally indicated in the acute evaluation of pediatric pelvic and genitourinary injuries. If there is severe allergy to IV contrast material, this modality can be considered in the trauma patient, but pediatric literature is lacking.

Imaging Findings

The child had an AP x-ray of the pelvis done. This image revealed multiple fractures, including fractures of the left iliac wing, the right symphysis pubis with diastasis of the symphysis pubis, fracture of the right inferior pubic ramus, and a right femoral neck fracture (Fig. 43.1). These findings, plus the presence of gross hematuria, prompted CT imaging with IV contrast and CT cystography. This study demonstrated a rupture at the dome of the urinary bladder, best appreciated on the delayed images. The contrast leaks out into the peritoneal space. The bladder wall is markedly irregular and thickened (Figs. 43.2–43.6).

Case Conclusion

The child was given packed red blood cells (15 cc/kg) and pain medication. In addition to the already mentioned injuries, she was found to have a right femoral neck fracture; Pediatric Orthopedics was consulted for this injury. She was taken to the operating room for exploratory laparotomy and repair of the bladder rupture, which was discovered during this procedure to involve the dome of the bladder. A Foley catheter was placed, and 1 week later, a cystourethrogram was performed. This demonstrated no extravasation, and the catheter was removed. She was ultimately discharged and followed closely.

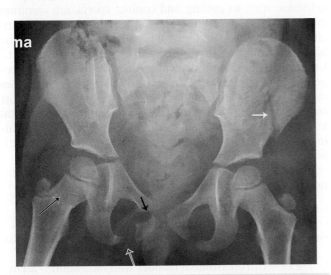

Fig. 43.1 Anteroposterior view of the pelvis demonstrates oblique fracture through the inferolateral left iliac wing *(white arrow)*; a fracture through the right symphysis pubis with widening of the symphysis pubis *(short black arrow)*; fracture of the right inferior pubic ramus, with a small displaced butterfly fragment at the ischio-pubic synchondrosis *(open white arrow)*; and a nondisplaced fracture of the right femoral neck *(long gray arrow)*.

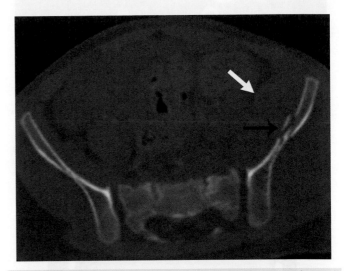

Fig. 43.3 Axial bone window computed tomography image demonstrates comminuted fracture of the left iliac wing *(black arrow)* and enlargement of the left iliacus muscle *(white arrow)* consistent with associated iliacus muscle hematoma.

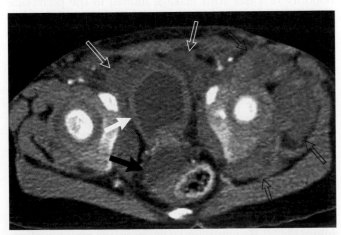

Fig. 43.2 Axial contrast-enhanced computed tomography image demonstrates bladder wall thickening *(white arrow)* and fluid, including higher density hemorrhagic fluid, seen in the perivesicle extraperitoneal space *(open white arrows)* and in the intraperitoneal cul-de-sac *(black arrow)*. Multiple soft tissue hematomas are also seen *(open black arrows)*.

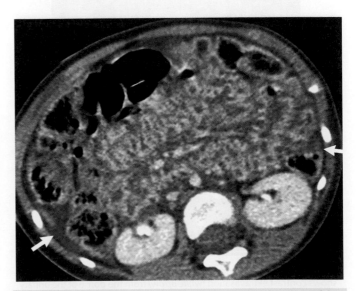

Fig. 43.4 Axial contrast-enhanced computed tomography image of the abdomen shows free intraperitoneal fluid, with fluid seen in bilateral paracolic gutters laterally *(arrows)*.

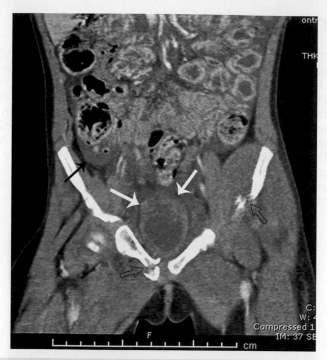

Fig. 43.5 Coronal contrast-enhanced computed tomography image demonstrates urinary bladder wall thickening that is greatest over the dome *(white arrows)* and free intraperitoneal fluid in the pericecal region *(black arrow)*. Pelvic fractures are again seen *(open arrows)*.

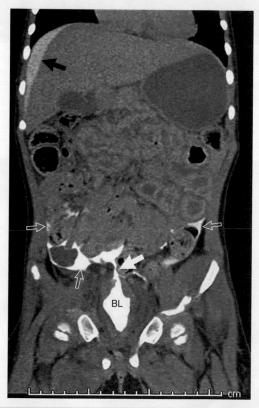

Fig. 43.6 Coronal image from a computed tomography cystogram shows contrast extravasation *(white arrow)* from the dome of the urinary bladder *(BL)*, consistent with intraperitoneal bladder rupture. Extravasated contrast is seen in the right lower quadrant and bilateral paracolic gutters *(open arrows)* and in the right perihepatic space *(black arrow)*.

Pelvic trauma is not common in the pediatric population, with a reported incidence of 2%–7%.[10–12] Mortality from pelvic trauma is usually due to associated injuries.[10] The pattern of pelvic injuries in pediatric patients differs from that of adults. While most pediatric pelvic fractures are less severe than in adults, they result from high-energy mechanisms (such as motor vehicle accidents and being struck by vehicles) and commonly have associated intraabdominal or genitourinary injuries.[13,14] Bladder injuries are associated with up to 15% of pediatric pelvic trauma.[10,11]

Pediatric urogenital injuries usually result from blunt, rather than penetrating, trauma, with motor vehicle collisions being a common mechanism.[9,14] Interestingly, sports activities, such as cycling and contact sports, are common causes of bladder rupture; martial arts has been an often-cited activity due to abdominal blow from kicking, since the bladder is an intraabdominal organ in the pediatric patient.[9] Urethral and bladder injuries are second to the kidney in urogenital injury frequency, and while liver and spleen injuries can accompany urogenital trauma, bowel injuries are most commonly seen.[14–16] Up to 50% of patients with urogenital injuries have associated abdominal injuries, and this increased risk of associated abdominal trauma is greater with bladder injury than with renal injury.[14,17]

Bladder injury is graded based on the American Association for the Surgery of Trauma:[15,18,19]

Grade I—Hematoma, partial-thickness laceration
Grade II—Extraperitoneal bladder wall laceration <2 cm
Grade III—Extraperitoneal bladder (>2 cm) or intraperitoneal (<2 cm) bladder laceration
Grade IV—Intraperitoneal bladder wall laceration >2 cm
Grade V—Intraperitoneal or extraperitoneal bladder wall laceration extending into the bladder neck or ureteric orifice

Bladder contusion, rupture, and a combination of both are potential injuries. Bladder contusions are benign in nature and require no treatment, but a careful assessment of other intraabdominal or genitourinary injuries should be made.[8,9] Bladder rupture may be extraperitoneal (the majority of cases with leakage limited to the perivesicle space) or intraperitoneal (caused by disruption of the peritoneal surface with resulting urinary extravasation into the peritoneal cavity).[9] Extraperitoneal bladder rupture is often accompanied by pelvic fractures,[9,10,20] and an estimated 80% of patients with bladder rupture have associated pelvic fractures. A distended bladder is a risk factor for bladder rupture.[9,10,20] Bladder rupture has been reported in patients who sustain significant blunt trauma and do not have pelvic fractures and occurs in 1.6% of pediatric blunt abdominal trauma.[8,9,14] Intraperitoneal bladder rupture usually occurs when a direct blow increases intravesicle pressure, injuring the weakest part of the bladder, which is the dome.[9]

Gross hematuria, as well as suprapubic abdominal pain and problems voiding, is a presenting symptom of bladder injury.[1,9,10,21] Hematuria may be gross (the majority of patients), microscopic, or even transient.[9,22]

The management of pediatric bladder injuries should involve not only the Pediatric Trauma Surgery team but also Pediatric Urology. While repair of intraperitoneal rupture is the standard of care, extraperitoneal rupture may be treated with catheter drainage alone, but repair is recommended if the patient is undergoing exploratory laparotomy for other injury management.[8,10,23,24] Repair has been shown to be associated with decreased complications and improved outcomes, including patients with extraperitoneal rupture.[15,23,25,26] A large national study of traumatic pediatric bladder injuries found that bladder injuries were more likely to be repaired if there was intraperitoneal rupture versus extraperitoneal rupture; however, repair of intraperitoneal rupture in their patient population was performed in 66% of patients with this injury, suggesting that the recommended standard of care (i.e., repair of intraperitoneal bladder rupture) was not followed in all cases.[23] Furthermore, they found an 82% decrease in-hospital mortality after repair, after controlling for overall bodily injury score, and reduced mortality regardless of type of bladder injury.[23]

IMAGING PEARLS

1. An AP view of the pelvis is not *routinely* indicated in pediatric trauma patients.
2. Imaging should be performed on patients with physical examination or laboratory findings suggestive of pelvis or genitourinary injury.
3. Consideration should be given to obtaining CT of the abdomen and pelvis if pelvic fractures are encountered on plain radiography. In some instances, for example, isolated acetabular fractures, this may not be indicated.
4. If CT is planned, plain radiography of the pelvis is not indicated.
5. IV contrast–enhanced CT of the abdomen and pelvis, even if performed with delayed bladder imaging, is not sufficient to exclude bladder rupture.
6. If bladder rupture is suspected, cystography should be obtained. This can be performed with plain radiography, fluoroscopy, or CT (the preferred modality to investigate this injury).

CT Cystography Procedure

(see "Detailed Instructions" if Needed)

After Complete Trauma CT of the Abdomen and Pelvis (or Hold Pelvis Scan for Full Bladder Cystography Imaging):

Drain the bladder by gravity through the Foley catheter.

Instill dilute contrast (instructions for dilution below) through the Foley catheter by gravity, with the bottom of the contrast bag 40 cm above the table.

Once the bladder is full, clamp the Foley catheter and perform CT scan of the pelvis. Scan is axial, but also perform coronal and sagittal reconstructions.

After scan, unclamp the Foley catheter and drain contrast from bladder (can lower the contrast bag to drain).

Reconnect the Foley to the urine bag drainage and be sure to unclamp the Foley catheter after the procedure is completed.

Detailed Instructions

Instructions for original contrast concentration around 300 (e.g., Isovue 300, Omnipaque 300, or Optiray 300, 320, or 350).

Using sterile technique, inject undiluted contrast into a bag of sterile NS: either 50 mL into a 1-L bag, 25 mL into a 500-mL bag, or 20 mL into a 300-mL bag. Shake bag to mix.

Insert vented IV tubing with Luer lock into the contrast saline bag; clear air from the line.

After draining the bladder, clamp the Foley catheter.

Insert a Christmas tree adapter (female IV connecter) into the Foley catheter to allow hookup of IV tubing from the contrast bag to the Foley. Unclamp the Foley catheter once connected securely.

Instill contrast by gravity, 40 cm above CT table. Clamp the catheter once the desired bladder volume is reached, then perform CT of the pelvis.

After the scan, unclamp the Foley catheter and drain contrast from the bladder (can lower the contrast bag to drain).

Clamp the catheter while reconnecting the Foley catheter to the urine bag.

Unclamp the Foley catheter at completion of the procedure and prior to the patient leaving the CT suite.

Bladder volume[a]:

Less than 2 years old: Weight (in kg) × 7 bladder volume (mL)
2 to 14 years old: (age in years × 30) + 30 bladder volume (mL)
Over 14 years old: 500 mL

[a]Frimberger D, Mercado-Deane MG. AAP Section on Radiology. Establishing a standard protocol for the voiding cystourethrography. *Pediatrics*. 2016 Nov;138(5):e20162590.

CT, Computed tomography; *IV*, intravenous; *NS*, normal saline.

References

1. Morgan DE, Nallamala LK, Kenney PJ, et al. CT cystography: radiographic and clinical predictors of bladder rupture. *AJR Am J Roentgenol.* 2000;174(1):89-95.
2. DeFrancesco CJ, Sankar WN. Traumatic pelvic fractures in children and adolescents. *Semin Pediatr Surg.* 2017;26(1):27-35.
3. Kwok MY, Yen K, Atabaki S, et al. Sensitivity of plain pelvis radiography in children with blunt torso trauma. *Ann Emerg Med.* 2015;65(1):63-71.
4. Guillamondegui OD, Mahboubi S, Stafford PW, et al. The utility of the pelvic radiograph in the assessment of pediatric pelvic fractures. *J Trauma.* 2003;55:236-239.
5. Deck AJ, Shaves S, Talner L, et al. Current experience with computed tomographic cystography and blunt trauma. *World J Surg.* 2001;25(12):1592-1596.
6. Wong AT, Brady KB, Caldwell AM, et al. Low-risk criteria for pelvic radiography in pediatric blunt trauma patients. *Pediatr Emerg Care.* 2011;27(2):92-96.
7. Haasz M1, Simone LA, Wales PW, et al. Which pediatric blunt trauma patients do not require pelvic imaging? *J Trauma Acute Care Surg.* 2015;79(5):828-832.
8. Gomez RG, Ceballos L, Coburn M, et al. Consensus statement on bladder injuries. *BJU Int.* 2004;94(1):27-32.
9. Guttmann I, Kerr HA. Blunt bladder injury. *Clin Sports Med.* 2013;32(2):239-246.
10. Desai AA, Gonzalez KW, Juang D. Pelvic trauma. *J Pediatr Intensive Care.* 2015;4(1):40-46.
11. Demetriades D, Karaiskakis M, Velmahos GC, et al. Pelvic fractures in pediatric and adult trauma patients: are they different injuries? *J Trauma.* 2003;54(6):1146-1151.

12. Pascarella R, Bettuzzi C, Digennaro V. Surgical treatment for pelvic ring fractures in pediatric and adolescence age. *Musculoskelet Surg.* 2013;97(3):217-222.
13. de la Calva C, Jover N, Alonso J, Salom M. Pediatric pelvic fractures and differences compared with the adult population. *Pediatr Emerg Care.* 2018 Jan 16. [Epub ahead of print].
14. Dokucu AI, Ozdemir E, Ozturk H, et al. Urogenital injuries in childhood: a strong association of bladder trauma to bowel injuries. *Int Urol Nephrol.* 2000;32(1):3-8.
15. Deibert CM, Glassberg KI, Spencer BA. Repair of pediatric bladder rupture improves survival: results from the National Trauma Data Bank. *J Pediatr Surg.* 2012;47(9):1677-1681.
16. McAleer IM, Kaplan GW, Scherz HC, et al. Genitourinary trauma in the pediatric patient. *Urology.* 1993;42(5):563-567.
17. Flancbaum L, Morgan AS, Fleisher M, Cox EF. Blunt bladder trauma: manifestation of severe injury. *Urology.* 1988;31(3):220-222.
18. Moore EE, Cogbill TH, Jurkovich GJ, et al. Organ Injury Scaling III: chest wall, abdominal vascular, ureter, bladder and urethra. *J Trauma.* 1992;33(3):337-339.
19. Bryk DJ, Zhao LC. Guideline of guidelines: a review of urological trauma guidelines. *BJU Int.* 2016;117(2):226-234.
20. Spiguel L, Glynn L, Liu D, Statter M. Pediatric pelvic fractures: a marker for injury severity. *Am Surg.* 2006;72(6):481-484.
21. Tarman GJ, Kaplan GW, Lerman SL, et al. Lower genitourinary injury and pelvic fractures in pediatric patients. *Urology.* 2002;59(1):123-126.
22. Brandes S, Borrelli J. Pelvic fracture and associated urologic injuries. *World J Surg.* 2001;25(12):1578-1587.
23. Deibert CM, Spencer BA. The association between operative repair of bladder injury and improved survival: results from the National Trauma Data Bank. *J Urol.* 2011;186(1):151-155.
24. Alperin M, Mantia-Smaldone G, Sagan ER. Conservative management of postoperatively diagnosed cystotomy. *Urology.* 2009;73(5):1163. e17-1163.e19.
25. Routh JC, Husmann DA. Long-term continence outcomes after immediate repair of pediatric bladder neck lacerations extending into urethra. *J Urol.* 2007;178(4):1816-1818.
26. Kotkin L, Koch MO. Morbidity associated with nonoperative management of extraperitoneal bladder injuries. *J Trauma.* 1995;38(6):895-898.

44   *Heads Up!: Head Trauma*

WINNIE WHITAKER, MD, FAAP and BHAIRAV PATEL, MD

Case Presentation

A 7-month-old child presents to the Emergency Department after rolling off a couch. The child's mother, who is visibly distraught and is worried that "her child's brain is ruined," reports that the child fell off the couch and struck the hardwood floor. The distance of the fall is approximately 2–3 feet. The child immediately cried and since the event, which occurred about 1 hour ago, has been at her baseline. There is no report of emesis.

The physical examination reveals age-appropriate vital signs. The child is alert, interactive, and smiling. There is a 3-cm right frontal hematoma with some ecchymoses but no step-off or laceration. The child is moving her neck well. There is no apparent abdominal or spine tenderness. The child is moving all of her extremities well and there is no other swelling, tenderness, or deformity.

Imaging Considerations

The majority of children with minor head trauma do not require neuroimaging. Injuries such as small nondepressed skull fractures are not clinically significant and would not lead to harm if they are unidentified. Rather, the decision to pursue radiological imaging should be made when history or physical examination findings lead to a high suspicion for clinically important traumatic brain injury that would require hospitalization or surgical intervention. Clinical prediction rules have been published to help determine which patients may or may not require neuroimaging, the most commonly used being those put forth by the Pediatric Emergency Care Applied Research Network (PECARN).[1]

PLAIN RADIOGRAPHY

The utility of plain radiographs in pediatric head trauma is limited. Skull radiographs can help diagnose fractures and delineate if a fracture is depressed but cannot detect intracranial injury. This is important for patient management, since there is often significant brain injury present without an associated skull fracture.[2] As such, most experts recommend forgoing plain radiography in favor of computed tomography (CT) scanning for patients with suspected head injury, as CT can identify intracranial injuries requiring surgical intervention.[2,3]

ULTRASOUND (US)

US may be useful in diagnosing skull fracture in children presenting with head trauma. Several studies have shown that US has high sensitivity and specificity in identifying skull fractures when compared to CT scan.[4–7] The advantage of US is that it may be performed at the bedside, without sedation, often by an emergency physician. A major limitation of US, similar to plain radiography, is the inability to identify clinically important intracranial injuries that may or may not be associated with skull fracture. US for this indication is also operator dependent.

COMPUTED TOMOGRAPHY

CT without contrast is the first-line imaging modality for diagnosing clinically important traumatic brain injuries.[1,3] It is relatively inexpensive and generally easily accessible and can quickly diagnose injuries that might require emergent intervention. CT can detect subarachnoid hemorrhage, subdural and epidural hematomas, pneumocephalus, ischemia, cerebral edema, midline shift, and signs of herniation, as well as scalp injuries and foreign bodies. However, subtle findings such as small hemorrhages or early cerebral edema may be difficult to detect, and study quality may be limited by motion artifact if patients are not completely still.[3] The benefits of the information obtained from a head CT must be weighed against the potential risk of cancer mortality from the radiation required to perform the study. The estimated lifetime risk due to radiation-induced malignancy from one head CT is approximately 1 in 1500 in a 1-year-old child and approximately 1 in 5000 in a 10-year-old child, with risk decreasing as patients get older.[8] This exposure risk can be mitigated by the implementation of pediatric-specific imaging protocols that adhere to the American College of Radiology radiation imaging dose guidelines.[9–11]

Angiography is utilized in patients with increased risk for injury to major vessels due to penetrating trauma to the head, but in practice, venography is typically done if the fracture crosses the expected location of the dural venous sinus. Children with facial or orbital entry wounds, transdural trajectory of penetration, or accompanying intracranial hemorrhage are more likely to have aneurysm development.[12]

MAGNETIC RESONANCE IMAGING (MRI)

MRI is an attractive alternative to CT in diagnosing clinically important traumatic brain injuries in children because it avoids ionizing radiation exposure while producing superior images. The disadvantages of MRI include cost, limited availability, time required for completion, and being highly sensitive to motion artifact, thus potentially increasing the need for sedation. Protocols with reduced acquisition times enable MRI to be a viable option in place of CT scans when available. These rapid, or fast-acquisition, MRIs have been determined to have similar sensitivity and specificity when compared with CT in diagnosing traumatic brain injuries.[13] MRI is more sensitive than CT in visualizing the brainstem and posterior fossa, as well as identifying subtle intraparenchymal insults such as diffuse axonal injury, cerebral edema, and contusion.[3] Because of this, MRI is a useful modality as a prognostic indicator once a patient has been stabilized and is often the preferred study for follow-up examinations.

Imaging Findings

The patient is low risk for acute intracranial injury requiring neurosurgical intervention based on the PECARN guidelines; therefore, no neuroimaging was obtained in this patient.

Case Conclusion

After discussion with the child's mother, including the indications, risks, and benefits of CT imaging, the decision was made to discharge the patient without neuroimaging. The mother was comfortable in discharging the child with close monitoring and strict return precautions.

Pediatric head trauma is a leading cause of injury and death in children. In the United States, it is estimated that there are over 800,000 emergency department visits a year due to head injuries in children less than 18 years of age.[14] The majority of pediatric patients with head trauma have minor injuries and do not require intervention. There are those patients, however, who have significant injury, and pediatric head trauma is the leading cause of death in patients above 1 year of age, accounting for more than 3000 deaths per year, and is a leading cause of significant morbidity.[15] The mechanism of head trauma differs among different ages of pediatric patients. Young children tend to sustain falls and are more often the victims of nonaccidental trauma, whereas older patients are more likely to sustain head trauma from penetrating injury, sports injuries, and motor vehicle crashes.[15]

The decision to obtain imaging is multifactorial and has been an area of fervent discussion. In some patients, the decision to obtain neuroimaging is straightforward (for example, a patient presenting with a concerning Glasgow Coma Scale [GCS] score [Tables 44.1–44.3] or those patients with a history and examination concerning for significant head trauma). However, there are a majority of patients in whom the decision to obtain neuroimaging is more nuanced. Several validated clinical decision rules have been developed. The PECARN decision rule is commonly used in practice in the United States. This clinical decision rule is useful to risk stratify patients who have sustained blunt head injury and guide the clinician regarding neuroimaging. This tool, along with history, physical examination (including the GCS), and provider experience, can be employed to determine which patients are not likely to require neuroimaging.

Management of head trauma depends on the patient's injury. General management considerations should be

Table 44.1 Glasgow Coma Scale (Modified), <2 Years of Age

Activity	Best Response	Score
Eye opening	Spontaneous	4
	To shout	3
	To pain	2
	None	1
Verbal	Smiles/coos	5
	Cries/inconsolable	4
	Persistent inappropriate crying	3
	Agitated, restless	2
	None	1
Motor	Smiles/coos	6
	Localizes pain	5
	Withdraws to pain	4
	Decorticate	3
	Decerebrate	2
	None	1
Total		**/15**

Table 44.2 Glasgow Coma Scale (Modified), 2–5 Years of Age

Activity	Best Response	Score
Eye opening	Spontaneous	4
	To verbal command	3
	To pain	2
	None	1
Verbal	Appropriate words/phrases	5
	Inappropriate words	4
	Persistent crying/screaming	3
	Grunts	2
	None	1
Motor	Normal/spontaneous	6
	Localizes pain	5
	Withdraws to pain	4
	Decorticate	3
	Decerebrate posture	2
	None	1
Total		**/15**

Table 44.3 Glasgow Coma Scale (Modified), >5 Years of Age

Activity	Best Response	Score
Eye opening	Spontaneous	4
	To verbal command	3
	To pain	2
	None	1
Verbal	Oriented	5
	Confused	4
	Inappropriate words	3
	Nonspecific sounds	2
	None	1
Motor	Normal/spontaneous	6
	Localizes pain	5
	Withdraws to pain	4
	Decorticate	3
	Decerebrate posture	2
	None	1
Total		**/15**

PECARN CT Clinical Decision Rule[1]

Younger Than 2 Years of Age

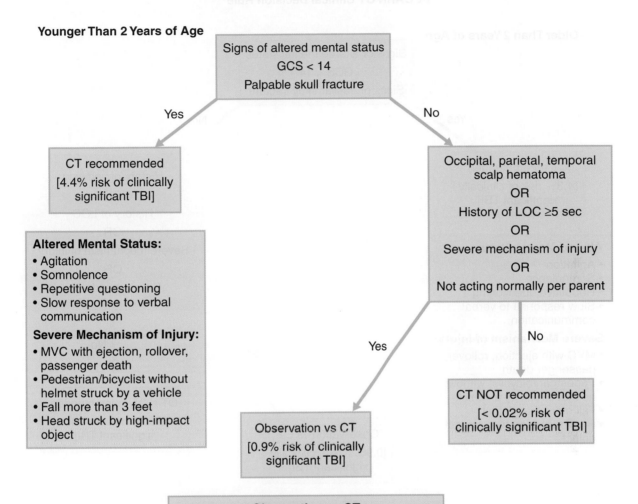

Signs of altered mental status
GCS < 14
Palpable skull fracture

Yes

CT recommended
[4.4% risk of clinically significant TBI]

No

Occipital, parietal, temporal scalp hematoma
OR
History of LOC ≥5 sec
OR
Severe mechanism of injury
OR
Not acting normally per parent

Altered Mental Status:
• Agitation
• Somnolence
• Repetitive questioning
• Slow response to verbal communication

Severe Mechanism of Injury:
• MVC with ejection, rollover, passenger death
• Pedestrian/bicyclist without helmet struck by a vehicle
• Fall more than 3 feet
• Head struck by high-impact object

Yes

No

Observation vs CT
[0.9% risk of clinically significant TBI]

CT NOT recommended
[< 0.02% risk of clinically significant TBI]

Observation vs CT

Decision based on:
• Physician experience
• Isolated vs multiple exam findings
• Clinical deterioration during observation period
• Age < 3 months
• Parental preference

Isolated findings: Isolated vomiting, isolated LOC, isolated headache, isolated certain scalp hematomas in infants > 3 months of age have a risk of clinically significant TBI < 1%.

PECARN CT clinical decision rule: younger than 2 years of age. *CT*, Computed tomography; *GCS*, Glasgow Coma Scale; *LOC*, loss of consciousness; *MVC*, motor vehicle crash; *PECARN*, Pediatric Emergency Care Applied Research Network; *TBI*, traumatic brain injury.

PECARN CT Clinical Decision Rule[1]

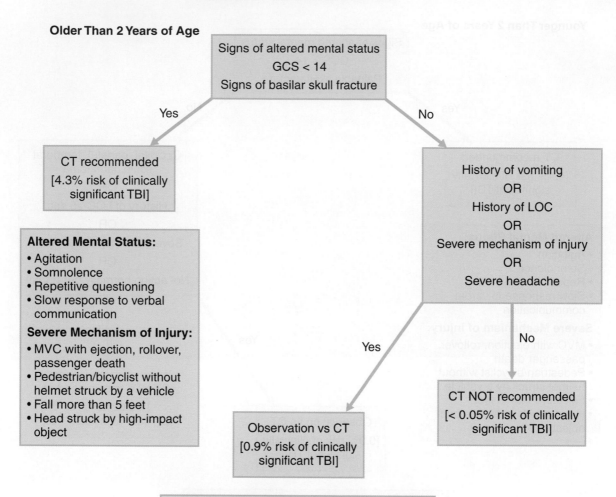

Older Than 2 Years of Age

Signs of altered mental status
GCS < 14
Signs of basilar skull fracture

Yes → CT recommended
[4.3% risk of clinically significant TBI]

No → History of vomiting
OR
History of LOC
OR
Severe mechanism of injury
OR
Severe headache

Altered Mental Status:
• Agitation
• Somnolence
• Repetitive questioning
• Slow response to verbal communication

Severe Mechanism of Injury:
• MVC with ejection, rollover, passenger death
• Pedestrian/bicyclist without helmet struck by a vehicle
• Fall more than 5 feet
• Head struck by high-impact object

Yes → Observation vs CT
[0.9% risk of clinically significant TBI]

No → CT NOT recommended
[< 0.05% risk of clinically significant TBI]

Observation vs CT

Decision based on:
• Physician experience
• Isolated vs multiple exam findings
• Clinical deterioration during observation period
• Parental preference

Isolated findings: Isolated vomiting, isolated LOC, isolated headache, isolated certain scalp hematomas in infants > 3 months of age have a risk of clinically significant TBI < 1%.

PECARN CT clinical decision rule: older than 2 years of age. *CT*, Computed tomography; *GCS*, Glasgow Coma Scale; *LOC*, loss of consciousness; *MVC*, motor vehicle crash; *PECARN*, Pediatric Emergency Care Applied Research Network; *TBI*, traumatic brain injury.

given to the Airway, Breathing, Circulation (ABC's) of trauma management. If there is suspicion for cervical spine injury, cervical spine precautions should be maintained in accordance with recommended trauma guidelines. Consultation with Pediatric Neurosurgery is appropriate for patients with skull fractures or intracranial hemorrhage.

SKULL FRACTURES

The presence of a skull fracture can be a sign of significant impact and does increase the potential for intracranial injury.[15] Patients with suspected skull fractures should have CT as their initial imaging study. If a skull fracture is identified initially by plain skull radiography, CT should be obtained. Management of skull fractures is dependent on the location and complexity of the facture. Complex fractures or fractures associated with intracranial injury require consultation with Pediatric Neurosurgery. Previous studies have demonstrated that many patients with isolated, linear skull fractures without intracranial injury due to blunt head trauma are hospitalized for observation.[16,17] However, children with these injuries can be discharged with close monitoring, since decompensation and development of a condition requiring neurosurgical intervention are not likely.[17–20] The majority of patients in one study (85%) were discharged within 1 day and the neurosurgical intervention rate was 0.2%; there were no deaths.[16] Nonaccidental trauma should also be considered in patients with skull fractures and should be appropriately addressed prior to discharge. A study of children 18 months and younger with isolated skull fractures not reported to be due to motor vehicle crashes or falls from shopping carts found that 6% of their study population had additional fractures on skeletal survey.[21]

GROWING SKULL FRACTURES

Special mention should be made of so-called growing skull fractures. These are uncommon complications of pediatric skull fractures but can also occur following cranial surgeries. They are thought to form due to the presence of a skull fracture with an underlying dural tear and intact arachnoid membrane.[22] They are more common in children under 3 years of age and a common presentation is parietal scalp swelling (associated with a linear parietal skull fracture); a low initial GCS is often seen.[22] Growing skull fractures can be difficult to diagnose. Patients who are at risk for developing this rare complication should be monitored by Pediatric Neurosurgery for 3 months following the initial injury.[22] Management of growing skull fractures depends on the size of the defect and the age of the patient.[22]

BASILAR SKULL FRACTURES

Basilar skull fractures classically are associated with hemotympanum, bruising behind the ear (Battle sign), bleeding/leakage of cerebrospinal fluid from the ear, and ecchymoses of the infraorbital regions (raccoon eyes). These fractures have a higher incidence of intracranial injury and increased association with meningitis, although this risk is low.[15] Due to the proximity to cranial nerve pathways, these fractures may be associated with cranial nerve deficits.

EPIDURAL HEMORRHAGE

These injuries are most commonly due to blunt trauma and are often associated with skull fractures (approximately 80% of cases), and the source of bleeding is identified as arterial in 30% of cases; venous bleeding is more common in pediatric patients.[15,23] The classically described loss of consciousness, followed by a lucid interval, and then clinical deterioration is not common in pediatric patients, in whom only about 20% experience loss of consciousness; persistent headache and vomiting are more common symptoms.[15] Epidural hematoma appears as a well-defined lens-shaped density on CT. Management involves consultation with Pediatric Neurosurgery; not all epidural hemorrhages require operative intervention, but admission for close monitoring is indicated.

SUBDURAL HEMORRHAGE

These injuries are commonly due to direct trauma and falls from significant heights and can be seen in nonaccidental trauma; bleeding occurs due to tearing of the bridging veins between the dura and the arachnoid membrane, although an associated fracture is usually not present.[15] Chronic subdural hemorrhage may be seen in children with coagulopathies,[15] but nonaccidental trauma should be considered in these patients as well. Subdural hemorrhage has a crescent shape on CT. Underlying brain injury is commonly associated.[15,23] Subdural hemorrhage is associated with long-term morbidity, such as seizures and developmental delay, particularly when the initial presentation consists of depressed mental status or CT imaging demonstrates underlying brain injury; associated mortality rates are between 10% and 20%.[15] Pediatric Neurosurgery should be promptly consulted in these patients.

SUBARACHNOID HEMORRHAGE

This injury results from tearing of the smaller vessels of the pia mater. Subarachnoid hemorrhage may be traumatic (associated with shear injuries) or nontraumatic (from ruptured aneurysms or arteriovenous malformations).[15] CT will typically demonstrate hyperintense blood within the basal cisterns and subarachnoid spaces.[15]

DIFFUSE AXONAL INJURY

This is injury to the white matter tracts, often from shear injuries, commonly seen with the forces involved in motor vehicle crashes, such as acceleration and deceleration.[23] Supportive management is indicated, but there is an associated mortality of up to 15% and neurologic dysfunction for survivors is present in approximately one-third of patients.[15]

Case Examples

Fig. 44.1 is a selected CT image of a 14-year-old pitcher who was struck in the head by a batted line drive. There is an epidural hematoma without midline shift. The patient was admitted for monitoring and did not require surgical intervention.

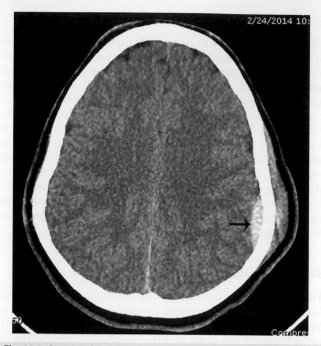

Fig. 44.1 Computed tomography axial image demonstrating an epidural hematoma *(black arrow)* without midline shift.

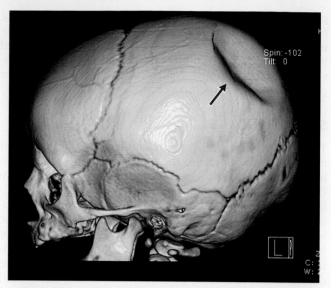

Fig. 44.3 A 3D reconstructed image of the skull from computed tomography imaging demonstrating a so-called "ping pong ball" fracture *(black arrow)*.

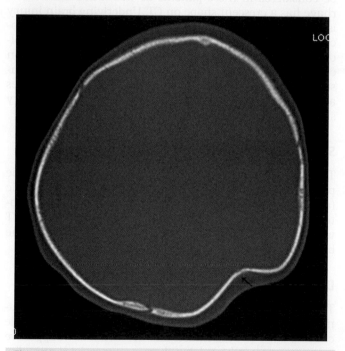

Fig. 44.2 Computed tomography axial bone window image demonstrating a so-called "ping pong ball" fracture *(black arrow)*.

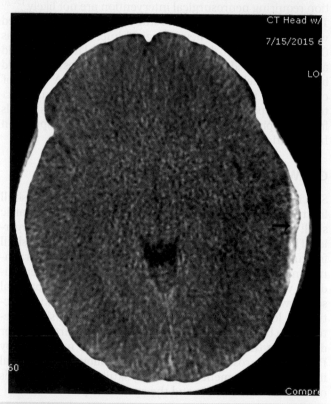

Fig. 44.4 Computed tomography axial image demonstrating subdural blood *(black arrow)* without mass effect or midline shift.

Figs. 44.2 and 44.3 are selected CT images demonstrating a so-called "ping pong ball" fracture. CT brain windows (not shown) demonstrated no intracranial hemorrhage, midline shift, or other intracranial injury. The patient, a 6-month-old baby, rolled off a bed and struck one of the legs of the bed, which was made of iron. The patient was taken to the operating suite for a craniotomy repair of the fracture, which was accomplished once the scalp swelling had subsided. A nonaccidental trauma evaluation was completed.

Fig. 44.4 is a selected CT image of a 3-year-old child who sustained a fall of approximately 4 feet from a high bar stool while sitting in her kitchen, landing on tile flooring. There is an extraaxial convexity hemorrhage that is crescent shape favoring subdural blood without mass effect or midline shift.

Fig. 44.5 is a selected CT image from a 15-year-old patient who was struck in the head by a thrown discus at track practice. There is a comminuted and depressed right parietal and temporal skull fracture. The patient was taken to the operating suite for elevation of the fracture and recovered well.

Fig. 44.6 is a selected CT image from a 3-month-old child presenting to the emergency department with altered mental status and found on physical examination to be in extremis, actively seizing, with depressed mental status and respiratory effort. There is a right-sided subdural hemorrhage with acute, subacute, and chronic components; there is marked mass effect and a left midline shift without fracture. The child was taken emergently to the operating suite for evacuation of the hematoma and placement of a subdural drain. A nonaccidental trauma evaluation was performed, during which numerous, multilayered retinal hemorrhages were discovered; his skeletal survey was normal. The lack of an explanation of the patient's clinical presentation, ophthalmologic findings, and radiographic findings were highly concerning for nonaccidental trauma.

IMAGING PEARLS

1. Plain radiography is not a first-line imaging modality in patients with head trauma. While simple skull fractures may be identified, complex fractures will not be well delineated, and this modality provides no information regarding associated intracranial injuries including intracranial hemorrhage.
2. Noncontrast CT is the imaging modality of choice for patients who have sustained head trauma. The ability of this test to identify fractures and intracranial hemorrhage, as well as the rapidity and availability of this examination, makes it ideal for this purpose.
3. MRI is utilized as a second-line imaging test in patients with injuries identified by CT when clinically indicated.
4. US can identify skull fractures; however, this modality has limited ability to evaluate the underlying brain for the presence of intracranial hemorrhage.

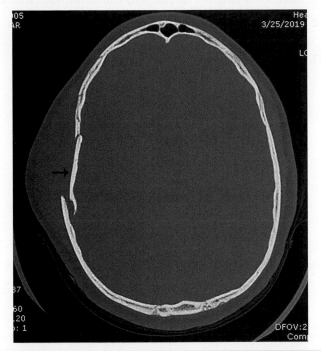

Fig. 44.5 Computed tomography axial bone window image demonstrating a comminuted depressed right parietal and temporal skull fracture *(black arrow)*.

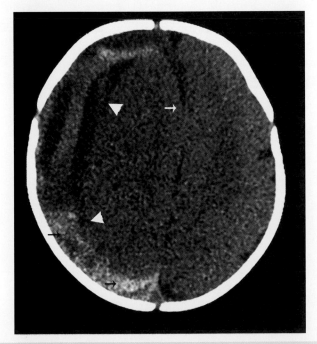

Fig. 44.6 Computed tomography axial image demonstrating a right-sided subdural hemorrhage *(white arrowheads)* with acute, subacute, and chronic components with internal membranes *(black arrows)*; there is marked mass effect and a left midline shift *(white arrow)*.

References

1. Kuppermann N, Holmes JF, Dayan PS, et al. Identification of children at very low risk of clinically-important brain injuries after head trauma: a prospective cohort study. *Lancet.* 2009;374 (9696):1160-1170.
2. Lloyd DA, Carty H, Patterson M, et al. Predictive value of skull radiography for intracranial injury in children with blunt head injury. *Lancet.* 1997;349(9055): 821-824.
3. Poussaint TY, Miller KK. Imaging of pediatric head trauma. *Neuroimaging Clin N Am.* 2002;12(2):271-294.
4. Niccolo P, Crosby BJ, Glass C, et al. Ability of emergency ultrasonography to detect pediatric skull fractures: a prospective, observational study. *J Emerg Med.* 2013;44(1):135-141.
5. Choi JY, Lim YS, Jang JH, et al. Accuracy of bedside ultrasound for the diagnosis of skull fractures in children aged 0 to 4 years. *Pediatr Emerg Care.* 2020;36(5):e268-e273.
6. Riera A, Chen L. Ultrasound evaluation of skull fractures in children: a feasibility study. *Pediatr Emerg Care.* 2012;28(5):420-425.
7. Rabiner JE, Friedman LM, Khine H, et al. Accuracy of point-of-care ultrasound for diagnosis of skull fractures in children. *Pediatrics.* 2013;131(6):e1757-e1764.
8. Brenner D, Elliston C, Hall E, et al. Estimated risks of radiation-induced fatal cancer from pediatric CT. *AJR Am J Roentgenol.* 2001;176(2):289-296.
9. Brinkman AS, Gill KG, Leys CM, et al. Computed tomography–related radiation exposure in children transferred to a level I pediatric trauma center. *J Trauma Acute Care Surg.* 2015;78(6):1134-1137.
10. Newman B, Callahan MJ. ALARA (as low as reasonably achievable) CT 2011—executive summary. *Pediatr Radiol.* 2011;41(suppl 2): 453-455.
11. Callahan MJ. CT dose reduction in practice. *Pediatr Radiol.* 2011;41(suppl 2):488-492.
12. Cotton BA, Nance ML. Penetrating trauma in children. *Semin Pediatr Surg.* 2004;13(2): 87-97.

13. Mehta H, Acharya J, Mohan AL, et al. Minimizing radiation exposure in evaluation of pediatric head trauma: use of rapid MR imaging. *AJNR Am J Neuroradiol.* 2016;37(1):11-18.

14. Centers for Disease Control and Prevention. *Surveillance Report of Traumatic Brain Injury-related Emergency Department Visits, Hospitalizations, and Deaths—United States, 2014.* Centers for Disease Control and Prevention, U.S. Department of Health and Human Services; 2019.

15. Schunk JE, Schutzman SA. Pediatric head injury. *Pediatr Rev.* 2012;33(9):398-411.

16. Mannix R, Monuteaux MC, Schutzman SA, et al. Isolated skull fractures: trends in management in US pediatric emergency departments. *Ann Emerg Med.* 2013;62(4):327-331.

17. Powell EC, Atabaki SM, Wootton-Gorges S, et al. Isolated linear skull fractures in children with blunt head trauma. *Pediatrics.* 2015;135(4): e851-e857.

18. Rollins MD, Barnhart DC, Greenberg RA, et al. Neurologically intact children with an isolated skull fracture may be safely discharged after brief observation. *J Pediatr Surg.* 2011;46(7): 1342-1346.

19. Blackwood BP, Bean JF, Sadecki-Lund C, et al. Observation for isolated traumatic skull fractures in the pediatric population: unnecessary and costly. *J Pediatr Surg.* 2016;51(4):654-658.

20. White IK, Pestereva E, Shaikh KA, et al. Transfer of children with isolated linear skull fractures: is it worth the cost? *J Neurosurg Pediatr.* 2016;17(5):602-606.

21. Laskey AL, Stump TE, Hicks RA, et al. Yield of skeletal surveys in children ≤18 months of age presenting with isolated skull fractures. *J Pediatr.* 2013;162(1):86-89.

22. Vezina N, Al-Halabi B, Shash H, et al. A Review of techniques used in the management of growing skull fractures. *J Craniofac Surg.* 2017;28(3):604-609.

23. Huisman TA. Intracranial hemorrhage: ultrasound, CT and MRI findings. *Eur Radiol.* 2005;15(3):434-440.

45 *Cruisin' for a Bruisin': Pulmonary Contusion*

GUYON HILL, MD

Case Presentation

A 13-year-old is brought to the Emergency Department after being struck by a large truck while attempting to cross a highway on his bicycle. There is no reported loss of consciousness. His vital signs show an afebrile patient with a heart rate of 120 beats per minute, respiratory rate of 28 breaths per minute, blood pressure of 100/70 mm Hg, and a pulse oximetry reading of 91% on room air. He is conversing on arrival and has bruising over the lower medial right side of his neck and upper- and mid-chest, bilaterally. He states his right collar bone hurts and he has bilateral chest pain, left more than the right, while taking deep breaths. There is no crepitus. He has some mild abdominal pain to the left upper quadrant. He also has an obvious deformity to his left lower extremity but is neurovascularly intact. His Glasgow Coma Scale score is 14.

Imaging Considerations

PLAIN RADIOGRAPHY

Plain radiographs are the most common imaging modality utilized to diagnose pediatric pulmonary trauma and should be obtained on every child when pulmonary contusion is suspected and in general on all seriously injured children.[1] When compared to advanced imaging such as computed tomography (CT), plain radiographs are the most appropriate first-line imaging modality to identify clinically significant pulmonary contusions, although plain radiography may underestimate the size of the injury.[2,3] Localized patchy opacities in nonanatomic distributions in the area of impact are the most frequently found abnormality when pulmonary contusions are present. Although radiographs obtained shortly after trauma may be negative for signs of pulmonary contusion, they may show other abnormal findings such as pneumothoraces or rib fractures, which will make contusions more likely.[2] It is not necessary to repeat radiographs if they are initially negative unless the child's respiratory status worsens.[1,2]

THORACIC ULTRASOUND (US)

US can be used to evaluate the pediatric lungs, although the findings associated with pulmonary contusions are nonspecific and should be interpreted by a skilled practitioner. Findings include what are commonly referred to as "B lines," which indicate interstitial edema, with an equivalent significance as Kerley B lines found on chest radiographs.[4]

Dynamic air bronchograms also may be seen,[4] similar to pneumonia, due to parenchymal consolidation, but with dynamic movement of air in the patent bronchi. Clinical context needs to be applied to differentiate B lines secondary to contusion versus other causes of sonographic B lines such as pulmonary edema or pneumonia.

COMPUTED TOMOGRAPHY

CT provides greater detail than either US or plain radiography; however, CT is not recommended for the sole purpose of diagnosing pulmonary contusion.[1] Pulmonary contusions appear as patchy localized opacities on CT. CT scans are more sensitive for the detection of pulmonary contusion than plain radiographs are, but this does not necessarily correlate with the patient symptoms or degree of injury. Small contusions may only be apparent on CT.

Imaging Findings

An initial, one-view chest radiograph was obtained. The image demonstrates abnormal lung opacities, left greater than right, suggestive of pulmonary contusion on the left. The opacity in the right lower lobe, predominantly retrocardiac, is thought more likely to represent atelectasis (Fig. 45.1).

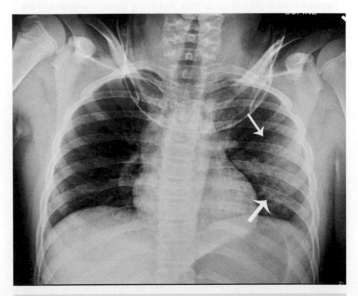

Fig. 45.1 One-view AP chest radiography demonstrating a left-sided pulmonary opacity consistent with a pulmonary contusion *(arrows)*.

Case Conclusion

The patient was placed on a non-rebreather mask for his hypoxia with improvement in his oxygen saturation. He underwent further imaging to evaluate his other physical examination findings: an intravenous contrast–enhanced CT scan of the abdomen and pelvis revealed a grade II splenic laceration and plain radiography of his left femur demonstrated a moderately displaced femur fracture. Given the neck bruising and concern for associated vascular injury, the patient underwent CT angiography of the vessels of the neck. No vessel injury or pneumothorax was noted, but a left pulmonary contusion was seen (Figs. 45.2 and 45.3). He was admitted to the hospital for further monitoring, closed reduction of the femur fracture, and pulmonary toilet. He had no worsening of his respiratory status and was discharged 2 days later without residual complications.

Pulmonary contusion is the most common injury resulting from thoracic trauma in children and may be caused by either blunt or high-speed penetrating mechanisms.[2,3,5,6] A high index of suspicion is necessary so that pulmonary contusion can be diagnosed early. Several factors make this injury more

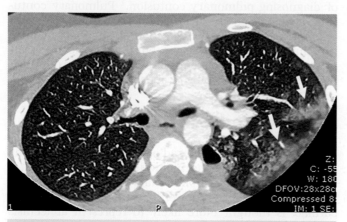

Fig. 45.2 Lung window axial image of the chest from the computed tomography angiogram of the neck demonstrates patchy consolidative opacities in the left upper lobe and in the superior segment of the left lower lobe *(arrows)*, most consistent with pulmonary contusion.

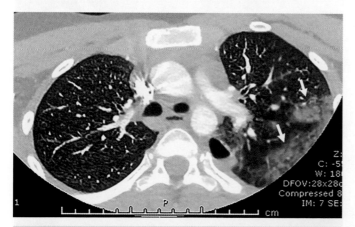

Fig. 45.3 Lung window axial image of the chest from the computed tomography angiogram of the neck demonstrates patchy consolidative opacities in the left upper lobe and in the superior segment of the left lower lobe *(arrows)*, most consistent with pulmonary contusion.

likely to occur in the pediatric population. In young patients, there is increased compliance of the chest wall from incomplete ossification of the ribs.[2,3,5,6] There is also decreased muscle mass when compared to adults, which allows for the greater transmission of force.[2,3,5,6] Patient presentations can range from asymptomatic with incidental findings on radiographs to tachypnea or hypoxia and even respiratory failure requiring mechanical ventilation. Most children will have some degree of symptoms, even if they are minor,[2,5,6] but may have minimal or no signs of external trauma.[2] Many of these patients will have associated injuries such as pneumothoraces, hemothoraces, pleural effusions, and other fractures, particularly of the extremities. It is more common for children to have pulmonary contusions without rib fractures, and the presence of a rib fracture implies a significant amount of force.[2,3,5–7] Extrathoracic injuries should also be considered.[2,3,7] While acute respiratory distress syndrome is a rare complication, when present, it is more often secondary to polytrauma or shock rather than direct injury to the lung.[2]

The initial management of symptomatic pulmonary contusion begins with supplemental oxygen to maintain oxygen saturation; this and close monitoring are all that is required for the majority of these injuries.[1,2] Aggressive pulmonary toilet and incentive spirometry are also beneficial.[1,2] For those patients who are more clinically unstable, noninvasive positive pressure ventilation can be of benefit.[1,2] In the case of severe injuries, intubation and ventilation while utilizing higher positive end-expiratory pressures may be necessary.[1,2] Patients with pulmonary contusion are typically hospitalized for monitoring of respiratory status and to ensure that there is no clinical deterioration.[2]

Pulmonary contusion in adults correlates with increased morbidity, but this is not necessarily the case for pediatric patients. The majority of children with isolated pulmonary contusions will have spontaneous resolution without any long-term effects and any morbidity associated with the event is generally associated with concomitant injuries.[2,5,6]

IMAGING PEARLS

1. Chest radiographs are the preferred method for diagnosing clinically significant pulmonary contusions in the pediatric population. Initial radiographs can be negative if obtained shortly after the injury, but repeat films are not warranted unless the patient's pulmonary status worsens.
2. The force necessary to cause a pulmonary contusion is significant, so it is important keep a wide differential of potential associated intrathoracic and extrathoracic injuries. Consider advanced imaging modalities, such as CT, when clinically indicated.
3. CT scan can be a helpful imaging modality to evaluate for other associated traumatic injuries but is not required for the diagnosis of pulmonary contusion or if it will not change clinical management. A pulmonary contusion seen on CT scan alone is not indicative of a clinically significant injury.
4. Chest ultrasonography is a potentially useful imaging modality in pediatric patients with suspected pulmonary contusion, but further research is needed in this area. The clinician should interpret the sonographic findings in the context of the patient's presentation as US signs may be indicative of a range of pulmonary processes.

References

1. Tenenbein M, Macias CG, Sharieff GQ, et al. *Strange and Schafermeyer's Pediatric Emergency Medicine*. 5th ed. New York: McGraw Hill Education; 2019.
2. Alemayehu H, Aguayo P. Pediatric blunt thoracic trauma. *J Pediatr Intensive Care*. 2015;4(1):35-39.
3. Cooper A, Barlow B, DiScala C, et al. Mortality and truncal injury: the pediatric perspective. *J Pediatr Surg*. 1994;29(1):33-38.
4. Stone MB, Secko MA. Bedside ultrasound diagnosis of pulmonary contusion. *Pediatr Emerg Care*. 2009;25(12):854-855.
5. Bonadio WA, Hellmich T. Post-traumatic pulmonary contusion in children. *Ann Emerg Med*. 1989;18(10):1050-1052.
6. Haxhija EQ, Nöres H, Schober P, et al. Lung contusion-lacerations after blunt thoracic trauma in children. *Pediatr Surg Int*. 2004;20(6):412-414.
7. Rodriguez RM, Friedman B, Langdorf MI, et al. Pulmonary contusion in the pan-scan era. *Injury*. 2016;47(5):1031-1034.

46 The Heart of the Matter: Ventricular Laceration

ROBERT VEZZETTI, MD, FAAP, FACEP

Case Presentation

A 12-year-old male presents with an injury to the chest. Apparently, he was "playing" with a nail gun and it went off, causing a nail to enter his chest. The child's vital signs show an afebrile patient, who looks apprehensive, pale, and diaphoretic. His heart rate is 112 beats per minute, respiratory rate is 22 breaths per minute, blood pressure is 112/62 mm Hg, and pulse oximetry reading is 95% on room air. He has what appears to be a wound to his right chest, just lateral to the sternum at the nipple line, without active bleeding. His breath sounds are equal. He does not have any other injuries.

Imaging Considerations

Pediatric penetrating chest trauma accounts for up to 8% of pediatric trauma cases.[1–3] The majority of cases are seen in adolescent populations.[2] Associated injuries include pneumothorax, hemothorax, cardiac, and great vessel injuries. When penetrating injury to the heart occurs, the right ventricle is more commonly involved and associated cardiac tamponade is often present.[4,5] Nail gun injuries in the pediatric population are uncommon. For a complete discussion on pediatric thoracic trauma, see Chapter 47 (Chest Pains: Pediatric Chest Trauma).

PLAIN RADIOGRAPHY

Plain radiography is an excellent first-line imaging modality to identify the presence of radiopaque foreign bodies involved in penetrating thoracic injury and can identify clinically significant associated injuries, such as pneumothorax and hemothorax. In one case series of penetrating thoracic injury due to a nail gun, chest radiography was diagnostic in all patients; no further imaging was performed and the patients in this series all underwent urgent operative intervention.[6]

ULTRASOUND

Echocardiogram can be used to identify pericardial effusions and assess ventricular function and can be useful in planning surgical intervention.[4,7] Retained foreign bodies can also be visualized and their location determined. Pericardial hemorrhage can be detected and alert the clinician to the presence of cardiac tamponade, which, in one review, was present in up to 73% of patients with cardiac nail gun injuries.[4] The advantages of lack of ionizing radiation and availability make this imaging modality particularly attractive.

COMPUTED TOMOGRAPHY (CT)

CT may be useful in pediatric penetrating thoracic injury, as concern for blood vessel injury is higher in patients who sustain this traumatic mechanism. Consider utilization of this modality in children with suspected cardiovascular injuries.[8,9] It is also reasonable to consider employing chest CT with angiography in children with abnormal initial chest radiographs suggestive of aortic injury.

Imaging Findings

The child underwent immediate plain radiography of the chest. These images demonstrated a linear metallic object measuring 5.7 cm long overlying the right side of the cardiac silhouette, in the anterior chest. The location and orientation of the object suggest that it is intracardiac (Figs. 46.1 and 46.2).

Case Conclusion

While preparations were made for operative intervention, the child had bedside echocardiography performed, which demonstrated a large pericardial effusion. Pediatric Cardiothoracic Surgery was consulted and the child was taken to the operating room for exploration and repair. A 12-mm

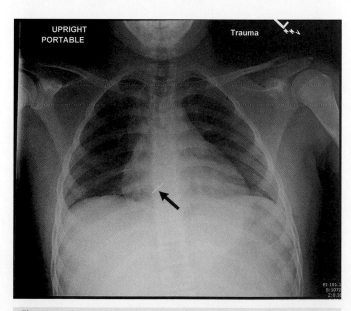

Fig. 46.1 Anterior-posterior view demonstrating a foreign object consistent with a nail, projecting over the right cardiac silhouette (arrow).

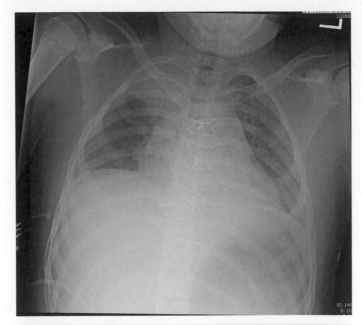

Fig. 46.3 Anterior-posterior view after median sternotomy shows the nail has been removed. There is postoperative atelectasis in the right upper lobe.

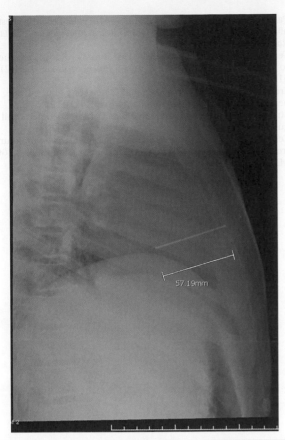

Fig. 46.2 Lateral view shows the nail to project intrathoracic, with location suggesting that the foreign body is intracardiac.

rent in the anterior wall of the right ventricle was noted; the nail was discovered in the right ventricle. The nail was removed and the ventricle was repaired without complication. Follow-up echocardiography showed no abnormalities. Postoperative plain radiography demonstrated atelectasis of the right upper lobe, but no pleural fluid or pneumothorax was identified (Fig. 46.3). These findings resolved. There were no residual effects from his ventricular injury.

Upon further exploration of the child's medical history, it was revealed there had been a history of depression without self-harm, and the mechanism of how the nail gun was discharged into the chest was not fully determined. In light of this history, Pediatric Psychiatry was consulted and it was felt the child was safe for discharge with close monitoring and follow-up; he was not suicidal and contracted for safety. The family was comfortable with this plan of care.

Cardiac injury due to trauma from a discharged nail gun has been previously reported.[4–7,10–12] Many of these injuries involve adults, and the exact incidence is not known. Described mechanisms producing nail gun injuries include accidental discharge, carelessness, inadequate training, and ricochet; many are reported to be self-inflicted.[4,10,13] Mortality from penetrating cardiac injury due to nail guns is similar to that of stab wounds—25%.[4,11]

Treatment of choice for the majority of these injuries is operative, and extraction of the nail should occur in a controlled setting, as circulatory decompensation is a possibility while removing the object. Thoracotomy is the accepted surgical intervention for penetrating thoracic injuries involving the heart. Hemodynamically unstable patients should undergo immediate operative intervention. However, if a patient has sustained a low-velocity injury and has stable vital signs and there are no signs of pericardial tamponade or ongoing bleeding, conservative, nonoperative management can be considered.[4,11]

IMAGING PEARLS

1. Hemodynamically unstable patients who have sustained penetrating thoracic trauma should undergo immediate operative exploration and repair. Do not delay treatment in unstable patients to obtain imaging.
2. Plain radiography is a reasonable first-line imaging modality in children who have sustained penetrating thoracic trauma.
3. Echocardiography, when available, is a rapid imaging test that can be employed in pediatric patients with penetrating thoracic trauma. This modality can detect and assess pericardial fluid, ventricular function, and cardiac tamponade.
4. CT may be employed in patients with suspected vessel or cardiac injury. CT angiography is especially useful in identifying vessel injury. Routine CT without CT angiographic technique is not recommended in cases of penetrating thoracic injury.

References

1. Holmes JF, Sokolove PE, Brant WE, Kuppermann N. A clinical decision rule for identifying children with thoracic injuries after blunt torso trauma. *Ann Emerg Med.* 2002;39(5):492-499.
2. Moore MA, Wallace EC, Westra SJ. Chest trauma in children: current imaging guidelines and techniques. *Radiol Clin North Am.* 2011;49(5):949-968.
3. Piccolo CL, Ianniello S, Trinci M, et al. Diagnostic imaging in pediatric thoracic trauma. *Radiol Med.* 2017;122(11):850-865.

4. Voswinkle JA, Bilfinger TV. Cardiac nail gun injuries: lessons learned. *J Trauma*. 1999;47:588-590.

5. Kulaylat AN, Chesnut CH III, Patel S, et al. Penetrating cardiac nail gun injury in a child. *Pediatr Emerg Care*. 2016;32(8):536-537.

6. Nolke L, Naughton P, Shaw C, et al. Accidental nail gun injuries to the heart: diagnostic, treatment, and epidemiological considerations. *J Trauma*. 2005;58:172-174.

7. Tuladhar S, Eltayeb A, Lakshmanan S, et al. Delayed presentation of right and left ventricle perforation due to suicidal nail gun injury. *Ann Card Anaesth*. 2009;12:136-139.

8. Golden J, Isani M, Bowling J, et al. Limiting chest computed tomography in the evaluation of pediatric thoracic trauma. *J Trauma Acute Care Surg*. 2016;81(2):271-277.

9. Patel RP, Hernanz-Schulman M, Hilmes MA, et al. Pediatric chest CT after trauma: impact on surgical and clinical management. *Pediatr Radiol*. 2010;40(7):1246-1253.

10. Temple AD, Fesmire FM, Seaberg DC, et al. Cardiac injury due to accidental discharge of nail gun. *J Emerg Med*. 2013;44(2): e161-e163.

11. Eren E, Keles C, Sareyyupoglu B, et al. Penetrating injury of the heart by a nail gun. *J Thorac Cardiovasc Surg*. 2004;127:598.

12. Straus JP, Woods RJ, McCarthy MC, et al. Cardiac pneumatic nail gun injury. *J Thorac Cardiovasc Surg*. 2006;132:702-703.

13. Centers for Disease Control and Prevention (CDC). Nail-gun injuries treated in emergency departments in the United States 2001–2005. *MMWR Morb Mortal Wkly Rep*. 2007;56:329-332.

47 Chest Pains: Pediatric Chest Trauma

ROBERT VEZZETTI, MD, FAAP, FACEP

Case Presentation

A 17-year-old male presents to the Emergency Department after being shot in the back. He reports chest pain and dyspnea. His vital signs are a heart rate of 110 beats per minute, a blood pressure of 110/75 mm Hg, and a respiratory rate of 25 breaths per minute. His physical examination is significant for an entry wound in his right axilla without any obvious exit wound. He also complains of right upper quadrant abdominal pain on palpation, although there is no external sign of injury.

Imaging Considerations

Imaging modality choice depends on the mechanism of injury and the clinical examination. Children with a reliable, unremarkable physical examination who have sustained isolated minor thoracic trauma generally do not require imaging. While there are no specific thoracic trauma clinical scenarios that mandate chest imaging, children who have sustained major thoracic trauma (such as penetrating injury); have significant associated injuries (such as femur fracture, intracranial hemorrhage); have multisystem trauma, significant hemothorax, or hemothorax that is not resolving or worsening; or have abnormal physical examination findings should undergo imaging. Particular attention should be given to abnormalities in blood pressure, Glasgow Coma Scale score, respiratory rate, focal chest findings, or the presence of femur fractures, as these findings have been shown to correlate with thoracic injury.[1] There are several imaging options available to the clinician.

PLAIN RADIOGRAPHY

Readily available, cost effective, and with minimal ionizing radiation exposure, plain radiography of the chest is the first-line imaging modality in the pediatric patient with thoracic trauma.[1-5] Clinically significant injuries are readily identified, such as hemothorax and pneumothorax. While anteroposterior (AP) and lateral views are helpful, an AP view is acceptable in a trauma scenario.[3]

COMPUTED TOMOGRAPHY (CT)

Guidelines for the use of CT in blunt or penetrating pediatric thoracic trauma are lacking. However, CT is generally not a first-line imaging modality in most pediatric thoracic trauma, and its routine use, particularly in blunt thoracic trauma, is not encouraged.

Blunt Thoracic Trauma

CT has been shown to be overused in pediatric blunt thoracic trauma.[2,6] While CT is superior to plain radiography in the diagnosis of pediatric thoracic injuries such as pulmonary contusion and pneumothorax, identification of these injuries by chest CT does not change management in most cases.[2,3] The mechanism of injury and an abnormal chest x-ray have been proposed as reliable predictors of significant thoracic injury in pediatric patients with blunt thoracic trauma, suggesting that routine chest CT in these patients is not indicated. CT use is better reserved for patients with concerning abnormal physical examination findings and/or initial plain radiography findings that need further clarification of identified pathology.[4,6,7] Clinical prediction rules for significant thoracic injury in pediatric patients have been developed[1,6] and show promise in reducing unnecessary ionizing radiation exposure by limiting the use of chest CT in pediatric patients who have sustained blunt thoracic trauma.

Penetrating Thoracic Trauma

There are clinical situations where chest CT imaging may be indicated and useful. Penetrating thoracic trauma can produce cardiac or vascular injuries, including the great vessels. Although this injury mechanism is rare in pediatric patients, such injuries are associated with higher mortality. Consider utilization of chest CT in children with suspected cardiovascular injuries or if there is concern for tracheobronchial tree injuries.[2,7] It is also reasonable to consider employing chest CT in children with abnormal initial chest radiographs suggestive of aortic injury, such as a widened mediastinum.[1] If CT imaging is employed, contrast-enhanced CT angiography is indicated to evaluate vessels for injury.[5]

THORACIC ULTRASOUND (US) AND ECHOCARDIOGRAPHY

Focused Assessment with Sonography for Trauma (FAST) is recognized by the American College of Surgeons as an adjunct in the evaluation of pediatric trauma patients but is an evolving technique in this population and is currently not supported as a routine imaging modality.[8,9] Thoracic sonography has, however, proven useful in the identification of pleural and pericardial fluid.[3,4] The use of thoracic US as a component of the eFAST (extended FAST) examination in adult populations has proven adept at the identification of pneumothorax with emerging applications in the identification of rib fractures and pulmonary contusions.[4,10] Echocardiography should be obtained in children with history or physical examination findings suggestive of cardiac injury, elevated cardiac biomarkers (e.g., troponin), or an abnormal electrocardiogram (ECG) to assess for pericardial effusion.

Imaging Findings

This patient had initial plain radiography of the chest (Fig. 47.1). There is a moderate-sized right pleural effusion, presumed to be a hemothorax given the history of trauma, with a metallic foreign body, presumed to be a bullet fragment. There is no pneumothorax. A chest tube was placed (Fig. 47.2) and a total of 600 mL of blood was ultimately obtained.

The patient continued to complain of right upper quadrant abdominal pain, and liver function tests were elevated. Abdominal CT imaging with intravenous (IV) contrast demonstrated the hemothorax (Fig. 47.3), gas-containing hypodense foci in the liver, as well as metallic density objects; these findings are consistent with a liver hematoma and metallic bullet fragments (Fig. 47.4).

Case Conclusion

The patient was admitted to the trauma service, where he was monitored for signs of further bleeding and decompensation. There was no evidence of worsening and his liver function tests normalized. The chest tube was removed and the child was discharged after several days in the hospital.

Pediatric thoracic trauma is not common, accounting for up to 8% of pediatric trauma cases, but is second only to brain injury as a cause of pediatric trauma-related deaths, accounting for mortality rates of 14% to 25%.[1,3,4] The presence of

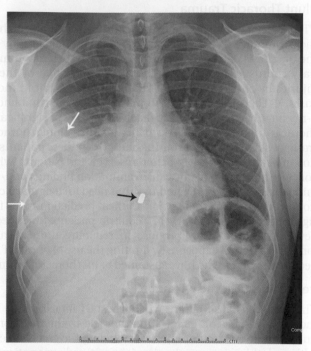

Fig. 47.1 Anterior-posterior chest radiograph shows a right pleural fluid collection consistent with hemothorax *(white arrows)* and a metallic foreign body consistent with a bullet fragment *(black arrow)*.

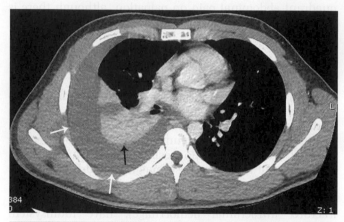

Fig. 47.3 Axial CT image with intravenous contrast demonstrates a moderately large right pleural fluid collection consistent with hemothorax *(white arrows)*, with atelectasis seen in the right lung *(black arrow)*.

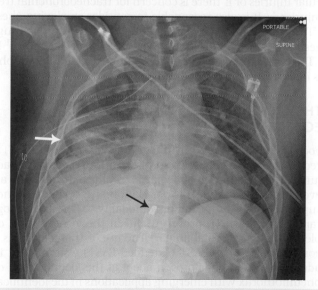

Fig. 47.2 Anterior-posterior view of the chest shows diminished size of right hemothorax *(white arrow)* following chest tube placement. Metallic bullet fragment is again seen *(black arrow)*

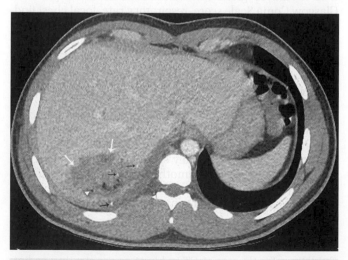

Fig. 47.4 Axial contrast-enhanced CT image shows a hypodense liver lesion consistent with a liver hematoma *(white arrows)*. Low density foci *(white arrowhead)* are consistent with gas due to bullet course through the chest, and dense foci are consistent with small bullet fragments *(black arrows)*

significant thoracic injury correlates with overall injury severity and increasing mortality.[3,5,10,11] Extrathoracic injury is commonly associated with thoracic injury.[5] The majority of these patients sustain blunt trauma (85%), often from motor vehicle accidents or nonaccidental trauma, whereas penetrating thoracic injury is often the result of gunshot wounds or stabbing.[3,4,11] Commonly used imaging protocols in the adult population do not directly translate to pediatric patients,[3] especially given that unique pediatric anatomy and physiology lead to differing injury patterns.[11]

BLUNT TRAUMA

Blunt thoracic trauma is commonly seen in younger patients, although it occurs at any age.[3,11] Associated injuries in pediatric patients include pulmonary contusion (most common), pneumothorax, hemothorax, and rib fractures. Rib fractures are less common in infants given the pliability of their bones, resulting instead in pulmonary contusions. One notable exception is in nonaccidental trauma, which often produces rib fractures, especially posterior rib fractures.[3,5]

PENETRATING TRAUMA

Penetrating trauma is seen almost exclusively in the teenage population.[3] Associated injuries are much like in blunt trauma, but pneumothorax and hemothorax are more common. Blood vessel, tracheobronchial tree, and cardiac injuries, although very rare in pediatric patients, are a concern with penetrating injuries[11]

IMAGING PEARLS

1. When imaging is indicated in pediatric thoracic trauma, the initial modality of choice should be plain radiography of the chest. In most trauma cases, an AP view alone is acceptable.
2. Plain radiography of the chest will identify the majority of clinically significant thoracic injuries in pediatric patients.
3. Pediatric patients with thoracic trauma generally do not require CT of the chest and CT is not indicated as first-line imaging for most patients.
4. IV contrast–enhanced CT should be considered in cases of penetrating trauma, if there is suspicion for vascular

injury on plain radiography, if further evaluation of an identified injury is indicated and CT will likely change management, or in cases of patient decompensation. Always consider other injuries in any child with thoracic trauma, which are common.
5. FAST and eFAST are evolving imaging techniques in pediatric trauma patients and are useful in identifying pleural or pericardial effusions. However, evidence of consistently reliable identification of other thoracic injuries using this modality in this patient population is lacking, and US should not, at this time, replace other imaging modalities, such as plain radiography.
6. Echocardiography should be employed in patients when a cardiac injury is suspected, either by history, physical examination, or abnormal laboratory/ECG findings.

References

1. Holmes JF, Sokolove PE, Brant WE, et al. A clinical decision rule for identifying children with thoracic injuries after blunt torso trauma. *Ann Emerg Med.* 2002;39(5):492-499.
2. Golden J, Isani M, Bowling J, et al. Limiting chest computed tomography in the evaluation of pediatric thoracic trauma. *J Trauma Acute Care Surg.* 2016;81(2):271-277.
3. Moore MA, Wallace EC, Westra SJ. Chest trauma in children: current imaging guidelines and techniques. *Radiol Clin North Am.* 2011;49(5):949-968.
4. Piccolo CL, Ianniello S, Trinci M, et al. Diagnostic imaging in pediatric thoracic trauma. *Radiol Med.* 2017;122(11):850-865.
5. Santorelli KH, Vane DW. The diagnosis and management of children with blunt injury of the chest. *Semin Pediatr Surg.* 2004;13:98-105.
6. Stephens CQ, Boulos MC, Connelly CR, et al. Limiting thoracic CT: a rule for use during initial pediatric trauma evaluation. *J Pediatr Surg.* 2017;52(12):2031-2037.
7. Patel RP, Hernanz-Schulman M, Hilmes MA, et al. Pediatric chest CT after trauma: impact on surgical and clinical management. *Pediatr Radiol.* 2010;40(7):1246-1253.
8. Bonasso PC, Dassinger MS, Deidre LW, et al. Review of bedside surgeon–performed ultrasound in pediatric patients. *J Pediatr Surg.* 2018;53(11): 2279-2289.
9. Holmes JF, Kelley KM, Wooton-Gorges SL, et al. Effect of abdominal ultrasound on clinical care, outcomes, and resource use among children with blunt torso trauma. *JAMA.* 2017;213:2290-2296.
10. Richards JR, McGahan JP. Focused assessment with sonography in trauma (FAST) in 2017: what radiologists can learn. *Radiology.* 2017;238(1):30-48.
11. Bliss D, Silen M. Pediatric thoracic trauma. *Crit Care Med.* 2002;30:S409-S415.

48 Check That Neck: Cervical Spine Imaging

ANNA SCHLECHTER, MD and BHAIRAV PATEL, MD

Case Presentation

A 12-month-old female presents following a motor vehicle accident. The child was reportedly secured in a rear car seat; however, the child was found outside of the vehicle lying on the pavement. The two-vehicle crash occurred at a high rate of speed (70–80 miles/hour), and there was considerable damage to both vehicles but no deaths at the scene.

In the Emergency Department, the child has a waxing and waning mental status, with her Glasgow Coma Scale (GCS) score varying between 8 and 12. She has some bruising to the right side of the forehead without crepitus or step-offs and her face seems uninjured; she is in a cervical collar applied by Emergency Medical Services prior to arrival. Examination of the neck shows no abnormalities, but the child seems to not want to move her neck and there appears to be some pain to palpation of cervical vertebrae, although it is hard to determine the exact spinal level. She is not moving her left leg well and there is swelling of the thigh.

Imaging Considerations

PLAIN RADIOGRAPHY

Plain cervical spine radiographs should be the initial radiologic study to evaluate for cervical spine injury in most children who require workup.[1] The three-view spine series (cross-table lateral, anterior-posterior [AP], and, when obtainable, open-mouth odontoid) should be obtained as the initial study.[2] Sensitivity for the cross-table lateral view for injury is 79% and increases to 90% with the addition of the AP or odontoid views.[3] It is necessary to review the images to ensure that all of the cervical vertebrae are visualized, as the most frequent cause of a missed injury of the vertebral body is an inadequate film series.[4]

COMPUTED TOMOGRAPHY (CT)

The sensitivity and specificity of CT for detecting cervical spine bony injury are ≥98%.[4] However, CT scan should be ordered judiciously, employing the principles of ALARA. Obtaining a cervical spine CT exposes a child to a greater radiation dose than a plain film series does. In 2002, a helical cervical spine CT was shown to expose a child's skin and thyroid to approximately 10 and 14 times the radiation, respectively, compared to five-view radiographs of the cervical spine.[5] With current newer CT technology, the exposure difference would not be as great but still would be

higher with CT than plain radiography. In children with a GCS score of ≤9, neurologic deficit on physical examination, or inadequate cervical spine radiographs (in the setting of a high likelihood of injury based on history and physical examination), imaging with CT of the cervical spine instead of plain radiographs is indicated.[6]

MAGNETIC RESONANCE IMAGING (MRI)

In patients with an abnormal neurologic examination, or when imaging of the spinal cord or other soft tissues of the spinal column is necessary, MRI should be obtained.[1] MRI is less sensitive than CT for the detection of bony injuries of the cervical spine and craniocervical junction but is better than CT for the identification of intervertebral disk herniation, ligamentous injuries, and spinal cord injuries as well as soft tissue trauma.[1]

Imaging Findings

Since the child underwent CT of the head, the cervical spine was imaged with this modality. Selected images of the cervical spine study are provided here. A cervical (C2) spine fracture with increased distance between C1 and C2, spinous process fractures. C1 and C2, and multiple spinous process fractures were demonstrated (Fig. 48.1).

Case Conclusion

The child continued to have a labile mental status and was subsequently intubated. MRI of the spine was obtained. These images demonstrated, in addition to the cervical spine fracture, several thoracic vertebral body compression fractures and complete disruption of the posterior atlanto-axial membrane (Fig. 48.2).

Multiple pediatric subspecialties were consulted during this child's care. Pediatric Neurosurgery and Spine Surgery brought the child to the operating suite and performed an occipitocervical fusion for the cervical vertebral injuries (Fig. 48.3). The thoracic vertebral compression fractures did not require operative intervention and were treated with thoracolumbosacral orthosis bracing. After a prolonged hospital stay, the patient was discharged with continued subspecialty follow-up and care. Her only remaining neurologic deficit was oral pharyngeal dysphagia, which was managed by Speech Pathology and Pediatric Otolaryngology specialists.

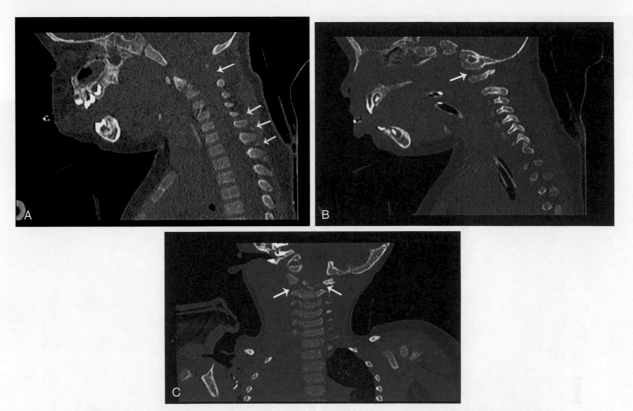

Fig. 48.1 (A) Sagittal computed tomography (CT) image demonstrating an angulated C2 fracture *(red arrow)*, abnormal widening between the C1 posterior arch and C2 spinous process indicative of ligamentous injury *(white arrow)*, and spinous process fractures *(yellow arrows)*. (B) Sagittal CT image demonstrating left atlantooccipital joint widening *(white arrow)*. (C) Coronal CT image demonstrating bilateral widening of the C1–C2 joints *(white arrows)*.

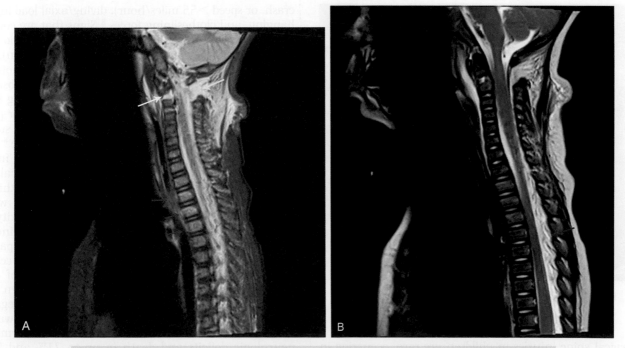

Fig. 48.2 (A) Sagittal magnetic resonance imaging (MRI) STIR (short tau inversion recovery) image demonstrating a C2 fracture *(white arrow)*, complete disruption of the posterior atlantoaxial membrane *(yellow arrow)*, and several upper thoracic spine compression fractures, evidenced by high-signal edema of the vertebral bodies with hematoma anterior to the spine at this level *(red arrows)*. (B) Sagittal MRI T2 image demonstrating a dorsal epidural hematoma *(red arrow)*.

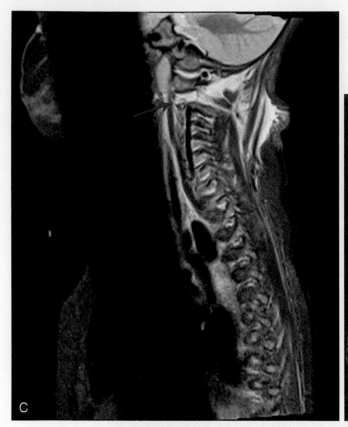

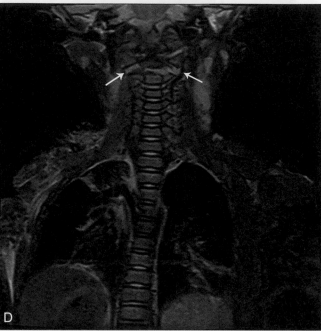

Fig. 48.2 cont'd (C) MRI Sagittal STIR image demonstrating left atlantooccipital joint widening *(red arrow)*. (D) MRI coronal image demonstrating widening of bilateral widening of the lateral C1–C2 joints *(white arrows)*.

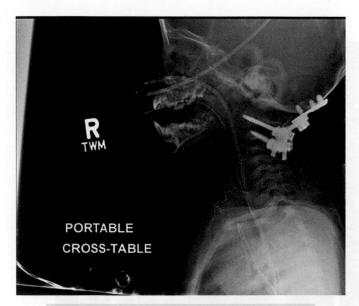

Fig. 48.3 Lateral cervical spine postoperative radiograph.

Cervical spine injuries in children are rare, occurring in only 1%–2% of pediatric blunt trauma.[7] The mechanisms that are considered high risk for cervical spine injury include motor vehicle collision with severe mechanism (head-on collision, rollover, ejection from the vehicle, death in the same

crash, or speed >55 miles/hour), diving/axial load injuries, hanging, and clotheslining forces.[8] Signs that are concerning for cervical spine injury include focal neurologic symptoms (even if they have resolved upon evaluation), neck symptoms (pain, torticollis, decreased range of motion or midline posterior pain), altered mental status, substantial coexisting injury (fractures of the face, pelvis, long bones, intracranial hemorrhage, or solid organ injury), or predisposing conditions such as history of cervical spine surgery, cervical arthritis, Ehlers-Danlos, or Down syndrome.[8]

Approximately 75% of cervical spine injuries in children younger than 8 years of age are axial cervical spine injuries (occiput to C2 region).[9] Children in this age group have relatively larger heads than bodies, weaker cervical musculature, increased ligamentous laxity, and immature vertebral joints and horizontally inclined articulating facets that facilitate sliding.[10] In comparison, children older than 8 years of age have subaxial cervical spine injury (C3 to C7) in approximately 50% of cases, with the most common injuries in older children being vertebral body and arch fractures.[9,11] It is integral to identify cervical spine injuries as they frequently warrant surgical intervention and are associated with permanent neurologic deficits and death in up to 21% and 7% of patients, respectively.[9] A child with a normal physical examination and an evaluation that otherwise indicates a low risk for cervical spine injury may be clinically cleared without diagnostic imaging.

IMAGING PEARLS

1. A child with no neck pain and full range of motion who is otherwise well, and without a history concerning for cervical spine injury, does not require imaging to clear the cervical spine.
2. A three-view spine series (cross-table lateral, AP, and, when obtainable, open-mouth odontoid) should generally be obtained as the initial screening test in most pediatric patients undergoing evaluation for cervical spine injury.
3. The most frequent cause of a missed injury of the vertebral body is an inadequate film series.
4. CT is extremely sensitive and specific for identification of cervical spine bony injury but exposes a child to a greater amount of ionizing radiation than plain radiography. CT imaging of the spine is often obtained if head imaging is obtained.
5. MRI is superior to CT for visualizing soft tissues, disk herniation, ligamentous injury, and injuries of the spinal cord, including hemorrhage.

References

1. Chung S, Mikrogianakis A, Wales PW, et al. Trauma association of Canada Pediatric Subcommittee National Pediatric Cervical Spine Evaluation Pathway: consensus guidelines. *J Trauma.* 2011;70(4):873-884.
2. Hernandez JA, Chupik C, Swischuk LE. Cervical spine trauma in children under 5 years: productivity of CT. *Emerg Radiol.* 2004;10(4):176-178.
3. Nigrovic LE, Rogers AJ, Adelgais KM, et al. Utility of plain radiographs in detecting traumatic injuries of the cervical spine in children. *Pediatr Emerg Care.* 2012;28(5):426-432.
4. Sanchez B, Waxman K, Jones T, et al. Cervical spine clearance in blunt trauma: evaluation of a computed tomography–based protocol. *J Trauma.* 2005;59(1):179-183.
5. Rybicki F, Nawfel RD, Judy PF, et al. Skin and thyroid dosimetry in cervical spine screening: two methods for evaluation and a comparison between a helical CT and radiographic trauma series. *AJR Am J Roentgenol.* 2002;179(4):933-937.
6. Borock EC, Gabram SG, Jacobs LM, et al. A prospective analysis of a two-year experience using computed tomography as an adjunct for cervical spine clearance. *J Trauma.* 1991;31(7):1001-1005.
7. Viccellio P, Simon H, Pressman BD, et al. A prospective multicenter study of cervical spine injury in children. *Pediatrics.* 2001;108(2):E20.
8. Leonard JC, Kuppermann N, Olsen C, et al. Factors associated with cervical spine injury in children after blunt trauma. *Ann Emerg Med.* 2011;58(2):145-155.
9. Leonard JR, Jaffe DM, Kuppermann N, et al. Cervical spine injury patterns in children. *Pediatrics.* 2014;133(5):e1179-e1188.
10. Orenstein JB, Klein BL, Gotschall CS, et al. Age and outcome in pediatric cervical spine injury: 11-year experience. *Pediatr Emerg Care.* 1994;10(3):132-137.
11. Brown RL, Brunn MA, Garcia VF. Cervical spine injuries in children: a review of 103 patients treated consecutively at a level 1 pediatric trauma center. *J Pediatr Surg.* 2001;36(8):1107-1114.

49 *My Achin' Back: Vertebral Compression Fractures*

ROBERT VEZZETTI, MD, FAAP, FACEP

Case Presentation

A 9-year-old female seeks care after falling from her bicycle. She states that she was riding her bike and attempted to "pop a wheelie." In doing so, she fell backward, separating herself from the bike, landing initially on her buttocks, but then onto her back. There is no reported loss of consciousness and she was wearing a helmet. She denies neck pain. She did not strike the handlebars and has no chest or abdominal pain.

Her physical examination reveals no fever, a heart rate of 100 beats per minute, a blood pressure of 105/54 mm Hg, and room air oxygen saturations of 99%. She has no outward signs of trauma. There is no chest or abdominal tenderness. Her pelvis is stable and nontender. She complains of diffuse tenderness around her mid-thoracic spine but cannot pinpoint a precise location of pain. There are no obvious external signs of trauma (i.e., no hematoma, bruising, or abrasion) and there are no step-offs, crepitus, or deformities. Her extremities have no signs of trauma. She is able to ambulate but complains of mid-thoracic back pain. She is grossly neurovascularly intact.

Imaging Considerations

PLAIN RADIOGRAPHY

Plain film radiography is the initial imaging modality of choice. A two-view study (anteroposterior and lateral) is sufficient,[1] and a complete view of the segment of interest is essential. Which spinal segments should be initially imaged can be based on history and clinical examination findings.

COMPUTED TOMOGRAPHY (CT)

CT is often utilized as an adjunct study to better visualize fractures identified on plain imaging, especially complex fractures, as CT gives excellent visualization of bony elements of the spine and depicts retropulsion of fracture fragments. CT is also used to evaluate the spine when a patient is undergoing body CT as part of a trauma evaluation. Reconstruction of the included spine is useful for fracture detection and is performed with no additional radiation exposure. In such cases, the reconstructed spine CT imaging will include only those areas included in the body scan. For example, spine reconstruction imaging from an abdomen and pelvis CT will include the lower thoracic spine, but not the upper thoracic spine. Routine use of CT as an initial imaging test should be discouraged.[1]

MAGNETIC RESONANCE IMAGING (MRI)

MRI is utilized when there are signs or concerns for spinal cord involvement and produces excellent visualization of the spinal canal, spinal cord, and the ligamentous elements of the vertebral bodies. Use of this modality should be reserved for patients with neurologic findings (paraesthesias, numbness, weakness, or paralysis).[1–3] MRI can also be used to confirm bone marrow edema related to vertebral fracture when imaging with other modalities is negative or equivocal. Loss of more than 50% of the anterior height of the vertebral body should prompt concern for posterior element disruption and MRI should be considered.[1,4] Availability and the need for sedation may be obstacles to the use of MRI in the urgent setting.

CT VERSUS MRI

One study specifically comparing CT and MRI for the identification of thoracic compression fractures found agreement between the two modalities with regard to fracture number and distribution.[5] In this study, all patients underwent CT and MRI. CT was found to be highly sensitive compared to MRI, and treatment decisions and outcomes were not changed by the addition of MRI in this study population, suggesting that information obtained from MRI should be weighed against the expense, time, and sedation need.[5]

Imaging Findings

Plain radiography of the thoracic spine was obtained. This demonstrated anterior vertebral body compression fractures of T5 through T8, with approximately 50% loss of anterior vertebral body height of T7, and more mild anterior compression fractures of T5, T6, and T8 (Figs. 49.1 and 49.2).

Case Conclusion

Once the fractures were identified, the child underwent additional imaging. Pediatric Orthopedics was consulted. Plain radiography of the cervical spine was obtained and no additional fractures were found. Since there was 50% loss of vertebral body height at T7, associated contiguous fractures, and no neurologic symptoms, the child underwent noncontrast CT of the thoracic and lumbar and a selected sagittal image is provided. CT confirmed the T5–T8 compression fractures, greatest at T7 with 50% height loss, with no retropulsion of fracture fragments (Fig. 49.3). The

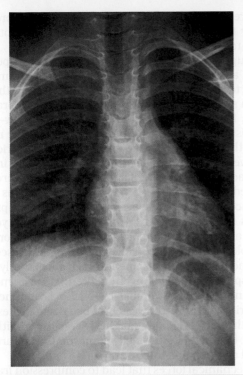

Fig. 49.1 Anteroposterior view of the thoracic spine shows no evidence of fracture.

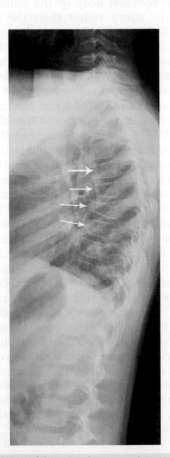

Fig. 49.2 Lateral view of the spine shows anterior vertebral body compression fractures of T5 through T8 *(arrows)*. There is 50% loss of anterior vertebral body height at T7 and 25% or less loss of vertebral body height at T5, T6, and T8.

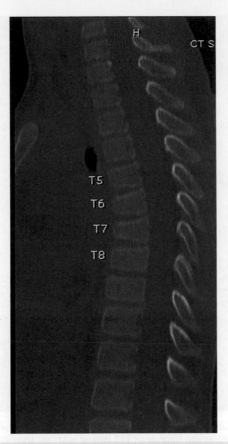

Fig. 49.3 Sagittal computed tomography reconstruction of the spine again demonstrates anterior vertebral body compression fractures of T5 through T8.

child was admitted for pain control and bedrest and was fitted with a thoracolumbosacral orthosis (TLSO) brace. She was discharged with careful follow-up and return precautions, specifically for the development of neurologic symptoms, such as incontinence, weakness, or numbness. She recovered uneventfully.

A comparison case is presented here, with a selected image. This child fell approximately 6 feet while playing on monkey bars. He landed on his buttocks and presented complaining of lower back pain only. There were no neurologic symptoms. Imaging revealed an anterior wedge compression fracture of T12 with less than 25% loss of vertebral body height and there is a possible subtle buckle of the anterior cortex of L1 (Fig. 49.4). He underwent further plain radiography of the spine, including cervical and thoracic segments and no further fractures were found. Pediatric Orthopedics was consulted and the child was admitted for pain control, bedrest, and TLSO bracing.

Another selected image is presented. This child had complaints of low back pain for 2 weeks without a known history of trauma. In these images, there is slight anterior wedging appearance of L1 (Fig. 49.5). Mild anterior wedging of vertebral bodies is commonly seen in pediatric patients, including those without a history of trauma, and is most often seen at the thoracolumbar junction.[6] Therefore, a mild decrease in anterior vertebral body height compared to posterior vertebral body height, especially in the thoracolumbar junction region, should be interpreted with caution

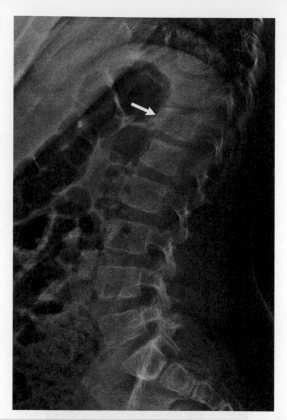

Fig. 49.4 Lateral view of the lumbar spine demonstrating an anterior wedge compression fracture of T12 *(arrow)* with less than 25% loss of vertebral body height.

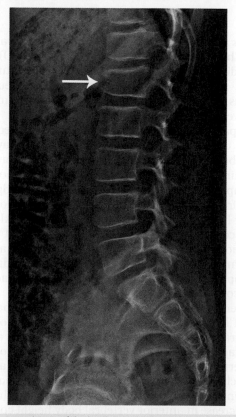

Fig. 49.5 Lateral view of the lumbar spine demonstrating mild anterior wedging of L1 *(arrow)*, likely physiologic.

and correlated closely with clinical history and presentation. For the patient in Fig. 49.5, the wedging noted was thought to be incidental, normal variation.

Although spine fractures are not common in pediatric patients, accounting for up to 4% of pediatric trauma injuries,[7] vertebral compression fractures are among the most common spinal injuries in this population.[8] Vertebral compression fractures are usually the result of low-energy mechanisms, such as a fall from a low height; the rest are due to other forms of injury, such as sports injuries.[1,8–10] More severe vertebral injuries, such as rotational injuries, burst fractures, and lateral compression fractures, are associated with high-speed mechanisms, such as motor vehicle accidents.[1,8–10] The age distribution of compression fractures is bimodal, with falls more common in younger children and high-energy or sports mechanisms more common in older children and adolescents.[1,8–10] Adolescent patients tend to have lower spine injuries, particularly of the lumbar spine, than do younger children.[1,9–11] The most frequently injured thoracic area is T4–T12.[12] Loss of height of the anterior cortex of the vertebral body, usually less than 20% of the vertebral body height, is consistent with compression fracture.[1] Neurologic compromise is rare with vertebral compression fractures.[1]

The mechanical forces that lead to compression fractures in the pediatric population are most often due to hyperflexion, rather than hyperextension or shear, injury.[8,12] In this population, the vertebral body of the immature spine is more inclined to injury rather than the intervertebral disc.[8,13] Spinal fracture without spinal cord involvement is more common in the pediatric population than the adult population.[9] However, spinal cord injury without radiographic abnormality (SCIWORA) has been described in the literature, first by Pang and Wilberger in 1982.[14] Since this time, the definition of SCIWORA has been debated, especially in the era of MRI. A proposed modification of the traditional SCIWORA definition has been the absence of abnormalities on both plain radiographs and MRI.[15] While SCIWORA is most commonly seen in cervical spine injuries, it has been reported in thoracic spine injuries, particularly in the context of a high-energy injury mechanism.[9,16] A recent study looking at SCIWORA defined this entity as "acute spinal cord injury associated with a sensory or motor deficit or both, with a symptom duration of at least 24 hours and without evidence of injury on plain radiographs or CT scans."[9,17] In this series of 250 pediatric patients with all levels of spine injury, there was a SCIWORA rate of 6%[9]; reported rates of SCIWORA in the literature range from 1% to almost 40%.[9,18] In a case series of 578 pediatric patients with vertebral trauma, 45 were found to have traumatic myelopathy, 3 had SCIWORA; of those patients, 2 had thoracic cord injuries from high-speed motor vehicle crashes and permanent neurologic deficits.[18]

An important management point is assessing the patient for other compression fractures, as where there is one vertebral fracture, multilevel involvement, both contiguous and noncontiguous, is not uncommon.[1,19–21] One study reported that 32% of patients with vertebral fractures had secondary fractures; of these, 6% had noncontiguous injury that was at least three levels away from the primary injury, with these secondary injuries in the thoracic and upper lumbar spine.[22] Another study reported a lower rate

(~12%) of patients with noncontiguous injury, with older children more likely to have these injuries and 44% had associated injuries (most often closed head injury).[23] Given this, it is reasonable to approach the patient with an identified spinal fracture, including compression fracture, as potentially having other spine fractures (both contiguous and noncontiguous) and evaluate the patient accordingly (i.e., additional plain radiography above and below the identified injury). Patients who have undergone a traumatic high-energy mechanism should be suspected as having additional noncontiguous fractures and associated injuries until proven otherwise.[1,9,11,19–23]

Treatment of vertebral compression fractures generally involves symptomatic care.[8] Bedrest, pain control, and nonoperative stabilization of the fracture are mainstays.[1,8,11,12,19] Bracing with TLSO and follow-up physical therapy have been shown to be well tolerated and to produce good outcomes.[1,12,24] Surgical intervention for compression fractures is rarely indicated, but there are instances where this treatment option may be considered. Neurologic symptoms are not commonly associated with compression fractures and are more likely seen in burst fractures of flexion-hyperextension injuries (e.g., chance fractures).[12,24,25] Operative management in these instances has been shown to be effective.[12,25]

IMAGING PEARLS

1. Plain radiography is the initial imaging modality in patients with suspected vertebral fractures. Two views (anteroposterior and lateral) are preferred.
2. CT should not be routinely obtained in patients with suspected vertebral fractures. Complex fractures that need better visualization can be imaged with this modality.
3. MRI should not be routinely utilized in patients with vertebral fractures. Although neurologic injury associated with compression fractures is not common, patients with neurologic findings or symptoms should have evaluation with MRI.
4. It is not uncommon for patients to have multilevel involvement of vertebral fractures. Strong consideration should be given to imaging several levels above and below an identified fracture, or to image the entire spine. Plain radiography is an appropriate initial imaging modality for this purpose.
5. Advanced imaging may be indicated in patients with multilevel fracture involvement or severe injury mechanisms, as associated injury is not uncommon, particularly with noncontiguous fractures.

References

1. Daniels AH, Sobel AD, Eberson CP. Pediatric thoracolumbar spine trauma. *J Am Acad Orthop Surg.* 2013;21(12):707-716.
2. Santiago R, Guenther E, Carroll K, Junkins Jr EP. The clinical presentation of pediatric thoracolumbar fractures. *J Trauma.* 2006;60(1):187-192.
3. Sledge JB, Allred D, Hyman J. Use of magnetic resonance imaging in evaluating injuries to the pediatric thoracolumbar spine. *J Pediatr Orthop.* 2001;21(3):288-293.
4. Reilly CW. Pediatric spine trauma. *J Bone Joint Surg Am.* 2007;89(suppl 1):98-107.
5. Franklin DB III, Hardaway AT, Sheffer BW, et al. The role of computed tomography and magnetic resonance imaging in the diagnosis of pediatric thoracolumbar compression fractures. *J Pediatr Orthop.* 2019;39(7):e520-e523.
6. Gaca AM, Barnhart HX, Bisset GS III. Evaluation of wedging of lower thoracic and upper lumbar vertebral bodies in the pediatric population. *AJR Am J Roentgenol.* 2010;194(2):516-520.
7. Martin BW, Dykes E, Lecky FE. Patterns and risks in spinal trauma. *Arch Dis Child.* 2004;89(9):860-865.
8. Reynolds R. Pediatric spinal injury. *Curr Opin Pediatr.* 2000;12(1):67-71.
9. Kim C, Vassilyadi M, Forbes JK, et al. Traumatic spinal injuries in children at a single level 1 pediatric trauma centre: report of a 23-year experience. *Can J Surg.* 2016;59(3):205-212.
10. Knox JB, Schneider JE, Cage JM, et al. Spine trauma in very young children: a retrospective study of 206 patients presenting to a level 1 pediatric trauma center. *J Pediatr Orthop.* 2014;34(7):698-702.
11. Dogan S, Safavi-Abbasi S, Chang SW, et al. Thoracolumbar and sacral spinal injuries in children and adolescents: a review of 89 cases. *J Neurosurg.* 2007;106:426-433.
12. Clark P, Letts M. Trauma to the thoracic and lumbar spine in the adolescent. *Can J Surg.* 2001;44(5):337-345.
13. Roaf R. Instrumentation and fusion technique for lumbar spine. Guidelines according to underlying pathology. *Orthop Rev.* 1986;15(1):56-57.
14. Pang D, Wilberger Jr JE. Spinal cord injury without radiographic abnormalities in children. *J Neurosurg.* 1982;57(1):114-129.
15. Yucesoy K, Yuksel KZ. SCIWORA in MRI era. *Clin Neurol Neurosurg.* 2008;110(5):429-433.
16. Trumble J, Myslinski J. Lower thoracic SCIWORA in a 3-year-old child: case report. *Pediatr Emerg Care.* 2000;16(2):91-93.
17. Grabb PA, Pang D. Magnetic resonance imaging in the evaluation of spinal cord injury without radiographic abnormality in children. *Neurosurgery.* 1994;35(3):406-414.
18. Trigylidas T, Yuh SJ, Vassilyadi M, et al. Spinal cord injuries without radiographic abnormality at two pediatric trauma centers in Ontario. *Pediatr Neurosurg.* 2010;46(4):283-289.
19. Srinivasan V, Jea A. Pediatric thoracolumbar spine trauma. *Neurosurg Clin N Am.* 2016;28(1):103-114.
20. Roche C, Carty H. Spinal trauma in children. *Pediatr Radiol.* 2001;31(10):677-700.
21. Rush JK, Kelly DM, Astur N, et al. Associated injuries in children and adolescents with spinal trauma. *J Pediatr Orthop.* 2013;33(4):393-397.
22. Mahan ST, Mooney DP, Karlin L, et al. Multiple level injuries in pediatric spinal trauma. *J Trauma.* 2009;67(3):537-542.
23. Firth GB, Kingwell SP, Moroz PJ. Pediatric noncontiguous spinal injuries: the 15-year experience at a level 1 trauma center. *Spine (Phila Pa 1976).* 2012;37(10):E599-E608.
24. Stadhouder A, Buskens E, Vergroesen DA, et al. Nonoperative treatment of thoracic and lumbar spine fractures: a prospective randomized study of different treatment options. *J Orthop Trauma.* 2009;23(8):588-594.
25. Satyarthee GD, Sangani M, Sinha S, et al. Management and outcome analysis of pediatric unstable thoracolumbar spine injury: large surgical series with literature review. *J Pediatr Neurosci.* 2017;12(3):209-214.

50 How'd That Happen? Nonaccidental Trauma

ROBERT VEZZETTI, MD, FAAP, FACEP

Case Presentation

A 3-month-old male presents with what the parents describe as fussiness since yesterday. The child has had nasal congestion over the past few days so they took him to an emergency department 1 day ago, where he had a respiratory syncytial virus test that was negative and a chest x-ray that was reported to be unremarkable, per the parents. The parents noted that, after discharge from the facility, the child appeared to have pain when his left leg was manipulated, and this has persisted over the past 24 hours.

Physical examination reveals a well-appearing child in no obvious distress. He is afebrile, with a heart rate of 150 beats per minute, a respiratory rate of 36 breaths per minute, and a room air oxygen saturation of 98%. Blood pressure was not obtained. He has no obvious signs of trauma and is moving all of his extremities without difficulty. The remainder of his physical examination is unremarkable until you palpate the proximal portion of his left lower leg—this action elicits crying from the child.

Imaging Considerations

Imaging plays a critical role in the evaluation of nonaccidental trauma (NAT). There are guidelines promulgated by the American College of Radiology (ACR) and the American Academy of Pediatrics that are designed to guide the clinician in choosing appropriate imaging for children who may have sustained NAT.[1–3]

After cutaneous findings, such as bruising, fractures are the second most common manifestation of NAT, especially in children under 18 months to 2 years of age.[3–8] Fractures in children with NAT can be seen in every location, and while no fracture is absolutely diagnostic of abuse,[9] there are radiographic patterns that suggest NAT. Any fracture raises the suspicion of abuse in the setting of an absent, inappropriate, or changing history.[9] Fractures with high specificity for abusive injury include rib fractures in young children, particularly posterior rib fractures; multiple fractures at various stages of healing without underlying metabolic bone disease or skeletal dysplasia; classic metaphyseal fractures; scapula fractures; sternum fractures; and spinous process fractures.[9–12] Metaphyseal fractures, colloquially called "bucket handle fracture" or "corner fracture," are the result of shearing forces applied to long bones and generally not the result of falls.[7,10,13] These injuries are highly specific for NAT in children under 1 year of age.[7–10,12,14] Common locations for these fractures include the distal femur, distal humerus, and proximal tibia and fibula.[7]

Posterior and lateral rib fractures have also been found to have high association with NAT in children under 1 year of age.[8–10,12] These injuries occur when the thorax is squeezed. One study found that posterior rib fractures have a positive predictive value of 95% for NAT that increased to 100% when clinical history was taken into account.[12,15] Interestingly, anterior rib fractures have been rarely reported in association with cardiopulmonary resuscitation (CPR),[16] and whether or not the two-thumb CPR technique commonly employed in infant CPR administration leads to an increase in posterior rib fractures remains to be determined.[17] The pliability of the pediatric rib cage makes rib fractures, outside of NAT, rare, and rib fractures in various stages of healing are highly specific for NAT, especially in the absence of metabolic or skeletal disease.[9]

Abusive head trauma is a common form of nonaccidental injury in the pediatric population and is a leading cause of death in children under 1 year of age.[7,8,10,18] Mechanisms of injury vary and can produce both fractures and intracranial hemorrhage, although a fracture may or may not be associated with intracranial hemorrhage. Neuroimaging, both computed tomography (CT) and magnetic resonance imaging (MRI), plays an important role in the acute management of a patient with suspected NAT as well as assists with patient prognosis.[10] Isolated, linear skull fractures or isolated intracranial injuries are not specific for NAT, and linear skull fractures occur in both accidental and abusive injuries. Therefore, correlation with the clinical history and evaluation are necessary, and one should consider further evaluation with a skeletal survey if there is a lack of a credible history to explain the injury.[7,10,18,19] Multiple skull fractures, fractures that cross suture lines, or bilateral skull fractures are radiographic features significantly associated with abusive head trauma.[18,20] Subdural hematomas are the most common intracranial finding associated with NAT but are not specific.[7,10,18] Correlation with history, physical examination, laboratory, and other radiographic findings is critical to help establish if the presence of an intracranial hemorrhage is due to NAT.

There are other underlying metabolic and genetic conditions that may mimic the radiographic findings of NAT. For example, patients with osteogenesis imperfecta are more susceptible to fractures. However, metabolic bone disease will have predictable patterns that can be seen on imaging.[10] Additionally, fractures due to NAT are far more likely to occur as opposed to fractures due to a metabolic abnormality.[9,11]

PLAIN RADIOGRAPHY

The radiographic skeletal survey is an initial, integral, imaging study utilized for the evaluation of children with suspected NAT. There are practice parameters that have been promulgated by the ACR and the Society for Pediatric Radiology recommending the views for a skeletal survey in children under the age of 2 years with suspected NAT.[2,7,10,19] Each anatomic region should be imaged separately, not combining separate regions such as the humerus and forearm and not obtaining views of the right and left extremities together. Further dedicated imaging of areas for clarification of initial imaging findings from the skeletal survey should be performed, for example, addition of lateral views and views coned down to a region of interest such as the wrist or knee. Complete skeletal survey views include the following:[2,10,12,19]

APPENDICULAR SKELETON VIEWS	AXIAL SKELETON VIEWS
Humeri (AP)	Skull (frontal and lateral, to include cervical spine)
Forearms (AP)	Cervical spine (lateral, if not included adequately on lateral skull)
Hands (PA)	Thorax (AP, lateral, and bilateral oblique, including ribs, spine)
Femurs (AP)	
Lower legs (AP)	Lumbosacral spine (lateral)
Feet (AP)	Abdomen to include the pelvis (AP)

AP, Anterior-posterior; PA, posterior-anterior.

A proper and complete skeletal survey has been shown to increase the detection of fractures.[4,7,12] A "babygram" (single view of the entire skeleton) is NOT adequate for proper visualization of fractures in the evaluation of NAT and should not be obtained.[7,12] In children who have equivocal findings or in whom NAT is strongly suspected, a follow-up skeletal survey should be performed 2 to 3 weeks after the initial survey, since this increases the chance of detecting occult fractures and increases the sensitivity and specificity for detecting healing fracture.[2,7,21,22] However, if the initial radiographic evaluation is unremarkable and there is low suspicion of NAT by other evaluation and investigation, repeat imaging is not indicated.[7]

COMPUTED TOMOGRAPHY

CT of the head is utilized in instances where there is suspected intracranial injury or if a skull fracture is suspected, either clinically or by history. CT increases sensitivity for detecting skull fractures.[7,10] Such injuries are often occult,[10,23] so a high index of suspicion for intracranial injury should always be maintained when evaluating children for NAT. Young children (<6 months of age) and any child with signs of trauma to the head, mental status changes, or focal neurologic findings should be considered candidates for neuroimaging.[2,19]

CT of the abdomen is employed if there is suspicion, either clinically or by laboratory findings, of an intraabdominal injury. Intravenous contrast should be utilized.[7,8,10]

MAGNETIC RESONANCE IMAGING (MRI)

MRI is often used as a follow-up study when there are abnormal findings on initial neuroimaging (CT) and can be used to assist in patient prognosis.[7,8,10,24] MRI may also be utilized in the nonacute setting to evaluate for the presence of parenchymal injury or hemorrhage.[7,8] This modality may not be readily available in the emergent setting and may require sedation to complete a meaningful study.

Imaging Findings

The chief complaint and physical examination findings prompted plain radiography of the left femur, tibia, and fibula. These images are presented here.

Two-view imaging of the left femur and left tibia-fibula demonstrated metaphyseal abnormalities of the distal femur and proximal tibia in a pattern consistent with classic metaphyseal lesions/fractures (Figs. 50.1–50.3).

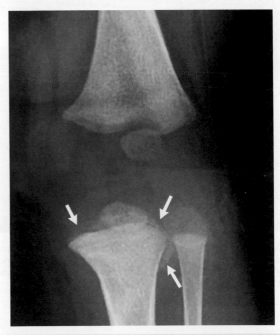

Fig. 50.1 Metaphyseal fractures of the distal left femur and proximal left tibia. It is not unusual for metaphyseal fractures to have a different appearance on different views, as a thin disk of bone is separated from the metaphysis and will often have a different appearance on different projections. This figure is a coned down anterior-posterior view of the knee from the left femur x-ray and shows a bucket handle appearance of the proximal left tibial metaphyseal fracture *(white arrows)*.

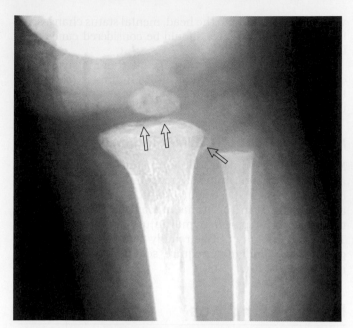

Fig. 50.2 Anterior-posterior view of the proximal left tibia and fibula with a slightly different projection from Fig 50.1. The tibial fracture *(open arrows)* appears as a horizontal linear lucency underlying the growth plate, with a bucket handle appearance laterally.

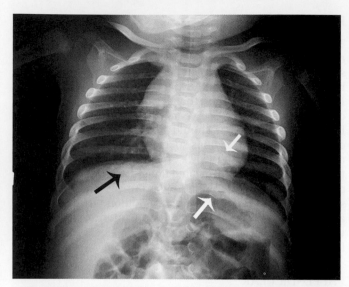

Fig. 50.4 Anterior-posterior view of the chest demonstrates healing fractures, with callus, of the left 8th and 10th posterior ribs *(white arrows)* and of the 9th posterior rib *(black arrow)*.

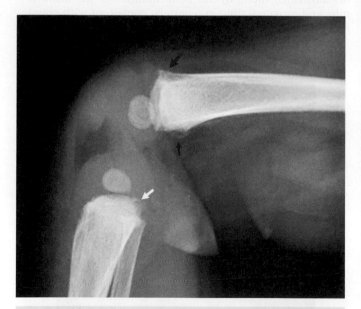

Fig. 50.3 A lateral view shows the left tibial metaphyseal fracture as an irregular bone fragment posteriorly *(white arrow)* and shows the distal femoral metaphyseal fracture to have a corner fracture appearance anteriorly and a bucket handle appearance posteriorly *(black arrows)*.

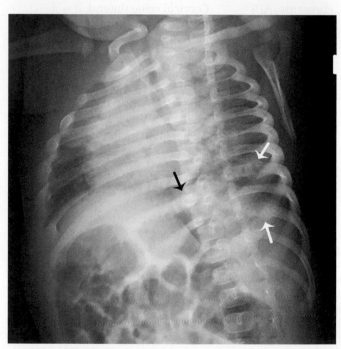

Fig. 50.5 Oblique view of the chest demonstrates healing fractures, with callus, of the left 8th and 10th posterior ribs *(white arrows)* and of the 9th posterior rib *(black arrow)*.

Case Conclusion

The initial imaging findings in this patient are concerning for NAT, as they are metaphyscal fractures, with high specificity for NAT. This, in combination with the lack of any credible history and the child's age, prompted additional imaging. A complete skeletal survey was obtained and selected images are provided.

There are subacute, healing fractures of the left posterior 8th, 10th, and right posterior 9th ribs (Figs. 50.4–50.6).

The usual skull views, as part of the skeletal survey, were not obtained, since the child also underwent cranial CT imaging, which did not show any fracture or hemorrhage. If a patient is undergoing CT of the head, it is reasonable to

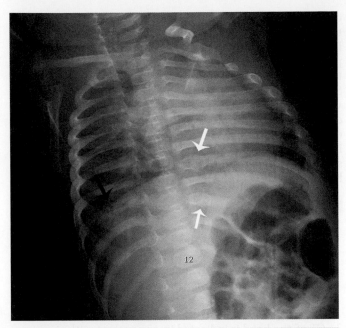

Fig. 50.6 Oblique view of the chest demonstrates healing fractures, with callus, of the left 8th and 10th posterior ribs *(white arrows)* and of the 9th posterior rib *(black arrow)*.

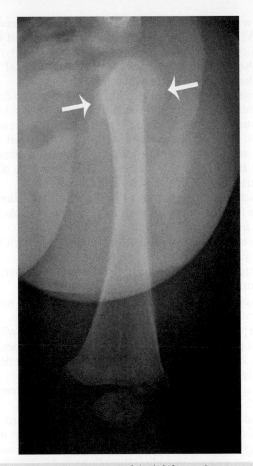

Fig. 50.7 Anterior-posterior view of the left femur shows metaphyseal fracture of the distal femur, seen medially and laterally *(black arrows)*, and callus formation about the proximal femur *(white arrows)* at the site of a proximal femur fracture. The proximal femur fracture is better seen on a frog lateral view (Fig 50.8).

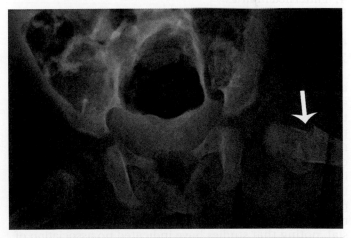

Fig. 50.8 Anterior-posterior view of the pelvis demonstrates a fracture of the left proximal femur *(arrow)*, with callus seen medial to the fracture.

not obtain additional plain radiographs of the skull; this will reduce radiation exposure, and CT is excellent in detecting skull fractures.

Pediatric Orthopedics and the Child Abuse Resource and Education (CARE) Team were consulted. Laboratory investigation was also performed, the results of which were unremarkable and not suggestive of a metabolic or genetic disorder predisposing the child to facture. Child Protective Services was notified and an investigation into the cause of the child's injuries was initiated. A follow-up skeletal survey at 2 weeks showed no additional fractures.

An additional case is presented here:

A 2-month-old child presented to the emergency department with left upper leg swelling and apparent pain. There was no history provided, other than the father of the child stating that he may have accidentally pulled the child's leg and heard a pop. Imaging of the left femur demonstrated a fracture of the proximal left femur (Figs. 50.7 and 50.8). A skeletal survey demonstrated callus formation, indicating healing fractures, of the posterior right 3rd, 4th, 5th, 8th, and 9th ribs and multiple bilateral metaphyseal fractures of the extremities (see Fig. 50.7).These injuries also prompted evaluation in the department by Pediatric Orthopedics and the CARE Team. Child Protective Services was notified and an investigation was initiated into the cause of the child's injuries.

There is no "typical" presentation of a child who has sustained NAT.[7] Risk factors for NAT vary by age and are multifactorial.[2] The rate of physical child abuse has been reported to be 1%–2% of the U.S. population, with children under the age of 2 years at highest risk for such an event.[9] Pediatric abusive injuries are likely underreported, with estimations that up to 20% of fractures due to NAT are attributed to other causes.[9,25] In addition, NAT may be underdetected, since studies have shown that the implementation of recommended laboratory and imaging testing to evaluate NAT is underutilized, as is referral to Child Protective Services.[10,26] Strikingly, up to 25% of children who have experienced an NAT event reexperience the event within 1 year, and many of these children present with previous injuries that are considered "minor"; NAT may not be the result of a single event but as part of a cycle of repeated injury.[27] Thirty percent of children who are hospitalized for nonaccidental head injuries have had a sentinel event.[27,28]

NAT evaluation consists of a through history as detailed as possible, the child's medical history, family history, events surrounding the injury (if an injury event is reported), and physical examination, noting that many children with fracture(s) do not have bruising associated with the fracture(s).[2,9,29] Between 10% and 40% of fractures found in NAT are not clinically suspected.[6]

Historical points suggestive of NAT include the following:[2]

1. There is either no explanation or a vague explanation given for a significant injury.
2. There is an explicit denial of trauma in a child with obvious injury.
3. An important detail of the explanation changes in a substantive way.
4. An explanation is provided that is inconsistent with the pattern, age, or severity of the injury or injuries.
5. An explanation is given that is inconsistent with the child's physical and/or developmental capabilities.
6. There is an unexplained or unexpected notable delay in seeking medical care.
7. Different witnesses provide markedly different explanations for the injury or injuries.

Physical examination findings should be considered in the context of the given history, or lack thereof. While there are few physical examination findings specific for NAT, there are findings that are suspect, including the following:[2]

1. ANY injury to a young, preambulatory infant, including bruises, mouth injuries, fractures, and intracranial or abdominal injury.
2. Injuries to multiple organ systems.
3. Multiple injuries in different stages of healing.
4. Patterned injuries
5. Injuries to nonbony or other unusual locations, such as over the torso, ears, face, neck, or upper arms.
6. Significant injuries that are unexplained.
7. Additional evidence of child neglect.

Laboratory testing is also utilized, and which studies are obtained is determined by historical and physical examination and radiographic findings. For example, if there is suspicion for abdominal injury, then liver and pancreatic enzymes levels are recommended, and recommended laboratory testing for intracranial hemorrhage or bruising includes coagulation studies and factor studies.[2] If bone mineralization normality is in question, then vitamin D level, calcium, alkaline phosphatase, and parathyroid hormone levels are recommended. While the routine use of vitamin D levels is somewhat controversial, noting that studies have indicated no association of low vitamin D levels and increased fracture risk in pediatric patients,[9,30,31] they are recommended by the American Academy of Pediatrics.[2] Many pediatric institutions have protocols recommending specific radiographic and laboratory tests depending on history and physical examination findings.

Adherence to published recommended imaging guidelines for NAT has been studied. Previously, there has been reported variability with national guideline compliance, both in the United States and other countries (with imaging guidelines similar to ACR guidelines), with overall poor compliance.[4,7,32,33] This has prompted multiple quality improvement initiatives with the goal of increasing imaging guideline compliance. Studies have reported an increase in compliance using various methods, including statewide distribution of educational materials to radiologists,[4] implementation of age-specific imaging and laboratory study protocols in the Emergency Department,[34] and routinely employed screening questionnaires for children admitted to the hospital for head injuries.[35]

IMAGING PEARLS

1. Adherence to published imaging guidelines is important for proper radiographic evaluation of patients in whom NAT is a concern.
2. A proper skeletal survey (including all the recommended views of the axial and appendicular skeleton) is essential. A "babygram" is NOT acceptable imaging for patients with suspected NAT.
3. CT of the head is indicated in any patient with signs of head trauma or neurologic findings. CT should also be strongly considered in young infants (i.e., those <6 months of age) as intracranial injury may not be clinically apparent.
4. CT of the abdomen is indicated when there is a clinical concern for abdominal trauma or if there are abnormal abdominal laboratory findings (i.e., elevated AST [aspartate transaminase], ALT [alanine aminotransferase], or abnormal urinalysis).
5. MRI is reserved for follow-up imaging of abnormal CT findings in nonacute cases. It is not a first-line imaging modality in the acute setting.
6. Dating fractures can be difficult, and while imaging can be helpful in establishing the degree of acuity (i.e., presence of a callus to indicate healing), caution should be exercised in providing such an interpretation in the urgent/emergent setting. Dating fractures is best left to radiologists with pediatric expertise and physicians specifically trained in child abuse pediatrics.

References

1. Wootton-Gorges SL, Soares BP, Alazraki AL, et al; Expert Panel on Pediatric Imaging. ACR Appropriateness Criteria® suspected physical abuse: child. *J Am Coll Radiol.* 2017;14(5S):S338-S349.
2. Christian CW, Committee on Child Abuse and Neglect, American Academy of Pediatrics. The evaluation of suspected child physical abuse. *Pediatrics.* 2015;135(5):e1337-e1354.
3. Flaherty EG, Perez-Rossello JM, Levine MA, et al. Evaluating children with fractures for child physical abuse. *Pediatrics.* 2014;133(2): e477-e489.
4. Wanner MR, Marine MB, Hibbard RA, et al. Compliance with skeletal surveys for child abuse in general hospitals: a statewide quality improvement process. *AJR Am J Roentgenol.* 2019;212(5):976-981.
5. Wood JN, Fakeye O, Mondestin V, et al. Development of hospital-based guidelines for skeletal survey in young children with bruises. *Pediatrics.* 2015;135(2):e312-e320.
6. Wood JN, French B, Song L, et al. Evaluation for occult fractures in injured children. *Pediatrics.* 2015;136(2):232-240.
7. Nguyen A, Hart R. Imaging of non-accidental injury; what is clinical best practice? *J Med Radiat Sci.* 2018;65(2):123-130.
8. Tiyyagura G, Beucher M, Bechtel K. Nonaccidental injury in pediatric patients: detection, evaluation, and treatment. *Pediatr Emerg Med Pract.* 2017;14(7):1-32.

9. Servaes S, Brown SD, Choudhary AK, et al. The etiology and significance of fractures in infants and young children: a multidisciplinary review. *Pediatr Radiol.* 2016;46(5):591-600.

10. Pfeifer CM, Hammer MR, Mangona KL, et al. Non-accidental trauma: the role of radiology. *Emerg Radiol.* 2017;24(2):207-213.

11. Leventhal JM, Martin KD, Asnes AG. Incidence of fractures attributable to abuse in young hospitalized children: results from analysis of a United States database. *Pediatrics.* 2008;122(3):599-604.

12. Dwek JR. The radiographic approach to child abuse. *Clin Orthop Relat Res.* 2011;469(3):776-789.

13. Lyons TJ, Oates RK. Falling out of bed: a relatively benign occurrence. *Pediatrics.* 1993;92(1):125-127.

14. Thackeray JD, Wannemacher J, Adler BH, et al. The classic metaphyseal lesion and traumatic injury. *Pediatr Radiol.* 2016;46(8):1128-1133.

15. Barsness KA, Cha ES, Bensard DD, et al. The positive predictive value of rib fractures as an indicator of nonaccidental trauma in children. *J Trauma.* 2003;54(6):1107-1110.

16. Maguire S, Mann M, John N, et al. Does cardiopulmonary resuscitation cause rib fractures in children? A systematic review. *Child Abuse Negl.* 2006;30(7):739-751.

17. Franke I, Pingen A, Schiffmann H, et al. Cardiopulmonary resuscitation (CPR)–related posterior rib fractures in neonates and infants following recommended changes in CPR techniques. *Child Abuse Negl.* 2014;38(7):1267-1274.

18. Fernando S, Obaldo RE, Walsh IR, et al. Neuroimaging of nonaccidental head trauma: pitfalls and controversies. *Pediatr Radiol.* 2008;38(8):827-838.

19. Wootton-Gorges SL, et al. *ACR Appropriateness Criteria Suspected Physical Abuse—Child.* 2016. Available at: https://acsearch.acr.org/docs/69443/Narrative/. Accessed December 20, 2019.

20. Meservy CJ, Towbin R, McLaurin RL, et al. Radiographic characteristics of skull fractures resulting from child abuse. *AJR Am J Roentgenol.* 1987;149(1):173-175.

21. Harper NS, Lewis T, Eddleman S, et al. Follow-up skeletal survey use by child abuse pediatricians. *Child Abuse Negl.* 2016;51:336-342.

22. Van Rijn RR, Sieswerda-Hoogendoorn T. Imaging child abuse: the bare bones. *Eur J Pediatr.* 2012;171(2):215-224.

23. Rubin DM, Christian CW, Bilaniuk LT, et al. Occult head injury in high-risk abused children. *Pediatrics.* 2003;111(6 pt 1):1382-1386.

24. Foerster BR, Petrou M, Lin D, et al. Neuroimaging evaluation of non-accidental head trauma with correlation to clinical outcomes: a review of 57 cases. *J Pediatr.* 2009;154(4):573-577.

25. Ravichandiran N, Schuh S, Bejuk M, et al. Delayed identification of pediatric abuse-related fractures. *Pediatrics.* 2010;125(1):60-66.

26. Taitz J, Moran K, O'Meara M. Long bone fractures in children under 3 years of age: is abuse being missed in emergency department presentations? *J Paediatr Child Health.* 2014;40(4):170-174.

27. Deans KJ, Thackeray J, Groner JI, et al. Risk factors for recurrent injuries in victims of suspected non-accidental trauma: a retrospective cohort study. *BMC Pediatr.* 2014;14:217.

28. Sheets LK, Leach M, Nugent M, Simpson P. Sentinel injuries precede abusive head trauma in infants. Pediatric Academic Societies Meeting; Baltimore, MD. 2009; E-PAS2009:5140.2.

29. Valvano TJ, Binns HJ, Flaherty EG, et al. Does bruising help determine which fractures are caused by abuse? *Child Maltreat.* 2009;14(4):376-381.

30. Schilling S, Wood JN, Levine MA, et al. Vitamin D status in abused and nonabused children younger than 2 years old with fractures. *Pediatrics.* 2011;127(5):835-841.

31. Contreras JJ, Hiestand B, O'Neill JC, et al. Vitamin D deficiency in children with fractures. *Pediatr Emerg Care.* 2014;30(11):777-781.

32. Kleinman PL, Kleinman PK, Savageau JA. Suspected infant abuse: radiographic skeletal survey practices in pediatric health care facilities. *Radiology.* 2004;233(2):477-485.

33. Patel H, Swinson S, Johnson K. Improving national standards of child protection skeletal surveys: the value of college guidance. *Clin Radiol* 2017 Mar;72(3):202-206.

34. Riney LC, Frey TM, Fain ET, et al. Standardizing the evaluation of nonaccidental trauma in a large pediatric emergency department. *Pediatrics.* 2018;141(1):e2017199.

35. Kim PT, McCagg J, Dundon A, et al. Consistent screening of admitted infants with head injuries reveals high rate of nonaccidental trauma. *J Pediatr Surg.* 2017;52(11):1827-1830.

Musculoskeletal

51 Growing Pains: Salter-Harris Classification of Physeal Injuries

ERIN MUNNS, MD

Case Presentation

A 15-year-old male presents to the emergency department with right wrist pain. The patient reports that he fell on his outstretched right hand while skateboarding. Physical examination is significant for mild swelling with tenderness to palpation over the distal right forearm. He has 2+ radial pulses with full range of motion and intact sensation in the radial, ulnar, and median distributions. Capillary refill in his fingers is normal. There is no shoulder or elbow pain, swelling, or deformity.

Imaging Considerations

PLAIN RADIOGRAPHY

Plain radiographs are the standard imaging modality for physeal fractures. Images should be obtained in at least two planes. Appropriate pain management is important in patients with potential fractures to help optimize positioning, making interpretation of the imaging study easier. There are cases in which a fracture may not be evident immediately on plain radiography. Nondisplaced Salter-Harris type I fractures will sometimes present with normal radiographs or have only subtle findings such as growth plate widening or surrounding soft-tissue swelling. Patients who continue to report tenderness over the growth plate on examination should be treated as if they have a Salter-Harris type I fracture with splinting of the extremity even in the setting of normal radiographs. These patients will require outpatient follow-up radiographs at 7 to 10 days, especially if they are still having pain, to assess for signs of bone healing response or other evidence of fracture that may not have been apparent on the original imaging studies.[1-3] Salter-Harris type II–V fractures are usually apparent on plain radiographs.

Forearm physeal fractures in children can have an associated supracondylar fracture, so the lateral forearm view should include the distal humerus or there should be accompanying elbow views. If wrist imaging shows an isolated distal ulnar physeal fracture, further evaluation of the proximal radius should be obtained to rule out associated radial fracture or dislocation, as isolated ulnar physeal fractures are uncommon.[1-3]

COMPUTED TOMOGRAPHY (CT)

Noncontrast CT imaging of physeal fractures is indicated only if needed for surgical planning or for further classification of Salter-Harris types III–V fractures depending on the site of injury. Discussion with an orthopedic specialist should occur before obtaining a CT in children with these fractures.

ULTRASOUND

Ultrasound is an emerging field for imaging pediatric fractures; however, plain radiographs continue to remain the gold standard for diagnosing physeal fractures. Ultrasound is currently indicated only as a first-line diagnostic modality in settings where plain radiography is not available. Ultrasound-guided forearm fracture reduction is also a rising trend, but more data are needed before this can be recommended over traditional reduction techniques.[4]

MAGNETIC RESONANCE IMAGING (MRI)

MRI can be useful in the outpatient setting to help differentiate acute injuries from chronic repetitive injuries in patients who have continued pain after expected healing, but it has limited diagnostic utility in the emergency department for suspected physeal injury.

Imaging Findings

The patient had a two-view x-ray of his right forearm and a three-view x-ray of his right wrist. Selected images of the wrist series are provided. There is a displaced growth plate–related fracture of the distal right radius, appearing to be a Salter-Harris type II fracture; there is a nondisplaced oblique fracture of the proximal right first metacarpal; there is an ulnar styloid process fracture (Figs. 51.1 and 51.2).

Case Conclusion

The patient was treated with closed reduction under ketamine sedation after consultation with Pediatric Orthopedics, who performed the reduction procedure (Figs. 51.3 and 51.4). The patient had a cast applied and follow-up scheduled with pediatric orthopedics seven days after his emergency department visit.

Physeal fractures are a unique consideration in pediatric patients as they involve the open growth plate. The growth plate represents an area of relative weakness and is more susceptible to injury compared to the surrounding bone and ligaments. Because the ligaments are stronger and

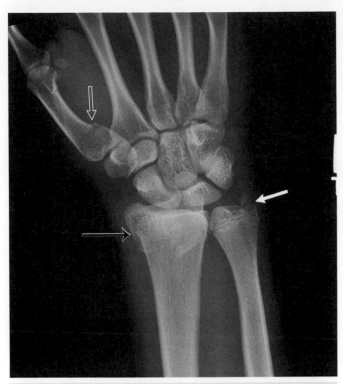

Fig. 51.1 Posterior-anterior view shows a displaced growth plate–related fracture of the distal right radius *(red arrow)*, better seen on subsequent lateral view; a nondisplaced oblique fracture of the proximal right first metacarpal *(open arrow)*; and a nondisplaced ulnar styloid process fracture *(white arrow)*.

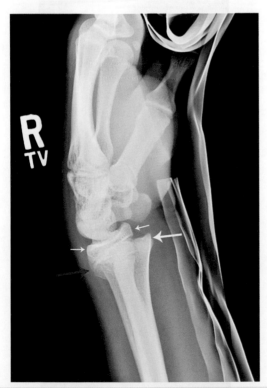

Fig. 51.2 Lateral view depicts the displaced Salter-Harris type II fracture of the distal right radius. The distal fracture fragment is comprised of the distal epiphysis of the radius *(small white arrows)* and the dorsal distal metaphyseal fragment *(red arrow)* and is displaced and rotated dorsally with respect to the proximal fracture fragment, which includes the volar metaphysis of the radius *(larger white arrow)*.

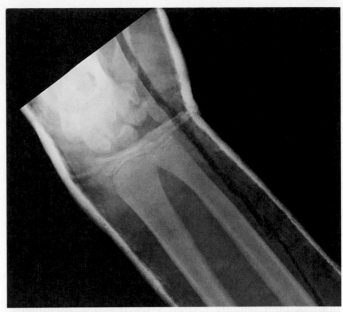

Fig. 51.3 Postreduction imaging of the Salter-Harris type II fracture.

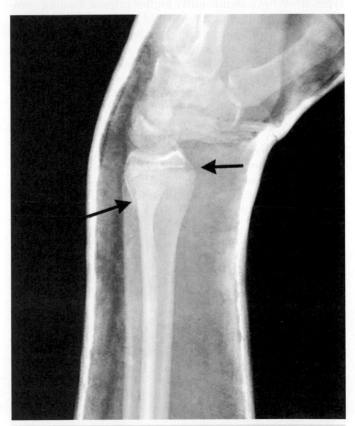

Fig. 51.4 Postreduction lateral view shows improved and near anatomic alignment of the Salter-Harris type II fracture *(arrows)*.

more flexible, pediatric patients are more likely to suffer a physeal fracture than a sprain.[3] Physeal fractures represent 18% of all pediatric fractures.[1,3] They occur most commonly in girls between ages 11 and 12 years and in boys between ages 12 and 14 years but can be seen at any point the physis remains open.[5]

The classic method for describing physeal injuries was first described in a paper by Salter and Harris in 1963.[6] The

Salter-Harris classification system divides physeal fractures into five types, labeled I–V (Fig. 51.5). This method can be broken down with the classic mnemonic:

S—"Straight or slipped," type I
A—"Above," type II
L—"Lower," type III
T—"Through," type IV
ER—"Erasure," type V

Type I involves a fracture "straight" through the growth plate. Type II involves the growth plate as well as the metaphysis "above" the growth plate. Types I and II can also be further described as displaced or nondisplaced. Type III involves the growth plate as well as the "lower" epiphysis. Type IV goes "through" the growth plate as well as both the metaphysis and epiphysis. Type V often involves a high mechanism injury and results in compression (or crush injury) of the growth plate.[1,7]

The physis heals rapidly in children, usually in 3 to 6 weeks, making early diagnosis and reduction of these fractures important to ensure appropriate healing.[2] Complications of poor healing include growth arrest, asymmetric growth, and decreased range of motion.[3,5] In general, types III–V have significantly higher rates of healing complications. Nondisplaced type I and II fractures can usually be treated with splinting and orthopedic follow-up. Displaced type I and II fractures often require closed reduction. Types III–V often require surgical repair.[1,2]

For comparison, imaging of a Salter-Harris type IV fracture is provided. This patient sustained a wrist injury while riding a motocross bike, falling off the bike and landing on his wrist. The wrist series is shown, demonstrating a Salter-Harris type IV fracture of the distal radius with dorsal displacement of the distal dorsal fragment (Figs. 51.6 and 51.7).

Finally, imaging from a 14-year-old female who fell out of a tree and landed on her left ankle shows a Salter-Harris type II fracture of the tibia and a Salter-Harris type I fracture of the distal fibula (Figs. 51.8–51.10). This is a fracture

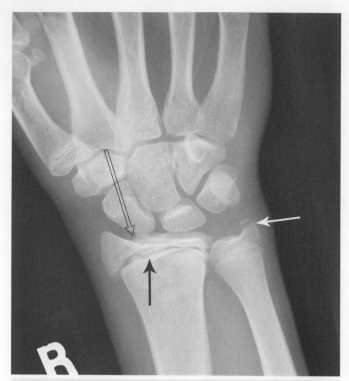

Fig. 51.6 Salter-Harris type IV fracture of the distal radius. Posterior-anterior view shows widening of the distal radial growth plate *(black arrow)*, fracture through the distal radial epiphysis *(open arrow)*, associated with lateral migration of the lateral distal epiphysis (styloid). There is also a fracture of the ulnar styloid *(white arrow)*.

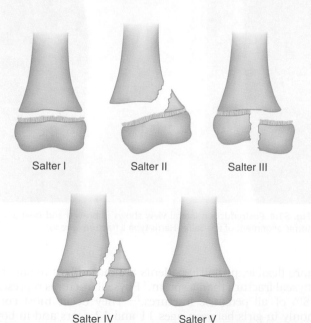

Fig. 51.5 Salter-Harris classification of physeal fractures. (From Shin EK. Fractures. In: Skirven TM, Feldscher SB, Amadio PC, et al., eds. *Rehabilitation of the Hand and Upper Extremity*. 7th ed. Philadelphia, PA: Elsevier; 2021: Fig. 22.5.)

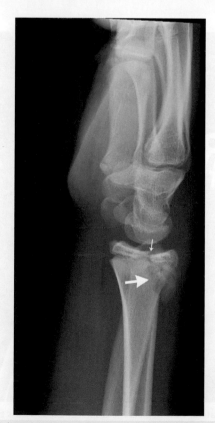

Fig. 51.7 Salter-Harris type IV fracture of the distal radius. Lateral view shows fracture through the growth plate *(red arrow)*, through the radial epiphysis *(small white arrow)*, and through the radial metaphysis *(large white arrow)*. There is mild dorsal displacement of the distal dorsal fracture fragment.

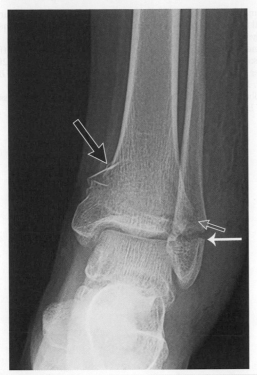

Fig. 51.8 Salter-Harris type II fracture of the distal tibia, through a closing physis, and Salter-Harris type I fracture of the distal fibula. Posterior-anterior view shows widening of the distal fibular physis with overlying soft tissue swelling *(white arrow)*, widening of the lateral distal tibial physis *(open arrow)*, and distal metaphysis fracture of the tibia *(black arrow)*.

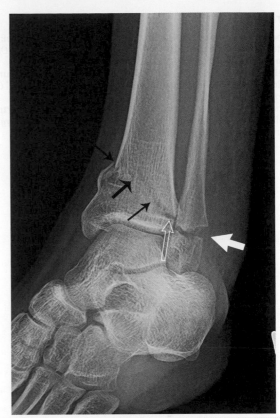

Fig. 51.10 Oblique view of the Salter-Harris type II fracture of the distal tibia *(black arrows)* and Salter-Harris type I fracture of the distal fibula *(white arrow)*. *Open arrow* points to fracture through the physis of the distal tibia.

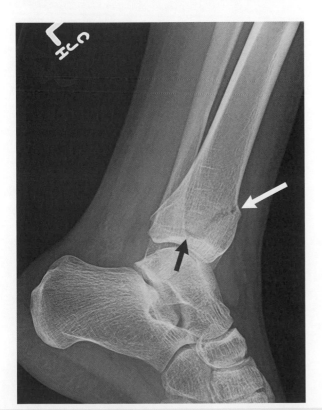

Fig. 51.9 Salter-Harris type II fracture of the distal tibia. Lateral view shows horizontally oriented fracture with widening of the mid to posterior physis of the distal tibia *(black arrow)* and oblique fracture through the distal tibial metaphysis *(white arrow)*.

through a tibial physis that is partially closed, due to osseous maturation. There is an oblique fracture of the distal left tibial metaphysis, propagating through the remaining open physis posteriorly and laterally, and there is widening of the distal fibular physis. Tibiotalar alignment appears maintained. She was treated with splinting, followed by casting and close follow-up.

IMAGING PEARLS

1. Plain radiography is the standard imaging modality for diagnosing physeal fractures in children.
2. Physeal fractures can be categorized into Salter-Harris types I–V, which helps with treatment and prognosis, as well as communication with pediatric orthopedic specialists.
3. Patients with continued tenderness over the growth plate should be treated as if they have a Salter-Harris type I fracture, even in the setting of normal radiographs, as pediatric patients are more likely to have an occult growth plate fracture compared to a ligamentous sprain.
4. In children with a physeal fracture, care should be taken to closely examine the surrounding bones and joints to ensure they do not have another associated fracture.

References

1. Capela DJ, Tartaglione JP, Dooley TP, et al. Classifications in brief: Salter-Harris Classification of Pediatric Physeal Fractures. *Clin Orthop Relat Res.* 2016;474(11):2531-2537.
2. Ho-Fun VM, Zapala MA, Lee EY. Musculoskeletal traumatic injuries in children: characteristic imaging findings and mimickers. *Radiol Clin North Am.* 2017;55(4):785-802.
3. Thornton MD, Della-Giustina K, Aronson PL. Emergency department evaluation and treatment of pediatric orthopedic injuries. *Emerg Med Clin North Am.* 2015;33(2):423-449.
4. Douma-den Hamer D, Blanker HM, Edens MA, et al. Ultrasound for distal forearm fracture: a systematic review and diagnostic meta-analysis. *PLoS One.* 2016;11(5):e0155659.
5. Levine RH, Foris LA, Waseem M. Salter Harris Fractures, StatPearls, https://www.statpearls.com/sp/rn/28713/. Accessed April 20, 2020.
6. Salter RB, Harris R. Injuries involving the epiphyseal plate. *J Bone Joint Surg.* 1963;45(3):587-622.
7. Tandberg D, Sherbring M. A mnemonic for the Salter-Harris Classification. *Am J Emerg Med.* 1999;17(3):321.

52 My Fracture Is Not Humerus: Supracondylar Fractures

ADA EARP, DO, FAAP

Case Presentation

A 5-year-old male is brought for right elbow pain and swelling after falling while playing on the monkey bars at school. The fall was witnessed by several teachers and friends, who reported no loss of consciousness or other injuries. He complains of right elbow pain but denies neck or back pain. His physical examination is remarkable for impressive right elbow swelling and pain. He is grossly neurovascularly intact and there is no other apparent injury.

Imaging Considerations

PLAIN RADIOGRAPHY

Proper evaluation of suspected supracondylar fractures requires anterior-posterior and lateral views of the elbow.[1,2] The lateral view is obtained with the elbow in flexion at a true 90-degree angle, or at least as close to this as possible.[1,2] Oblique views are not typically required but can be used to further identify minimally displaced fractures if there is strong clinical suspicion for a fracture.[2] The clinician should bear in mind the possibility of additional associated fractures with a supracondylar fracture. Associated fractures of the wrist and forearm are most common, but fractures of the proximal humerus or clavicle also occur. Therefore, when a supracondylar fracture is present, one should have a low threshold to image other sites of clinical concern, such as the wrist or forearm, when clinically indicated by physical examination, or when physical examination is difficult, especially in young children.[1,2]

There are several key elements to address when evaluating a plain radiograph for supracondylar fractures, as not all are readily evident. The lateral view is particularly important for this purpose:[1]

ELEMENT	COMMENTS
Fat pad	Normally visualized but elevated
Anterior	with joint effusion
Posterior	Visualization associated with joint effusion
Anterior humeral line	Runs from the anterior cortex of the humerus and usually passes through the middle third of the capitellum; exceptions under age 5[a]
Diaphyseal-condylar angle	Angle between humeral and humeral condyle axes, normally 30–45 degrees

ELEMENT	COMMENTS
Coronoid line	Tangential line joining the anterior coronoid edge with the front edge of the lateral condyle

[a]The anterior humeral line in children: when <4 years can pass through the anterior third (31%), middle third (52%), or posterior third (18%) of the capitellum without any pathology.[1,3]

The elbow fat pads are an important element, as they may be the only indication of a fracture. Fat pads may be seen in either a posterior location or anterior location.[1,4] The posterior fat pad is always associated with a joint effusion when it is seen on the lateral view with the elbow flexed (hence the importance of the 90-degree lateral elbow radiograph).[2,4] The presence of a posterior fat pad is associated with an occult elbow fracture in 76% of cases when no fracture is identified on the initial radiographs.[5] The presence of a posterior fat pad is not exclusive to supracondylar fractures, however. One series reported that the presence of a posterior fat pad was associated with a supracondylar fracture in 53% of cases, proximal ulna in 26% of cases, lateral condyle in 12% of cases, or radial-neck in 9% of cases.[5] The anterior fat pad is normally visualized on a lateral flexed elbow view but can be elevated due to the presence of an elbow joint effusion.

ULTRASONOGRAPHY

Ultrasonography has the advantage of lacking ionizing radiation and general availability, but skill is required in order to produce a meaningful study. This modality has a reported sensitivity of up to 96% and specificity up to 90% for detecting pediatric elbow fractures when performed by providers in the emergency setting who are specifically trained in sonographic musculoskeletal imaging.[4]

COMPUTED TOMOGRAPHY (CT)

Routine use of CT is not indicated for suspected pediatric supracondylar fractures. However, this modality has excellent sensitivity and specificity for the detection of these injuries.[4,6] CT may be utilized if there is a complex injury but subspecialty consultation is appropriate prior to obtaining such a study.

MAGNETIC RESONANCE IMAGING (MRI)

Routine use of MRI is not indicated for suspected pediatric supracondylar fractures. This imaging modality does have the ability to detect soft tissue and cartilage injuries.[6,7]

Imaging Findings

After administration of intranasal fentanyl, plain radiography is obtained of the elbow and the forearm. Selected images are seen here, demonstrating a severely displaced supracondylar fracture (Figs. 52.1 and 52.2).

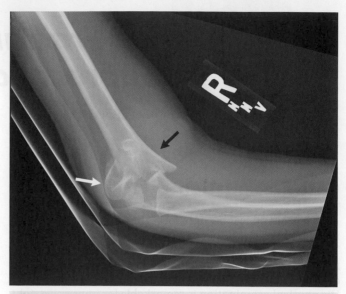

Fig. 52.2 Lateral radiograph of the elbow demonstrates a Gartland type III supracondylar fracture, with posterior displacement of the distal fracture fragment *(white arrow)* compared to the proximal fracture fragment *(black arrow)*, as well as overriding of fracture fragments.

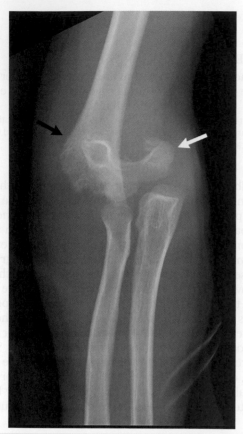

Fig. 52.1 Anterior-posterior radiograph of the elbow demonstrates a Gartland type III supracondylar fracture, with medial displacement of the distal fracture fragment *(white arrow)* compared to the proximal fracture fragment *(black arrow)*, as well as overriding of fracture fragments.

Case Conclusion

Pediatric Orthopedics was consulted to evaluate the patient, who was placed in a posterior long arm splint without any attempt at reduction. He was taken to the operating suite several hours later for closed reduction and percutaneous pinning of the fracture and recovered without complications.

Supracondylar fractures are common in the pediatric population, representing 3% of all fractures.[1,2] The usual mechanism of injury is a fall from an outstretched arm and can result from extension and flexion injuries, with the majority being extension-type injuries.[1,2,8] Extension injuries are classified according to the Gartland Classification System (Fig. 52.3), which classifies these fractures based on the degree of fracture displacement seen on the lateral view plain radiograph:[1,2]

GARTLAND TYPE	FINDINGS	STABLE?	MANAGEMENT
I	Minimal (<2 mm) to no displacement Intact anterior humeral line	Yes	Conservative—immobilization for 3–4 weeks
II	Slight displacement (>2 mm) with a posterior angulation of the distal fragment Anterior humeral line does not bisect the capitellum correctly Intact posterior cortex	Maybe	Controversial
III	Posteromedial or posterolateral displacement of the distal fragment Loss of integrity of the posterior cortex	No	Closed reduction and fixation with K wires
IV	No specific radiographic findings but multidirectional instability noted during surgical reduction.	No	Operative technique varies

A posterior fat pad may be the only radiographic indication of a type I supracondylar fracture. A type IV fracture can be diagnosed during surgical reduction; this represents multidirectional instability but is not diagnosed radiographically. See Fig. 52.3.

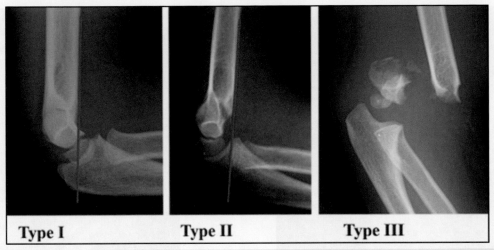

Fig. 52.3 Lateral radiographs depicting the modified Gartland classification of supracondylar humeral fractures. Type I fractures are nondisplaced. The anterior humeral line *(red)* intersects the capitellum. Type II fractures have loss of cortical continuity anteriorly with an intact posterior cortex. The anterior humeral line *(red)* does not intersect the capitellum that is displaced posteriorly. Type III fractures have complete loss of anterior and posterior cortical continuity and are unstable. (From Douglas RR, Ho CA. Fractures of the pediatric elbow and shoulder. In: Abzug JM, Neiduski R, Kozin SH, eds. *Pediatric Hand Therapy*. Elsevier, 2020. Figure 19.2)

The degree of swelling and pain with supracondylar fractures can vary depending on the severity of the fracture and the pain tolerance of individual patients. Prior to obtaining radiography, appropriate pain management should be provided. This can easily be accomplished with intranasal fentanyl, which is efficacious and safe, prior to intravenous access. Once intravenous access is established, morphine or fentanyl are good choices.

Physical examination may be difficult due to pain and anxiety. Manipulation of obvious deformities should be kept to a minimum during the physical examination and can potentiate neurovascular injury.[1,9] Attention should be paid to the neurovascular status of the injured extremity, since supracondylar fractures can have accompanying injuries to nearby structures either by direct injury or due to compression from swelling. Neurovascular injuries are most common in type III injuries, with an incidence of 10% to 15%.[2] The most common injury involves the anterior interosseous nerve branch of the median nerve, which, if injured, prevents thumb opposition to the second finger (i.e., an inability to make an "ok" sign).[1,2] Management of supracondylar fractures is based on fracture type.[1,3,9,10]

There is consensus among authors regarding the management of type I and type III fractures. Type II fracture management is somewhat controversial. Some authors recommend a conservative approach for fractures that do not have malrotation or displacement,[1,11] while those fractures that are displaced should have closed reduction and pinning with K wires.[1,9] Type II fractures that are initially treated conservatively may require operative repair and are monitored closely by an orthopedic specialist. In addition to K wires, which have been traditionally used for operative repair, elastic stable intramedullary nails, and external fixator devises have been used.[12,13] The American College of Orthopedic Surgery Guidelines for the treatment of pediatric humeral supracondylar fractures recommends closed reduction and fixation with pinning for type II and type III

fractures.[14] The guidelines do not specify the optimal timing of repair in patients who do not have neurovascular compromise, but it is reasonable to obtain prompt orthopedic consultation prior to patient disposition in any patient with type II and type III injuries. Some authors recommend an approach of splinting and repair within 12 to 18 hours of injury, with admission and careful monitoring of neurovascular status, provided there is no neurovascular compromise.[9] Others recommend reduction and repair emergently (<8 hours) or urgently (<24 hours).[2] Regardless of when operative repair takes place, the extremity should be splinted in a position of comfort until the procedure takes place. Additionally, there are no recommendations regarding the duration of pinning and the timing of pin removal, but removal typically occurs 3 to 4 weeks postoperatively.[2,9] Open reduction is not typically necessary.[2]

Surgical complications with pin placement are not common (4%) but can include infection, nerve injury, pin migration, and rarely compartment syndrome.[9,15] Cubitus varus malformation is the most common complication of treatment with either immobilization or pinning and results in the "gunstock" appearance of arm.[9]

Compartment syndrome is rare with supracondylar fractures. In pediatric patients, the need for increasing narcotic pain medication is the most reliable indicator of compartment syndrome.[9,15] Patients who require repair of a vascular injury are also at an increased risk for the development of compartment syndrome.[9,16,17]

For comparison, two other cases with selected imaging are presented here:

The 5-year-old male in Figs. 52.4 and 52.5 sustained a nondisplaced right supracondylar fracture after falling while chasing a dog. He was initially placed in a posterior long arm splint and followed up with Pediatric Orthopedics. He was then placed in a long arm cast for 3 weeks and recovered.

The 2-year-old female in Figs. 52.6 and 52.7 fell from a playscape, injuring her right elbow. Imaging revealed a

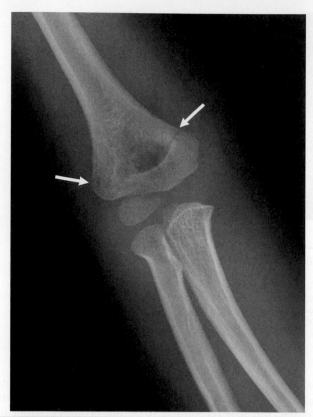

Fig. 52.4 Anterior-posterior radiograph of the elbow demonstrating a nondisplaced Gartland type I supracondylar fracture *(white arrows).*

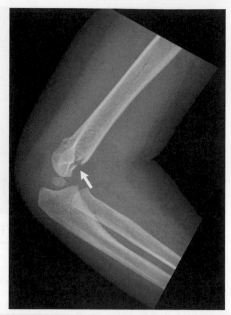

Fig. 52.6 Lateral radiograph of the elbow demonstrating a Gartland type II supracondylar fracture *(white arrow),* with mild posterior angulation of the distal fracture fragment.

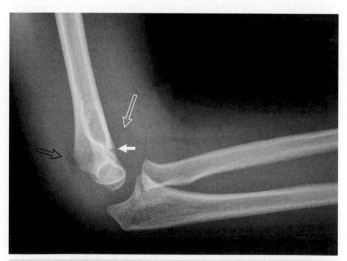

Fig. 52.5 Lateral radiograph of the elbow demonstrating a nondisplaced Gartland type I supracondylar fracture *(white arrow).* On this view, the posterior fat pad is visualized *(open black arrow)* and the anterior fat pad is elevated *(open white arrow),* and these findings are consistent with elbow joint effusion.

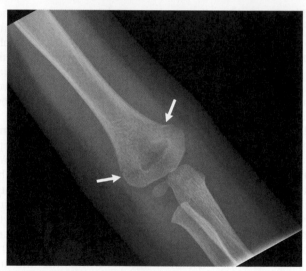

Fig. 52.7 Anterior-posterior radiograph of the elbow demonstrating a Gartland type II supracondylar fracture *(white arrows).*

IMAGING PEARLS

1. Plain radiography is the imaging modality of choice in pediatric patients with suspected supracondylar fractures.
2. Elbow imaging should consist of a two-view study including a 90-degree lateral elbow view.
3. There are several elements, including the presence of a posterior fat pad and the anterior humeral line, that can assist the clinician in determining the presence of a fracture and subsequent management.
4. Always consider the possibility of additional fractures, especially of the forearm or wrist. If there is suspicion of additional fracture, then a separate dedicated series of that part should be obtained.

supracondylar fracture of the distal humerus, with mild posterior angulation of the distal fracture fragment. The patient was taken to the operating suite for closed reduction and percutaneous pinning after consultation with Pediatric Orthopedics.

References

1. Zorrilla S de Neira J, Prada-Cañizares A, Marti-Ciruelos R, et al. Supracondylar humeral fractures in children: current concepts for management and prognosis. *Int Orthop.* 2015;39(11):2287-2296.
2. Sherman SC. Pediatric supracondylar fracture. *J Emerg Med.* 2011;40(2):e35-e37.
3. Ladenhauf HN, Schaffert M, Bauer J. The displaced supracondylar humerus fracture: indications for surgery and surgical options: a 2014 update. *Curr Opin Pediatr.* 2014;26(1):64-69.
4. Lee SH, Yun SJ. Diagnostic performance of ultrasonography for detection of pediatric elbow fracture: a meta-analysis. *Ann Emerg Med.* 2019;74(4):493-502.
5. Skaggs DL, Mirzayan R. The posterior fat pad sign in association with occult fracture of the elbow in children. *J Bone Joint Surg Am.* 1999;81(10):1429-1433.
6. Rabiner JE, Khine H, Avner JR, et al. Accuracy of point-of-care ultrasonography for diagnosis of elbow fractures in children. *Ann Emerg Med.* 2013;61(1):9-17.
7. Pudas T, Hurme T, Mattila K, et al. Magnetic resonance imaging in pediatric elbow fractures. *Acta Radiol.* 2005;46(6):636-644.
8. Omid R, Choi PD, Skaggs DL. Supracondylar humeral fractures in children. *J Bone Joint Surg Am.* 2008;90(5):1121-1132.
9. Abzug JM, Herman MJ. Management of supracondylar fractures in children: current concepts. *J Am Acad Orthop Surg.* 2012;20(2):69-77.
10. Howard A, Mulpuri K, Abel MF, et al. American Academy of Orthopaedic Surgeons. The treatment of pediatric supracondylar humerus fractures. *J Am Acad Orthop Surg.* 2012;20(5):320-327.
11. Moraleda L, Valencia M, Barco R, et al. Natural history of unreduced Gartland type-II supracondylar fractures of the humerus in children: a two to thirteen-year follow-up study. *J Bone Joint Surg Am.* 2013;95(1):28-34.
12. Lacher M, Schaeffer K, Boehm R, et al. The treatment of supracondylar humeral fractures with elastic stable intramedullary nailing (ESIN) in children. *J Pediatr Orthop.* 2011;31(1):33-38.
13. Slongo T. Radial external fixator for closed treatment of type III and IV supracondylar humerus fractures in children. A new surgical technique. *Oper Orthop Traumatol.* 2014;26(1):75-97.
14. Mulpuri K, Hosalkar H, Howard A. AAOS clinical practice guideline: the treatment of pediatric supracondylar humerus fractures. *J Am Acad Orthop Surg.* 2012;20(5):328-330.
15. Bashyal RK, Chu JY, Schoenecker PL, et al. Complications after pinning of supracondylar distal humerus fractures. *J Pediatr Orthop.* 2009;29(7):704-708.
16. Bae DS, Kadiyala RK, Waters PM. Acute compartment syndrome in children: contemporary diagnosis, treatment, and outcome. *J Pediatr Orthop.* 2001;21(5):680-688.
17. Choi PD, Melikian R, Skaggs DL. Risk factors for vascular repair and compartment syndrome in the pulseless supracondylar humerus fracture in children. *J Pediatr Orthop.* 2010;30(1):50-56.

53 Elbow Grease: Lateral and Medial Condyle Fractures of the Humerus

ROBERT VEZZETTI, MD, FAAP, FACEP

Case Presentation

A 4-year-old male presents with right elbow pain and swelling. He was playing on his school's monkey bars when he fell, landing on his right arm and elbow. He fell approximately 3 feet. There was no reported loss of consciousness and the child immediately cried. He complained of elbow pain and was brought directly for evaluation.

The child is afebrile and has age-appropriate vital signs. He has no signs of trauma to his head. He has no neck or back pain, crepitus, swelling, or deformity and is ambulatory. He does not appear to have any injury to his shoulders or his left arm. He initially refuses to move his right arm at the elbow, which is swollen. With some coaxing, he has movement at the elbow but this is limited secondary to pain. There is not any upper arm, forearm, wrist, hand, or digit pain, swelling, or deformity. He is grossly neurovascularly intact.

Imaging Considerations

PLAIN RADIOGRAPHY

Anteroposterior (AP) and lateral views of the elbow are usually performed to evaluate for fracture. In general, these views will suffice but an internal oblique view is useful to assess the degree of displacement for condyle fractures. One study reported significant discrepancies between the apparent displacement of lateral condyle fracture fragments on AP and lateral views, compared to an internal oblique view.[1] This study showed that a majority of fractures that were detected on AP and lateral views had a different degree of displacement and fracture pattern on an internal oblique view, and the authors recommended adding an internal oblique view to the AP and lateral views to assess lateral condyle fractures.[1,2] Internal oblique radiography has also been recommended by some authors at follow-up after initial two-view radiography, as useful for detecting displacement in initially nondisplaced or minimally displaced lateral condyle fractures.[3]

As with lateral condyle fractures, two-view imaging of medial condyle fractures is usually utilized. Some have suggested utilization of internal oblique views in these fractures,[4] although in another case series, the authors identified all fractures with AP and lateral views.[5]

Medial epicondyle fractures are visualized with AP and lateral views. Oblique views, however, can help determine fracture fragment displacement and should be obtained.[6]

COMPUTED TOMOGRAPHY (CT)

CT is not indicated as a first-line test in the evaluation of most elbow injuries. In cases where an injury is particularly complex, noncontrast CT can provide additional information about the anatomy of the injury. Pediatric Orthopedic consultation should be considered prior to obtaining CT.

MAGNETIC RESONANCE IMAGING (MRI)

MRI is also not a first-line imaging test for acute elbow injury. It has proven useful for follow-up imaging in cases where the detection of displacement by plain radiography is difficult.[7] MRI has also been utilized in nondisplaced fractures to better delineate whether a fracture is complete or not.[8]

Imaging Findings

The child initially had two-view imaging of the right elbow. These images demonstrate a fracture of the lateral condyle, not significantly displaced. An elbow joint effusion is present, as evidenced by subtle visualization of the posterior fat pad (Figs. 53.1 and 53.2). Due to the presence of the lateral condyle fracture, an internal oblique view was also obtained. The fracture is again seen, without significant displacement. (Fig. 53.3).

Case Conclusion

Pediatric Orthopedics was consulted, and due to the minimal displacement of the fracture, the child was treated with casting immobilization. Follow-up was arranged for 1 week and repeat imaging at that time demonstrated that the displacement had not worsened. He recovered uneventfully.

LATERAL CONDYLE FRACTURES

Lateral condyle fractures are among the most common humeral injuries in pediatric patients, second only to supracondylar fractures, accounting for 10%–20% of humeral fractures in this population; however, these are Salter-Harris type IV fractures, with fracture occurring across a metaphyseal and epiphyseal equivalent, the latter being cartilaginous.[1,9] Lateral condyle fractures are most commonly caused by falls,

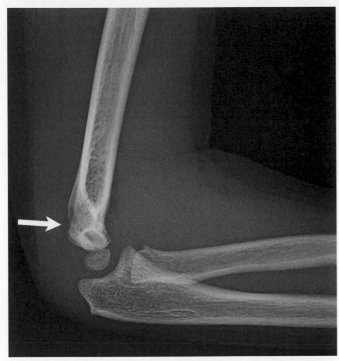

Fig. 53.1 Lateral view of the elbow with a fracture of distal humerus lateral condyle. The fracture is not well visualized on this lateral view, but there is subtle visualization of the posterior fat pad *(arrow)*, consistent with an elbow joint effusion.

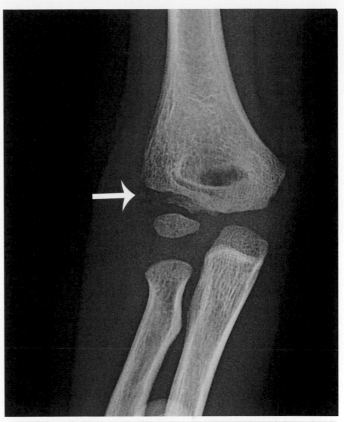

Fig. 53.3 Lateral condyle fracture visualized on the oblique view *(arrow)*, with minimal, but not significant, displacement.

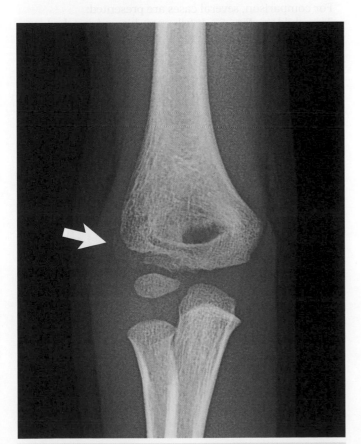

Fig. 53.2 Anteroposterior view demonstrates the lateral condyle fracture fragment *(arrow)* separated slightly from the underlying humerus, but not significantly displaced.

and associated injuries include ipsilateral dislocations and ipsilateral upper limb fractures.[9–12]

There are multiple classification systems used to describe lateral condyle fractures and assist in management guidance. These systems include the Milch, Jakob, Rutherford, and Badelon systems.[9,13–15] These classification systems advocate closed reduction and immobilization as long as the fracture remains stable; otherwise, operative repair is indicated.[9,13–15]

Management of lateral condyle fractures is determined by the degree of displacement. Complications rates are low in patients who have displacement less than 2 mm.[9,16–19] Therefore, most authors suggest that factures with less than 2-mm displacement can be managed nonoperatively (type I fracture), fractures between 2-mm and 4-mm displacement often exhibit worsening displacement and may need closed reduction and pinning (type II fracture), and fractures greater than 4 mm benefit from open reduction and internal fixation (type III fracture); intact articular cartilage can be useful as a predictor for closed pinning versus open reduction and internal fixation.[2,9,16–19]

Follow-up radiography at 1 week is recommended to assess for fracture displacement.[9,20] One study found a displacement rate of almost 15%, usually occurring within the first week following the injury, with nonunion, malunion, and decreased motion as complications.[20] Another study found a displacement rate of around 10%; displacement was detected by subsequent radiographs at follow-up within 1 week in all but one case.[21] Operative intervention was suggested with displacement of more than 2 mm, and follow-up radiography beyond the first week was not indicated until after approximately 3 weeks of immobilization.[21] Treatment compliance can also factor into the management of minimally displaced lateral condyle fractures. While these fractures may not require operative fixation, if noncompliance with follow-up is a concern, reduction and fixation may be indicated to ensure proper healing and maximize return to normal function.[12]

Operative repair is most often accomplished with wiring.[9–11,22,23] Most fractures heal well, but there are cases of delayed union or nonunion. In these cases, patients were either treated nonoperatively or had inadequate operative management.[9,16,21] Malunion has also been reported, and common causes of this complication include inadequate initial reduction or subsequent displacement.[9,10,12,18]

MEDIAL CONDYLE FRACTURES

Medial condyle fractures are uncommon, comprising 1%–2% of elbow fractures in the pediatric population.[4,24] These injuries are Salter-Harris type IV fractures, and nonunion and physeal damage are concerns.[4,24] Due to later ossification of the trochlea, these fractures can be difficult to detect radiographically.[4,24–26] Previous literature has suggested that medial condyle fractures are seen primarily in older age children (average age of 9 years old) with minimally displaced fractures occurring in younger children;[5] but a more recent study found an average age of almost 5 years old, with no difference noted between age and severity of the fracture.[4] Interestingly, medial condyle fractures have been reported in patients as young as 6 months of age.[27]

Medial condyle fractures, like lateral condyle fractures, are managed based on degree of displacement and generally heal well. Minimally displaced fractures (less than 2 mm) should be immobilized, and functional results are usually good.[4,24,26,27] Surgical management is usually accomplished with wiring and is recommended for fractures with greater than 2-mm displacement.[4]

MEDIAL EPICONDYLE FRACTURES

Medial epicondyle fractures represent essentially all epicondylar fractures in the pediatric population.[6,28] An important feature of these injuries is the association with joint dislocation, which, if present, can incarcerate the displaced epicondylar fragment within the joint either before or after a reduction.[6,28]

Medial epicondyle fractures generally heal well, even in cases of fibrous nonunion (which occurs in up to 90% of patients), with little to no sequelae; traditional management has been immobilization with casting.[6,28,29] More controversial is the amount of displacement present to indicate operative intervention. Some authors suggest that fractures with less than 5-mm displacement can be managed with immobilization,[6,28–30] and some have suggested nonoperative treatment in patients with fracture displacement up to 15 mm,[29] with great variability in management.[6,28,30] Incarceration of a medial epicondyle fracture fragment within the joint is an absolute indication for operative intervention to prevent painful sequelae; ulnar nerve palsy (the most commonly affected nerve with these injuries) is not an absolute indication for surgery.[6,28,31]

ELBOW OSSIFICATION CENTERS

Knowledge of the order of ossification of the bones of the pediatric elbow is helpful when interpreting elbow imaging. This is especially useful to avoid mistakenly diagnosing an elbow fracture. The six ossification centers of the elbow appear and ossify in a predicable manner based on age.[32,33] A helpful mnemonic for remembering this order is CRITOE:[32,33]

OSSIFICATION CENTER	APPEARANCE AGE	PHYSEAL FUSION AGE
Capitellum	1 year	14 years
Radial head	4–5 years	16 years
Internal (medial) epicondyle	6–7 years	15 years
Trochlea	8–10 years	14 years
Olecranon	10 years	14 years
External (lateral) epicondyle	11 years	16 years

This is a general guideline. Notably, these ossification centers have been shown to appear earlier in females than males, and there is variation in the age of appearance and ossification for both sexes.[34]

For comparison, several cases are presented:

The child in Fig. 53.4 fell onto his outstretched arm while running, resulting in a displaced lateral condyle

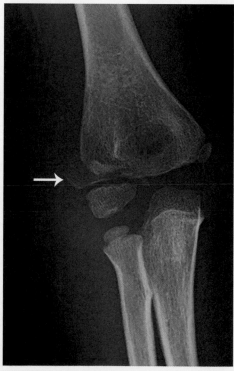

Fig. 53.4 Anteroposterior view shows a displaced lateral condyle fracture. The distal fracture fragment *(arrow)* is displaced laterally with respect to the humerus.

fracture. After consultation with Pediatric Orthopedics, the child was taken to the operating room for closed reduction and fixation.

The child in Figs. 53.5 and 53.6 fell from a tree, resulting in an elbow joint dislocation and a displaced lateral condylar fracture, requiring operative reduction and pinning.

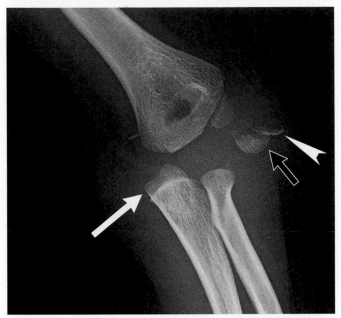

Fig. 53.5 Anteroposterior view demonstrates elbow joint dislocation, with medial dislocation of the proximal ulna *(white arrow)* and radius with respect to the humerus. A fracture through the lateral condyle is present with marked distal and lateral displacement and rotation of the distal lateral condyle fracture fragment *(arrowhead)*, including the lateral fracture fragment of the ossified capitellum *(black arrow)*.

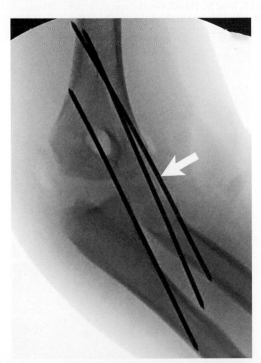

Fig. 53.6 Anteroposterior view after reduction and pinning shows near anatomic alignment, with the capitellum *(arrow)* in the expected location.

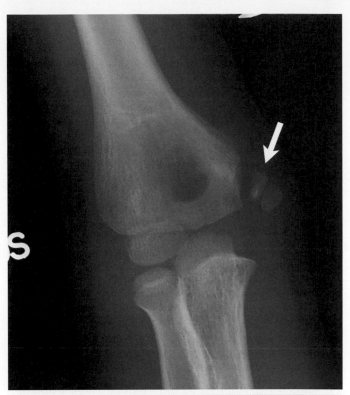

Fig. 53.7 Anteroposterior view of an avulsion fracture of the medial epicondyle *(arrow)*, with a mild degree of displacement.

The selected image in Fig. 53.7 demonstrates a medial epicondyle fracture with mild displacement. The child was managed with immobilization only and did well.

IMAGING PEARLS

1. Plain radiography is the imaging modality of choice for suspected condylar and epicondylar injuries in pediatric patients.
2. Images should include AP, lateral, and oblique views of the elbow. If AP and lateral views are initially obtained and a condylar or epicondylar fracture is discovered, then oblique views should be obtained.
3. Consider imaging of the areas above and below the suspected injury (i.e., humerus and/or forearm), as associated injury is not uncommon.
4. CT can help further define a fracture but should not be a first-line test for acute elbow injury, and consultation with Pediatric Orthopedics prior to obtaining CT is reasonable.
5. MRI can be utilized to visualize fractures that are difficult to detect with plain radiography but is not a first-line imaging test for acute elbow injuries.

References

1. Song KS, Kang CH, Min BW, et al. Internal oblique radiographs for diagnosis of nondisplaced or minimally displaced lateral condylar fractures of the humerus in children. *J Bone Joint Surg Am.* 2007;89(1):58-63.
2. Pannu GS, Eberson CP, Abzug J, et al. Common errors in the management of pediatric supracondylar humerus fractures and lateral condyle fractures. *Instr Course Lect.* 2016;65:385-397.

3. Kurtulmuş T, Safülam N, Saka G, et al. Paediatric lateral humeral condyle fractures: internal oblique radiographs alter the course of conservative treatment. *Eur J Orthop Surg Traumatol.* 2014;24(7): 1139-1144.

4. Leet AI, Young C, Hoffer MM. Medial condyle fractures of the humerus in children. *J Pediatr Orthop.* 2002;22(1):2-7.

5. Bensahel H, Csukonyi Z, Badelon O, et al. Fractures of the medial condyle of the humerus in children. *J Pediatr Orthop.* 1986;6(4): 430-433.

6. Pathy R, Dodwell ER. Medial epicondylar fractures in children. *Curr Opin Pediatr.* 2015;27(1):58-66.

7. Haillotte G, Bachy M, Delpont M, et al. The use of magnetic resonance imaging in management of minimally displaced or nondisplaced lateral humeral condyle fractures in children. *Pediatr Emerg Care.* 2017;33(1):21-25.

8. Thévenin-Lemoine C, Salanne S, Pham T, et al. Relevance of MRI for management of non-displaced lateral humeral condyle fractures in children. *Orthop Traumatol Surg Res.* 2017;103(5):777-781.

9. Tan SHS, Dartnell J, Lim AKS, et al. Paediatric lateral condyle fractures: a systematic review. *Arch Orthop Trauma Surg.* 2018;138(6):809-817.

10. Skak SV, Olsen SD, Smaabrekke A. Deformity after fracture of the lateral humeral condyle in children. *J Pediatr Orthop B.* 2001;10(2): 142-152.

11. Wirmer J, Kruppa C, Fitze G. Operative treatment of lateral humeral condyle fractures in children. *Eur J Pediatr Surg.* 2012;22(4):289-294.

12. Launay F, Leet AI, Jacopin S, et al. Lateral humeral condyle fractures in children: a comparison of two approaches to treatment. *J Pediatr Orthop.* 2004;24(4):385-391.

13. Jakob R, Fowles JV, Rang M, et al. Observations concerning fractures of the lateral humeral condyle in children. *J Bone Joint Surg Br.* 1975;57(4):430-436.

14. Rutherford A. Fractures of the lateral humeral condyle in children. *J Bone Joint Surg Am.* 1985;67(6):851-856.

15. Badelon O, Bensahel H, Mazda K, et al. Lateral humeral condylar fractures in children: a report of 47 cases. *J Pediatr Orthop.* 1988;8(1):31-34.

16. Foster DE, Sullivan JA, Gross RH. Lateral humeral condylar fractures in children. *J Pediatr Orthop.* 1985;5(1):16-22.

17. Flynn JC, Richards Jr JF, Saltzman RI. Prevention and treatment of non-union of slightly displaced fractures of the lateral humeral condyle in children. An end-result study. *J Bone Joint Surg Am.* 1975; 57(8):1087-1092

18. Weiss JM, Graves S, Yang S, et al. A new classification system predictive of complications in surgically treated pediatric humeral lateral condyle fractures. *J Pediatr Orthop.* 2009;29(6):602-605.

19. Marcheix PS, Vacquerie V, Longis B, et al. Distal humerus lateral condyle fracture in children: when is the conservative treatment a valid option? *Orthop Traumatol Surg Res.* 2011;97(3):304-307.

20. Knapik DM, Gilmore A, Liu RW. Conservative management of minimally displaced (≤2 mm) fractures of the lateral humeral condyle in pediatric patients: a systematic review. *J Pediatr Orthop.* 2017;37(2):e83-e87.

21. Pirker ME, Weinberg AM, Höllwarth ME, et al. Subsequent displacement of initially nondisplaced and minimally displaced fractures of the lateral humeral condyle in children. *J Trauma.* 2005;58(6): 1202-1207.

22. Li WC, Xu RJ. Comparison of Kirschner wires and AO cannulated screw internal fixation for displaced lateral humeral condyle fracture in children. *Int Orthop.* 2012;36(6):1261-1266.

23. McGonagle L, Elamin S, Wright DM. Buried or unburied K-wires for lateral condyle elbow fractures. *Ann R Coll Surg Engl.* 2012;94(7):513-516.

24. Fernandez FF, Vatlach S, Wirth T, et al. Medial humeral condyle fracture in childhood: a rare but overlooked injury. *Eur J Trauma Emerg Surg.* 2019;45(5):757-761.

25. Fowles JV, Kassab MT. Displaced fractures of the medial humeral condyle in children. *J Bone Joint Surg Am.* 1980;62(7):1159-1163.

26. Papavasiliou V, Nenopoulos S, Venturis T. Fractures of the medial condyle of the humerus in childhood. *J Pediatr Orthop.* 1987;7(4):421-423.

27. DeBoeck H, Casteleyn PP, Opdecam P. Fracture of the medial humeral condyle: report of a case in an infant. *J Bone Joint Surg Am.* 1987;69(9): 1442-1444.

28. Firth AM, Marson BA, Hunter JB. Paediatric medial humeral epicondyle fracture management: 2019 approach. *Curr Opin Pediatr.* 2019;31(1):86-91.

29. Farsetti P, Potenza V, Caterini R, Ippolito E. Long-term results of treatment of fractures of the medial humeral epicondyle in children. *J Bone Joint Surg Am.* 2001;83(9):1299-1305.

30. AO Foundation. *AO Surgery Reference. Paediatric Distal Humerus.* 2016. Available at: https://www2.aofoundation.org/wps/portal/ surgery?showPage=diagnosis&bone=PediatricHumerus&segment= Distal. Accessed March 20, 2020.

31. Dodds SD, Flanagin BA, Bohl DD, et al. Incarcerated medial epicondyle fracture following pediatric elbow dislocation: 11 cases. *J Hand Surg Am.* 2014;39(9):1739-1745.

32. Kim HH, Gauguet JM. Pediatric elbow injuries. *Semin Ultrasound CT MR.* 2018;39(4):384-396.

33. Delgado J, Jaramillo D, Chauvin NA. Imaging the injured pediatric athlete: upper extremity. *Radiographics.* 2016;36(6):1672-1687.

34. Patel B, Reed M, Patel S. Gender-specific pattern differences of the ossification centers in the pediatric elbow. *Pediatr Radiol.* 2009; 39(3):226-231.

54 Rough Trip: Scapula Fracture

ROBERT VEZZETTI, MD, FAAP, FACEP

Case Presentation

A 17-year-old male presents with right shoulder pain after falling while playing soccer. The patient tripped while running and landed on his shoulder. He was able to continue playing the game but now complains of vague right shoulder pain. When asked to localize the pain, he points to his back, at the inferior portion of the scapula. He has no neck pain, other back pain, abdominal pain, numbness, weakness, or other injury.

Imaging Considerations

PLAIN RADIOGRAPHY

Plain radiography is the first-line imaging modality to employ in patients with extremity injuries, including the shoulder. A "shoulder series" is generally a two- or three-view study of the glenohumeral joint. Standard projections are an anteroposterior (AP) view and an orthogonal view such as a lateral scapular Y view. There are many variations and modifications on this basic series that can be used in the setting of trauma, but the scapular Y view provides a profile view of the scapula and is useful for suspected scapular fractures. A scapular series can also be utilized and usually consists of AP and lateral (scapular Y) views. Clinically significant fractures are identified, relative exposure to ionizing radiation is low, and the wide availability of plain radiography makes this technique an attractive choice.

ULTRASOUND (US)

US is a useful imaging modality to detect fractures in the pediatric patient. There have been reports of the identification of scapular fractures using this imaging technique, but more study is needed before this method can be routinely employed.[1] The main concern is the operator-dependent nature of US. Scapular fractures can be difficult to detect, and if US is used to detect fractures, an experienced operator should perform the study.

COMPUTED TOMOGRAPHY (CT)

CT may have a role in the evaluation of pediatric patients with scapular fractures. Children who sustain significant blunt force trauma may require CT to evaluate for other life-threatening thoracic injuries. In such patients, pulmonary or great vessel injuries may be present, necessitating imaging beyond plain radiography. Clinical history and physical examination should direct further radiographic evaluation.

Imaging Findings

The patient had plain radiography performed. There is a transverse lucency along the lateral border of the body of the scapula, confirmed on multiple views, consistent with a nondisplaced fracture (Figs. 54.1–54.3).

Case Conclusion

Once a scapular fracture was diagnosed, a careful reevaluation for co-injury was performed. No other injuries were found and the patient maintained normal vital signs. Consultation with Pediatric Orthopedics was performed, and a sling was placed. The family and child were instructed to follow up with Pediatric Orthopedics in 3–5 days for reevaluation. Pain management and rest were recommended.

Scapular fractures are uncommon.[2] The majority of these fractures are secondary to high-energy mechanisms, such as motor vehicle accidents. As such, many patients with scapular fractures have associated injuries, including thoracic (pulmonary contusions and rib fractures), ipsilateral upper extremity injury (acromion and coracoid process fractures), spine fractures (particularly involving the thoracic spine), and pelvic ring fractures. Upper extremity, thoracic, and pelvic ring injuries have been found to be more frequently associated with scapula fractures, but patients with increased injury severity have also been reported to have an increased association of scapular fractures.[3] In the pediatric patient population, those children involved in high-energy motor vehicle accidents who had scapular fractures did not have an associated higher mortality rate but did have an association with increased morbidity, including intracranial hemorrhage, thoracic injury, upper extremity fractures, and spine fractures.[4] Isolated scapular fractures have been reported.[5] In any case, when a clinician diagnoses a scapular fracture, a careful history and physical examination should be performed.

Great vessel injuries have a reported association with scapular fractures, particularly in patients with high Injury Severity Scores (ISS).[2,6] A scapular fracture that occurs in the context of high force, blunt thoracic trauma should prompt consideration of additional imaging for associated thoracic injury. At a minimum, plain chest radiography should be performed and CT imaging of the chest with intravenous contrast should be considered, based on history (i.e., high-speed motor vehicle crashes, complaints of chest pain, complaints of difficulty breathing), clinical examination findings (i.e., low oxygen saturation, tachypnea, difficulty breathing, signs of chest trauma), and the results of

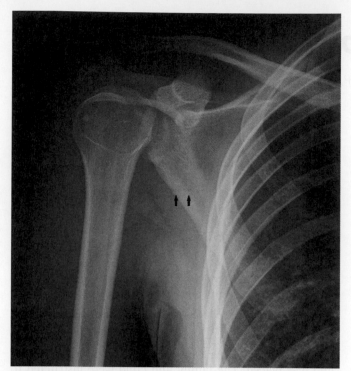

Fig. 54.1 AP radiographic view of the right shoulder shows a linear lucency *(arrows)* present along the lateral aspect of the body of the scapula.

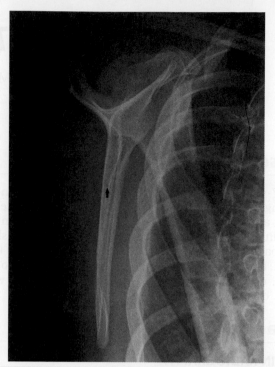

Fig. 54.3 Lateral view confirms transverse lucency in the scapular body consistent with nondisplaced fracture *(arrow)*.

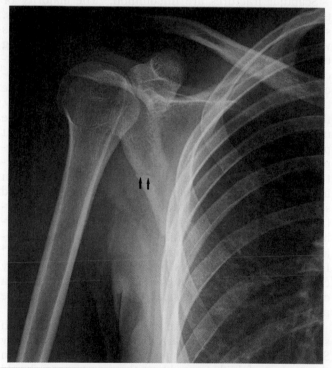

Fig. 54.2 AP radiographic view of the right shoulder shows a linear lucency *(arrows)* present along the body of the scapula.

chest radiography (if abnormal, such as a widened mediastinum or aortic knob, consider CT).[6]

IMAGING PEARLS

1. Scapular fractures are uncommon in pediatric patients. These fractures have been reported in high-energy blunt trauma and are often associated with additional thoracic, upper extremity, and spine injuries. The presence of a scapular fracture should prompt the clinician to perform a careful history and physical examination looking for concurrent injury.

2. Plain radiography is the first-line imaging modality in pediatric patients with a low-risk injury mechanism and no other physical examination findings to suggest a life-threatening thoracic injury. AP and lateral or scapular Y views, either as a shoulder or scapular series, are standard views for the evaluation of suspected scapular fracture.

3. Chest CT may be indicated in patients with historical or physical examination findings suggestive of significant injury. Plain radiography should be obtained prior to chest CT. The decision to obtain chest CT should be based on history, physical examination, and plain chest radiography.

References

1. McCrady BM, Schaefer MP. Sonographic visualization of a scapular body fracture: a case report. *J Clin Ultrasound*. 2011;39(8):466-468.
2. Veysi VT, Mittal R, Agarwal S, et al. Multiple trauma and scapula fractures: so what? *J Trauma*. 2003;55(6):1145-1147.
3. Baldwin KD, Ohman-Strickland P, Mehta S, et al. Scapula fractures: a marker for concomitant injury? A Retrospective review of data in the National Trauma Database. *J Trauma*. 2008;65(2):430-435.
4. Shannon SF, Hernandez NM, Sems SA, et al. High-energy pediatric scapula fractures and their associated injuries. *J Pediatr Orthop*. 2019;39(7):377-381.
5. Donovan M, Attia MW. An unusual cause of an isolated scapula fracture. *JAAPA*. 2018;31(3):26-28.
6. Abd El-Shafy I, Rosen LM, Prince JM, et al. Blunt traumatic scapular fractures are associated with great vessel injuries in children. *J Trauma Acute Care Surg*. 2018;85(5):932-935.

55 *Humeral Shaft Fractures: Nothing Funny About That!*

ROBERT VEZZETTI, MD, FAAP, FACEP

Case Presentation

A 6-year-old boy presents with right upper arm and shoulder pain after falling off a horse while riding at a brisk trot. There is no reported loss of consciousness and he denies neck pain, abdominal pain, back pain, or elbow pain. His vital signs are age appropriate and there is no obvious injury other than mild edema and tenderness of his proximal right humerus. There is no apparent weakness or numbness. He has brisk capillary refill and a strong radial pulse. Sensation is intact. There are no lacerations or abrasions of the skin.

Imaging Considerations

PLAIN RADIOGRAPHY

The classification of humerus fractures depends on their location: proximal physeal fractures are classified using the Salter-Harris Classification, with the majority being Salter-Harris type I or II fractures, whereas humeral shaft fractures are classified by angulation, displacement, and location.[1] A child may not be able to indicate exactly where the source of their pain might be and shoulder imaging may be obtained rather than dedicated imaging of the humerus if a shoulder injury is initially suspected. The proximal humerus can be visualized with a shoulder series and typical views include anteroposterior (AP), scapular Y, and axillary views.[2,3] Two-view imaging (AP and lateral projections) of the affected extremity is generally sufficient when evaluating pediatric long bone injuries[4] and is appropriate to diagnose humeral shaft fractures in these patients.[1,2] Comparative views are generally not indicated. Consideration should be given to imaging joints above and below an injury; humeral radiographs will generally adequately visualize the elbow and shoulder joints, but dedicated imaging of those sites should be performed if clinically indicated.

Prior to obtaining imaging, adequate pain control should be provided. Intranasal fentanyl (a dose of 2 μg/kg) has been proven to be effective pain control with minimal side effects, allowing for imaging of the patient.[5]

COMPUTED TOMOGRAPHY (CT)

CT is not indicated in the evaluation of humeral shaft fractures. In cases of complex fractures, there may be a role,[3] but consultation with Pediatric Orthopedics or an orthopedist comfortable with the management of these fractures in the pediatric patient is reasonable prior to advanced imaging.

MAGNETIC RESONANCE IMAGING (MRI)

As with CT, MRI is generally not indicated in the initial evaluation of proximal humerus fractures. If there is a complex fracture or concern for neurovascular injury, MRI may have a role,[3] but consultation with Pediatric Orthopedics or an orthopedist comfortable with the management of these fractures in the pediatric patient is reasonable prior to advanced imaging.

Imaging Findings

Shoulder imaging was obtained revealing a proximal humerus shaft fracture with 2 cm of overlap; the humeral head is aligned with the glenoid (Figs. 55.1 and 55.2). In this view, the complete humerus is not visualized and full humeral imaging is indicated to assess for associated distal humeral injury. Two views of the humerus are obtained, again demonstrating the fracture; note that there is overriding of fracture fragments with posterior and lateral displacement of the distal facture fragment (Figs. 55.3 and 55.4).

Case Resolution

Since there was no evidence of an open fracture, an underlying pathologic etiology, or vascular injury, this child was treated with sling application and good pain control. Referral to Pediatric Orthopedics was arranged and the child was seen as an outpatient in follow-up clinic. Healing was monitored with serial examinations and follow-up plain radiography. The fracture healed well and did not require operative intervention (Figs. 55.5 and 55.6).

Pediatric proximal humerus fractures are not common, comprising approximately 2% of all pediatric fractures.[1-3,6] In pediatric patients, boys are more likely to sustain proximal humerus fractures and two injury mechanisms dominate: direct trauma to the shoulder (fall, sports injury, or motor vehicle crash; horse-related injuries are also a common mechanism) and falling with the arm in an outstretched position, with the arm abducted and internally rotated.[1-3,6,7] These fractures may occur either in the metaphysis or through the physis; adolescent patients tend to fracture the physis, while younger children tend to fracture the metaphysis.[1] Injury to the physis, which contains elements of chrondrocyte activity, by either direct or indirect means, has the potential to adversely affect future bone growth, and identifying such injuries is important.[8]

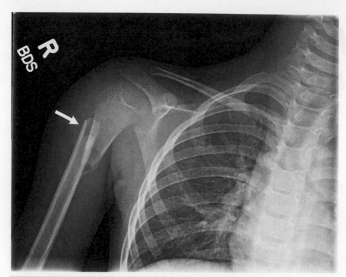

Fig. 55.1 Anteroposterior view of the shoulder. There is a proximal humeral shaft fracture *(arrow)*.

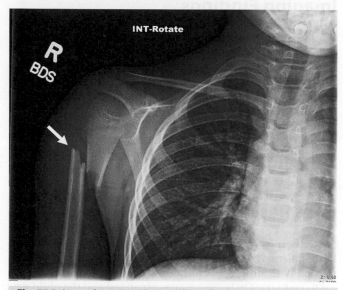

Fig. 55.2 Internal rotation AP view of the shoulder again demonstrating the right humerus fracture. There is overriding of fracture fragments with lateral displacement of the distal fragment *(arrow)*.

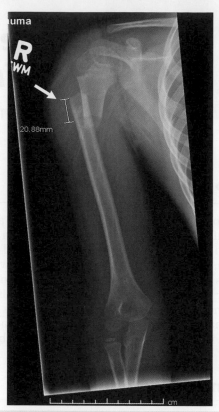

Fig. 55.3 Anteroposterior humerus view demonstrating overriding of fracture fragments and lateral displacement of the distal fracture fragment *(arrow)*.

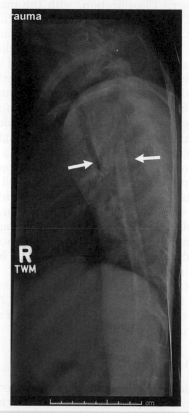

Fig. 55.4 Lateral humerus view demonstrating overriding of fracture fragments and posterior displacement of the distal fracture fragment *(arrows)*.

Humeral shaft fractures, as with proximal humeral fractures, are also uncommon in pediatric patients, accounting for less than 10% of all humerus fractures.[1] Mechanisms of injury, as with proximal humeral fractures, are usually a direct blow or a fall on an outstretched hand.[1] Most occur in the middle third of the humerus, followed by the proximal third.

The blood supply to the proximal humerus derives from the axillary artery and the nerve supply is the axillary nerve, and vascular injuries are rare. Nerve injury is also uncommon in pediatric patients and, if present, often will resolve spontaneously.[1,6]

Consideration of the child's developmental age, medical history, and mechanism of injury should be part of the

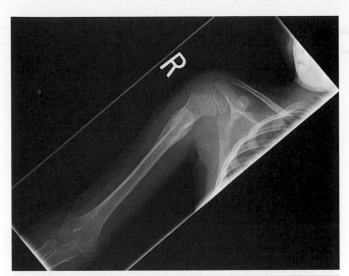

Fig. 55.5 Follow-up AP view of the humerus 2 months later. There is callus formation and remodeling of the bone without functional impairment.

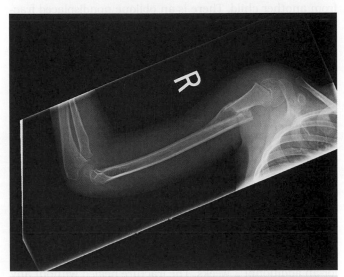

Fig. 55.6 Follow-up lateral humerus view 2 months later. There is callus formation and remodeling of the bone without functional impairment.

evaluation of children with any fracture; if concern for nonaccidental trauma arises, an appropriate evaluation should take place (see Chapter 50: Nonaccidental Trauma).

The vast majority of pediatric humeral shaft fractures require nothing more than the application of a sling (with or without swathe), pain control, and monitoring by Pediatric

Orthopedics. The remodeling potential in pediatric patients is great and surgical intervention is rarely, if ever, indicated.[1–3] If surgical intervention is considered, the age of the child and the amount of displacement/angulation are taken into consideration, with no absolute criteria for displacement or angulation dictating the need for operative intervention.[1,3,6,9] It is reasonable to consult Pediatric Orthopedics prior to disposition of the patient to ensure appropriate follow-up and definitive treatment.

IMAGING PEARLS

1. Plain radiography is the imaging modality of choice in the evaluation of proximal humerus fracture with a shoulder series, including AP and trans-scapular or axillary views.
2. Ensure adequate pain control prior to obtaining imaging. While pain protocols are often institution dependent, intranasal medications such as fentanyl have proven to be effective.
3. Comparison views of the contralateral extremity are generally not indicated.
4. Consider imaging the joints above and below a bone shaft fracture. The decision to image these areas should be based on historical and physical examination findings. In the absence of trauma or if the developmental history of a child does not match the mechanism of injury, consider a nonaccidental trauma evaluation.

References

1. Arora R, Fichadia U, Hartwig E, et al. Pediatric upper-extremity fractures. *Pediatr Ann*. 2014;43(5):196-204.
2. Lieber J, Schmittenbecher P. Developments in the treatment of pediatric long bone shaft fractures. *Eur J Pediatr Surg*. 2013;23(6):427-433.
3. Popkin CA, Levine WN, Ahmad CS. Evaluation and management of pediatric proximal humerus fractures. *J Am Acad Orthop Surg*. 2015;23(2):77-86.
4. Shrader MW. Proximal humerus and humeral shaft fractures in children. *Hand Clin*. 2007;23(4):431-435, vi.
5. Lefèvre Y, Journeau P, Angelliaume A, et al. Proximal humerus fractures in children and adolescents. *Orthop Traumatol Surg Res*. 2014;100(suppl 1):S149-S156.
6. Delavan A and Fenton LZ. Pediatric fractures. In: *Pediatric Radiology*. Oxford: Oxford University Press; 2014:265-273.
7. Graudins A, Meek R, Egerton-Warbutron D, et al. The PITCHFORK (Pain in Children Fentanyl or Ketamine) trial: a randomized controlled trial comparing intranasal ketamine and fentanyl for the relief of moderate to severe pain in children with limb injuries. *Ann Emerg Med*. 2015;65(3):248-254.
8. Nguyen JC, Markhardt BK, Merrow AC, et al. Imaging of pediatric growth plate disturbances. *Radiographics*. 2017;37(6):1791-1812.
9. Ghosh A, Di Scala C, Drew C, et al. Horse-related injuries in pediatric patients. *J Pediatr Surg*. 2000;35(12):1766-1770.

56 In Pieces: Clavicle Fracture

SUJIT IYER, MD

Case Presentation

A 12-year-old male presents after a direct fall onto his right arm and shoulder while playing soccer. He is comfortable and prefers to hold the arm close to his body and is supporting the injured arm with his opposite hand. There is an obvious bulge at the midshaft of the clavicle with no abrasion or breaks in the skin seen. There is no tenting of the skin.

Imaging Considerations

Plain radiography is the imaging modality of choice in children with suspected clavicle fractures. These fractures can readily be seen on a shoulder series or a chest x-ray. A shoulder series is sufficient if there is no concern for associate pulmonary injury. If there is concern for accompanying thoracic injury, then plain chest radiography should be obtained.

PLAIN RADIOGRAPHY

A single anteroposterior (AP) view is usually sufficient to diagnose most midshaft clavicle fractures and define the angle of displacement. The AP cephalic tilt view (angled 15–45 degrees) is often used in conjunction with the standard AP view to project the clavicle above the ribs, facilitating visualization of fractures and associated displacement. Oblique clavicle views may be added when trying to distinguish between an acromioclavicular (AC) joint injury and a fracture to the distal clavicle, or when the medial clavicle is of greater concern.

COMPUTED TOMOGRAPHY (CT)

CT scan is rarely needed for most clavicle fractures. However, medial clavicle fractures and sternoclavicular joint disruption can be missed on plain radiography and CT may be warranted to detect these injuries, as well as to evaluate for other major thoracic injuries in these cases.[1] In select cases where accurate measurement of shortening may influence the decision of operative management, CT scan may be used but should be balanced with the risk for exposure to ionizing radiation in a young patient.[2]

ULTRASOUND (US)

A small pediatric study showed that bedside US had high positive and negative predictive values (95% and 96%) without any added pain or discomfort when compared to plain radiographs for clavicle fractures. In resource-limited settings, this may be an accurate modality to confirm the diagnosis when clinical suspicion is high and providers have sufficient training in performing musculoskeletal US.[3]

Imaging Findings

Selected clavicle images for this child are provided. There is an acute, transverse fracture of the mid clavicle, with mild inferior displacement of the distal fracture fragment, with only minimal superior angulation of the fracture apex (Fig. 56.1). An image of the healing fracture, with callus formation, is shown in Fig. 56.2; this is the fracture 3 weeks later.

For comparison, Fig. 56.3 shows a distal clavicle fracture from another child. There is an oblique nondisplaced fracture of the lateral right clavicle, just medial to the AC joint.

In Fig. 56.4, a more complex clavicle fracture is seen from another child who was involved in a motor vehicle crash. These images demonstrate a comminuted segmental fracture of the left clavicle, with the lateral fracture fragment displaced inferiorly with respect to the proximal/medial fracture fragment, and an intervening central fracture fragment is rotated perpendicular to the long axis of the bone.

Case Conclusion

A single AP view demonstrated a transverse nondisplaced midshaft clavicle fracture. The patient was put in a sling for comfort and given instructions to immobilize the area for 3 weeks with recommendations to avoid contact sports for an additional 2 weeks. The fracture healed without any residual pain, restriction of motion, or limitations.

The child with the distal clavicle fracture was also treated with a sling and pain management. His fracture healed well without apparent complication. The child involved in the motor vehicle crash required operative intervention and did well (Figs. 56.5 and 56.6).

Clavicle fractures are a common injury in children, and 90% will occur in the middle third of the clavicle, with young children (less than 10 years old) usually having nondisplaced fractures.[4] In a young child, the history usually involves a direct fall onto the shoulder, and examination findings often include a localized hematoma with a preference to not raise or abduct the affected arm. Tenting of the skin, or signs of an open fracture (abrasions or puncture marks), should warrant emergent orthopedic referral. Distal clavicle fractures are less common and may appear clinically similar to AC separations with signs of localized pain and increased pain with adduction of the arm across the chest. Distal clavicle fractures may be suspected if pain is more medial to the AC joint and may require oblique clavicle views. Proximal clavicle fractures are the least common and

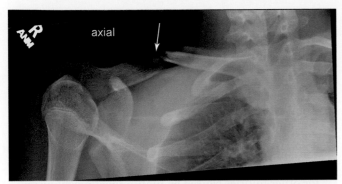

Fig. 56.1 AP radiographic view shows a midshaft clavicle fracture with almost one shaft width inferior displacement of the lateral/distal fracture fragment *(arrow)* and minimal superior angulation of the fracture apex.

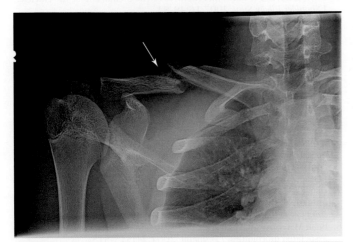

Fig. 56.2 AP radiographic view shows a healing midshaft clavicle fracture. Note the callus formation *(arrow)*.

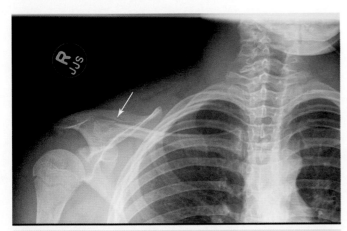

Fig. 56.3 AP radiographic view shows a nondisplaced oblique fracture of the distal clavicle *(arrow)*.

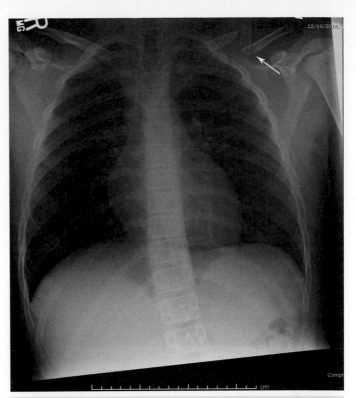

Fig. 56.4 AP view of the chest shows a comminuted segmental clavicle fracture, with inferior displacement of the lateral fracture fragment *(white arrow)*, and an intervening central fracture fragment *(black arrow)* that is rotated perpendicular to the long axis of the bone.

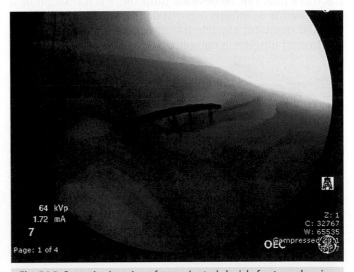

Fig. 56.5 Operative imaging of comminuted clavicle fracture, showing near anatomic alignment after plate and screw fixation.

classically seen after a high-impact force such as a motor vehicle accident. These fractures warrant greater consideration of major injuries to the head, neck, lungs, and abdomen due to the high velocity needed to cause these injuries.

Although most midshaft clavicle fractures can be managed nonoperatively, more recent adult evidence has supported earlier surgical intervention in comminuted and completely displaced clavicle factures to reduce nonunion and improve function. In smaller pediatric studies, this has led to a trend of earlier surgical intervention in adolescent children.[5,6]

Clavicle fractures are the most common skeletal fractures in neonates, with incidences ranging from 0.5% to 1.6%.[7,8] Classic risk factors include difficult vaginal delivery, large birth weight, and shoulder dystocia. Displaced fractures are

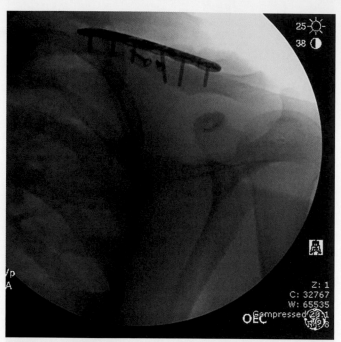

Fig. 56.6 Operative imaging of comminuted clavicle fracture, showing near anatomic alignment after plate and screw fixation.

usually more obvious in the immediate postpartum period, with signs of restricted movement of the arm, crying when trying to swaddle the patient, or local edema. Nondisplaced fractures may not be obvious until there is formation of a visible callus as infants are usually asymptomatic. Overall, isolated neonatal clavicle fractures from birth delivery do not impart long-term complications.

IMAGING PEARLS

1. When clinical suspicion is high, a single AP view is sufficient to diagnose most clavicle fractures. If the AP view is normal, consider an AP view with greater cephalic angulation.
2. Distal clavicle fractures may be hard to distinguish from AC joint injuries without the use of radiographs and may warrant oblique views.
3. CT has limited use in most clavicle injuries, but when the clinical suspicion is high, it may be warranted to elucidate proximal clavicle fractures and also evaluate for other injuries caused by high-impact mechanisms.

References

1. Throckmorton T, Kuhn JE. Fractures of the medial end of the clavicle. *J Shoulder Elbow Surg.* 2007;16:49-54.
2. Omid R, Kidd C, Yi A, Villacis D, et al. Measurement of clavicle fracture shortening using computed tomography and chest radiography. *Clin Orthop Surg.* 2016;8:367-372.
3. Cross KP, Warkentine FH, Kim IK, et al. Bedside ultrasound diagnosis of clavicle fractures in the pediatric emergency department. *Acad Emerg Med.* 2010;17:687-693.
4. Postacchini F, Gumina S, et al. Epidemiology of clavicle fractures. *J Shoulder Elbow Surg.* 2002;11:452-456.
5. Yang S, Werner BC, Gwathmey FW. Treatment trends in adolescent clavicle fractures. *J Pediatr Orthop.* 2015;35:229-233.
6. Suppan CA, Bae DS, Donohue KS, et al. Trends in the volume of operative treatment of midshaft clavicle fractures in children and adolescents: a retrospective, 12-year, single-institution analysis. *J Pediatr Orthop B.* 2016;25:305-309.
7. Hsu TY. Hung FC, Lu JY, et al. Neonatal clavicular fracture: clinical analysis of incidence, predisposing factors, diagnosis, and outcome. *Am J Perinatol.* 2002;19:17-21.
8. Beall MH, Ross MG. Clavicle fracture in labor: risk factors and associated morbidities. *J Perinatol.* 2001;21:513-515.

57 *Let's Play! Forearm Fractures*

SUJIT IYER, MD

Case Presentation

A 4-year-old child presents after falling on an outstretched hand while running at school. He complains of pain to the right forearm and is splinted by the school nurse and given pain medicine by paramedics. There is no open abrasion or puncture to the skin. His vital signs are all age appropriate. There does not appear to be any injury to the head, neck, back, shoulder, upper arm, or wrist. He is grossly neurovascularly intact.

Imaging Considerations

Most forearm fractures result from a fall onto an outstretched hand, and immediate pain control is key to completing a thorough examination as well as obtaining adequate radiographs.[1] Intranasal fentanyl (2 mcg/kg, maximum single-dose 100 mcg) delivered via a mucosal atomizer device can achieve pain control within 10 minutes while radiographs and intravenous access are obtained.

PLAIN RADIOGRAPHY

This is the imaging modality of choice when evaluating patients with suspected forearm fractures. A true anteroposterior view (AP) and lateral view of the forearm should include the wrist and distal humerus. A true lateral view of the forearm will illustrate partial overlapping of the radius and ulna at the proximal and distal ends and the elbow will be flexed at 90 degrees. If there is concern about an elbow fracture or dislocation, dedicated elbow radiographs should be obtained.

ULTRASOUND (US)

US has been shown to be a feasible method to diagnose isolated forearm fractures in resource-limited settings and has been used to guide reductions.[2] The combination of US with clinical decision instruments has also been used in resource-rich settings to diagnose and manage treatment of distal forearm fractures with the intent to reduce radiograph use.[3] Most studies have shown that time to train emergency physicians in diagnosing straightforward forearm fractures is short (i.e., 1 hour).[4] The utility of US is more limited when evaluating midshaft and proximal forearm fractures that involve the elbow or more complicated injuries.

ADVANCED IMAGING (COMPUTED TOMOGRAPHY AND MAGNETIC RESONANCE IMAGING)

These imaging modalities are not indicated for the initial evaluation of forearm injuries. However, for complex fractures or if the extent of the fracture is not clear, these modalities may be utilized. Consultation with a Pediatric Orthopedic specialist is appropriate prior to employing these modalities.

Imaging Findings

After appropriate pain medication administration, the patient had two-view imaging of the forearm. This demonstrated mid radial and ulnar diaphyseal fractures with mild volar angulation of the distal fracture fragments; the visualized portions of the elbow and distal humerus appear normal (Figs. 57.1 and 57.2).

Case Conclusion

Pediatric Orthopedics was consulted and the child was placed in a cast. Although the fracture did not require reduction, the fracture was molded during the cast application, and, due to good pain control, the patient tolerated this well. Follow-up was arranged. Imaging 2 months later demonstrated callous formation with near anatomic alignment (Figs. 57.3 and 57.4).

Forearm fractures are the most common fractures in children, accounting for almost 50% of all childhood fractures.[5] The radius and ulna are uniquely connected by an interosseous membrane longitudinally and by articulations at both the elbow and the wrist. If, by examination or radiograph, one bone is fractured, special attention should be paid to the other bone as well as proximal and distal joints for concurrent injuries. Physical examination should pay special attention for punctures to the skin with oozing blood, which may be a sign of an open fracture with a retracted segment. Sensory and motor examinations are important to assess for median, radial, and ulnar nerve neurapraxias. Forearm fractures can rarely have a complicating supracondylar fracture (also called a "floating elbow"), so providers should thoroughly examine the elbow and also evaluate for signs of compartment syndrome in these cases.[6]

Distal forearm fractures should be evaluated by radiograph for physeal injuries and correlated for risk of Salter-Harris type I injuries by localized tenderness on examination. Buckle fractures (torus fracture) commonly occur at the distal metaphysis and are important to differentiate from nondisplaced greenstick fractures by radiograph. An ulnar styloid fracture is a distal avulsion fracture that often has a concurrent radial fracture, but avulsions at the base of the styloid itself may warrant surgical intervention.

Management of these injures depends on several factors, including the age of the child and severity of the fracture. Traditional management of displaced forearm fractures

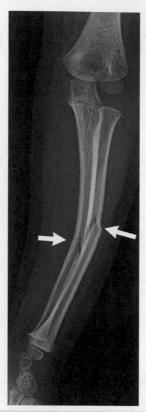

Fig. 57.1 Nondisplaced radial and ulnar diaphyseal fractures *(arrows)*, with mild volar angulation of the distal fracture fragments. The visualized portions of the elbow and distal humerus look normal.

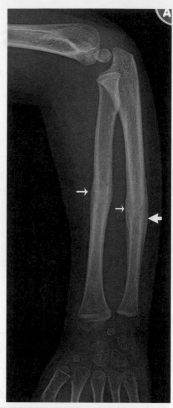

Fig. 57.3 Follow-up imaging demonstrating callous formation and near anatomic alignment *(arrows)*.

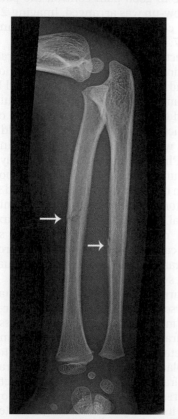

Fig. 57.2 Nondisplaced radial and ulnar diaphyseal fractures *(arrows)*, with mild volar angulation of the distal fracture fragments. The visualized portions of the elbow and distal humerus look normal.

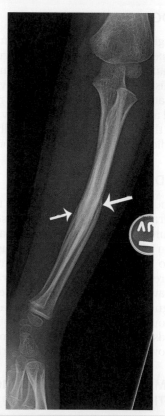

Fig. 57.4 Follow-up imaging demonstrating callous formation and near anatomic alignment *(arrows)*.

included closed reduction followed by immobilization with casting.[7,8] Fractures that are treated with closed reduction and immobilization do have a reported risk of radiographic loss of reduction of 5% to 75%; this risk is related to the amount of initial displacement and the inability to achieve anatomic alignment after reduction, among other factors.[9,10] Surgical management should be performed in patients with open fractures, fractures with neurovascular compromise, and fractures that have failed attempted closed reduction.[11,12] The most commonly utilized surgical technique is intramedullary fixation or internal fixation with plates/screws.[11,12]

Special consideration should be given to bowing and greenstick fractures. Plastic deformities (or bowing fractures) will show bowing on radiograph without a clear fracture. Greenstick fractures are unique to pediatrics and will show a complete fracture on one side of the cortex and a buckling or bowing or the other side. Bowing fractures may be initially missed during radiographic interpretation. The management of these fractures varies, with some authors advocating that all bowing deformities should undergo reduction and others citing age and degree of deformity as criteria for reduction.[12,13] Greenstick fractures are generally treated with closed reduction and immobilization, although controversy exists as to whether the fracture should be completed and then reduced.[12] Consultation with a pediatric orthopedic specialist is appropriate and helpful in determining management options in these patients.

For comparison, additional cases are presented here:

The patient in Figs. 57.5 and 57.6 fell off the monkey bars while playing at a park. Imaging of the forearm

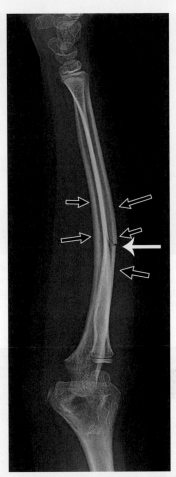

Fig. 57.6 Plastic bowing *(black arrows)* fractures of the shafts of the radius and ulna, with apex posterior bowing. A nondisplaced greenstick fracture of the proximal shaft of the radius *(white arrow)* is also seen.

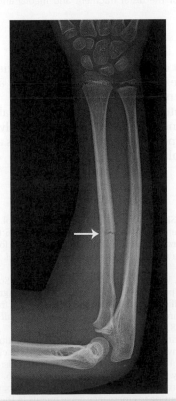

Fig. 57.5 Plastic bowing fractures of the shafts of the radius and ulna, with apex posterior bowing, but with bowing fractures best seen on Fig. 57.6. A nondisplaced greenstick fracture of the proximal shaft of the radius *(white arrow)* is also seen.

demonstrates plastic bowing fractures of the shafts of the radius and ulna, with apex posterior bowing. A nondisplaced greenstick fracture of the proximal shaft of the radius is also seen. Pediatric Orthopedics was consulted and spoke at length with the family, offering casting with close monitoring or reduction in the operating room. After the risks and benefits of each course of action were discussed, they family elected casting.

The patient in Figs. 57.7 and 57.8 jumped from a playground swing, landing on his arm. Imaging demonstrates a Salter-Harris type IV fracture of the proximal radius and an intraarticular fracture of the olecranon. Pediatric Orthopedics was consulted and the patient underwent reduction in the emergency department, as well as casting, and was discharged with close follow-up.

The patient in Fig. 57.9 fell while running, landing on her outstretched arm. Images demonstrated angulated and displaced distal radius and ulna fractures. This patient had the fractures reduced to anatomic alignment under sedation in the emergency department by Pediatric Orthopedics. Reduction was maintained and operative intervention was not required.

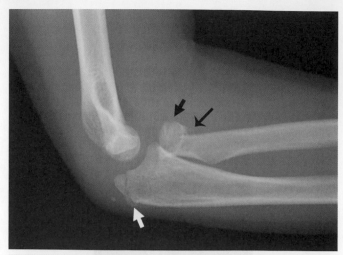

Fig. 57.7 Salter-Harris type IV fracture of the radius and olecranon fracture. Lateral view demonstrates fractures of the radial metaphysis (neck) and epiphysis (head) *(black arrows)* and an intraarticular fracture through the proximal ulna *(white arrow).*

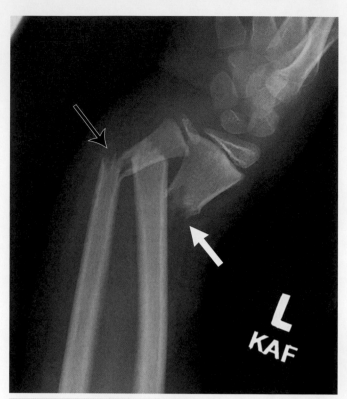

Fig. 57.9 The anteroposterior view demonstrates transverse fractures of the distal radius *(white arrow)* and ulna *(black arrow).* The radial fracture demonstrates overriding of fracture fragments, lateral displacement of the distal fracture fragment, and medial angulation of the fracture apex. The ulnar fracture also demonstrates mild lateral displacement of the distal fragment and medial angulation of the fracture apex.

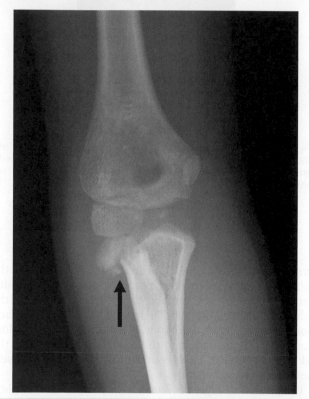

Fig. 57.8 Salter-Harris type IV fracture of the radius and olecranon fracture. The anteroposterior (AP) view again shows the fracture of the proximal radius *(arrow),* with medial displacement of the distal fracture fragment, and medial angulation of the fracture apex. The ulna fracture is not well visualized on the AP view.

concurrent dislocations, and injuries proximal and distal to the point of contact as these may alter management.

3. An adequate forearm radiograph should always include the wrist and distal humerus to completely evaluate the proximal and distal portions of the radius and ulna and their articulations.

References

1. Chia B, Kozin SH, Herman MJ, et al. Complications of pediatric distal radius and forearm fractures. *Instr Course Lect.* 2015;64:499-507.
2. Wellsh BM, Kuzma JM. Ultrasound-guided pediatric forearm fracture reductions in a resource-limited ED. *Am J Emerg Med.* 2016;34(1): 40-44.
3. Ackermann O, Wojciechowski P, Dzierzega M, et al. Sokrat II—an international, prospective, multicenter, phase IV diagnostic trial to evaluate the efficacy of the wrist SAFE algorithm in fracture sonography of distal forearm fractures in children. *Ultraschall Med.* 2019; 40(3):349-358.
4. Epema AC, Spanjer MJB, Ras L, et al. Point-of-care ultrasound compared with conventional radiographic evaluation in children with suspected distal forearm fractures in the Netherlands: a diagnostic accuracy study. *Emerg Med J.* 2019;36(10):613-616.
5. Naranje SM, Erali RA, Warner WC, et al. Epidemiology of pediatric fractures presenting to emergency departments in the United States. *J Pediatr Orthop.* 2016;36(4):e45-e48.
6. Koche MS, Waters PM, Micheli, LJ. Upper extremity injuries in the paediatric athlete. *Sports Med.* 2000;30(2):117-135.

IMAGING PEARLS

1. Pain control is key to obtaining adequate AP and lateral views for forearm fractures.
2. Injury to both the radius and ulna is common. Special attention should be made for signs of open fracture,

7. Bohm ER, Bubbar V, Yong Hing K, et al. Above and below-the-elbow plaster casts for distal forearm fractures in children. A randomized controlled trial. *J Bone Joint Surg Am.* 2006;88:1-8.
8. Webb GR, Galpin RD, Armstrong DG. Comparison of short and long arm plaster casts for displaced fractures in the distal third of the forearm in children. *J Bone Joint Surg Am.* 2006;88:9-17.
9. Goldstein RY, Otsuka NY, Egol KE. Re-displacement of extraphyseal distal radius fractures following initial reduction in skeletally mature patients. *Bull Hosp Jt Dis.* 2013;71:132-137.
10. Alemdargou KB, Iltar S, Cimen O, et al. Risk factors in redisplacement of distal radial fractures in children. *J Bone Joint Surg Am.* 2008;90:1224-1230.
11. Garg NK, Ballal MS, Malek RA, et al. Use of elastic stable intramedullary nailing for treating unstable forearm fractures in children. *J Trauma.* 2008;65(1):109-115.
12. Bae DS. Pediatric distal radius and forearm fractures. *J Hand Surg.* 2008;33(10):1911-1923.
13. Vorlat P, De Boeck H. Bowing fractures of the forearm in children: a long-term follow-up. *Clin Orthop Relat Res.* 2003;413:233-237.

58 Italian Twins: Monteggia and Galeazzi Fractures

ROBERT VEZZETTI, MD, FAAP, FACEP

Case Presentation

A 4-year-old male presents with right forearm pain after falling while in a "bouncy house." Apparently, the child was in the house with several other children and had a witnessed fall onto the arm. The parents noted that he had swelling to his right elbow. There is no other reported injury, and Emergency Medical Services applied a temporary splint and gave the child intranasal fentanyl (2 µg/kg) for pain management.

His physical examination is significant for right elbow pain and swelling. He has limited range of motion of the forearm at the elbow but he does not appear to have shoulder, upper arm, wrist, hand, or digit injury. He is grossly neurovascularly intact.

Imaging Considerations

PLAIN RADIOGRAPHY

Plain radiography is an appropriate imaging modality to utilize in patients with suspected skeletal injury. It is important to obtain adequate imaging, which includes anterior-posterior (AP) and lateral views of the entire forearm and elbow (important for suspected Monteggia fracture) and wrist (important for suspected Galeazzi fracture).[1,2]

COMPUTED TOMOGRAPHY (CT)

CT does not generally play a role in the evaluation of patients with suspected Monteggia or Galeazzi fracture. CT may be indicated if injury at either the radiocapitellar or radioulnar joints is suspected but not confirmed on initial plain radiographs or if the injury is complex (e.g., comminuted fracture).

MAGNETIC RESONANCE IMAGING (MRI)

This modality is generally not indicated in the initial evaluation of musculoskeletal injury. If there is a complex injury or neurologic symptoms, then MRI may be indicated; consultation with a pediatric orthopedic specialist would be advisable in these cases.

Imaging Findings

Plain radiographs of the patient's right forearm, including AP and lateral views, were obtained and are provided here. There is a transverse fracture through the proximal to mid diaphysis of the right ulna, superimposed upon a bowing

fracture of the ulnar diaphysis. There is an accompanying radial head dislocation (Figs. 58.1 and 58.2).

While the presence of the splint does obscure some detail, the process of removing the splint was challenging, leading to difficulties imaging the child. If a splint is applied prior to radiography, it should be removed if possible; if this is not able to be accomplished, then imaging should be performed with the best views that the clinical situation will allow.

For comparison, two additional cases are presented here:

The child in Figs. 58.3–58.5 fell while riding her bicycle. These images demonstrate a nondisplaced fracture of the proximal third of the ulnar diaphysis, with anterior dislocation of the radial head, consistent with a Monteggia fracture. Note that the dislocation of the radial head is seen on the lateral view (Fig. 58.3) and not adequately seen on the

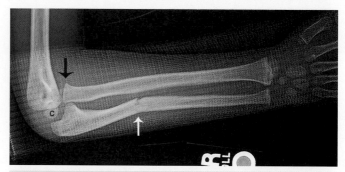

Fig. 58.1 Radiographic view of the forearm in a splint demonstrates a nondisplaced transverse fracture of the junction of the proximal to middle thirds of the diaphysis of the ulna *(white arrow)*, superimposed upon a bowing fracture of the ulna. A radiocapitellar dislocation is also seen, with anterior dislocation of the radial head *(black arrow)*, with respect to the capitellum *(c)*.

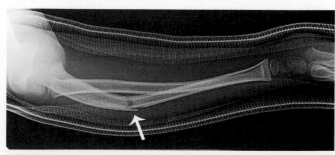

Fig. 58.2 Radiographic view in a splint demonstrates a nondisplaced transverse fracture of the junction of the proximal to middle thirds of the diaphysis of the ulna *(white arrow)*, superimposed upon a bowing fracture of the ulna, with bowing directed posterolaterally.

258

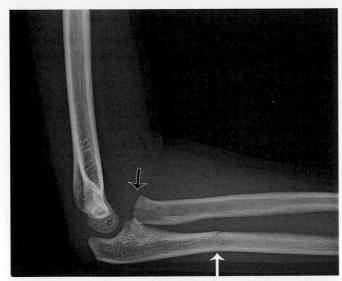

Fig. 58.3 Lateral radiographic view demonstrates a transverse, nondisplaced fracture of the proximal diaphysis of the ulna *(white arrow)*, with minimal anterolateral angulation of the fracture apex. Note anterior dislocation of the radial head *(black arrow)* with respect to the capitellum *(c)*.

oblique and frontal views (Figs. 58.4 and 58.5). This demonstrates the importance of obtaining a good-quality lateral view of the elbow region.

Fig. 58.6 provides a single view demonstrating a Monteggia fracture. Note the dislocated radial head. It is helpful to draw the radiocapitellar line, which is a line drawn

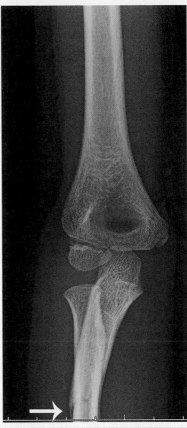

Fig. 58.5 AP radiographic view demonstrates a transverse, nondisplaced fracture of the proximal diaphysis of the ulna *(white arrow)*.

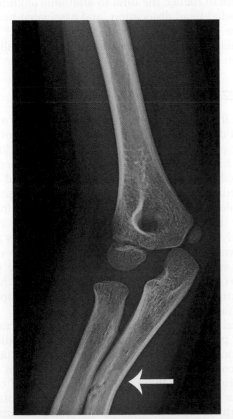

Fig. 58.4 Oblique radiographic view demonstrates a transverse, nondisplaced fracture of the proximal diaphysis of the ulna *(white arrow)*, with minimal anterolateral angulation of the fracture apex.

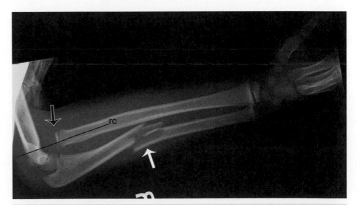

Fig. 58.6 A single lateral view demonstrating a Monteggia fracture, with a mildly displaced ulna fracture *(white arrow)*. Note the dislocated radial head *(black arrow)*. The radiocapitellar line is shown *(rc)*.

centrally in the radius, along the longitudinal axis of the proximal radius, and especially the neck, which should usually intersect the capitellum on all views, but especially on the lateral view; if it does not, this is suggestive of a radiocapitellar dislocation. However, in some normal elbows, and especially in younger patients with lesser ossification of the capitellum, the radiocapitellar line can miss intersection with or be tangential to the ossified capitellum. Therefore, clinical correlation with the injury and clinical evaluation are important.

Case Conclusion

Pediatric Orthopedics was consulted and the child underwent closed reduction of the radial head dislocation, which was accomplished without complication. A cast was placed and follow-up was arranged. Figs. 58.7 and 58.8 demonstrate the appearance of the child's injuries 3 months postinjury. There is osseous union and continuing remodeling at the ulnar fracture site.

MONTEGGIA FRACTURE

The Monteggia facture was first described by Giovanni Batista Monteggia in 1814 and named for him subsequently in 1909.[3,4] Monteggia fracture describes a fracture dislocation: there is a fracture of the ulna associated with disruption of the proximal radioulnar joint and radial head dislocation. Subsequently, the terms *Monteggia lesion* and *Monteggia equivalent injury* have been coined and described.[4,5] Bado's classification was based on the direction of the radial head dislocation, generally associated with the type of ulnar fracture: type I (anterior), type II (posterior), type III (lateral), and type IV (presence of a concomitant radial diaphyseal fracture, in addition to the ulnar fracture).[5,6] Pediatric patients tend to have anterior-lateral, rather than posterior, fracture-dislocation injuries.[6] The distribution of the various types of Monteggia fracture has been found to correlate with age, with Bado type I fractures occurring evenly in preschool and school-age children and type II or III occurring primarily in preschool-age children; overall, type I fractures are the most common.[7]

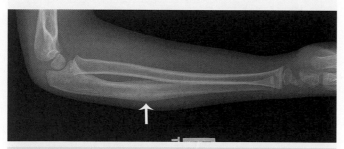

Fig. 58.7 Lateral view shows a healing fracture of the ulna, with mature callus contributing to remodeling *(white arrow)*, with osseous union, 3 months postinjury. No dislocation is seen.

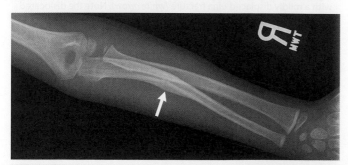

Fig. 58.8 AP view shows a healing fracture of the ulna, with mature callus contributing to remodeling *(white arrow)*, with osseous union, 3 months postinjury.

The ulna fracture may be a plastic deformation, a metaphyseal buckle fracture, a greenstick fracture, or a complete displaced fracture.[6] Treatment usually consists of closed reduction of the ulnar fracture and radial head dislocation followed by immobilization.[6,8,9] Loss of reduction or instability has been reported in approximately 20% of cases, and there is variability in the management of these injuries.[8,10] Some authors have proposed a treatment strategy based on the ulna fracture component with closed reduction recommended for incomplete ulnar fracture and open reduction for complete ulnar fractures, oblique/transverse fractures, comminuted fractures or if the radial head is not able to be reduced.[8–11] It appears that a treatment strategy based on the ulnar fracture component results in excellent outcomes in pediatric patients.[8] Overall complication rate is low, but malunion of the ulna and injury of the interosseous nerve (the most commonly injured nerve in Monteggia fracture) or other nerves are the most commonly reported adverse outcomes.[9]

Monteggia fracture can be difficult to detect, particularly if the ulnar fracture is not complete. In up to 50% of patients, the diagnosis is not made at the initial evaluation and management is controversial in these missed injuries with delayed diagnosis.[12–14] While conservative treatment has been advocated in the past, many authors recommend open reduction since a radial head that has not been reduced is associated with pain and outcomes are good with open reduction, although residual movement restriction has been reported.[14,15]

There are several factors associated with a poor prognosis. Failure to reduce the ulna to anatomic alignment, persistent radial head dislocation, and associated nerve damage have been implicated in poor outcome.[9] Chronic Monteggia fracture-dislocation should be surgically treated with open reduction.[9]

GALEAZZI FRACTURE

This is a fracture of the radius associated with a radioulnar joint dislocation. This fracture is not common in the pediatric population.[7,16] The fracture is named for Italian surgeon Riccardo Galeazzi. Galeazzi fractures account for a reported 1% to 3% of forearm fractures and often go unrecognized;[16,17] in one series, 41% of these injuries went undetected.[17] The location of the radius fracture is typically the distal to middle third of the bone. The most commonly used classification of this fracture is the Letts and Rowani classification system, which also describes Galeazzi variants.[9,18,19] In skeletally immature patients, there is a Galeazzi equivalent fracture, in which the associated disruption at the distal radioulnar joint appears as distal ulnar epiphysiolysis.[19]

Galeazzi injuries are generally treated conservatively in pediatric patients (as opposed to the adult population, in whom conservative management is often associated with poor outcomes), with closed reduction followed by immobilization. However, if there is instability, failure of closed reduction or if there is suspected extensor tendon entrapment, then operative repair is indicated.[1,9,16] Complications are not common, but there is a small risk of radial nonunion or recurrent subluxation; the complication rate is increased with delayed diagnosis or improper immobilization.[1,9]

IMAGING PEARLS

1. Plain radiography is the imaging modality of choice for musculoskeletal trauma.
2. Two views, anterior-posterior and lateral, should be obtained of the forearm.
3. Ensure adequate pain control in order to optimize imaging. If a splint has been applied, removal prior to imaging should be done if possible.
4. A Monteggia injury involves an ulna fracture with radial head dislocation, while a Galeazzi injury involves a radial fracture (typically distal third) with radioulnar joint dislocation. As such, the elbow and wrist should be adequately visualized on imaging to evaluate for these injury patterns.

References

1. Giannoulis FS, Sotereanos DG. Galeazzi fractures and dislocations. *Hand Clin.* 2007;23(2):153-163.
2. Nicolaidis SC, Hildreth DH, Lichtman DM. Acute injuries of the distal radioulnar joint. *Hand Clin.* 2000;16(3):449-459.
3. Andjelković S, Vučković Č, Milutinović S, et al. Giovanni Battista Monteggia (1762–1815). *Srp Arh Celok Lek.* 2015;143(1-2):105-107.
4. Rehim SA, Maynard MA, Sebastin SJ, et al. Monteggia fracture dislocations: a historical review. *J Hand Surg Am.* 2014;39(7):1384-1394.
5. Bado JL. The Monteggia lesion. *Clin Orthop Relat Res.* 1967;50:71-86.
6. Ring D. Monteggia fractures. *Orthop Clin North Am.* 2013;44(1):59-66.
7. Joeris A, Lutz N, Blumenthal A, et al. The AO pediatric comprehensive classification of long bone fractures (PCCF). *Acta Orthop.* 2017;88(2):123-128.
8. Ramski DE, Hennrikus WP, Bae DS, et al. Pediatric Monteggia fractures: a multicenter examination of treatment strategy and early clinical and radiographic results. *J Pediatr Orthop.* 2015;35(2):115-120.
9. Rodríguez-Merchán EC. Pediatric fractures of the forearm. *Clin Orthop Relat Res.* 2005;4(32):65-72.
10. Leonidou A, Pagkalos J, Lepetsos P, et al. Pediatric Monteggia fractures: a single-center study of the management of 40 patients. *J Pediatr Orthop.* 2012;32(4):352-356.
11. Ring D, Rhim R, Carpenter C, et al. Isolated radial shaft fractures are more common than Galeazzi fractures. *J Hand Surg Am.* 2006;31(1):17-21.
12. Gleeson AP, Beattie TF. Monteggia fracture-dislocation in children. *J Accid Emerg Med.* 1994;11(3):192-194.
13. David-West KS, Wilson NI, Sherlock DA, et al. Missed Monteggia injuries. *Injury.* 2005;36(10):1206-1209.
14. Lincoln TT, Mubarak SJ. 'Isolated' traumatic radial head dislocation. *J Pediatr Orthop.* 1994;14(4): 454-457.
15. Freedman L, Luk K, Leong JC. Radial head reduction after a missed Monteggia fracture: brief report. *J Bone Joint Surg Br.* 1988;70(5):846-847.
16. Eberl R, Singer G, Schalamon J, et al. Galeazzi lesions in children and adolescents: treatment and outcome. *Clin Orthop Relat Res.* 2008;466(7):1705-1709.
17. Walsh HP, McLaren CA, Owen R. Galeazzi fractures in children. *J Bone Joint Surg Br.* 1987;69(5):730-793.
18. Letts M, Rowhani N. Galeazzi-equivalent injuries of the wrist in children. *J Pediatr Orthop.* 1993;13(5):561-566.
19. Little JT, Klionsky NB, Chaturvedi A, et al. Pediatric distal forearm and wrist injury: an imaging review. *Radiographics.* 2014;34(2):472-490.

59 Bones Out of Place? Wrist Fractures

ANNA SCHLECHTER, MD

Case Presentation

An 11-year-old male presents with left wrist pain and swelling 3 days after he fell while playing soccer. Apparently, in the course of the game, he fell on his outstretched left arm. After the injury, he continued to play but later in the day he noted pain and swelling to the left wrist. He denies neck, shoulder, elbow, upper arm, hand, or digit pain. He denies back pain.

Physical examination reveals a well-appearing patient, in no distress, with age-appropriate vital signs. He has obvious swelling to the left wrist and there is pain with palpation of the distal radius and ulna; this pain is reproduced with movement of the wrist. He has no shoulder, upper arm, elbow, or hand tenderness or swelling and there is full range of motion at these areas. His radial pulse is strong with good capillary refill. He is grossly neurovascularly intact.

Imaging Considerations

PLAIN RADIOGRAPHY

This is the initial imaging testing of choice for suspected wrist fractures. Exposure to ionizing radiation is low and the modality is readily and widely available. Two views (anteroposterior and lateral) should be obtained, although an oblique view may be helpful if a fracture is suspected but cannot be completely visualized on two-view imaging.

ULTRASOUND

This modality is advantageous given the lack of radiation and rapidity. Ultrasound has been demonstrated to be effective in identifying wrist fractures, including when performed by physicians with minimal ultrasound experience.[1]

COMPUTED TOMOGRAPHY

This modality is not initially employed but may be utilized to better visualize complex fractures. Consultation with a pediatric orthopedic specialist is appropriate prior to obtaining computed tomography imaging.

MAGNETIC RESONANCE IMAGING (MRI)

This modality is not a first-line imaging test. If there is a complex fracture, concern for neurovascular compromise, concern for an infectious process, or concern for an oncologic process, use of MRI may be appropriate. Consultation with a pediatric orthopedic specialist is appropriate prior to obtaining MRI.

Imaging Findings

The patient had plain radiography of his wrist, including anteroposterior, lateral, and oblique views. These images demonstrate a subtle Salter-Harris type II fracture of the distal left radius with minimal posterior displacement of the distal fragment; there is also a Salter-Harris type I fracture of the distal left ulna that is anatomically aligned. Soft tissue swelling surrounds the fracture sites (Figs. 59.1 and 59.2).

Case Conclusion

The patient was placed in a sugar tong splint and arrangements were made to follow-up with Pediatric Orthopedics. He kept his appointment 1 week later and at that time was placed in a short arm cast. Four weeks later, the cast was removed and a Velcro wrist splint was applied, which was worn for several weeks more. He recovered uneventfully. Interestingly, he was seen approximately 1 year later for a

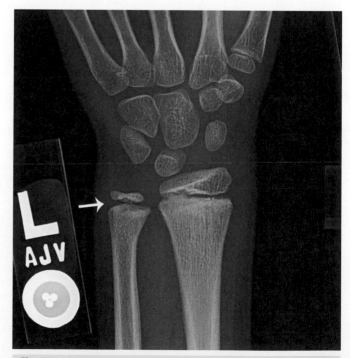

Fig. 59.1 Anteroposterior view shows Salter-Harris type I fracture of the distal ulna, with widening of the growth plate *(arrow)*. The distal radial fracture is not well seen on this view.

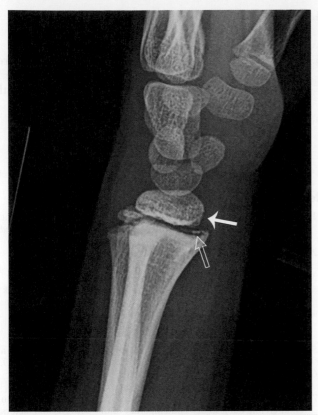

Fig. 59.2 Lateral view shows Salter-Harris type II fracture of the distal radius, with subtle fracture lucency in the distal radial metaphysis *(open arrow)* and mild dorsal/posterior displacement of the distal radial epiphysis *(white arrow)* compared to the metaphysis.

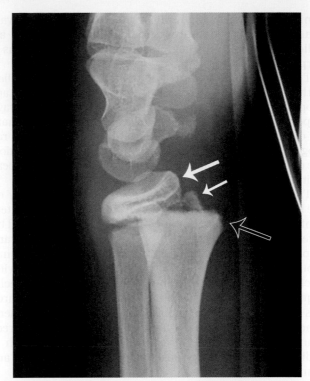

Fig. 59.3 Lateral view demonstrates a Salter-Harris type II fracture of the distal radius. The distal fracture fragment is displaced posteriorly and rotated and consists of the distal radial epiphysis *(large white arrow)* and the triangular-shaped distal metaphyseal fragment *(small white arrow)*. The donor site for the metaphyseal fragment, and the site of metaphyseal fracture, is marked by the *open arrow*.

second left wrist injury he sustained while falling during a football game. Imaging at this visit demonstrated a new, acute Salter-Harris type II fracture of the left distal radius with posterior displacement of the distal fragment (Fig. 59.3). This time, the fracture was reduced in the emergency department by Pediatric Orthopedics under sedation, a cast was placed, and the patient was discharged with close observation and follow-up.

Wrist fractures include fractures of the distal radial metaphysis, fractures of the radial physis, distal ulnar fractures, and carpal fractures including scaphoid (navicular) fractures, triquetral fractures, and hamate fractures.

Fractures of the distal radius are the most common fracture in children and adolescents, accounting for approximately 45% of wrist fractures.[2] This type of fracture occurs most frequently during early adolescence. The mechanism of injury is usually a fall on a hyperextended wrist. The most common type of distal radial metaphyseal fracture is the torus (buckle) fracture, wherein a single cortex buckles or has plastic deformation. Greenstick fractures—wherein one cortex breaks completely while the other has plastic deformation—are also frequently seen. Metaphyseal chip or "corner fractures" of the radius in infants are highly specific for child abuse and warrant further investigation.[3]

Physeal fractures of the radius are uncommon but should be considered during the adolescent growth spurt.[4] These are especially important to identify as they may lead to premature closure and growth arrest at the injury site.

Patients with nondisplaced Salter-Harris type I physeal fractures of the distal radius or ulna will have normal radiographs initially but have bony tenderness and may have displacement or obscuration of the volar fat pad on the lateral view. Radiographs obtained 7–10 days after injury may show irregularity of osseous margins adjacent to the physis consistent with bone resorption or may show periosteal new bone. With time, sclerosis often develops in the adjacent metaphysis, these signs of a healing response confirming the diagnosis.

Distal ulnar fractures usually occur in conjunction with a distal radial fracture, which dictates management. Two important variations to be aware of are fractures through the base of the ulnar styloid that can be associated with triangular fibrocartilage complex instability and the Galeazzi equivalent, wherein a distal ulnar physeal fracture occurs with a radial shaft fracture (*without* disruption of the distal radioulnar joint as is seen in a Galeazzi fracture-dislocation).[5,6] The Galeazzi equivalent injury frequently requires operative management (see Chapter 58 on Galeazzi fractures).

The most common type of carpal fracture is fracture of the scaphoid (navicular). These usually occur in the older adolescent, as the carpal bones remain predominantly cartilaginous until late childhood and early adolescence, and are associated with tenderness in the anatomic snuffbox and pain with radial deviation. About one-third will initially present with chronic nonunion.[7] These fractures may not be visualized in a standard wrist series, and a posteroanterior scaphoid view with 30 degrees of ulnar deviation may aid in visualization. If radiographs remain normal but clinical suspicion is high, MRI or bone scan may be warranted.[8] Hamate fractures should be assessed with an oblique view with 45 degrees of supination as well as a carpal tunnel view.

The majority of fractures of the wrist can be identified with adequate history, physical examination, and the appropriate plain radiographs as delineated earlier. It is always important to obtain multiple views of the wrist to evaluate for displacement and angulation of fractures.[9] If initial radiographs are normal but history and physical examination are concerning for fracture, appropriate splinting and repeat of imaging in 1–2 weeks are warranted.

Treatment of these injuries depends on the severity of the fracture. Most injuries heal well without operative intervention, but consideration for surgical treatment should be given to those patients with open fractures or significant displacement.[10] Attempts at reduction and fracture manipulation should be kept to a minimum.[10] Patients with buckle fractures heal extremely well; immobilization techniques vary from Velcro wrist splints to casting, but regardless of the method of immobilization, further displacement is not the norm and follow-up imaging is not routinely recommended with these injuries.[11,12] Consultation with a pediatric orthopedic specialist is appropriate when there are management questions.

IMAGING PEARLS

1. Fractures of the distal radius are the most common fracture seen in children and adolescents.
2. Metaphyseal chip or "corner" fractures in infants are highly specific injuries for child abuse and warrant further investigation.
3. Physeal fractures of the radius can lead to premature closure and impaired growth at the injury site. Salter-Harris type I fractures may not be visible on initial x-rays. Children with suspected Salter-Harris type I fractures should be splinted and have repeat imaging performed in approximately 1 week.

4. The Galeazzi equivalent is a distal radius fracture with concomitant distal ulnar physeal fracture that frequently requires surgical intervention.
5. Scaphoid fractures are the most common carpal fracture and may be missed on a standard wrist series. They are best imaged with a posterior-anterior scaphoid view with 30 degrees of ulnar deviation.
6. For nearly all wrist fractures, if history and physical examination are concerning for fracture but none is visualized on x-ray, the patient should be splinted and have repeat images performed in 1–2 weeks.

References

1. Hedelin H, Tingstrom C, Hebelka H, et al. Minimal training sufficient to diagnose pediatric wrist fractures with ultrasound. *Crit Ultrasound J.* 2017;9(1):11.
2. Rodríguez-Merchán EC. Pediatric fractures of the forearm. *Clin Orthop Relat Res.* 2005;432:65-72.
3. Swischuk LE. Radiographic signs of skeletal trauma. In: Ludwig S, Korbnerg A, eds. *Child Abuse: A Medical Reference.* 2nd ed. New York Churchill-Livingstone, 1992.
4. Gill TJ IV, Micheli LJ. The immature athlete. Common injuries and overuse syndromes of the elbow and wrist. *Clin Sports Med.* 1996;15(2):401-423.
5. Abid A, Accadbled F, Kany J, et al. Ulnar styloid fracture in children: a retrospective study of 46 cases. *J Pediatr Orthop B.* 2008;17(1):15-19.
6. Bae DS, Waters PM. Pediatric distal radius fractures and triangular fibrocartilage complex injuries. *Hand Clin.* 2006;22(1):43-45.
7. Gholson JJ, Bae DS, Zurakowski D, Waters PM. Scaphoid fractures in children and adolescents: contemporary injury patterns and factors influencing time to union. *J Bone Joint Surg Am.* 2011;93(13):1210-1219.
8. Guly HR. Injuries initially misdiagnosed as sprained wrist (beware the sprained wrist). *Emerg Med J.* 2002;19(1)19:41-42.
9. Parmelee-Peters K, Eathorne SW. The wrist: common injuries and management. *Prim Care.* 2005;32(1):35-70.
10. Liao JCY, Chong AKS. Pediatric hand and wrist fractures. *Clin Plast Surg.* 2019;46(3):425-436.
11. Riera-Alvarez L, Pons-Villanueva J. Do wrist buckle fractures in children need follow-up? Buckle fractures' follow-up. *J Pediatr Orthop B.* 2019;28(6):553-554.
12. Pulos N, Kalar S. Hand and wrist injuries: common problems and solutions. *Clin Sports Med.* 2018;37(2):217-243.

60 *Snuffbox? Scaphoid Fractures*

GUYON HILL, MD, and MARY TEELER, BS

Case Presentation

A 16-year-old female presents to the emergency department with complaints of right wrist and hand pain following a fall on an outstretched hand during sports practice after school. Vital signs are age appropriate and her physical examination is significant for tenderness in the anatomic snuffbox and the radial portion of the wrist. Grip strength and range of motion in the wrist are both reduced in the injured hand. She is neurovascularly intact in the right upper extremity and has no other significant findings on physical examination.

Imaging Considerations

Imaging is often obtained in acute traumatic orthopedic injuries. Plain radiographs are often the first-line imaging modality, although additional modalities including computed tomography (CT) and magnetic resonance imaging (MRI) may be required.

PLAIN RADIOGRAPHY

In the case of a possible scaphoid fracture, a standard wrist series should be obtained. Plain radiographs should be the initial imaging modality; however, scaphoid fractures may go undetected on initial plain radiography, with false-negative reads on the initial imaging reported as high as 20%–54%.[1–3] Scaphoid fractures may not be visualized on a standard three-view wrist series but are best seen on specialized scaphoid views; one of these is an anteroposterior scaphoid view taken with the wrist in full pronation and with 30 degrees of ulnar deviation, but other scaphoid views include posteroanterior views, also with ulnar deviation.

MAGNETIC RESONANCE IMAGING

MRI has greater sensitivity and specificity for scaphoid fracture than CT does and MRI shows greater accuracy than other modalites do.[4,5] MRI can detect bone marrow edema within hours of the injury. MRI is also able to accurately detect injuries in the other surrounding osseous and soft tissues.

COMPUTED TOMOGRAPHY

CT is sensitive and highly specific for the diagnosis of scaphoid fractures. This imaging technique can be used immediately following the trauma; however, CT is not as sensitive as MRI or bone scan for scaphoid fracture and cannot as conclusively rule out a scaphoid fracture.[5] CT can be useful in patients who have contraindications to receiving an MRI.

BONE SCAN (BONE SCINTIGRAPHY)

While skeletal scintigraphy is an additional option for identifying a scaphoid fracture, it must be performed at least 72 hours postinjury. It is also important to consider that while bone scan sensitivity for scaphoid fracture is the highest at 99%, it only has an 86% specificity.[5] Bone scan also requires the injection of radioactive material and has the highest radiation exposure of the imaging options, which is a significant consideration, especially in the pediatric population. Bone scans have the benefit of being able to detect other bony injuries.

Case Conclusion

Plain radiographs of the wrist were obtained in the emergency department. These images demonstrate a nondisplaced transverse fracture of the scaphoid (Figs. 60.1–60.3). The other visualized bones are normal.

The patient was placed in a thumb spica splint and referred to Pediatric Orthopedics. Follow-up imaging demonstrated satisfactory healing of the fracture.

The scaphoid (navicular) bone is the most commonly fractured carpal bone and one of the most common injuries of the upper extremities. The size and shape of the bone as well as the location in the proximal portion of the hand can make diagnosis more difficult. In addition, the unique and tenuous blood supply of the bone can predispose it to chronic nonunion if there is a delay in diagnosis. In the pediatric population, scaphoid fractures are less common in children less than 10 years old.[6] The classic clinical presentation consists of tenderness of the scaphoid or anatomic snuffbox, decreased range of motion in flexion and extension of the wrist, decreased grip strength, and pain with radial deviation of the wrist. Patients can also have pain with axial loading of the thumb or resisted supination of the forearm. The most common mechanism of injury is a fall on an outstretched hand, but fractures of the scaphoid can also occur with direct axial compression.

Plain radiographs should be the first study of choice; however, initial radiographs may be normal. If there is a clinical suspicion of a scaphoid fracture based on tenderness in the anatomic snuffbox, the extremity should be splinted and follow-up plain radiographs obtained in 10–14 days, at which time a fracture should be evident. Mounting evidence suggests that obtaining advanced imaging early can avoid unnecessary immobilization and improve outcomes while

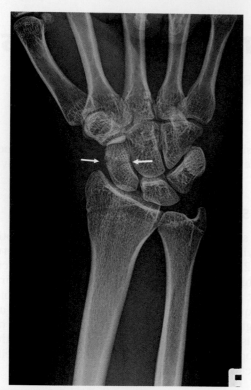

Fig. 60.1 Posteroanterior (PA) radiographic view of the wrist demonstrates a nondisplaced transverse scaphoid fracture, through the distal waist *(arrows)*. The fracture is seen well here on PA view and on oblique images (Fig. 60.3), but not visualized on the lateral view (Fig 60.2).

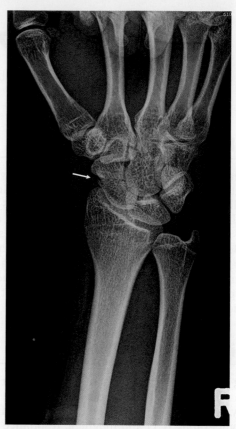

Fig. 60.3 Oblique view of the wrist demonstrates a nondisplaced transverse scaphoid fracture, through the distal waist *(arrow)*. The fracture is seen well on the PA (Fig. 60.1) image and here on the oblique image, but not visualized on the lateral view (Fig 60.2).

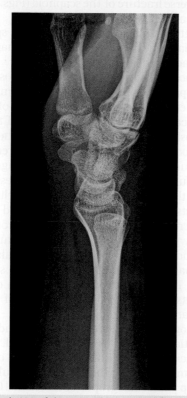

Fig. 60.2 Lateral view of the wrist. The scaphoid fracture is seen well on PA (Fig. 60.1) and oblique images (Fig. 60.3), but not visualized here on the lateral view.

reducing overall cost.[1,7–9] If available, a CT, MRI, or bone scan may make a definitive diagnosis earlier, but each modality has benefits as well as limitations.[10] Both CT and MRI can be conducted immediately after the injury while bone scan should not be used until 72 hours postinjury. Early diagnosis or suspicion of a scaphoid fracture is crucial as delayed treatment makes nonunion more likely to occur. Up to one-third of pediatric patients will be found to have a chronic nonunion at initial presentation.[11] Other complications of scaphoid fracture include carpal instability and avascular necrosis, which is less common in children than adults.[12]

Management options for scaphoid fracture include operative treatment, immobilization, and direct functional treatment.[10] If a patient has imaging that does not reveal a fracture, early functional treatment can be started using an elastic bandage or orthosis, with repeat imaging if clinically indicated.[10] Immobilization is indicated for stable fractures, although this can be difficult owing to the bone's location, as extremity movement will directly impact the bone.[10] There are several appropriate options for immobilization, with and without thumb inclusion, and no one method has proven superior over the others; duration of immobilization is generally 6 weeks.[10] Operative treatment is indicated for unstable fractures.[10]

IMAGING PEARLS

1. Initial plain radiographs are helpful if they clearly indicate a scaphoid fracture but a significant portion may be normal.
2. If initial radiographs are negative but a scaphoid fracture is suspected, immobilization should be provided until either repeat imaging or advanced imaging such as CT, MRI, or a bone scan can confirm or exclude the diagnosis.
3. Early use of advanced imaging such as MRI, CT, or bone scan to make a definitive diagnosis of scaphoid fracture is a cost-effective means to reduce unnecessary immobilization.
4. MRI is overall the most accurate method to definitively diagnose a scaphoid fracture if initial radiographs are negative but there are limitations in terms of cost and availability.

References

1. Sabbagh MD, Morsy M, Moran SL. Diagnosis and management of acute scaphoid fractures. *Hand Clin.* 2019;35(3):259-269.
2. Waeckerle JF. A prospective study identifying the sensitivity of radiographic findings and the efficacy of clinical findings in carpal navicular fractures. *Ann Emerg Med.* 1987;16(7):733-737.
3. Jørgsholm P, Thomsen N, Besjakov J, et al. MRI shows a high incidence of carpal fractures in children with posttraumatic radial-sided wrist tenderness. *Acta Orthop.* 2016;87(5):533-537.
4. Carpenter CR, Pines JM, Schuur JD, et al. Adult scaphoid fracture. *Acad Emerg Med.* 2014;21(2):101-121.
5. Mallee WH, Wang J, Poolman RW, et al. Computed tomography versus magnetic resonance imaging versus bone scintigraphy for clinically suspected scaphoid fractures in patients with negative plain radiographs. *Cochrane Database Syst Rev.* 2015;2015(6):CD010023.
6. Ahmed I, Ashton F, Tay WK, et al. The pediatric fracture of the scaphoid in patients aged 13 years and under: an epidemiological study. *J Pediatr Orthop.* 2014;34(2):150-154.
7. Karl JW, Swart E, Strauch RJ. Diagnosis of occult scaphoid fractures: a cost-effectiveness analysis. *J Bone Joint Surg Am.* 2015;97(22):1860-1868.
8. Rua T, Malhotra B, Vijayanathan S, et al. Clinical and cost implications of using immediate MRI in the management of patients with a suspected scaphoid fracture and negative radiographs results from the SMaRT trial. *Bone Joint J.* 2019;101-B(8):984-994.
9. Yin ZG, Zhang JB, Gong KT. Cost-effectiveness of diagnostic strategies for suspected scaphoid fractures. *J Orthop Trauma.* 2015;29(8):e245-e252.
10. Rhemrev SJ, Ootes D, Beeres FJ, et al. Current methods of diagnosis and treatment of scaphoid fractures. *Int J Emerg Med.* 2011;4:4.
11. Gholson JJ, Bae DS, Zurakowski D, et al. Scaphoid fractures in children and adolescents: contemporary injury patterns and factors influencing time to union. *J Bone Joint Surg Am.* 2011;93(13):1210-1219.
12. Stoner MJ, Dietrich AM. Injuries of the upper extremities. In: Tenenbein M, Macias CG, Sharieff QG, Yamamoto LG, Schafermeyer R, eds. *Stange and Schafermeyer's Pediatric Emergency Medicine*, 5th ed. New York: McGraw-Hill Education, 2019:197-208.

61 Punchin' Out: Fifth Metacarpal (Boxer's) Fracture

ROBERT VEZZETTI, MD, FAAP, FACEP

Case Presentation

A 15-year-old male presents with left hand pain after becoming angry and punching a wall. He did this several hours ago and his only complaint is medial hand pain; he denies digit, wrist, forearm, or elbow pain. He denies numbness or weakness. This is the second time he has sustained this injury. However, he was not seen the first time because he and his parents felt the injury was minimal but they both want to make sure that "nothing is broken this time."

Imaging Considerations

PLAIN RADIOGRAPHY

A complete hand series consisting of posteroanterior (PA), lateral, and oblique views is standard when evaluating pediatric hand injuries. Important considerations are the degree of angulation, any associated injuries, and if rotation is present, as rotational deformities can result in significant long-term deformities. Intraarticular extension or involvement of a growth plate should also be noted. Plain radiographs of the affected hand are generally sufficient to identify the degree of metacarpal injury. If clinically indicated, appropriate radiographs of the wrist, forearm, and elbow should also be obtained.

Consideration should be given to physeal injuries when reviewing pediatric hand imaging. The physis is a vulnerable location in pediatric bones, particularly in young children, who tend to injure the physis by shear forces, whereas older patients (such as adolescents) tend to have compressive injuries, preserving the physis and injuring the shaft.[1] If there is question regarding the presence of a fracture, comparative hand imaging may be employed but is rarely necessary.

ULTRASOUND (US)

US has become increasingly utilized in the acute care setting to identify fractures in the adult population.[2] In one prospective study, US identified 38 of 39 fifth metacarpal fractures with a sensitivity of 97.4% and a specificity of 92.9%.[3] However, patients included in this study were all over the age of 14 years. In another study of approximately 200 children aged 2 to 17 years, reported sensitivity and specificity for detecting hand fracture by US were 91% and 97%, respectively.[4] Several studies in the adult population have obtained similar results[5]; large prospective studies in the pediatric population are lacking. While US has potential for evaluating suspected hand fractures, further study is needed in the pediatric population.

COMPUTED TOMOGRAPHY (CT) AND MAGNETIC RESONANCE IMAGING (MRI)

While CT and MRI may be utilized to evaluate for specific injuries of the hand and wrist (e.g., occult scaphoid fracture) in the outpatient setting, these are of limited utility in the acute setting for suspected metacarpal fractures.

Imaging Findings

Plain radiography of the left hand, including posteroanterior, lateral, and oblique views, is obtained. The hand series demonstrates an acute fracture of the fifth metacarpal (Figs. 61.1–and 61.3) with volar angulation of the distal fracture fragment. There is a callus noted, evidence of a healing previous fracture.

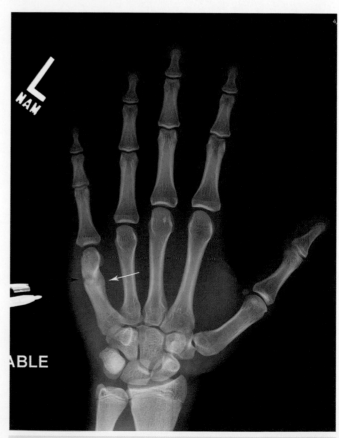

Fig. 61.1 Posteroanterior view of the left hand demonstrates a fifth metacarpal fracture *(red arrow)*, with adjacent callus indicating a prior healed fracture *(yellow arrow)*.

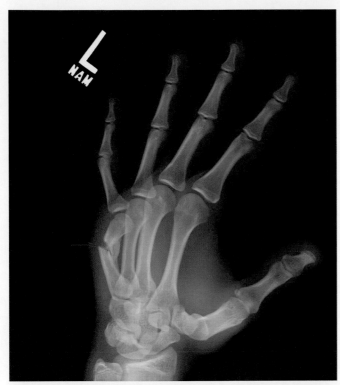

Fig. 61.2 Oblique view demonstrates an acute fracture *(arrow)* with volar angulation of the distal fracture fragment, superimposed upon a healing previous fracture.

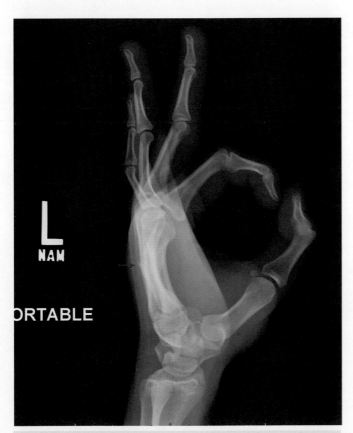

Fig. 61.3 Lateral view of the injured hand. The fifth metacarpal fracture is minimally evident *(arrow)* but there is no sign of gross displacement.

Case Conclusion

The patient was placed in an ulnar gutter splint and follow-up with Pediatric Hand Surgery was arranged. Adequate pain control was ensured. Prior to his discharge, the patient was screened for any potential psychiatric issues, such as suicidal ideation. The patient was seen in the Hand Clinic and was treated with cast immobilization and did not require operative reduction.

Boxer's fractures are far more common in males of this age group, typically in the late teenage years and early twenties, and is the most common hand fracture.[6] A typical mechanism, as the name implies, is punching a wall or hard object or when a patient is involved in a fistfight, although accidental trauma is also reported.[6–8] In pediatric patients, hand fractures are not uncommon and have increased in frequency; many times, the mechanism involves high-impact sports.[8–11] These fractures may be subcapital (neck), diaphyseal, or basal in location.

Most boxer's fractures can be treated conservatively.[12–14] Splinting with an ulnar gutter splint is indicated, along with referral to a qualified hand or orthopedic surgeon. Reduction, when clinically indicated, may be achieved surgically with K (Kirschner) wires and often is performed once edema has improved.[13] Compliance with splint or casting varies among pediatric patients and should be tailored to the developmental age of the child, but in most instances, compliance with immobilization can be achieved.[1,15]

> **IMAGING PEARLS**
>
> 1. Plain radiography, including PA, lateral, and oblique views of the affected hand is sufficient in the majority of patients with suspected fifth metacarpal (boxer's) fractures.
> 2. US has proven effective in the identification of fifth metacarpal fractures, but studies in younger pediatric populations are lacking.
> 3. Most boxer's fractures can be treated with immobilization. Referral to a qualified orthopedic or hand surgeon for definitive management is recommended.

References

1. Nellans KW, Chung KC. Pediatric hand fractures. *Hand Clin.* 2013;29(4):569-578.
2. Champagne N, Eadie L, Regan L, et al. The effectiveness of ultrasound in the detection of fractures in adults with suspected upper and lower limb injury: a systematic review and subgroup meta-analysis. *BMC Emerg Med.* 2019;19(1):1-15.
3. Aksay E, Yesilaras M, Kılıc TY, et al. Sensitivity and specificity of bedside ultrasonography in the diagnosis of fractures of the fifth metacarpal. *Emerg Med J.* 2015;32(3):221-225.
4. Neri E, Barbi E, Rabach I, et al. Diagnostic accuracy of ultrasonography for hand bony fractures in paediatric patients. *Arch Dis Child.* 2014;99(12):1087-1090.
5. Kocaoglu S, Ozhasenekler A, Icme F, et al. The role of ultrasonography in the diagnosis of metacarpal fractures. *Am J Emerg Med.* 2016;34(9):1868-1871.
6. Gudmundsen TE, Borgen L. Fractures of the fifth metacarpal. *Acta Radiol.* 2009;50(3):296-300.
7. Altizer L. Boxer's fracture. *Orthop Nurs.* 2006;25:271-273.

8. Sanjna SS, Lynne R, Smith GA. Epidemiology of pediatric hand injuries presenting to United States emergency departments, 1990 to 2009. *J Trauma Acute Care Surg*. 2012;72(6):1688-1694.
9. Williams AA, Lochner HV. Pediatric hand and wrist fractures. *Curr Rev Musculoskelet Med*. 2013;6(1):18-25.
10. Bredan, K. Another angry adolescent: another boxer's fracture? *Pediatr Emerg Care*. 2014;30(8):558-560.
11. Chew EM, Chong AKS. Hand fractures in children: epidemiology and misdiagnosis in a tertiary referral hospital. *J Hand Surg Am*. 2012;37(8):1684-1688.
12. Galanakis I, Aligizakis A, Kantonis P, et al. Treatment of closed metacarpal fractures using percutaneous transverse fixation with Kirschner wires. *J Trauma*. 2003;55(3):509-513.
13. Malik S, Rosenberg N. *Fifth Metacarpal Fractures (Boxer's Fracture)*. Treasure Island, FL: StatPearls; 2019.
14. Dunn JC, Kusnezov N, Orr JD, et al. The boxer's fracture: splint immobilization is not necessary. *Orthopedics*. 2016;39(3):188-192.
15. Liao JCY, Chong AKS. Pediatric hand and wrist fractures. *Clin Plast Surg*. 2019;46(3):425-436.

62 Pfunny Pfingers: Phalanx Fractures (Dislocations, Etc.)

ROBERT VEZZETTI, MD, FAAP, FACEP

Case Presentation

A 12-year-old male presents with a left fifth phalanx injury (his "pinky" finger). He was jumping on a trampoline and somehow injured the digit; he believes he landed on the digit. Since then, he has had pain and swelling.

His examination reveals a patient complaining of digit pain. There is swelling and tenderness of the left fifth digit at the proximal interphalangeal (PIP) joint with limited range of motion secondary to the pain. He is grossly neurovascularly intact and there is no apparent wrist, forearm, elbow, upper arm, or shoulder injury. He does state he has "hand pain" as well, proximal to his swollen finger.

Imaging Considerations

PLAIN RADIOGRAPHY

This is the imaging modality of choice for the evaluation of phalanx injuries. A minimum of two views (posterior-anterior and lateral) should be utilized, although an oblique view may be useful as well, as some injuries may not easily be visible in two planes; the clinician should consider obtaining an oblique view if there is a strong clinical suspicion and two-view imaging does not demonstrate a fracture.[1]

ULTRASOUND (US)

There has been interest in point-of-care US (POCUS), done at the bedside by emergency physicians, for detecting fractures of the phalanges and hand. This imaging modality has proven to be sensitive and specific in the detection of phalanx fractures in adult patients. Ultrasonography has been shown to be efficacious at detecting other hand fractures such as metacarpal fractures, with reported sensitivities and specificities of 92% and 87%, respectively, in patients aged 5 to 55.[2,3] One study, done in adult patients, demonstrated a sensitivity of 79% and a specificity of 90% utilizing POCUS for proximal and middle phalanx fractures; although, in this study, smaller fractures were more difficult to detect, particularly middle phalanx volar fractures.[4]

Large-scale studies specifically evaluating the efficacy of phalanx fracture detection in the pediatric population using US are lacking. However, the lack of ionizing radiation, availability, and apparent efficacy in the adult population at fracture detection make this modality an attractive imaging option.

COMPUTED TOMOGRAPHY

While computed tomography may be helpful to assess complex fracture injury extent and anatomy, this modality is not indicated for phalanx fractures. If there is an associated complex metacarpal or carpal fracture that requires better radiographic visualization, then computed tomography may be indicated to assist with the management of those fractures.

MAGNETIC RESONANCE IMAGING (MRI)

This modality is not indicated as an initial imaging test for suspected phalanx fractures.

Imaging Findings

Imaging of the left fifth finger was obtained. The images are provided. There is a Salter-Harris type II fracture of the fifth proximal phalanx. There is fracture of the proximal metaphysis of the proximal phalanx, seen as a buckling of the cortex. Although the fracture is nondisplaced, there is volar and radial angulation of the fracture apex (Figs. 62.1–62.3).

Case Conclusion

The child was placed in an ulnar gutter splint and follow-up was arranged with Hand Surgery, after closed reduction. The injury did not require operative intervention.

Phalanx fractures are among the most frequent hand fractures in pediatric patients.[1,5,6] With an incidence of 27 per 1000 patients, these fractures make up the second most common reason to seek fracture care in an emergency setting.[5,7] Injury patterns are associated with age; toddlers and school-age children are more likely to sustain phalanx fractures (often from crush injuries or lacerations) in a home location, whereas older children often have injuries associated with sports activities.[1,5,8]

Management of phalanx fractures depends on fracture location, displacement, and orientation.[5] Fracture type, including the Salter-Harris classification system for fractures involving the growth plate, can aid in management. Most phalanx injuries in pediatric patients can be managed nonoperatively.[6] Generally, lower-grade fractures, such as Salter-Harris types I and II, are managed nonoperatively with closed reduction; types III and IV may require either

271

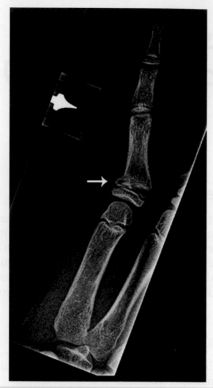

Fig. 62.1 PA view demonstrates a Salter-Harris type II fracture of the fifth proximal phalanx. There is fracture of the proximal metaphysis of the proximal phalanx *(arrow)*. Although the fracture is nondisplaced, there is volar and radial angulation of the fracture apex.

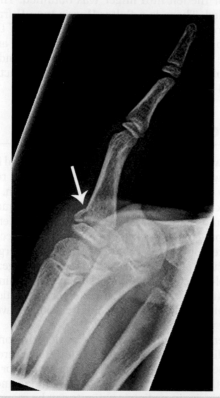

Fig. 62.2 Lateral view demonstrates a Salter-Harris type II fracture of the fifth proximal phalanx. There is fracture of the proximal metaphysis of the proximal phalanx *(arrow)*, seen as a buckling of the dorsal cortex. Although the fracture is nondisplaced, there is volar and radial angulation of the fracture apex.

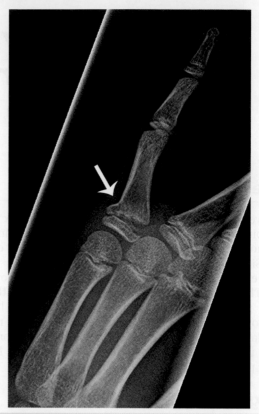

Fig. 62.3 Oblique view demonstrates a Salter-Harris type II fracture of the fifth proximal phalanx. There is fracture of the proximal metaphysis of the proximal phalanx *(arrow)*, seen as a buckling of the cortex medially. Although the fracture is nondisplaced, there is volar and radial angulation of the fracture apex.

closed or open reduction; and type V injuries require surgical consultation.[1] Buddy taping versus splinting has been investigated. A study comparing buddy taping and splinting for fracture management demonstrated that the risk for secondary displacement of extraarticular phalanx fractures (both those requiring closed reduction and those not requiring closed reduction) was low in both groups, with patient satisfaction and comfort higher in the buddy taping group.[9]

Fractures of the base of the phalanx are often Salter-Harris type II fractures[1,5,10] and are among the most common hand injuries in the pediatric population. Due to excellent bone remodeling, these fractures tend to heal quite well. Displaced fractures should have closed reduction attempted, while severe comminution, ligament disruption, and flexor tendon interposition at the fracture site are indications for open operative reduction and fixation.[1,5] Most phalanx fractures are immobilized for 3 weeks.[1] Some authors recommend follow-up plain radiography 3 to 7 days after reduction to ensure that the fracture has not displaced.[1] Proximal phalanx fractures that are displaced and have failed closed reduction should be operatively repaired with pinning, although patient age, along with fracture type and displacement, is a factor in deciding if operative repair is warranted.[11] Pediatric patients who have undergone closed reduction and percutaneous pinning (after failing closed reduction) have been shown to have good functional and cosmetic outcomes.[11]

Fractures of the phalangeal shaft with no or minimal displacement are often treated by buddy taping for several weeks, followed by gradual return to normal range of motion and activity.[1,5,12] Displaced fractures should be reduced (typically by closed reduction), followed by immobilization (often with splinting then casting).[1,5,13] These fractures are usually Salter-Harris type III and typically are immobilized for 3 weeks.[1] Referral for follow-up care to a qualified hand or orthopedic specialist is appropriate.

Fractures that involve the neck of the phalanx are managed based on the degree of displacement. Nondisplaced fractures may be splinted and followed closely, while displaced fractures, due to inherent instability, are usually managed surgically, most often with closed reduction and percutaneous pinning.[5,6,10,14] Interestingly, a small study comparing closed reduction and immobilization versus operative intervention in children demonstrated similar outcomes between the two groups.[15] These injuries occur almost exclusively in the pediatric population.[14,16] In addition to being unstable, these fractures have poor remodeling potential, and if malunion occurs, overlapping of the digits during flexion can occur.[14] Distal finger fractures are usually Salter-Harris type I or II and open fractures are not uncommon, as there are often associated nail injuries, including lacerations of the nailbed and nail avulsion.[1] Consultation with a qualified hand specialist is appropriate for these patients for follow-up care.

Complications of phalanx fractures include cosmetic deformities and impairment of function, including growth arrest (associated with physeal injury), avascular necrosis (if blood supply is disrupted), infection, and arthofibrosis.[1,17] Some fracture types are associated with higher complication rates, including Salter-Harris type IV fractures and Seymour fractures.[18] Phalanx fractures that have malunion may be treated with osteotomy.[1,19]

One particular fracture worth mentioning is the Seymour fracture, first described in 1966.[20,21] This often overlooked fracture, typically a Salter-Harris type I or II, involves the distal phalanx and an associated laceration of the nail matrix with avulsion of the proximal nail plate. This most commonly is due to an axial load injury and often involves the middle finger.[6,14,20,21] This injury results in exposure of the cuticle seal and there is potential for infection. While radiography demonstrates a physeal injury, there may only be dorsal widening of the physis.[14] These fractures should be thoroughly explored and oral antibiotics initiated. Consultation with a qualified hand surgeon is appropriate in these cases.

Another fracture deserving special mention is the volar plate avulsion fracture. This injury occurs when the PIP joint is hyperextended, and the volar plate ligament produces an avulsion fracture at the volar base of the middle phalanx. This fracture is usually managed initially with splinting for a short duration (7 to 10 days is sufficient), followed by early range of motion exercises.[6,22] Prolonged immobilization should be avoided, since healing occurs not by bony union but by fibrous nonunion, and prolonged casting can lead to joint contracture.[6,22]

For comparison, several images of phalanx injuries are provided:

The 17-year-old patient in Figs. 62.4 and 62.5 was involved in a motor vehicle collision. The vehicle's airbag

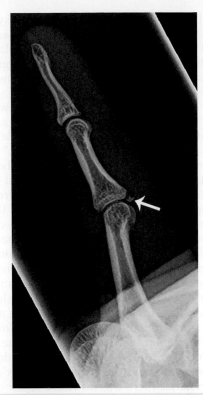

Fig. 62.4 Lateral view shows a volar plate avulsion fracture *(arrow)* of the middle phalanx of the fifth finger at the proximal interphalangeal joint.

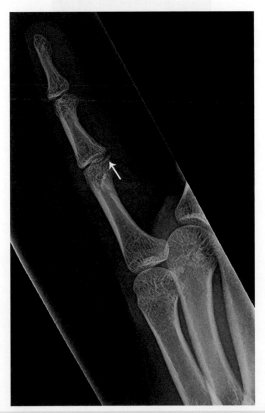

Fig. 62.5 Oblique view shows a volar plate avulsion fracture *(arrow)* of the middle phalanx of the fifth finger at the proximal interphalangeal joint.

deployed and caused his left fifth digit (the "pinky finger") to hyperextend. He presented with pain to the volar side of the digit. Lateral and oblique views show a volar plate avulsion fracture of the middle phalanx of the fifth finger at the PIP joint. He was placed in a finger splint and followed up with Hand Surgery 1 week later.

A 12-year-old had his right index finger "twisted" by a classmate 1 week prior to presentation (Figs. 62.6 and 62.7). He stated that the finger "went to the side" at the PIP joint and the patient "pushed it back into place." Since then, he has had continued swelling and pain at the PIP joint. Imaging demonstrates soft tissue swelling and there is no joint dislocation. A mildly comminuted fracture is seen of the distal diaphysis of the proximal phalanx of the right index finger, with a transverse and an oblique component. There is a small volar separated cortical fragment and surrounding soft tissue swelling, but no significant displacement or angulation of major fracture fragments. This patient was treated with an aluminum splint and buddy taping.

The 2-year-old child in Figs. 62.8 and 62.9 slammed her ring finger in a door. Imaging demonstrates an amputation injury of the soft tissues of the distal tip of the fourth finger, as well as amputation of the distal tuft of the left fourth distal phalanx. The wound was cleaned and dressed, oral antibiotics were initiated, and the child was referred to Hand Surgery, since there was no viable repair option. The patient did well and the wound healed well.

The 16-year-old patient in Figs. 62.10 and 62.11 was attempting to catch a football when his "finger jammed"; he

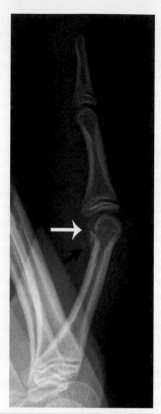

Fig. 62.7 Lateral view shows a mildly comminuted fracture *(white arrow)* of the distal diaphysis of the proximal phalanx of the right index finger, with a transverse and an oblique component. There is a small volar separated cortical fragment *(black arrow)* and surrounding soft tissue swelling, but no significant displacement or angulation of major fracture fragments.

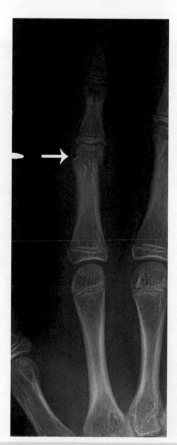

Fig. 62.6 PA view demonstrates a mildly comminuted fracture *(white arrow)* of the distal diaphysis of the proximal phalanx of the right index finger, with a transverse and an oblique component.

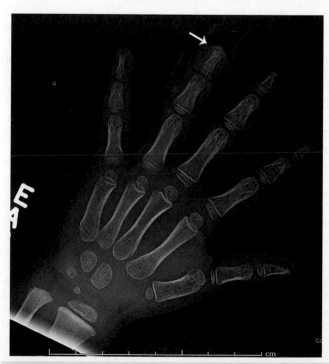

Fig. 62.8 PA view demonstrates an amputation injury of the soft tissues of the distal tip of the fourth finger *(arrow)*, as well as amputation of the distal tuft of the left fourth distal phalanx.

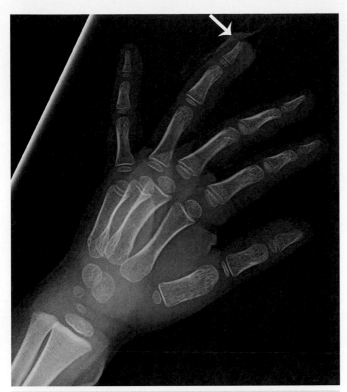

Fig. 62.9 Oblique view shows an amputation injury of the soft tissues of the distal tip of the fourth finger *(arrow)*, as well as amputation of the distal tuft of the left fourth distal phalanx.

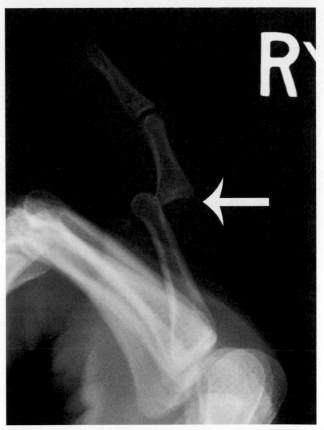

Fig. 62.11 Lateral view shows a dislocation of the little finger proximal interphalangeal joint *(arrow)*, with the middle phalanx dislocated in a dorsal direction. No definite fractures are seen.

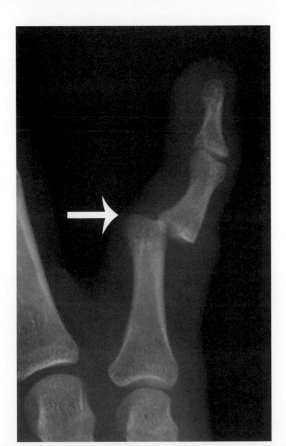

Fig. 62.10 PA view shows a dislocation of the little finger proximal interphalangeal joint *(arrow)*, with the middle phalanx dislocated in a medial direction. No definite fractures are seen.

is unsure exactly in which direction the digit was moved but now has swelling and pain. Imaging demonstrates a dislocation of the little finger PIP joint, with the middle phalanx dislocated in a medial and dorsal direction. No definite fractures were seen. Reduction was performed and subsequent imaging confirmed the finger in anatomic alignment and the presence of a small volar avulsion fracture fragment at the PIP joint. The patient was splinted (ulnar gutter splint) and referred to Hand Surgery.

IMAGING PEARLS

1. Plain radiography is the imaging modality of choice for suspected phalanx fractures.
2. Two views of the involved digit (posteroanterior and lateral) are required. An oblique view may be helpful as well, particularly if a fracture is suspected but not well visualized on the other views.

References

1. Papadonikolakis A, Li Z, Smith BP, et al. Fractures of the phalanges and interphalangeal joints in children. *Hand Clin.* 2006;22(1):11-18.
2. Kozaci N, Ay MO, Akcimen M, et al. The effectiveness of bedside point-of-care ultrasonography in the diagnosis and management of metacarpal fractures. *Am J Emerg Med.* 2015;33(10):1468-1472.
3. Aksay E, Yesilaras M, Kılıc TY, et al. Sensitivity and specificity of bedside ultrasonography in the diagnosis of fractures of the fifth metacarpal. *Emerg Med J.* 2015;32(3):221-225.

4. Aksay E, Kilic TY, Yeşilaras M, et al. Accuracy of bedside ultrasonography for the diagnosis of finger fractures. *Am J Emerg Med.* 2016;34(5):809-812.

5. Abzug JM, Dua K, Bauer AS, et al. Pediatric phalanx fractures. *J Am Acad Orthop Surg.* 2016;24(11):e174-e183.

6. Cornwall R, Ricchetti ET. Pediatric phalanx fractures: unique challenges and pitfalls. *Clin Orthop Relat Res.* 2006;445:146-156.

7. Naranje SM, Erali RA, Warner Jr WC, et al. Epidemiology of pediatric fractures presenting to emergency departments in the United States. *J Pediatr Orthop.* 2016;36(4):e45-e48.

8. Vadivelu R, Dias JJ, Burke FD, Stanton J. Hand injuries in children: a prospective study. *J Pediatr Orthop.* 2006;26(1):29-35.

9. Weber DM, Seiler M, Subotic U, et al. Buddy taping versus splint immobilization for paediatric finger fractures: a randomized controlled trial. *J Hand Surg Eur Vol.* 2019;44(6):640-647.

10. Al-Qattan MM, Al-Zahrani K, Al-Boukai AA. The relative incidence of fractures at the base of the proximal phalanx of the fingers in children. *J Hand Surg Eur Vol.* 2008;33(4):465-468.

11. Boyer JS, London DA, Stepan JG, et al. Pediatric proximal phalanx fractures: outcomes and complications after the surgical treatment of displaced fractures. *J Pediatr Orthop.* 2015;35(3):219-223.

12. Nellans KW, Chung KC. Pediatric hand fractures. *Hand Clin.* 2013;29(4):569-578.

13. Oetgen ME, Dodds SD. Non-operative treatment of common finger injuries. *Curr Rev Musculoskelet Med.* 2008;1(2):97-102.

14. Cornwall R. Pediatric finger fractures: which ones turn ugly? *J Pediatr Orthop.* 2012;32(suppl 1):S25-S31.

15. Park KB, Lee KJ, Kwak YH. Comparison between buddy taping with a short-arm splint and operative treatment for phalangeal neck fractures in children. *J Pediatr Orthop.* 2016;36(7):736-742.

16. Al-Qattan M. Phalangeal neck fractures in children: classification and outcome in 66 cases. *J Hand Surg Br.* 2001;26(2):112-121.

17. Huelsemann W, Singer G, Mann M, et al. Analysis of sequelae after pediatric phalangeal fractures. *Eur J Pediatr Surg.* 2016;26(2):164-171.

18. Lankachandra M, Wells CR, Cheng CJ, et al. Complications of distal phalanx fractures in children. *J Hand Surg Am.* 2017;42(7):574.e1-574.e6.

19. Waters PM, Taylor BA, Kuo AY. Percutaneous reduction of incipient malunion of phalangeal neck fractures in children. *J Hand Surg Am.* 2004;29(4):707-711.

20. Seymour N. Juxta-epiphysial fracture of the terminal phalanx of the finger. *J Bone Joint Surg Br.* 1966;48:347-349.

21. Krusch-Mandi I, Kottstorfer J, Thalhamer G, et al. Seymour fractures: retrospective analysis and therapeutic considerations. *J Hand Surg Am.* 2013;38(2):258-264.

22. Weber DM, Kellenberger CJ, Meuli M. Conservative treatment of stable volar plate injuries of the proximal interphalangeal joint in children and adolescents: a prospective study. *Pediatr Emerg Care.* 2009;25(9):547-549.

63 Can't Move Your Hips: Pelvic Fractures

ROBERT VEZZETTI, MD, FAAP, FACEP

Case 1 Presentation

A 14-year-old male presents with a complaint of acute right hip pain. The patient is an avid soccer player and was kicking a ball "pretty hard." Immediately upon full extension of the right leg, he felt a "pop." Thereafter, he began to experience pain that was radiating to the right upper thigh. He was unable to continue the game. He denies other injury and denies numbness or weakness involving the right leg.

His physical examination reveals appropriate-for-age vital signs. He weighs 59 kg (body mass index of 18.7—normal for his height of 180 cm). He has a completely unremarkable examination, with the exception of his right hip. He has mild tenderness to palpation of the anterior superior iliac spine. While he has full range of motion of the right leg at the hip joint, flexion and extension produce pain. He has no spine tenderness, deformity, or crepitus. He is able to ambulate but does so with a slight limp. There is no lower extremity tenderness, swelling, deformity, or crepitus. He is grossly neurovascularly intact.

IMAGING CONSIDERATIONS: LOW-ENERGY MECHANISMS

Imaging is often employed in the evaluation of children with musculoskeletal complaints, including hip issues, although not all patients require radiographic testing. A thorough history and physical examination can help identify which patients would benefit from imaging.

Plain Radiography

This modality is the initial test of choice for the majority of patients in whom imaging is indicated. Previous studies have shown plain radiography to be generally effective in identifying pelvic avulsion fractures.[1,2] In a large study of 228 patients with pelvic avulsion fractures, 99% were identified by plain radiography; only two patients required advanced imaging (such as computed tomography [CT] or magnetic resonance imaging); fracture displacement and fracture size were identified in 90% and 97% of cases, respectively.[1,2] Patients with acute onset of pain or pain that is continuous, not improving, or worsening should have plain radiography performed.[2,3]

Ultrasound (US)

The use of US to detect fractures is controversial. Studies have indicated US as an effective imaging modality for the identification of hip avulsion fractures,[2,4] but other studies have not supported these findings, especially when compared to more advanced imaging modalities.[2,5] US may show a widened physis on the injured side, compared to the nonaffected side.[6] US can also detect nondisplaced or minimally displaced fractures, which may be difficult to see radiographically.[4,7]

US is attractive because of the lack of ionizing radiation and general availability, but expertise is required to obtain a meaningful study and interpret the images obtained.

Computed Tomography

CT is not a first-line imaging modality when there is a low-energy mechanism or an avulsion fracture is suspected. CT may be employed as a secondary imaging modality when plain radiography does not reveal a fracture but clinical suspicion for a fracture remains high.

This modality is often employed when a patient is involved in a high-energy mechanism, such as a motor vehicle accident or significant fall and is typically part of an abdomen/pelvis study for trauma (see later, "High Energy Mechanisms").

Magnetic Resonance Imaging (MRI)

Persistent or worsening symptoms may warrant advanced imaging with MRI, particularly if other imaging modalities have not demonstrated any abnormal findings. As such, this modality is generally not a first-line imaging test in the emergent setting.

CASE 1 IMAGING FINDINGS

Plain radiographic imaging of the pelvis was obtained, including anteroposterior and frog leg views. It is helpful to obtain a full view of the pelvis, rather than a hemipelvis view, as both right and left sides can be visualized together. An avulsion fracture is seen at the right anterior superior iliac spine. There is no dislocation and no signs of a slipped capital femoral epiphysis (Figs. 63.1 and 63.2).

CASE 1 CONCLUSION

Pediatric Orthopedics was consulted and they recommended discharge with non–weight-bearing instructions, crutch use, and supportive care. Follow-up was arranged with the Pediatric Orthopedic Clinic. Operative intervention was not required.

Pediatric pelvis apophyseal avulsion fractures are commonly related to adolescent sports activity, especially soccer, football, and gymnastics and are the result of a forceful contraction through muscle-tendon unit and bone interaction, at the cartilaginous growth plate.[2,7–9] The most common locations for this injury include the anterior inferior

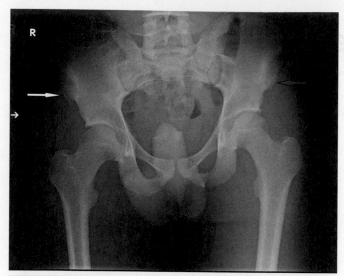

Fig. 63.1 Anterior-posterior view demonstrating a right anterior superior iliac spine avulsion fracture *(white arrow)*, with minimal displacement. Note comparison to the normal, nonavulsed left anterior superior iliac spine *(open arrow)*.

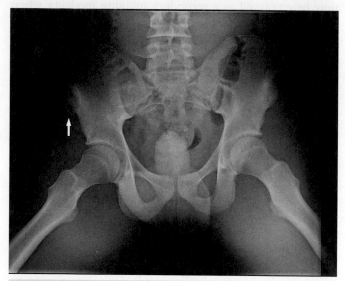

Fig. 63.2 Frog lateral view demonstrating avulsion fracture of the right anterior superior iliac spine *(arrow)*. There is no evidence of slipped capital femoral epiphysis or hip dislocation.

iliac spine, the anterior superior iliac spine, the ischial tuberosity, and insertion of the hamstring.[1,2,7] It is common for patients with this injury to report a sudden "crack" or "pop" in the hip, followed by pain, and such symptoms should raise suspicion for this injury when reported.[2] History and physical examination are important to help distinguish an avulsion fracture from other causes of hip pain that may produce similar symptoms, as treatment differs according to the underlying etiology. The sudden onset of the pain while engaged in sports activity points to a musculoskeletal etiology; fever is suggestive of an infectious etiology; and chronic pain is suggestive of an overuse injury or apophysitis.

Plain radiography is usually diagnostic for hip avulsion fractures, showing the fracture fragment and any displacement.[1-3,6]

This is particularly true for avulsion fractures of the ischial tuberosity, but some fractures, such as that of the anterior inferior iliac spine, may be difficult to visualize on an anterior-posterior (AP) view and may require either additional views or advanced imaging for visualization.[2,10]

The majority of patients with pelvic avulsion fractures are treated conservatively, with nonoperative management, although which fractures require operative treatment is a matter of some controversy.[2,7,11,12] The site of the fracture, grade of displacement, and athlete preference can be taken into account when a treatment plan is considered, which may involve rest and nonsteroidal antiinflammatory drug use, with gradual return to weight bearing and activity, along with physical therapy exercises.[2,7,12,13] Some authors recommend conservative treatment for minimally displaced fractures and operative intervention for fractures with greater than 15–20 mm displacement, or patients with persistent symptoms or activity limitations.[2,7,12] Whether operative intervention allows a patient to return to normal activity sooner is debated in the literature.[7] It is appropriate to consult pediatric orthopedics for treatment recommendations and to arrange appropriate follow-up.

Complications due to hip avulsion fractures arise when these injuries are not identified. A patient with a hip avulsion fracture who undergoes stretching exercise and/or physical activity risks further displacement of the fracture fragment and nonunion.[2,3] Ischial tuberosity fractures have a higher risk and rate of nonunion.[1,2] Displacement of more than 20 mm has shown to increase the likelihood of nonunion by 26 times.[1] Widely separated fracture fragments will heal but have been associated with persistent/chronic pain, instability and sports activity limitations, culminating in disability.[2,14]

HIGH-ENERGY PEDIATRIC PELVIC FRACTURES

In contrast to pelvic avulsion fractures, high-energy pediatric pelvic fractures are not common and are usually the result of motor vehicle collision (MVC), often the result of being struck by a motor vehicle as a pedestrian; the location of impact is typically the side of the body.[15,16] These fractures themselves are typically not life-threatening but may be associated with other injuries, such as head or abdominal trauma, which may be life-threatening.[15] Injury patterns are related to the age of the child, since initially, the pelvic ring is more cartilaginous, the periosteum is thicker, and the sacroiliac and other pelvic joints are wider and thicker, allowing the child to absorb more force compared to an adult.[15] Over time, injury patterns become more like an adult as the child's pelvic structures mature. Also, unlike adults, children who sustain pelvic fractures have an overall lower mortality and less significant hemorrhage.[15,17,18]

IMAGING CONSIDERATIONS: HIGH-ENERGY MECHANISMS

The decision facing the clinician when evaluating high-energy pelvic injuries is whether to employ plain radiography or CT. Additional consideration should be given to whether screening plain radiographs are effective or indicated in pediatric patients.

Plain Radiography

The overall sensitivity of pelvic radiographs for detecting pelvic fractures has been found to be 54% to 78%.[19,20] Routine pelvic radiography is commonly obtained in adult trauma patients.[19,21] Routine radiography may not be indicated in all pediatric patients, however. Studies have sought to identify factors to risk stratify patients who might need radiography. One study reported a screening tool combining eight high-risk clinical findings (pelvic tenderness, laceration, ecchymosis, abrasion, Glasgow Coma Scale score <14, positive urinalysis, abdominal pain/tenderness, femur fracture) and five high-risk mechanisms of injury (unrestrained MVC, MVC with ejection, MVC rollover, auto vs. pedestrian, auto vs. bicycle) to be effective in ruling out (but not detecting) pelvic fractures in pediatric patients.[22] Children with major trauma who did not have any of these high-risk criteria may safely forego pelvic imaging.[22] Another study reported that pelvic contusions and abrasions, hip/pelvic pain, abdominal pain and distension, back pain, the hip held in rotation at presentation, and femur deformity/pain were independently predictive of pelvic fracture, which were helpful in determining the need for pelvic radiography.[23] One study found that the lack of lower extremity injury, lack of an abnormal physical examination of the pelvis, and no need for abdominopelvic CT can exclude pelvic fracture and obviate the need for imaging.[24] Some authors recommend no imaging in patients with no or low suspicion of pelvic fracture or intraabdominal injury based on mechanism and physical examination and a screening pelvic radiograph (AP) view in patients with suspicion for pelvic fracture injury but in whom CT is not indicated.[19,21,25]

Computed Tomography

Although CT has been reported to be more sensitive in detecting pelvic fractures, the routine use of CT for pelvic fracture evaluation is not recommended.[19,26] Studies have reported pelvic fractures that were identified by plain radiographs and CT found no difference in classification and management of the fractures, suggesting that most pediatric pelvic fractures can be managed based on plain radiography findings.[26,27]

CT is indicated if there is suspected instability, significant disruption, or when posterior ring disruption is suspected based on plain films.[19] Acetabular fractures should be evaluated with CT imaging as well.[19] If a patient requires CT to evaluate intraabdominal injury, then the pelvis will be adequately visualized, obviating the need for plain pelvic radiography.

Magnetic Resonance Imaging

This modality is not a first-line imaging modality in pediatric trauma patients. MRI has been noted to be useful in the evaluation and treatment planning of fractures in which plain radiography or CT underestimate the extent of injury.[28]

Case 2 Presentation

Presented here are selected images from a 4-year-old child involved in a high-speed motor vehicle accident. The child was a backseat passenger and was not restrained. She had complaints of abdominal pain and mild tenderness throughout. An initial pelvis x-ray revealed multiple fractures (Fig. 63.3). Due to the apparent complexity of the fractures noted on plain imaging, a CT scan was ordered. Interestingly, no liver, spleen, or apparent bowel injuries were identified and the child had normal AST (aspartate aminotransferase) and ALT (alanine transaminase) values. Selected imaging from the CT is presented here. There is a comminuted fracture of the anterior aspect of the right iliac bone with buckling of the iliac wing and several adjacent small fracture fragments; there is a mildly displaced, minimally comminuted fracture through the anterior aspect of the left iliac wing; there is a mildly displaced fracture through the pubis just to the left of the symphysis extending caudally through the ischiopubic ramus (Figs. 63.4–63.6).

CASE 2 CONCLUSION

This child was admitted to the Pediatric Trauma Service and Pediatric Orthopedics was consulted. No operative intervention was required and the child did well with physical therapy and close monitoring.

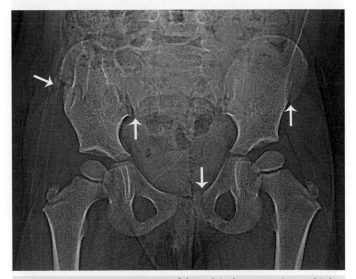

Fig. 63.3 Anterior-posterior view of the pelvis demonstrating multiple fractures (arrows).

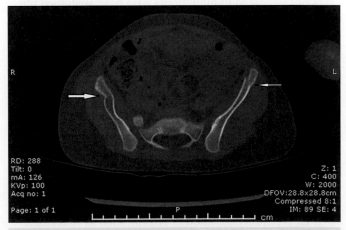

Fig. 63.4 Computed tomography axial image (bone window) shows bilateral anterior iliac wing fractures (arrows).

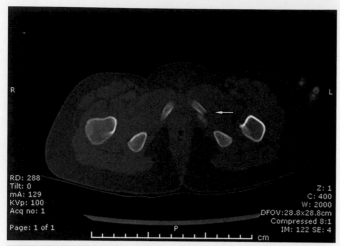

Fig. 63.5 Computed tomography axial image (bone window) shows a left inferior pubic ramus fracture *(arrow)*.

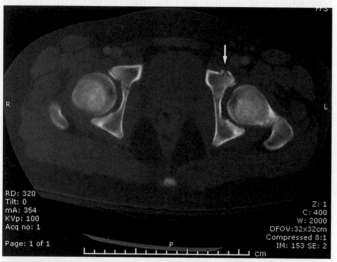

Fig. 63.6 Computed tomography axial image (bone window) shows fracture of the left superior pubic ramus/anterior column of acetabulum *(arrow)*.

IMAGING PEARLS

1. Routine imaging, either with plain radiography or CT, is not indicated in all patients who have sustained hip or other pelvic trauma. The presence or absence of historical and clinical findings may help determine if imaging is required. Ultimately, the decision to obtain imaging is based on clinical examination findings.
2. Plain radiography is the imaging modality of choice in patients with low-energy mechanisms. This is an excellent modality to visualize apophyseal avulsion fractures.
3. CT is more sensitive in detecting pelvic fractures. However, CT use does not change management in the majority of pediatric patients with pelvic fractures identified on plain radiography.
4. CT may be indicated if there is a suspected complex pelvic fracture, including disruption of the posterior pelvic ring and acetabular fractures.
5. If CT is required for another reason, such as to evaluate for intra-abdominal injury, the pelvis can be adequately visualized on CT, obviating the need for plain radiography.

References

1. Schuett DJ, Bomar JD, Pennock AT. Pelvic apophyseal avulsion fractures: a retrospective review of 228 cases. *J Pediatr Orthop.* 2015;35:617-623.
2. Ghanem IB, Rizkallah M. Pediatric avulsion fractures of pelvis: current concepts. *Curr Opin Pediatr.* 2018;30(1):78-83.
3. Singer G, Eberl R, Wegmann H, et al. Diagnosis and treatment of apophyseal injuries of the pelvis in adolescents. *Semin Musculoskelet Radiol.* 2014;18:498-504.
4. Martinoli C, Valle M, Malattia C, et al. Paediatric musculoskeletal US beyond the hip joint. *Pediatr Radiol.* 2011;41(suppl 1):S113-S124.
5. Koulouris G, Connell D. Evaluation of the hamstring muscle complex following acute injury. *Skeletal Radiol.* 2003;32:582-589.
6. Davis KW. Imaging pediatric sports injuries: lower extremity. *Radiol Clin North Am.* 2010;48(6):1213-1235.
7. McKinney BI, Nelson C, Carrion W. Apophyseal avulsion fractures of the hip and pelvis. *Orthopedics.* 2009;32(1):42-48.
8. Rossi F, Dragoni S. Acute avulsion fractures of the pelvis in adolescent competitive athletes: prevalence, location and sports distribution of 203 cases collected. *Skeletal Radiol.* 2001;30:127-131.
9. Martinoli C, Garello I, Marchetti A, et al. Hip ultrasound. *Eur J Radiol.* 2012;81(12):3824-3831.
10. Ali E, Khanduja V. Adolescent avulsion injuries of the pelvis: a case study and review of the literature. *Orthop Nurs.* 2015;34:21-26.
11. Pogliacomi F, Calderazzi F, Paterlini M, et al. Surgical treatment of anterior iliac spines fractures: our experience. *Acta Biomed.* 2014;85(suppl 2):52-58.
12. Eberbach H, Hohloch L, Feucht MJ, et al. Operative versus conservative treatment of apophyseal avulsion fractures of the pelvis in the adolescents: a systematical review with meta-analysis of clinical outcome and return to sports. *BMC Musculoskelet Disord.* 2017;18(1):162.
13. Schiller J, DeFroda S, Blood T. Lower extremity avulsion fractures in the pediatric and adolescent athlete. *J Am Acad Orthop Surg.* 2017;25:251-259.
14. Moeller JL. Pelvic and hip apophyseal avulsion injuries in young athletes. *Curr Sports Med Rep.* 2003;2:110-115.
15. Amorosa LF, Kloen P, Helfet DL. High-energy pediatric pelvic and acetabular fractures. *Orthop Clin North Am.* 2014;45(4):483-500.
16. Silber JS, Flynn JM. Changing patterns of pediatric pelvic fractures with skeletal maturation: implications for classification and management. *J Pediatr Orthop.* 2002;22:22-26.
17. Grisoni N, Connor S, Marsh E, et al. Pelvic fractures in a pediatric level I trauma center. *J Orthop Trauma.* 2002;16(7):458-463.
18. Ismail N, Bellemare JF, Mollitt DL, et al. Death from pelvic fracture: children are different. *J Pediatr Surg.* 1996;31(1):82-85.
19. Guillamondegui OD, Mahboubi S, Stafford PW, et al. The utility of the pelvic radiograph in the assessment of pediatric pelvic fractures. *J Trauma.* 2003;55(2):236-239.
20. Obaid AK, Barleben A, Perral D, et al. Utility of plain film pelvic radiographs in blunt trauma patients in the emergency department. *Am Surg.* 2006;72(10):951-954.
21. Rees MJ, Aickin R, Kolbe A, et al. The screening pelvic radiograph in pediatric trauma. *Pediatr Radiol.* 2001;31(7):497-500.
22. Lagisetty J, Slovis T, Thomas R, et al. Are routine pelvic radiographs in major pediatric blunt trauma necessary? *Pediatr Radiol.* 2012;42(7):853-858.
23. Ramirez DW, Schuette JJ, Knight V, et al. Necessity of routine pelvic radiograph in the pediatric blunt trauma patient. *Clin Pediatr (Phila).* 2008;47(9):935-940.
24. Wong AT, Brady KB, Caldwell A, et al. Low-risk criteria for pelvic radiography in pediatric blunt trauma patients. *Pediatr Emerg Care.* 2011;27(2):92-96.
25. Kevill K, Wong AM, Goldman HS, et al. Is a complete trauma series indicated for all pediatric trauma victims? *Pediatr Emerg Care.* 2002;18(2):75-77.
26. Silber JS, Flynn JM, Katz MA, et al. Role of computed tomography in the classification and management of pediatric pelvic fractures. *J Pediatr Orthop.* 2001;21(4):446-450.
27. Bent MA, Hennrikus WL, Latorre JE, et al. Role of computed tomography in the classification of pediatric pelvic fractures—revisited. *J Orthop Trauma.* 2017;31(7):e200-e204.
28. Hearty T, Swaroop VT, Gourineni P, et al. Standard radiographs and computed tomographic scan underestimating pediatric acetabular fracture after traumatic hip dislocation: report of 2 cases. *J Orthop Trauma.* 2011;25:e68 e73.

64 All Fun and Games: Femoral Fractures

ROBERT VEZZETTI, MD, FAAP, FACEP

Case Presentation

A 2-year-old male presents with acute right leg pain after falling while jumping on a trampoline. Apparently, he fell off the trampoline onto the ground and landed on his left leg. The distance was estimated at 3 ft (approximately 1 m) and the incident was witnessed by his parents and two older siblings. There is no reported loss of consciousness. The child is unable to ambulate secondary to pain. His vital signs are age appropriate except for a heart rate of 120 beats per minute. He is crying even before his examination from what appears to be left thigh pain. His physical examination shows no obvious injury, other than left thigh edema and he is tender on palpation. He has no neck or back pain. He is neurovascularly intact.

Imaging Considerations

Children who sustain extremity injuries may need imaging. The decision to image is based on history and physical examination findings. Proper imaging technique is essential if imaging is employed.

PLAIN RADIOGRAPHY

Plain radiography of the injured extremity is all that is generally required to properly evaluate the presence of fractures. A two-view study is preferred, consisting of anteroposterior (AP) and lateral views.[1] Appropriate pain control is paramount in order to obtain clinically useful images of the injured extremity. The clinician should also consider imaging of the area above and below the involved bone if injury is suspected. For example in this child, consideration should be given to imaging the pelvis, lower extremity (tibia-fibula), ankle, and foot if clinically indicated. There are times when a complete imaging series is not practical (e.g., deformity preventing full range of motion and positioning for two views). In these situations, a single AP view will suffice. Of particular concern are patients with neurovascular compromise; do not delay treatment in these patients to obtain imaging. Once the situation has stabilized, appropriate imaging studies can be obtained.

COMPUTED TOMOGRAPHY (CT)

Ipsilateral femoral neck fractures are associated with adult femoral shaft fractures in up to 9% of patients, prompting utilization of CT to detect these fractures.[2] However, in the pediatric population, this association is quite low.[2] In pediatric patients, routine CT imaging to look for associated femoral neck fracture with femoral shaft fractures is not recommended. CT utilization should be based on clinical examination and mechanism of injury, as well as concern for other injuries.[2]

Imaging Findings

This child had a two-view study of the injured leg. There is a spiral, mid to distal diaphyseal femur fracture with minimal degree of displacement of the distal fragment (Figs. 64.1 and 64.2). The second set of images shows a nondisplaced, oblique distal femur metaphyseal fracture in a different patient, extending toward the physis, consistent with a Salter-Harris type II fracture (Figs. 64.3 and 64.4).

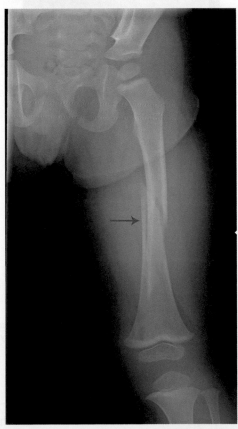

Fig. 64.1 AP view shows a spiral fracture of the mid to distal diaphysis of the femur with very mild medial displacement of the distal fracture fragment *(red arrow)*.

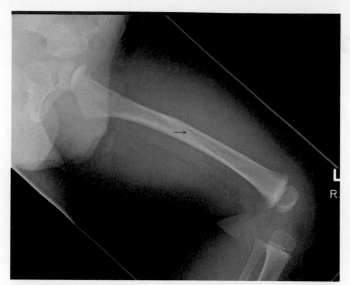

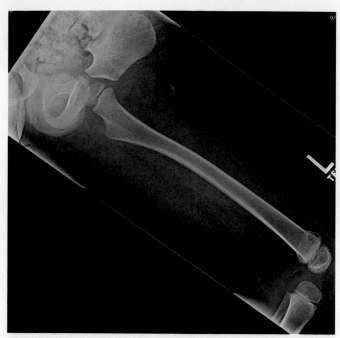

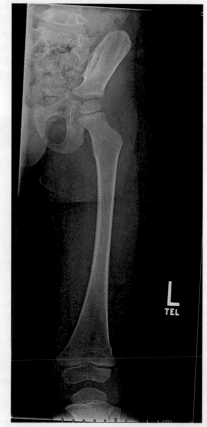

Fig. 64.2 The fracture is visualized *(red arrow)* but difficult to see on this lateral view.

Fig. 64.4 Lateral view of the distal femoral Salter Harris type II fracture seen in Fig. 64.3.

Fig. 64.3 AP view of a different patient with an oblique fracture of the distal femoral metaphysis *(arrows)*, extending toward the physis, consistent with a Salter-Harris type II fracture.

Case Conclusion

Pediatric Orthopedics was consulted and the child was taken to the operating room for closed reduction of the fracture and application of a spica cast. He was in the cast for 8 weeks and recovered without complications.

Femoral shaft fractures are not uncommon in pediatric patients and account for approximately 1% to 2% of all pediatric fractures[3,4] and 4% of all long bone pediatric fractures.[5] The location of the fracture can be described as the proximal end segment (epiphysis and metaphysis), diaphyseal segment, and distal end segment (epiphysis and metaphysis).[6] Treatment of these fractures depends on the age of the patient and the severity of the fracture.[7,8] Traditionally, younger patients may be treated with a spica cast or Pavlik harness (typically employed in children under the age of 5 years old), while older children may be treated with a spica cast or intramedullary fixation using flexible or rigid nails.[3,5,9] There have been documented trends for operative management in older children (above 5 years of age).[3] Nonoperative treatment is preferred in younger children due to the excellent remodeling potential in this age group, with treatment recommendations consisting of early spica casting or traction with delayed spica casting.[5,9] Pediatric Orthopedic consultation is appropriate in these patients and management does vary, despite the existence of management guidelines. This was demonstrated in one study where published American Academy of Orthopedic Surgery guidelines had little direct impact on pediatric femur fracture management.[10]

Consideration should also be given to the possibility of nonaccidental trauma in young patients with femur fractures, especially if children are nonambulatory or when a given history of injury does not match the developmental capabilities of a child.[4,8,9] In these cases, a complete skeletal survey should be performed and appropriate laboratory testing (liver enzymes, urinalysis, etc.) obtained, noting that most pediatric centers have age-specific nonaccidental trauma protocols based on the medical literature and professional association guidelines (such as the American

Academy of Pediatrics) to aid in the evaluation of children with suspected nonaccidental injury (see Chapter 50, Nonaccidental Trauma).[11–13] This child was developmentally capable of sustaining this injury, no other injuries or concerning physical examination findings were noted, and no additional workup was indicated.

IMAGING PEARLS

1. Provide adequate pain control to aid in obtaining the best images possible.
2. Pediatric femur fractures can be adequately visualized with two-view radiographic imaging (AP and lateral) of the injured extremity.
3. Consider imaging areas above and below the injured bone if clinically indicated.
4. A complete skeletal survey is indicated in children under the age of 1 year with a femur fracture. Children older than 1 year may require a complete skeletal survey based on history and physical examination findings and further imaging can be selectively employed.

References

1. Delavan A, Fenton LZ. Pediatric fractures. *Pediatric Radiology*. In: Reid J, Lee E, Paladin A, Carrico C, Davros W (eds). Oxford: Oxford University Press; 2014:265-273.
2. Caldwell L, Chan CM, Sanders JO, et al. Detection of femoral neck fractures in pediatric patients with femoral shaft fractures. *J Pediatr Orthop*. 2017;37(3):e164-e167.
3. Naranje SM, Stewart MG, Kelly DM, et al. Changes in the treatment of pediatric femoral fractures: 15-year trends from United States Kids' Inpatient Database (KID) 1997 to 2012. *J Pediatr Orthop*. 2016;36(7):e81-e85.
4. Hubbard EW, Riccio AI. Pediatric orthopedic trauma: an evidence-based approach. *Orthop Clin North Am*. 2018;49(2):195-210.
5. Rapp M, Kaiser MM, Grauel F, et al. Femoral shaft fractures in young children (<5 years of age): operative and non-operative treatment in clinical practice. *Eur J Trauma Emerg Surg*. 2016;42(6):719-724.
6. Joeris A, Lutz N, Blumenthal A, et al. The AO Pediatric Comprehensive Classification of Long Bone Fractures (PCCF). *Acta Orthop*. 2017;88(2):129-132.
7. Rickert KD, Hosseinzadeh P, Edmonds EW. What's new in pediatric orthopaedic trauma: the lower extremity. *J Pediatr Orthop*. 2018;38(8):e434-e439.
8. Kocher MS, Sink EL, Blasier DR, et al. Treatment of pediatric diaphyseal femur fractures. *J Am Acad Orthop Surg*. 2009;17(11):718-725.
9. Jevsevar DA, Shea KG, Murray J, et al. AAOS Clinical Practice Guideline on the treatment of pediatric diaphyseal femur fractures. *J Am Acad Orthop Surg*. 2015;23(12):e101.
10. Oetgen ME, Blatz AM, Matthews A. Impact of clinical practice guideline on the treatment of pediatric femoral fractures in a pediatric hospital. *J Bone Joint Surg Am*. 2015;97:1641-1646.
11. Riney LC, Frey TM, Fain ET, et al. Standardizing the evaluation of nonaccidental trauma in a large pediatric emergency department. *Pediatrics*. 2018;141(1):1-9.
12. Christian CW, Committee on Child Abuse and Neglect. The evaluation of suspected child physical abuse. *Pediatrics*. 2015;135(5):e1337-e1354.
13. Flaherty EG, Perez-Rossello JM, Levine MA, et al. Evaluating children with fractures for child physical abuse. *Pediatrics*. 2014;133(2):e477-e489.

65

Knee Pain: It's Not Always the Knee—Slipped Capital Femoral Epiphysis

ROBERT VEZZETTI, MD, FAAP, FACEP

Case Presentation

A 9-year-old female presents with 5 weeks of progressively worsening left knee pain. There has been no known trauma and the family denies fever, rash, knee swelling or erythema, weakness, numbness, or incontinence. She is able to ambulate but, due to her pain, has been excused from physical education classes at school. She has seen numerous physicians, and multiple plain radiographs of the left knee were reported as "normal" according to the family. Her primary care provider obtained bloodwork (a complete blood count, erythrocyte sedimentation rate, and C-reactive protein), and the family was told this also was "normal."

The child is afebrile and has normal, age-appropriate vital signs; her weight is 60 kg, with a height of 142 cm (body mass index of 22.5). Her examination shows a child who is not in distress until you ask her to ambulate. She complies and you notice a demonstrable limp to her left side. Her pelvis is stable and unremarkable. Your examination does not show any signs of trauma and there is no edema, erythema, warmth, or tenderness of her left knee. You perform range-of-motion maneuvers of the knee, which are normal. You examine her left thigh, which also appears unremarkable. Range of motion of her left leg at the hip produces knee pain and mild left hip pain. Her lower leg examination, including her ankle and foot, is unremarkable, including distal pulses. She has no cervical, thoracic, or lumbar findings. Her neurologic examination is nonfocal; she has equal strength of her lower extremities.

Imaging Considerations

PLAIN RADIOGRAPHY

Plain radiography is the initial imaging modality of choice for most pediatric orthopedic complaints and remains the initial modality of choice for slipped capital femoral epiphysis (SCFE).[1–6] The exposure to ionizing radiation is minimal, sedation is not required, and plain radiography is widely available. Proper technique is essential. For suspected hip pathology, pediatric plain radiographs of the pelvis should include anteroposterior (AP) and frog leg lateral views.[1,3–6] Signs of SCFE on plain radiography include posterior and medial slippage of the femoral head, decreased craniocaudal height of the femoral head, evidence of posterior lip of the epiphysis superimposed on the metaphysis, widening and irregularity of the growth plate, and an abnormal relationship of the lateral femoral head to the Klein line.[3,6] The Klein line is drawn along the superolateral border of the femoral neck and should intersect the lateral proximal femoral epiphysis. Although the Klein line can be used to detect slippage, recent studies have called into question the utility of this line, especially in subtle SCFE or cases of preslippage.[3,7–9]

It is not adequate to obtain a hemipelvis view in pediatric patients, as both femoral heads and the complete pelvis should be visualized. Subtle findings of SCFE, Legg-Calve-Perthes disease, or other pathology can be overlooked if only a hemipelvis view is utilized. Evaluation of the contralateral hip is also indicated as bilateral SCFE is common and occurs in greater frequency in patients with endocrine disorders, who have a higher incidence of SCFE.[3,10] If a patient cannot perform the frog lateral view due to pain, cross-table lateral views can be obtained. The role of other imaging modalities is controversial and generally indicated on an individual case basis. Options include the following.

ULTRASOUND (US)

The utilization of sonography for pediatric musculoskeletal complaints has risen in recent years. This modality has been well established in the detection of developmental dysplasia of the hip and is the imaging modality of choice for these patients.[2,3,11] The use of US for the detection of SCFE has been described previously with a reported accuracy of 93%.[2,11,12] Common findings of SCFE on US include displacement of the proximal femoral epiphysis compared to the metaphysis, referred to as a physeal step-off, and joint effusion.[2,11]

US for SCFE has the advantage of avoiding ionizing radiation, but expertise in specialized pediatric orthopedic US is required to produce meaningful images and provide correct interpretation. Therefore, at this time, US evaluation for SCFE is not widely available.

MAGNETIC RESONANCE IMAGING (MRI)

Without the use of ionizing radiation, MRI can detect early SCFE, prior to anatomic slippage of the femoral head. Additionally, MRI has the advantage of detecting other pathology, especially inflammatory processes and avascular necrosis. MRI is also used as an adjunctive test, after treatment for SCFE, to monitor disease progression or complications, especially the development of avascular necrosis of the femoral head.[3] Limitations include institutional availability and the need for possible sedation.

COMPUTED TOMOGRAPHY (CT)

CT is not an initial imaging modality of choice but may be used for pre- or postoperative planning.[3,13] Proximal femoral deformities can be evaluated, assisting in osteotomy if indicated. Postoperative intra-articular penetration of femoral hardware can also be assessed with CT.[3,13] A limiting factor in its use is exposure to ionizing radiation.

Imaging Findings

In this patient, one could repeat films of the knee (AP, lateral, and a patellar view). This may be appropriate if access to the prior images or their interpretation is not available, or if there are concerning physical examination findings that warrant repeat imaging of the knee. However, physical examination elicited primarily left hip pain, with radiation to the left upper knee. In light of the history and physical examination findings, plain radiography of the pelvis is indicated, including AP and frog leg views.

There is widening and irregularity of the left proximal femoral physis, with mild posterior and medial slippage of the left proximal femoral epiphysis, best visualized on the frog leg view (Figs. 65.1 and 65.2). These findings are consistent with SCFE. A useful method to detect the presence of an SCFE is the Klein line. This is a line drawn along the superior edge of the neck of the femur. This line should intersect the lateral portion of the superior femoral epiphysis (Fig. 65.3).

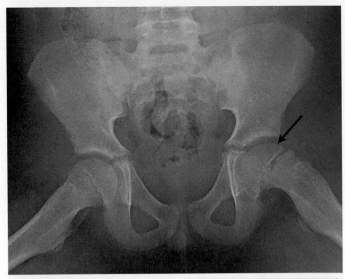

Fig. 65.2 Medial and posterior slippage of the left femoral head epiphysis is best seen on the frog lateral view (*arrow*).

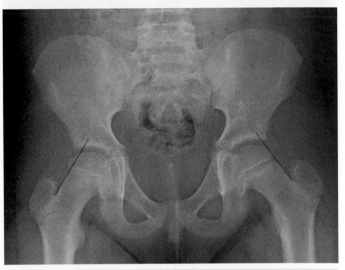

Fig. 65.3 Klein line. Note the lack of intersection of the left Klein line with the lateral aspect of the left superior femoral epiphysis compared to the right. Findings are consistent with a left slipped capital femoral epiphysis.

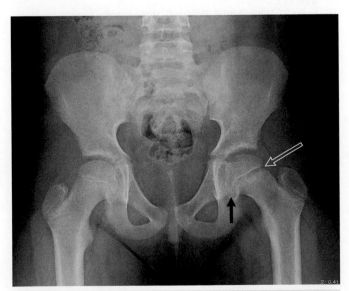

Fig. 65.1 AP view of the pelvis shows widening and irregularity of the left proximal femoral physis (*white arrow*), with subtle medial slippage of the proximal left femoral epiphysis (*black arrow*).

Case Conclusion

Pediatric Orthopedic consultation was obtained and the child was taken to the operating room for pinning of the slippage (Figs. 65.4 and 65.5). She underwent physical therapy and rehabilitation, with a gradual return to physical activity.

Etiologies of pediatric hip complaints vary by age.[1] A careful history and physical examination are required to help narrow what could otherwise be a wide differential diagnosis. A history of fever should always prompt concerns for osteomyelitis, myositis, or a septic joint. Always consider referred pain; children with hip pathology will often complain of knee pain, as this child did. SCFE is more common in obese children.[14–16]

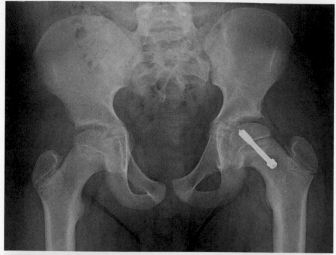

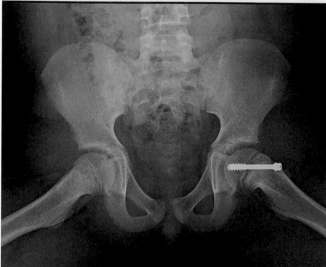

Figs. 65.4 and 65.5 Postoperative images demonstrate pinning of the left femur and normal appearance of the right hip.

Initial treatment for SCFE is having the child non—weight-bearing with urgent Pediatric Orthopedic evaluation. Surgical pinning is the treatment for most patients with SCFE; most patients with mild to moderate disease have an excellent prognosis.[6,17] Even with prompt surgical stabilization, though, complications can arise, the most serious of which is avascular necrosis, which is more common in patients with unstable SCFE.[4,6,11,17] Prompt consultation with Pediatric Orthopedic Surgery is indicated to determine the best management for these patients.

IMAGING PEARLS

1. Consider imaging of the hip in pediatric patients with knee complaints. Pain from hip pathology, such as in SCFE, is often referred to the knee.

2. Plain radiography is the preferred imaging modality.
3. Imaging of pediatric hip pain should include the pelvis and both hips, not hemipelvis views of the affected side. Comparison of both hips is required, as subtle pathology can be missed if only one side is imaged. Also, imaging of the contralateral hip is indicated due to the high incidence of bilateral SCFE.
4. A lateral (either frog leg or cross-table lateral) view should be included when imaging pediatric patients with hip pain. Subtle forms of SCFE can be missed with one-view (AP) pelvis imaging.
5. If plain radiography is negative with clinically suspected SCFE, consider MR imaging for further evaluation.

References

1. Gill KG. Pediatric hip: pearls and pitfalls. *Semin Musculoskelet Radiol.* 2013;17(3):328-338.
2. Vanderhave KL, Brighton B, Casey V, et al. Applications of musculoskeletal ultrasonography in pediatric patients. *J Am Acad Orthop Surg.* 2014;22(11):691-698.
3. Georgiadis AG, Zaltz I. Slipped capital femoral epiphysis: how to evaluate with a review and update of treatment. *Pediatr Clin North Am.* 2014;61(6):1119-1135.
4. Otani T, Kawaguchi Y, Marumo K. Diagnosis and treatment of slipped capital femoral epiphysis: recent trends to note. *J Orthop Sci.* 2018;23(2):220-228.
5. Aronsson DD, Loder RT, Breur GJ, et al. Slipped capital femoral epiphysis: current concepts. *J Am Acad Orthop Surg.* 2006;14(12):666-679.
6. Peck D. Slipped capital femoral epiphysis: diagnosis and management. *Am Fam Physician.* 2010;82(3):258-262.
7. Klein A, Joplin RJ, Rediy JA, et al. Roentgenopraghic features of slipped capital femoral epiphysis. *Am J Roentgenol Radium Ther.* 1951;66(3):361-374.
8. Pinkowsky GJ, Hennrikus WL. Klein line on the anteroposterior radiograph is not a sensitive diagnostic test for slipped capital femoral epiphysis. *J Pediatr.* 2013;162(4):804-807.
9. Geeen DW, Mogekwu N, Scher DM, et al. A modification of Klein's Line to improve sensitivity of the anterior-posterior radiograph in slipped capital femoral epiphysis. *J Pediatr Orthop.* 2009;29(5):449-453.
10. Loder RT, Wittenberg B, DeSilva G. Slipped capital femoral epiphysis associated with endocrine disorders. *J Pediatr Orthop.* 1995;15(3):349-356.
11. Asad I, Lee MS. Point-of-care ultrasound diagnosis of slipped capital femoral epiphysis. *Clin Pract Cases Emerg Med.* 2019;22(3):81-82.
12. Kalio PE, Lequesne GW, Paterson DC, et al. Ultrasonography in slipped capital femoral epiphysis: diagnosis and assessment of severity. *J Bone Joint Surg Br.* 1991;73(6):884-889.
13. Senthi S, Blyth P, Metcalf R, et al. Screw placement after pinning of slipped capital femoral epiphysis: a postoperative CT scan study. *J Pediatr Orthop.* 2011;31(4):388-392.
14. Poussa M, Schlenzka D, Yrjonen T. Body mass index and slipped capital femoral epiphysis. *J Pediatr Orthop.* 2003;12(6):369-371.
15. Manoff EM, Banffy MB, Winell JJ. Relationship between body mass index and slipped capital femoral epiphysis. *J Pediatr Orthop.* 2005;25(6):744-746.
16. Schmitz MR, Blumberg TJ, Nelson SE, et al. What's new in pediatric hip? *J Pediatr Orthop.* 2018;38(6):e300-e304.
17. Loder RT, Stames T, Dikos G, et al. Demographic predictors of severity of stable slipped capital femoral epiphysis. *J Bone Joint Surg Am.* 2006;88(1):97-105.

Weak in the Knees: Patellar Dislocation

MALIA J. MOORE, MD

Case Presentation

A 14-year-old female is brought to the Emergency Department following a basketball game. She pivoted to take a shot and felt a tearing sensation, followed by a pop, then fell to the ground. She presents with an obvious right knee deformity. Her vital signs are normal for her age, and on examination, her knee is held in flexion at 30 degrees with a laterally palpable patella. She is grossly neurovascularly intact and there are no other injuries. Interestingly, the patient tells you she had the same injury twice in the past, most recently 5 months ago, involving the left knee, but never on the right. She is otherwise healthy.

Imaging Considerations

Imaging is often employed in the evaluation of children with orthopedic complaints. Generally, imaging begins with plain radiography and progresses to other modalities based on history and physical examination. In the case of patellar dislocation, imaging may not be necessary prior to reduction unless there is concern for alternate diagnosis, as dislocation is often clinically apparent.[1] Postreduction imaging is advised to evaluate for an osteochondral fracture, which is considered an indication for operative management[1,2]

PLAIN RADIOGRAPHY

The initial preferred imaging modality for a suspected patellar fracture is plain radiography. Anterior-posterior (AP), lateral, and oblique films should be requested, with the addition of a "sunrise view," in the setting of concern for patellar injury.[2] Prereduction imaging is likely unnecessary, as the diagnosis is usually clinically apparent, and the presence of fracture does not impact success of reduction.[3–5] If prereduction radiographs are obtained, the dislocation can be readily identified; the patella tends to dislocate laterally.[6] Postreduction imaging should be obtained on all patients to assess for fracture; however, plain radiography may have poor sensitivity for fracture. Multiple studies have revealed that fractures were present on arthroscopy in up to 70% of patients, which were not identified on plain radiography.[4] Plain radiographs are also useful to evaluate patients who may have a predisposition to patellar dislocation, such as abnormal anatomy.[7]

MAGNETIC RESONANCE IMAGING (MRI)

MRI is superior to plain radiography in identifying fracture and is the study of choice to detect injuries due to patellar dislocations that have spontaneously reduced.[3,8,9] However, this is not a first-line imaging modality. MRI may be employed during follow-up evaluations, as it is useful for evaluating the articular cartilage, soft tissue injury, and medial patellofemoral ligament injury.

ULTRASOUND (US)

US is not a first-line imaging modality for patellar dislocation; however, it may be used to detect medial patellofemoral ligament injury during the postreduction follow-up period.[10]

COMPUTED TOMOGRAPHY (CT)

CT is not a first-line imaging modality for diagnosing patellar dislocation. Use of this technology may be indicated in children with severe pain or associated complex fracture or when the diagnosis is uncertain. Primarily, CT is useful to assess the anterior tibial tubercle–trochlear groove distance, of which an abnormal measurement is an indication of patellar instability.[7]

Imaging Findings

Prior to reduction, the patient had one view imaging of the right knee. This image shows a laterally displaced patella without apparent fracture (Fig. 66.1).

Case Conclusion

The child's clinical history, examination, and knee radiography were suggestive of patellar dislocation. She had a reduction performed immediately, which was successful. Postreduction imaging showed a reduced patella and no patellar fracture; there was remaining mild laxity (Figs. 66.2–66.4). She was discharged in a knee immobilizer with planned outpatient orthopedic follow-up. At this evaluation, the patient and her family were presented with surgical and nonsurgical management options, given the multiple episodes of dislocation. Nonsurgical management was chosen, and the patient began a physical therapy regimen.

Patellar dislocation is one of the most common pediatric orthopedic injuries presenting to Emergency Departments in the United States, and the knee is the most commonly injured joint among adolescent athletes.[6,11] Mechanism varies by age, with age less than 5 more likely to be injured by falls off of structures within or adjacent to the home, such as stairs, beds, trampolines, and play structures; however,

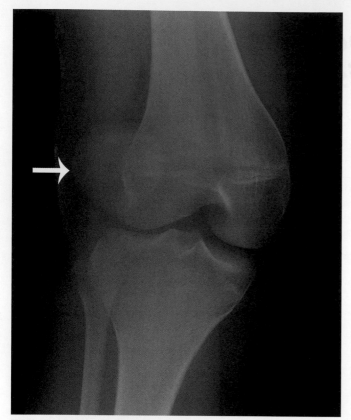

Fig. 66.1 AP radiographic view of the injured knee demonstrating a laterally displaced right patella *(arrow)*.

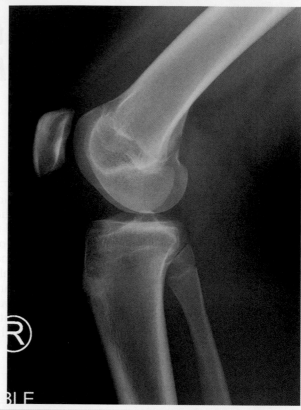

Fig. 66.3 Postreduction lateral view demonstrating a reduced patellar dislocation.

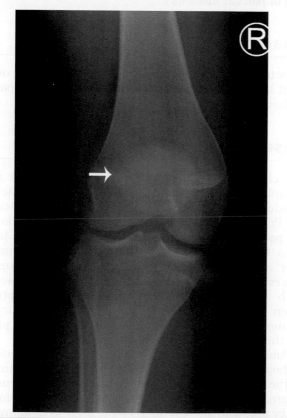

Fig. 66.2 Postreduction AP view demonstrating a reduced patellar dislocation *(arrow)*.

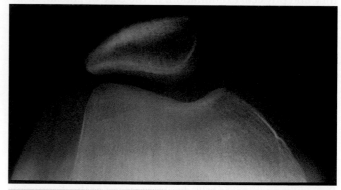

Fig. 66.4 Postreduction "sunrise" view demonstrating a reduced patellar dislocation.

patellar dislocation is uncommon in this age group. Children older than age 5 are predominantly injured playing sports, particularly football, basketball, and soccer.[6,11] A common mechanism of injury is the athlete who makes a sharp or sudden turn (a "cut") or is struck at the knee while the knee is in the flexed position; a dislocation can also occur when the knee is in full extension and a valgus stress is applied during rotation.[6] While high-energy mechanisms are commonly associated with primary dislocations, ligamentous laxity or patella alta (a congenital condition that produces a higher than normal patellar position) may be a contributing cause to low-energy dislocations.[6,12]

Initial treatment for an acute dislocation consists of reduction. While the maneuver is very rapid to perform and generally discomfort is quite brief, providing analgesia or anxiolysis should be considered. This can be accomplished quite easily with intranasal formulations of midazolam and fentanyl. The dose for midazolam is 0.2 mg/kg (typically a maximum dose of 10 mg), and for fentanyl, it is 2 µg/kg (up to a maximum of 100 µg), providing effective analgesia and anxiolysis with minimal adverse effects.[13] To perform a reduction, the clinician slowly extends the knee while applying gentle medial pressure to the lateral aspect of the dislocated patella. Successful reduction is indicated by the return of the patella to the tibiofemoral tract and normal flexion and extension of the knee.[6] Postreduction plain radiographs are recommended to ensure proper reduction and to assess for associated fractures.[6]

Long-term management consists of nonoperative and operative options. Nonoperative management usually involves immobilization for a period of several weeks, followed by physical therapy.[6] Operative management is considered if osteochondral fragments are present, if there is cartilage damage, or if there is ligamentous injury with recurrent subluxation events.[2,6,14] Referral to Pediatric Orthopedics is appropriate.

IMAGING PEARLS

1. Children with a clinical diagnosis of patellar dislocation do not need prereduction imaging.
2. Postreduction imaging with plain radiography is recommended to assess for the presence of accompanying fractures.
3. CT is not a first-line imaging modality for acute patellar dislocation but may be useful to assess for the risk of patellar instability.
4. MRI is not a first-line imaging modality for acute patellar dislocation. However, MRI may be employed during follow-up evaluations, as it is useful for evaluating soft tissue injury, medial patellofemoral ligament injury, and the articular cartilage.

5. US is not indicated in acute patellar dislocation but may be employed as a follow-up study, although this is not commonly the case.

References

1. Krause EA, Lin CW, Ortega HW, et al. Pediatric lateral patellar dislocation: is there a role for plain radiography in the emergency department? *J Emerg Med.* 2013;44(6):1126-1131.
2. Stefancin JJ, Parker RD. First-time traumatic patellar dislocation: a systematic review. *Clin Orthop Relat Res.* 2007;455:93-101.
3. Desai N, Caperell KS. Joint dislocations in the pediatric emergency department. *Clin Pediatr Emerg Med.* 2016;17(1):53-66.
4. Beasley LS, Vidal AF. Traumatic patellar dislocation in children and adolescents: treatment update and literature review. *Curr Opin Pediatr.* 2004;16(1):29-36.
5. Lu DW, Wang EE, Self WH, et al. Patellar dislocation reduction. *Acad Emerg Med.* 2010;17(2):226-226.
6. Ramponi D. Patellar dislocations and reduction procedure. *Adv Emerg Nurs J.* 2016;38(2):89-92.
7. Koh JL, Stewart C. Patellar instability. *Orthop Clin North Am.* 2015; 46(1):147-157.
8. Seeley M, Bowman KF, Walsh C, et al. Magnetic resonance imaging of acute patellar dislocation in children: patterns of injury and risk factors for recurrence. *J Pediatr Orthop.* 2012;32(2):145-155.
9. Tuite MJ, Kransdorf MJ, Beaman FD, et al. ACR appropriateness criteria acute trauma to the knee. *J Am Coll Radiol.* 2015 Nov;12(11): 1164-1172.
10. Zhang GY, Zheng L, Ding HY, et al. Evaluation of medial patellofemoral ligament tears after acute lateral patellar dislocation: comparison of high-frequency ultrasound and MR. *Eur Radiol.* 2015;25(1):274-281.
11. Gage BE, McIlvain NM, Collins CL, et al. Epidemiology of 6.6 million knee injuries presenting to United States emergency departments from 1999 through 2008. *Acad Emerg Med.* 2012;19(4):378-385.
12. Shah JN, Howard JS, Flanigan DC, et al. A systematic review of complications and failures associated with medial patellofemoral ligament reconstruction for recurrent patellar dislocation. *Am J Sports Med.* 2012;40(8):1916-1923.
13. Ryan PM, Kienstra AJ, Cosgrove P, et al. Safety and effectiveness of intranasal midazolam and fentanyl used in combination in the pediatric emergency department. *Am J Emerg Med.* 2019;37(2):237-240.
14. Meyers AB, Laor T, Sharafinski M, et al. Imaging assessment of patellar instability and its treatment in children and adolescents. *Pediatr Radiol.* 2016;46(5):618-636.

It's the Way You (Don't) Walk: Fractures of the Tibia and Fibula

ANNA SCHLECHTER, MD

Case Presentation

A 7-year-old male is brought in for evaluation. A few hours prior to presentation, he was jumping up and down on a couch when he jumped off, landing on his right leg. He states he heard a "pop" and then began to experience pain and difficulty with ambulation secondary to the pain. There is no reported loss of consciousness; he denies neck pain, back pain, hip pain, weakness, numbness, or other symptoms.

His physical examination reveals an afebrile child who is complaining of right lower leg pain. His heart rate is 91 beats per minute, respiratory rate is 20 breaths per minute, and blood pressure is 118/62 mm Hg. There is mild swelling to the anterior surface of the midshaft of the right tibia and fibula. There is no obvious deformity. There is no abrasion, laceration, or ecchymoses. His anterior tibial and posterior tibial pulses are intact. He has no pain, swelling, or tenderness to the ipsilateral hip, knee, ankle, or foot. He has normal range of motion at these joints. He is grossly neurologically intact. There is no back tenderness, crepitus, step-off, or deformity.

Imaging Considerations

PLAIN RADIOGRAPHY

Plain radiographs typically suffice when assessing acute tibial injuries in children and include anterior-posterior (AP) and lateral views. These should incorporate the entire length of the lower leg and include both knee and ankle.

COMPUTED TOMOGRAPHY (CT)

This modality is rarely indicated for midshaft fractures. Tibia or fibular fractures that involve the knee (e.g., tibial plateau) or ankle joint may require use of non-contrast CT to evaluate the extent of the fracture.

MAGNETIC RESONANCE IMAGING (MRI)

This modality is not indicated in the initial evaluation of tibia or fibula fractures. In instances where the fracture may involve the knee or ankle joint, MRI may be helpful to evaluate associated ligamentous or meniscal injuries.

Imaging Findings

Two-view imaging of the right tibia and fibula was obtained. There is a nondisplaced spiral fracture of the distal tibia with an intact fibula, with visualized joints that are normal and no abnormal bone density; the visualized portions of the knee and foot appear normal (Figs. 67.1 and 67.2).

Case Conclusion

Pediatric Orthopedics was consulted and recommended application of a posterior long leg splint, with follow-up in 1 week, since this injury was an isolated, nondisplaced tibia fracture. Strict return precautions were provided and included symptoms of compartment syndrome. Follow-up imaging several months later demonstrates a progressively healing right distal tibia fracture noted in stable alignment (Figs. 67.3 and 67.4).

Tibial shaft fractures are the third most common fracture in children—only fractures of the femur and forearm are more prevalent.[1,2] Approximately 30% of cases of tibial fracture have an associated fibula fracture.[3] Adolescent patients are more likely to have combined fractures of the tibia and fibula than other pediatric age groups.[4,5]

A few unique types of pediatric tibia and fibula fractures are important to identify:

Transverse fractures of the tibia/fibula result from a direct blow, and while they are frequently seen in sports injuries, they are also the most common type of long bone fracture associated with nonaccidental trauma.[6]

Bowing fractures are caused by axial loading and may be subtle on radiographs.

Buckle fractures occur when compressive forces lead to buckling of the cortex. Findings on radiographs may be subtle, especially on the AP view.

Stress fractures present as gradual onset of pain and limp and are much more common in older adolescents and young adults. Only 9% occur in children younger than 16 years old, 32% in adolescents aged 16 to 19 years old, and 59% in patients over 20 years old; the proximal third of the tibia is the most often region affected.[7] Radiographs may be normal or may show limited cortical changes or subperiosteal bone formation.[7]

Isolated fibula fractures may also occur when there is a direct blow to the lateral lower leg; however, prior to diagnosis, it is important to closely examine the distal tibial physis, as concomitant fractures to this location are frequently present.

Spiral (toddler's) fracture/oblique fractures often occur with minor trauma. These fractures are frequently

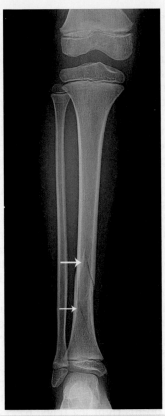

Fig. 67.1 AP view demonstrates a nondisplaced spiral fracture of the distal tibia *(arrow)* with an intact fibula.

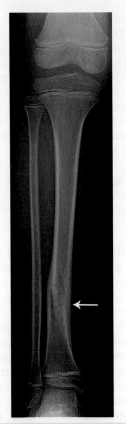

Fig. 67.3 AP view demonstrates a progressively healing right distal tibia fracture *(arrow)* noted in stable alignment.

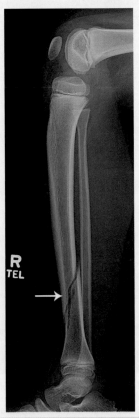

Fig. 67.2 Lateral view demonstrates a nondisplaced spiral fracture of the distal tibia *(arrow)* with an intact fibula.

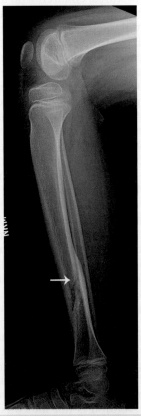

Fig. 67.4 Lateral view demonstrates a progressively healing right distal tibia fracture *(arrow)* noted in stable alignment.

not seen on lateral radiographs, and the appearance of the fracture on AP view can also be subtle and difficult to visualize.[8] Internal oblique views may also aid in identifying the fracture, although sometimes the fracture can only be visualized over a week after the injury, when bone resorption at the fracture site, periosteal reaction and callous have developed.[9] In this case, the lower leg should be immobilized and made non–weight bearing until repeat imaging is performed.[10] Such fractures commonly occur in the distal half to third of the tibia. Although operator dependent, extremity ultrasound has also been described as a possible imaging modality. Ultrasound may show a hypoechoic hematoma along the tibial cortex or elevated periosteum indicative of a fracture, despite negative radiographs.[11]

Spiral fractures should be considered suspicious for non-accidental trauma when they occur when the patient is too young to walk or cruise. Pathognomonic findings for abuse include metaphyseal fractures that can be seen as corner fractures and bucket handle fractures.[12]

Treatment of tibia fractures is dependent on several factors. Consultation with a qualified pediatric orthopedic surgeon is appropriate if there are questions regarding management. There are accepted parameters with respect to angulation, displacement, translation, and degree of shortening that guide surgical versus nonsurgical treatment.[13–15] There are myriad surgical intervention techniques that are available for use; which technique is utilized is largely individualized to each patient and clinical situation.[16] Surgical intervention is most often indicated for patients with open fractures, children who are difficult to cast or are at risk for compartment syndrome (such as obese children), segmental fractures, or fracture patterns that are not able to be well controlled with casting.[14] One study examining closed reduction versus operative management of closed tibia fractures found no difference in outcome, but patients with associated fibula facture or more severe initial fracture displacement (>20%) were more likely to fail closed reduction treatment.[17] As a general rule, combined tibia and fibula fractures, displaced Salter-Harris type I–III fractures, and Salter-Harris type IV fractures mandate immediate orthopedic consultation.[18] Nondisplaced Salter-Harris type I–III fractures of the tibia may be managed conservatively with immobilization and timely pediatric orthopedic follow-up (usually within 1 week).[18]

Distal fibular fractures are commonly reported in pediatric patients, and the majority of these are Salter-Harris type I and II injuries or distal avulsion injuries; more severe Salter-Harris Classification fractures (i.e., III–V) rarely occur as isolated injuries.[18] Isolated distal fibula fractures are stable and usually can be treated with immobilization. Interestingly, the traditional management of casting for several weeks has been challenged, given the low likelihood of complications associated with these injuries. Options that have been explored include a walking cast/boot, ankle bracing, and elastic stockinettes, along with crutch use; patients managed with these have been shown to have good outcomes, faster return to activities, and overall improved satisfaction.[18–20]

If surgical intervention is not indicated, casting can be accomplished in the emergency department setting utilizing

procedural sedation (previously known as "conscious sedation").[14] Use of fluoroscopy is helpful to ensure proper alignment after reduction and cast application.[14] Many authors recommend admission for observation after reduction to ensure appropriate pain control and to monitor for the development of compartment syndrome, although this is often institution dependent.[2,14] Compartment syndrome is not common in the pediatric population compared to the adult population, and the risk of this complication is even lower in children under the age of 8 years.[2,21,22] Reported rates of compartment syndrome in pediatric patients are between 0.2% and 8%, although the rate is lower in preadolescent patients.[2,15,21,23] Patients with certain injury mechanism histories appear to be at higher risk for the development of compartment syndrome: high-energy mechanisms (for example, skiing accidents, falls from significant height, and motor vehicle accidents), significantly displaced fractures, the presence of an associated fibula fracture, and open fractures.[2,24] One study has suggested that children under the age of 12 years old with closed, minimally displaced, tibia-only fractures that resulted from a low-energy mechanism can be discharged if pain is adequately controlled, careful return precautions are given, and timely follow-up is ensured.[2]

For comparison, several other cases are provided:

A 14-year-old male presented to the Emergency Department with right leg pain and swelling after jumping from a horse, landing on his right leg (Figs. 67.5 and 67.6). He

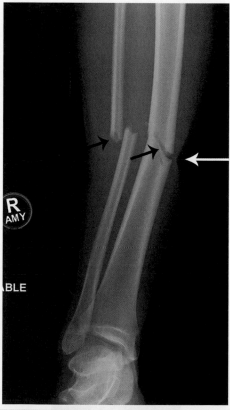

Fig. 67.5 AP view demonstrates acute fractures of the mid tibial and fibular diaphyses *(black arrows)* with lateral angulation of the distal fracture fragments. Note the skin dimpling *(white arrow)* overlying the tibial fracture.

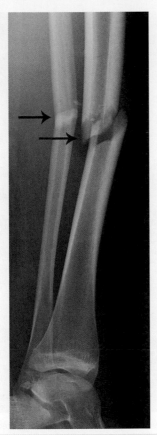

Fig. 67.6 Lateral view demonstrates acute fractures of the mid tibial and fibular diaphyses *(black arrows)*.

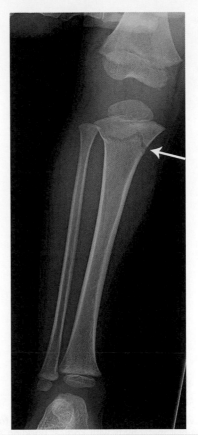

Fig. 67.7 AP view demonstrates a transverse nondisplaced proximal right tibial metaphyseal fracture *(arrow)*.

had no other injury. His examination demonstrated skin dimpling at the site of the presumed fracture; this dimpling can be seen on the images, which demonstrate an acute, oblique fracture of mid tibial shaft and a transverse fracture of mid fibular shaft. Pediatric Orthopedics was consulted and the fracture was reduced and splinted. IV antibiotics (cefazolin) were administered. He was admitted to the hospital and underwent intramedullary nailing without complication.

A 5-year-old male reported bilateral leg pain after a motor vehicle accident (Figs. 67.7–67.10). Due to difficulty with pain localization, the child had imaging of his entire legs, bilaterally. Images of his femurs and ankles were unremarkable. However, tibia-fibula images revealed bilateral nondisplaced proximal tibial metaphyseal fractures, the fracture on the left extending to the growth plate consistent with a Salter-Harris type II fracture. Proximal tibial metaphyseal injuries can be associated with later development of tibial valgus deformities. He was placed in bilateral leg casts and was admitted to the Pediatric Trauma Service with continued Pediatric Orthopedic consultation.

The patient in Fig. 67.11 is a 14-year-old female who was struck by a car while riding her bike and reported pain in her right lower leg. At presentation, there was a 3-cm laceration noted with swelling and tenderness. She was grossly neurovascularly intact. These images demonstrate a markedly comminuted fracture of the proximal tibial diaphysis

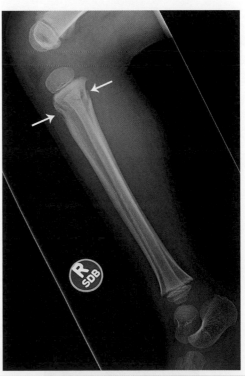

Fig. 67.8 Lateral view demonstrates a transverse nondisplaced proximal right tibial metaphyseal fracture *(arrows)*.

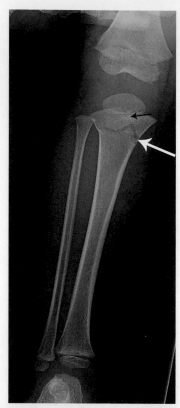

Fig. 67.9 AP view shows a nondisplaced transverse fracture of the proximal left tibial metaphysis with cortical buckling *(white arrow)*. There is also an oblique fracture plane *(black arrow)* extending to the growth plate, consistent with a Salter-Harris type II injury.

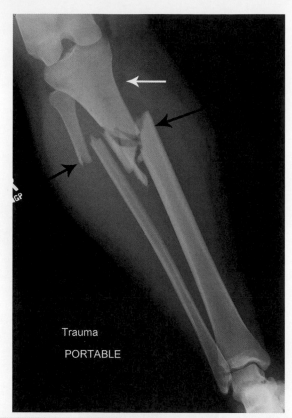

Fig. 67.11 AP view shows a markedly comminuted fracture of the proximal tibial diaphysis and transverse fracture of the proximal fibular diaphysis *(black arrows)*, with medial displacement and proximal migration of the distal fragments. Gas bubbles are seen in the soft tissues *(white arrow)*.

and a transverse fracture of the proximal fibular diaphysis, with medial displacement of the distal fragments. Knee and ankle joint alignments are maintained. There are small collections of gas in the soft tissue. This child was taken emergently to the operating room for debridement and intramedullary pinning of the fracture.

IMAGING PEARLS

1. Initial images of the tibia and fibula should include AP and lateral views and include views of both the knee and ankle.
2. Spiral fractures may be difficult to visualize. Oblique radiographs can be helpful, but patients with suspected fractures based on history and physical but normal imaging should be immobilized and made non-weightbearing until they can follow up with an orthopedist and have repeat radiography in approximately 7 days.
3. Spiral fractures are especially concerning for nonaccidental trauma when the child is not yet walking or cruising.
4. If a patient appears to have an isolated fibula fracture, evaluate for a distal tibial physeal injury.

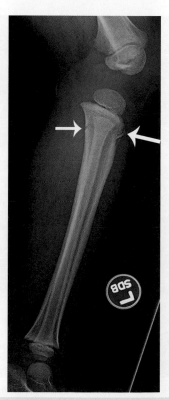

Fig. 67.10 Lateral view shows a nondisplaced transverse fracture of the proximal left tibial metaphysis with cortical buckling *(arrows)*.

References

1. Heinrich SD, Mooney JF. Fractures of the shaft of the tibia and fibula. In: Rockwood CA, Wilkins KE, Beaty JH, eds. *Rockwood and Wilkins' Fractures in Children*, 4th ed. Philadelphia: Lippincott-Raven Publishers; 2006:1033.

2. Malhotra K, Pai S, Radcliffe G. Do minimally displaced, closed tibial fractures in children need monitoring for compartment syndrome? *Injury*. 2015;46(2):254-258.

3. Mashru RP, Herman MJ, Pizzutillo PD. Tibial shaft fractures in children and adolescents. *J Am Acad Orthop Surg*. 2005;13(5):345-552.

4. Audigé L, Slongo T, Lutz N, et al. The AO Pediatric Comprehensive Classification of Long Bone Fractures (PCCF). *Acta Orthop*. 2017; 88(2):133-139.

5. Joeris A, Lutz N, Blumenthal A, et al. The AO Pediatric Comprehensive Classification of Long Bone Fractures (PCCF). *Acta Orthop*. 2017 Apr;88(2):123-128.

6. Loder RT, Bookout C. Fracture patterns in battered children. *J Orthop Trauma*. 1991;5(4):428-433.

7. Coady CM, Micheli LJ. Stress fractures in the pediatric athlete. *Clin Sports Med*. 1997;16(2):225-238.

8. Shravat BP, Harrop SN, Kane TP. Toddler's fracture. *J Accid Emerg Med*. 1996;13(1):59-61.

9. Tenenbein M, Reed MH, Black GB. The toddler's fracture revisited. *Am J Emerg Med*. 1990;8(3):208-211.

10. Mellick LB, Milker L, Egsieker E. Childhood accidental spiral tibial (CAST) fractures. *Pediatr Emerg Care*. 1999;15(5):307-309.

11. Lewis D, Logan P. Sonographic diagnosis of toddler's fracture in the emergency department. *J Clin Ultrasound*. 2006;34(4):190-194.

12. Swischuk LE. Radiographic signs of skeletal trauma. In: Ludwig S, Korbnerg A, eds. *Child Abuse: A Medical Reference*. 2nd ed. New York Churchill-Livingstone; 1992.

13. Sarmiento A. On the behavior of closed tibial fractures: clinical/radiological correlations. *J Orthop Trauma*. 2000;14:199-205.

14. Ho CA. Tibia shaft fractures in adolescents: how and when can they be managed successfully with cast treatment? *J Pediatr Orthop*. 2016; 36(suppl 1):S15-S18.

15. Rickert KD, Hosseinzadeh P, Edmonds EW. What's new in pediatric orthopaedic trauma: the lower extremity. *J Pediatr Orthop*. 2018; 38(8):e434-e439.

16. Lieber J, Schmittenbecher P. Developments in the treatment of pediatric long bone shaft fractures. *Eur J Pediatr Surg*. 2013;23(6):427-433.

17. Kinney MC, Nagle D, Bastrom T, et al. Operative versus conservative management of displaced tibial shaft fracture in adolescents. *J Pediatr Orthop*. 2016;36(7):661-666.

18. Boutis K. Common pediatric fractures treated with minimal intervention. *Pediatr Emerg Care*. 2010;26(2):152-157.

19. Boutis K, Willan AR, Babyn P, et al. Randomized controlled trial of casting vs. air-stirrup ankle brace in children with acute low risk ankle fractures. *Pediatrics*. 2007;119(6):e1256-e1263.

20. Gleeson AP, Stuart MJ, Wilson B, et al. Ultrasound assessment and conservative management of inversion injuries of the ankle in children: plaster of Paris versus Tubigrip. *J Bone Joint Surg Br*. 1996; 78(3):484-487.

21. McQueen MM, Gaston P, Court-Brown CM. Acute compartment syndrome. Who is at risk? *J Bone Joint Surg Br*. 2000;82(2):200-203.

22. Ferlic PW, Singer G, Kraus TR, et al. The acute compartment syndrome following fractures of the lower leg in children. *Injury*. 2012; 43(10):1743-1746.

23. Erdos J, Dlaska C, Szatmary P, et al. Acute compartment syndrome in children: a case series in 24 patients and review of the literature. *Int Orthop*. 2011;35(4):569-575.

24. Grottkau BE, Epps HR, Di Scala C. Compartment syndrome in children and adolescents. *J Pediatr Surg*. 2005;40(4):678-682.

25. Pandya NK, Edmonds EW, Mubarak SJ. The incidence of compartment syndrome after flexible nailing of pediatric tibial shaft fractures. *J Child Orthop*. 2011;5(6):439-447.

68 Tough Day: Triplane Fracture

ROBERT VEZZETTI, MD, FAAP, FACEP

Case Presentation

A 12-year-old male presents to the emergency department with left ankle pain. Two hours ago, he was jumping on a trampoline when he "landed wrong, twisting" the ankle. He cannot remember in which direction the ankle twisted but he states he developed swelling to the ankle and had difficulty ambulating due to pain. He denies neck pain, back pain, numbness, and weakness, and there is no other injury. His examination reveals a pleasant patient with vital signs that are appropriate for his age. There is swelling and tenderness to the left lateral malleolus. He has diminished range of motion secondary to pain and does not want to bear weight. He has good dorsalis pedis and posterior tibial pulses with brisk capillary refill. He is neurologically intact. The rest of the extremity has no signs of injury.

Imaging Considerations

PLAIN RADIOGRAPHY

Plain radiography is the imaging modality of choice to evaluate suspected bony injuries. For suspected Tillaux and triplane fractures, plain radiography is the recommended initial imaging modality.[1] The modality is widely available and relatively inexpensive, and ionizing radiation exposure is minimal compare to other modalities. Tillaux fractures demonstrate a distinct pattern: an anterior lateral physeal separation with fracture extension through the epiphysis into the joint.[2,3] Lack of fracture involvement of the metaphysis in the coronal plane distinguishes this fracture from a triplane fracture.[2,3]

COMPUTED TOMOGRAPHY (CT)

CT is usually not a first-line imaging modality in the evaluation of fractures in general. However, CT may be indicated to better define an injury when the clinical picture is not clear or the fracture appears particularly complex. CT has been shown to accurately identify the anatomic characteristics of a fracture and is advocated by some authors to assist in planning appropriate fracture management.[1,4–6] CT has been shown to impact fracture classification and management decisions in patients with intraarticular fractures (especially of the partially closed distal tibial physis) who initially underwent plain radiography.[7] CT scanning has also been shown to be accurate in the estimation of intraarticular displacement in Tillaux fractures.[8] Some authors suggest obtaining CT imaging only if there is less than 2 mm of displacement of fracture fragments on radiography, voicing concerns that plain radiography may underestimate the amount of displacement,[5] and other authors promulgate routine use of CT with these injuries.[9] However, another study found that additional imaging with CT scanning did not significantly change fracture impression or management when compared to plain radiography.[10]

CT has been shown to impact management in patients with triplane fractures as well.[11] As with Tillaux fractures, this is a matter of debate, and some studies have indicated that the additional use of CT did not change the management of such fractures as much as previously thought.[10] CT use does involve greater exposure to ionizing radiation. However, after consultation with an orthopedic specialist, it is reasonable to obtain a CT scan.

MAGNETIC RESONANCE IMAGING (MRI)

While usually not a first-line imaging modality, MRI can be utilized as a follow-up study. MRI is excellent at detecting ligamentous injuries and osteochondral fractures.[4] Consultation with an orthopedic specialist is appropriate if consideration is given to emergent MRI imaging.

Imaging Findings

Plain radiography was obtained. These images demonstrate a Salter-Harris type IV fracture of the distal tibia (Figs. 68.1–68.3).

Case Conclusion

Due to the results of initial imaging, a noncontrast CT scan of the ankle was obtained. This study demonstrated a triplane fracture of the distal tibia. The epiphyseal fracture shows 2–3 mm of diastasis. The distal fibula and tarsal bones are intact (Figs 68.4 and 68.5). Pediatric Orthopedics was consulted and the patient was taken to the operating suite for open reduction and internal fixation.

Tillaux and triplane fractures occur when portions of the distal tibial physis have closed but portions of the physis remain open. The distal tibial physis closes in a distinct pattern—the middle physis closes first, followed by the medial physis, then the lateral physis. When a rotational force is applied to the partially closed physis, the open lateral physis is most vulnerable to injury.[2,3,8] These fractures traverse the antero-lateral physis to the distal epiphysis, causing it to fracture, thus producing the Tillaux and triplane fracture patterns.[2] Because the physis has to have begun closure for

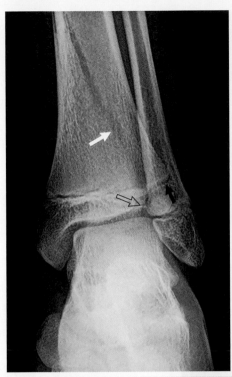

Fig. 68.1 AP radiographic view demonstrates a Salter-Harris type IV fracture of the distal tibia, a triplane fracture. Fracture components include a long, oblique, coronally oriented fracture of the distal tibial diaphysis and metaphysis *(white arrow)*; a horizontal fracture through the anterolateral physis, seen as widening of the growth plate *(black arrow)*; and a subtle vertical, sagittal fracture through the distal tibial epiphysis *(open arrow)*.

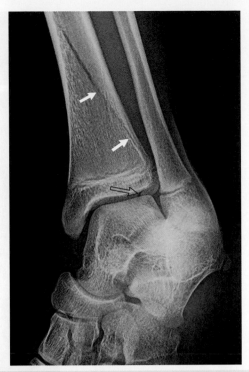

Fig. 68.3 Oblique view demonstrates a Salter-Harris type IV fracture of the distal tibia, a triplane fracture. Fracture components include a long, oblique, coronally oriented fracture of the distal tibial diaphysis and metaphysis *(white arrows)*; a horizontal fracture through the anterolateral physis, not seen well on this projection; and a subtle vertical, sagittal fracture through the distal tibial epiphysis *(open arrow)*.

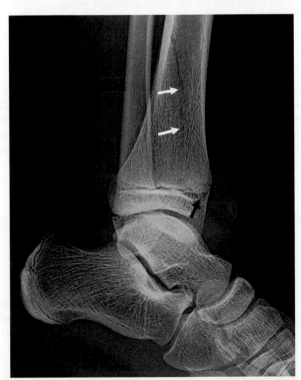

Fig. 68.2 Lateral view demonstrates a Salter-Harris type IV fracture of the distal tibia, a triplane fracture. Fracture components include a long, oblique, coronally oriented fracture of the distal tibial diaphysis and metaphysis *(white arrows)*; and a horizontal fracture through the anterolateral physis, seen as widening of the growth plate *(black arrow)*.

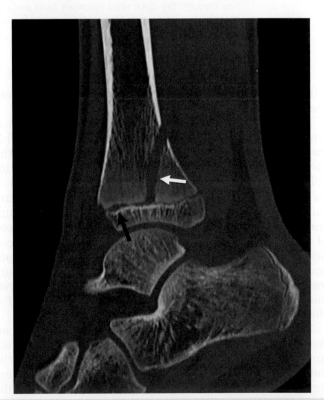

Fig. 68.4 Sagittal reconstructed computed tomography image demonstrates the coronally oriented fracture of the distal tibial metaphysis and diaphysis *(white arrow)* and widening of the anterior physis of the tibia *(black arrow)*, the latter consistent with growth plate fracture.

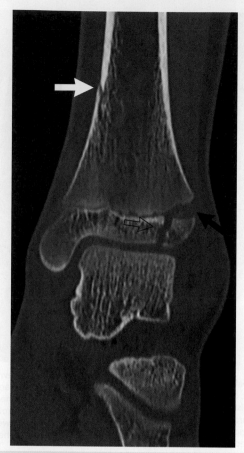

Fig. 68.5 Coronal reconstructed computed tomography image demonstrates the vertically oriented, sagittal fracture through the distal tibial epiphysis *(open arrow)*; widening of the lateral physis *(black arrow)*, consistent with growth plate fracture; and the metadiaphyseal fracture is partially seen *(white arrow)*.

a Tillaux or triplane fracture to occur, these injuries are seen in adolescents.

The Tillaux fracture was named for Paul Jules Tillaux, who first described this fracture pattern in 1982.[2,3,6] This fracture is a Salter-Harris type III fracture, involving the distal tibia physis with an intraarticular component involving the distal epiphysis.[2,3] Triplane fractures are similar to Tillaux fractures, but with an additional fracture through the metaphysis (Fig. 68.6). Triplane fractures are complex Salter-Harris type IV fractures and are comprised of three fracture planes—an epiphyseal sagittal fracture, a horizontal fracture through the physis, and an oblique/coronal fracture through the metaphysis.[9,10,12] Like Tillaux fractures, triplane fractures require a partially open physis and occur in the adolescent population, although at a slightly younger age.[9,10,13]

Treatment of triplane and Tillaux fractures depends on the amount of displacement present. Nondisplaced fractures or fractures with less than 2 mm displacement can be managed with closed reduction, immobilization in a long leg cast, and close orthopedic follow-up.[2,3,12,13] While there is practice variation, there is general agreement that displacement of 2 mm or more requires open reduction and internal fixation, followed by casting, and orthopedic

follow-up.[2,3,5,6,8,12,13] In one study of patients with Tillaux fracture and 2–4 mm of fracture displacement, all underwent open reduction and fixation (without prior closed reduction attempt) and had excellent outcomes.[5] Tillaux and triplane fractures that are not properly reduced have been associated with postinjury pain, joint stiffness, and the development of arthritis.[3,6,8,12,13]

IMAGING PEARLS

1. Plain radiography should be the first-line imaging modality when evaluating patients with suspected fractures, including those with suspected Tillaux or triplane fractures.
2. The role of CT is somewhat controversial. This modality is often utilized to better define fracture extent and anatomy, after plain radiography has demonstrated the fracture.
3. It is appropriate to obtain a CT after orthopedic consultation.
4. MRI is not employed as an initial imaging modality but may be used as a follow-up study if clinically indicated.

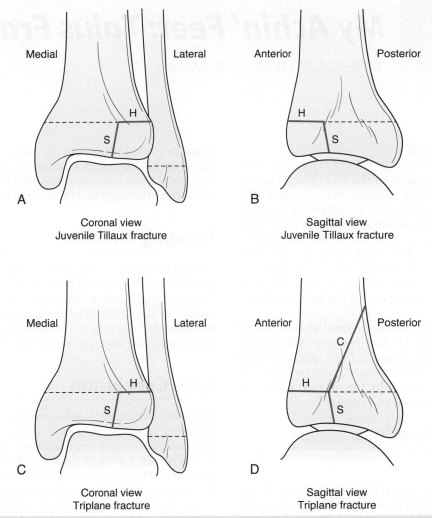

Fig. 68.6 Comparison of Tillaux (A, B) and triplane (C, D) fractures. Both fractures include a horizontal fracture through the anterolateral distal tibial physis *(H)* and a vertical, usually sagittal, fracture through the epiphysis *(S)*. The triplane fracture also includes a fracture through the distal tibial metaphysis, usually in the coronal plane *(C)*.

References

1. Wuerz TH, Gurd DP. Pediatric physeal ankle fracture. *J Am Acad Orthop Surg.* 2013;21(4):234-244.
2. Habusta SF, Griffin EE. *Tillaux Fracture. StatPearls* [Internet]. Treasure Island, FL: StatPearls Publishing; 2019.
3. Koury SI, Stone CK, Harrell G, et al. Recognition and management of Tillaux fractures in adolescents. *Pediatr Emerg Care.* 1999;15(1):37-39.
4. Kim JR, Song KH, Song KJ, et al. Treatment outcomes of triplane and Tillaux fractures of the ankle in adolescence. *Clin Orthop Surg.* 2010;2(1):34-38.
5. Kaya A, Altay T, Ozturk H, et al. Open reduction and internal fixation in displaced juvenile Tillaux fractures. *Injury.* 2007;38(2):201-205.
6. Ali Al-Ashhab ME, Mahmoud Mohamed AA. Treatment for displaced Tillaux fractures in adolescent age group. *Foot Ankle Surg.* 2020; 26(3):295-298.
7. Nenopoulos A, Beslikas T, Gigis I, et al. The role of CT in diagnosis and treatment of distal tibial fractures with intra-articular involvement in children. *Injury.* 2015;46(11):2177-2180.
8. Horn BD, Crisci K, Krug M, et al. Radiologic evaluation of juvenile Tillaux fractures of the distal tibia. *J Pediatr Orthop.* 2001;21(2):162-164.
9. Crawford AH. Triplane and Tillaux fractures: is a 2 mm residual gap acceptable? *J Pediatr Orthop.* 2012;32(suppl 1):S69-S73.
10. Liporace FA, Yoon RS, Kubiak EN, et al. Does adding computed tomography change the diagnosis and treatment of Tillaux and triplane pediatric ankle fractures? *Orthopedics.* 2012;35(2): e208-e212.
11. Eismann EA, Stephan ZA, Mehlman CT, et al. Pediatric triplane ankle fractures: impact of radiographs and computed tomography on fracture classification and treatment planning. *J Bone Joint Surg Am.* 2015;97(12):995-1002.
12. Schnetzler KA, Hoernschemeyer D. The pediatric triplane ankle fracture. *J Am Acad Orthop Surg.* 2007;15(12):738-747.
13. Su AW, Larson AN. Pediatric ankle fractures: concepts and treatment principles. *Foot Ankle Clin.* 2015;20(4):705-719.

ROBERT VEZZETTI, MD, FAAP, FACEP

Case Presentation

A 14-year-old male is brought to the Emergency Department after being involved in a motor vehicle crash. The patient was a restrained front seat passenger in a vehicle that was struck by another car while stopped at a red light.

The patient did not lose consciousness and has no complaint of head pain, neck pain, back pain, or abdominal pain. He states he feels that his right foot "was twisted" and "slammed into the floorboard" of the car. He complains of pain to the dorsal aspect of the foot. He denies numbness.

His physical examination reveals normal vital signs and is generally unremarkable. He has swelling and pain on palpation of the dorsal-lateral aspect of his right foot. There is no obvious deformity. The joint appears to be stable. He has brisk capillary refill and both the dorsalis pedis and posterior tibial pulses are equal and strong.

Imaging Considerations

PLAIN RADIOGRAPHY

This is the first-line imaging modality in patients with suspected bone injury. Patients with injuries that are suspected to involve the talus should have anterior-posterior, lateral, and oblique views of the ankle (an ankle series); if the talus head is not fully visualized, consideration should be given to obtaining an anterior-posterior view of the foot.[1] Radiography has been shown to have difficulty in detecting talar dome fractures and lateral process fractures.[2,3]

COMPUTED TOMOGRAPHY (CT)

This imaging modality is often used as a follow-up to plain radiography. CT can provide excellent bony detail, and if there is a complex fracture, the diagnosis of a talus fracture is in question, or there is strong clinical suspicion of a talus fracture with negative plain radiography, utilization of CT is appropriate. This is especially true as some talus fractures may be occult or not well depicted on plain radiographs, making CT useful in these cases.[1] CT has been found to improve detection of talar dome fractures, improve talus fracture classification, and detect fractures of the lateral process of the talus, which can be difficult to visualize with plain radiography.[2,3]

MAGNETIC RESONANCE IMAGING (MRI)

This is not a first-line imaging modality for the evaluation of fractures but can be useful when there are significant symptoms and a strong clinical suspicion of injury with negative plain radiography or equivocal CT. MRI is especially useful for the evaluation for osteochondral injury (e.g., talar dome osteochondral injury), ligamentous injury, acute or chronic physeal injury, and stress fracture.

Imaging Findings

Three-view plain radiography of the right ankle (anterior-posterior, lateral, and mortise views) was obtained. These images demonstrate a thin, curvilinear ossification dorso-lateral to the distal talar neck consistent with an acute avulsion chip fracture of the talus neck. The ankle mortise is normal in appearance (Figs. 69.1–69.3).

Case Conclusion

Pediatric Orthopedics was consulted. The patient was placed in an ankle boot, given crutches, and advised to be non–weight bearing until follow-up with Pediatric Orthopedics within 1 week of discharge from the Emergency Department. The injury healed well and the patient did not develop complications from his injury.

Fractures of the talus are not common and are the result of an axial loading injury to the anterior portion of the tibia with the foot in dorsiflexion.[4] The reported incidence of talus fracture in the pediatric population is 0.1%–0.8%.[5,6] Previously reported etiologies causing talus fractures include motor vehicle accidents and falls from significant heights.[5,7] The neck of the talus is the most common fracture site, followed by the body.[4]

Talar neck fractures represent 50% of all talus fractures and are well described in the litertature.[1] Talar body fractures are the second most common fracture of the talus and are seen in high-energy mechanism injuries and activities that involve landing on one's feet (e.g., cheerleading and gymnastics injuries) resulting in shear fractures of the talar body.[1] Fractures of the talar head are uncommon and there is sparse literature on this injury. Less than 10% of talus fractures involve the head, and outcomes are not well documented; often, this fracture is associated with other fractures, typically from high-energy injuries.[1] A unique fracture is a lateral process fracture, also known as "snowboarder's fracture" since this fracture is more common in participants of this sport; the injury occurs when the foot is in a dorsiflexed and inverted position.[1] These fractures are frequently missed.[1,8]

Talus fractures have associated complications, including avascular necrosis (AVN) (7%), arthrosis (17%), delayed union (3%), neurapraxia (7%), and the need for further surgery (10%). These complications have been found to be more common in adolescent boys.[4,5,7] AVN is more

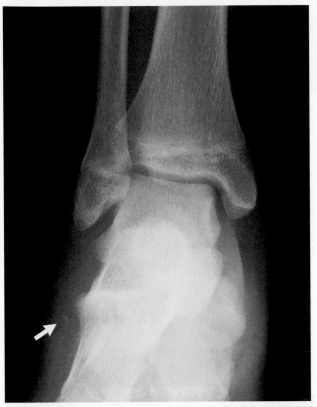

Fig. 69.1 Anterior-posterior view of the ankle demonstrates a <6-mm curvilinear ossification projecting in the soft tissues lateral to the distal talus, suggesting an acute, mildly displaced, chip fracture *(arrow)*.

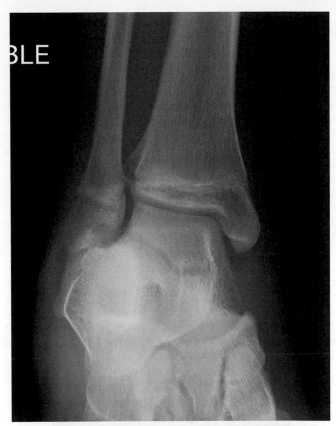

Fig. 69.3 Mortise view demonstrating a normal appearance.

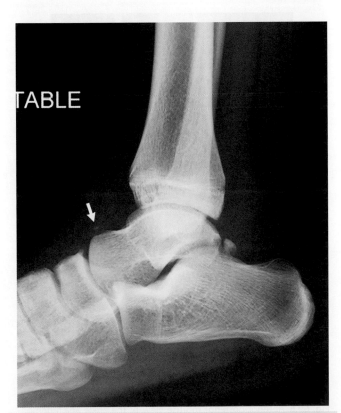

Fig. 69.2 Lateral view of the ankle demonstrates a <6-mm curvilinear ossification dorsal to the distal neck of the talus, confirming a cortical avulsion fracture of the talar neck *(arrow)*.

commonly associated with fracture-dislocations, and while the exact mechanism that leads to the development of AVN is not well understood, dislocation is a risk factor.[4–6,9] One study found that older patients (above the age of 12 years) had a higher incidence of fracture-dislocations, which were more likely to be associated with vascular injury.[7] Another study found low rates of AVN, but like previously reported series AVN was seen in patients with displaced fractures.[5] This older group also was more likely to require operative intervention.[7] AVN has been reported in patients with minimally displaced fractures, so prompt follow-up and monitoring are important for patients with fracture-dislocation injuries.[6,9] A review of reported talus fracture series since 1985 in pediatric patients found an incidence of AVN of 16% in 83 cases of nondisplaced talus fractures and 51% in 49 cases of displaced and comminuted talus fractures.[6]

The Hawkins Classification System has been used to describe talus fractures[10]:

TYPE	DESCRIPTION
I	Talar neck fracture with no to minimal displacement
II	Talar neck fracture with subtalar dislocation
III	Talar neck fracture with subtalar and tibiotalar dislocations
IV	Talar neck fracture with subtalar, tibiotalar, and talonavicular dislocations.

Worsening fracture type increases the risk for AVN; avulsion fractures are extremely low risk for this complication.[10]

Guidelines for the management of talus fractures in the pediatric population have not been definitively established.[4,5,7,11] There are management guidelines for adult patients that many authors adhere to for the pediatric population, which consist of cast immobilization without weight bearing for 6 to 8 weeks in nondisplaced fractures and reduction and operative fixation for displaced fractures.[7,12] In this patient, there was an avulsion injury, which was at low risk for complications and expected to heal quite well with conservative management, hence the utilization of an orthopedic boot and not a cast. Providers should consult with Pediatric Orthopedics or an orthopedic specialist who is comfortable managing pediatric factures to assist in the formulation of a plan of care.

A comparison case is presented here:

An 8-year-old male who was jumping off of a playground apparatus is shown in Figs. 69.4–69.6. Shortly after doing this, he began to complain of left hindfoot pain and swelling. These images demonstrate a nondisplaced talar neck fracture. This patient was placed in a short leg cast, was followed closely by Pediatric Orthopedics, and did well.

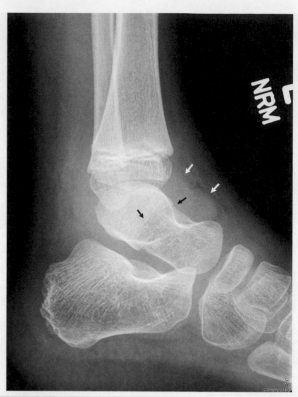

Fig. 69.5 Lateral view of the ankle shows a transverse nondisplaced fracture through the proximal neck of the talus *(black arrows)* with associated soft tissue swelling and ankle joint effusion *(white arrows)*.

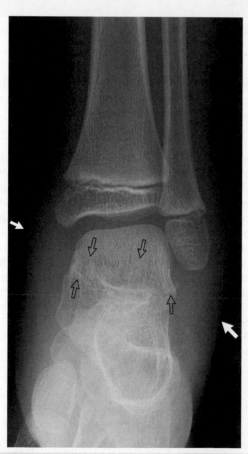

Fig. 69.4 Anterior-posterior (AP) view of the ankle demonstrates an obliquely oriented transverse fracture through the talus *(open arrows)*. Undulating course of the fracture through the talus causes the fracture to be seen in more than one location on an AP projection. Surrounding soft tissue swelling is seen medially and laterally *(white arrows)*.

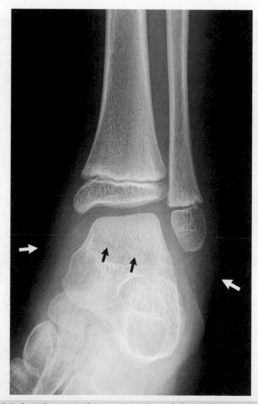

Fig. 69.6 Anterior-posterior mortise view of the ankle again demonstrates obliquely oriented transverse fracture through the talus *(black arrows)*. Soft tissue swelling is again seen medially and laterally *(white arrows)*.

IMAGING PEARLS

1. Plain radiography is the imaging modality of choice with bony injuries, including suspected talus fractures.
2. Non–contrast-enhanced CT may be indicated for talus fractures in certain clinical situations. These include complex fractures, cases in which the extent of the injury needs to be better delineated, and if there is strong clinical suspicion for a talus fracture and plain radiographs are not revealing.
3. MRI is not first-line imaging for the routine diagnosis of talus injuries but can be useful when there is strong clinical suspicion of injury with negative plain radiography or equivocal CT. If there is concern for either tendon/ligamentous injury or neurologic injury, then MRI may be appropriate.

References

1. Early JB. Talus fracture management. *Foot Ankle Clin.* 2008;13(4):635-657.
2. Dale JD, Ha AS, Chew FS. Update on talar fracture patterns: a large level I trauma center study. *AJR Am J Roentgenol.* 2013;201(5):1087-1092.
3. Wu Y, Jiang H, Wang B, et al. Fracture of the lateral process of the talus in children: a kind of ankle injury with frequently missed diagnosis. *J Pediatr Orthop.* 2016;36(3):289-293.
4. Byrne AM, Stephens M. Paediatric talus fracture. *BMJ Case Rep.* 2012;2012:bcr1020115028.
5. Smith JT, Curtis TA, Spencer S, et al. Complications of talus fractures in children. *J Pediatr Orthop.* 2010;30(8):779-784.
6. Rammelt S, Zwipp H, Gavlik JM. Avascular necrosis after minimally displaced talus fracture in a child. *Foot Ankle Int.* 2000;21(12):1030-1036.
7. Eberl R, Singer G, Schalamon J, et al. Fractures of the talus—differences between children and adolescents. *J Trauma.* 2010;68(1):126-130.
8. von Knoch F, Reckord F, von Knoch M, et al. Fracture of the lateral process of the talus in snowboarders. *J Bone Joint Surg Br.* 2007;89:772-777.
9. Talkhani IS, Reidy D, Fogarty EE, et al. Avascular necrosis of the talus after a minimally displaced neck of talus fracture in a 6 year old child. *Injury.* 2000;31(1):63-65.
10. Alton T, Patton DJ, Gee AO. Classifications in brief: the Hawkins Classification for Talus Fractures. *Clin Orthop Relat Res.* 2015;473(9):3046-3049.
11. Michel-Traverso A, Ngo TH, Bruyere C, et al. Talus fracture in a 4-year-old child. *BMJ Case Rep.* 2017;2017:bcr2016215063.
12. Jensen I, Wester JU, Rasmussen F, et al. Prognosis of fracture of the talus in children. 21 (7–34)-year follow-up of 14 cases. *Acta Orthop Scand.* 1994;65:398-400.

70 *My Achin' Back! Spondylolysis/Spondylolisthesis*

ROBERT VEZZETTI, MD, FAAP, FACEP

Case Presentation

A 15-year-female presents with low back pain for 2 months. She had no trauma preceding the pain but is very active and plays soccer. The pain increases with activity. She has tried ibuprofen multiple times, with some relief. Her mother took her to her primary care provider last week where a urine test was performed, which was unremarkable. She has not had fever, vomiting, abdominal pain, vaginal bleeding, vaginal discharge, numbness, or weakness.

Her physical examination reveals a well-appearing child who is afebrile. Her heart rate is 65 beats per minute, respiratory rate is 20 breaths per minute, blood pressure is 125/75 mm Hg, and pulse oximetry is 100% on room air. Her weight is 44 kg. She has an unremarkable examination except for mild midspinal lumbar tenderness without crepitus, warmth, or deformity to palpation. She ambulates with a steady gait. Her neurologic examination is benign, with equal tone and strength throughout.

Imaging Considerations

Not every pediatric patient with nontraumatic back pain requires imaging. Imaging should be considered in patients with localized pain, neurologic deficits, worsening pain, or persistent pain.[1-4] Feldman et al. devised an algorithm for the evaluation of nontraumatic pediatric back pain utilizing history, physical examination, complete blood count (recommended in children under 10 years of age in this study due to the association of back pain and leukemia in younger patients), and imaging (plain radiography and magnetic resonance imaging [MRI]).[4] In this group of close to 100 patients, if radiographs were positive and correlated with historical and physical examination findings, then the patient was treated accordingly; if the radiographs were negative and concerning pain was reported (such as constant pain or night pain) or there was an abnormal neurological examination, an MRI study was obtained and positive findings on MRI were treated accordingly.[4] Patients who had negative radiographs and intermittent pain were treated for presumed overuse syndromes or sprains with rest, physical therapy, and nonsteroidal antiinflammatory medications.[4] Using this algorithm, 36% of the patients in the study group were diagnosed with a specific condition, 68% of these patients had a positive finding on initial radiographs, and the remaining patients in this group who had negative initial radiographs had positive findings on MRI.[4]

A study by Ramirez et al. had similar results when examining the utility of MRI in patients after employing the Feldman et al. algorithm of history, physical examination, and plain radiography. These investigators found that 34% of patients in their study had an identifiable cause of back pain, with diagnostic yield increasing from 8.8% (based on history, physical examination, and plain radiographs) to 36% with the use of MRI. Of the 89 patients who had confirmed pathology, 26% were discovered with plain radiographs and 74% with MRI.[2]

Bhatia et al. also employed an algorithm similar to Feldman et al. utilizing history, physical examination, laboratory investigation, and plain radiography in 73 patients; 57 (78%) of the patients in this study had no identifiable cause of back pain and none of these had abnormal radiologic or laboratory findings.[3] Of the remaining 16 patients, 9 were diagnosed with spondylolysis (with or without spondylolisthesis), with the remaining patients having another diagnosis (osteoid osteoma and disk herniation).[3] Thirteen patients (nearly 18%) in this study had a definitive diagnosis, and of those patients, 10 had abnormal plain radiography, 8 of whom were diagnosed with spondylolysis with or without spondylolisthesis (scoliosis was not considered an etiology of back pain).[3]

PLAIN RADIOGRAPHY

Plain radiography is an excellent first-choice imaging study due to its low cost and widespread availability, but this is not without controversy, as some authors report low diagnostic yield with plain radiographic imaging for pediatric patients with back pain.[1,3-6] Notably, plain radiographs appear normal in the majority of patients with non-concerning histories and physical examinations.[3-5] There is also controversy regarding the optimal number of views to obtain. Postero-anterior (PA) or anteroposterior (AP) and lateral views of the spine appear to be sufficient in most cases, as an oblique view has not been shown to increase diagnostic accuracy,[1,5,7,8] although some authors advocate its use.[9] There are stages in the development of spondylolysis, including early stress reaction without fracture, progression to fracture, and if healing and union do not occur, where there is nonunion and a wider osseous defect at the pars.[10] Much of the historical plain film literature in spondylolysis has been in adults, who often have advanced, terminal spondylolysis; however, pediatric patients are more likely than adults to present with early or progressive spondylolysis that may be amenable to healing with conservative management but is more difficult to detect on plain film evaluation, including on oblique views.[11] It is reasonable to obtain two views of the spine (PA and lateral), and, if symptoms persist or worsen, consideration can be given to obtaining oblique views or advanced imaging modalities.[3,5]

COMPUTED TOMOGRAPHY (CT)

CT has been shown to be sensitive and specific for detecting spondylolysis and spondylolisthesis.[12,13] Computerized tomography can also help to characterize other pathology of the posterior elements of the spine, the vertebral end plates, and facet joints.[7,10] Single photon emission CT (SPECT/CT) combines nuclear medicine bone scan imaging with low-dose CT and detects spondylolysis and other vertebral pathology but also shows increased radionucleotide uptake of a stress reaction in the pars interarticularis prior to the development of fracture.[10] SPECT/CT is useful if there is a strong clinical suspicion of spondylolysis and plain radiography is unremarkable.[9,10] However, this is not an imaging technique utilized in the emergency care setting and is most often ordered in outpatient follow-up, frequently by an orthopedic surgeon. There is radiation exposure with SPECT/CT imaging; most of this is the exposure of a nuclear medicine bone scan with a very small additional contribution to dose by low-dose CT.[10]

MAGNETIC RESONANCE IMAGING

Patients may benefit from MRI if further clarification of plain radiography findings is needed, or if there is concern for an infectious, inflammatory, or neoplastic process, as these alternative diagnoses can be readily detected with this modality. MRI is more sensitive than CT scan for the detection of stress reactions in the pars and can detect stress reactions in the pars prior to the development of an osseous defect.[7,14] T2-weighted images may demonstrate an abnormal signal that can be observed in the pars interarticularis and the adjacent pedicles, suggesting pathology.[5,15] MRI may also be useful if there are associated neurologic symptoms.[9] There have been proposed algorithms for the utilization of MRI in patients with persistent or worsening symptoms or an abnormal neurologic examination.[2,4]

Imaging Findings

Plain radiography of the lumbar spine (AP and lateral views) was obtained. These images demonstrate a grade I spondylolisthesis of L5 on S1 associated with bilateral spondylolysis at L5. There is no other pathology of the lumbosacral spine noted (Figs. 70.1 and 70.2).

For comparison, two additional cases are provided:

The images in Figs. 70.3–70.6 are of a 13-year-old competitive gymnast who was found to have an L5 spondylolysis with a grade I spondylolisthesis. The patient was managed with physical therapy and nonsteroidal antiinflammatory medications (NSAIDs), along with rest, and recovered without operative intervention.

The images in Figs. 70.7–70.9 are of a 15-year-old competitive swimmer with an L4 spondylolysis with a grade I spondylolisthesis, who, despite physical therapy, continued to have pain interfering with her athletic activity. She underwent operative intervention and recovered.

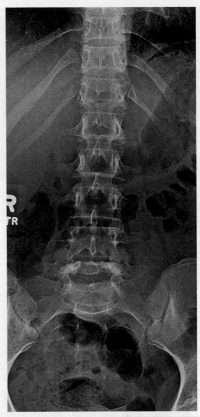

Fig. 70.1 Anteroposterior view of the lumbosacral spine shows no discernible abnormality. (Image courtesy of Brian Kaufman, MD (Pediatric Orthopedics, DCMC).)

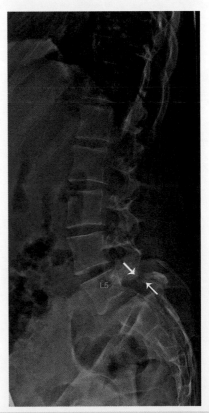

Fig. 70.2 Lateral view demonstrates a grade I spondylolisthesis of L5 on S1 associated with bilateral spondylolysis at L5 *(arrows)*. (Image courtesy of Brian Kaufman, MD (Pediatric Orthopedics, DCMC).)

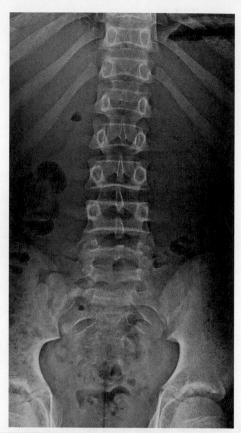

Fig. 70.3 Anteroposterior view of the lumbar spine shows no discernible abnormality. (Image courtesy of Brian Kaufman, MD (Pediatric Orthopedics, DCMC).)

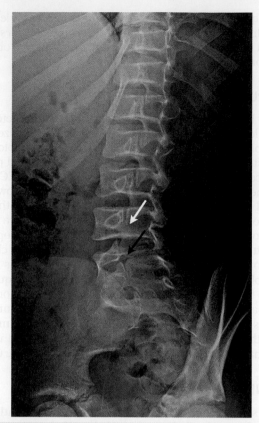

Fig. 70.5 Oblique view demonstrates a right-sided pars defect at L5 *(black arrow)*. Compare to the intact pars interarticularis at L4 *(white arrow)*. (Image courtesy of Brian Kaufman, MD (Pediatric Orthopedics, DCMC).)

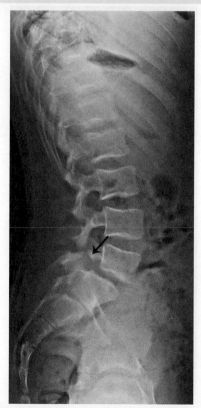

Fig. 70.4 Lateral view demonstrates bilateral spondylolysis defects *(arrow)* at L5 with grade I spondylolisthesis, with L5 subluxed anteriorly with respect to S1. (Image courtesy of Brian Kaufman, MD (Pediatric Orthopedics, DCMC).)

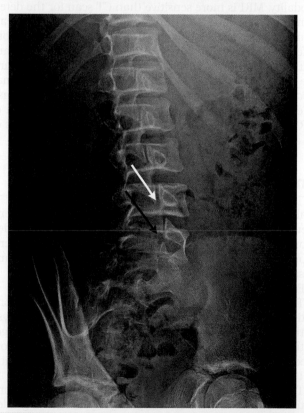

Fig. 70.6 Oblique view demonstrates a left-sided pars defect at L5 *(black arrow)*. Compare to the intact pars interarticularis at L4 *(white arrow)*. (Image courtesy of Brian Kaufman, MD (Pediatric Orthopedics, DCMC).)

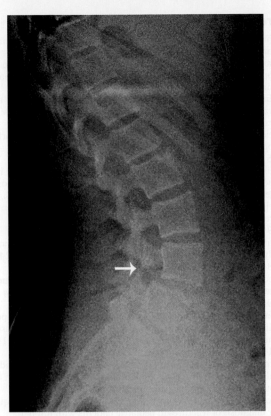

Fig. 70.7 Lateral view demonstrates an L4 spondylolysis with a grade I spondylolisthesis *(arrow)*. (Image courtesy of Brian Kaufman, MD (Pediatric Orthopedics, DCMC).)

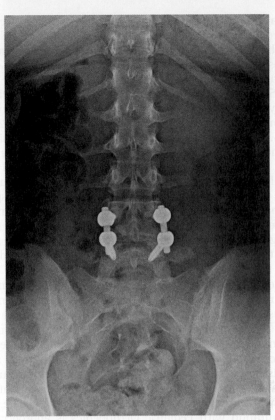

Fig. 70.9 L4 spondylolysis with a grade I spondylolisthesis, postoperative imaging, anteroposterior view. (Image courtesy of Brian Kaufman, MD (Pediatric Orthopedics, DCMC).)

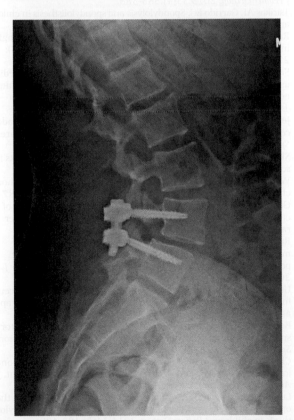

Fig. 70.8 L4 spondylolysis with a grade I spondylolisthesis, postoperative imaging, lateral view. (Image courtesy of Brian Kaufman, MD (Pediatric Orthopedics, DCMC).)

Case Conclusion

The patient was referred to Pediatric Orthopedics. A physical therapy program was initiated and NSAIDs were prescribed for pain as needed. The patient was advised to refrain from soccer while she was treated. She was asked to return to the clinic in 2 months for a repeat evaluation, or sooner if symptoms worsened.

Back pain in the pediatric population has many causes, including direct trauma, overuse syndromes, spondylolysis, spondylolisthesis, vertebral osteomyelitis, urinary tract infection, and neoplasm. No one symptom can reliably be used to determine whether back pain is from serious or less serious etiologies. The incidence of back pain in this population varies and has been reported to be between approximately 12% and 33%, although some studies have reported an incidence as low as 2%.[1,2,16] Pediatric back pain has been increasing in recent years and may be due to several factors, including obesity and backpack use.[1,3,17,18] It has been previously reported in the literature that the majority of pediatric patients have an identifiable cause of back pain at follow-up examinations,[7] although this has been challenged recently.[3,6,7,19]

Spondylolysis is a common cause of lower back pain in the pediatric population.[5,7] Spondylolysis is a pars interarticularis defect. If bilateral there can be progression to spondylolisthesis, where the upper vertebral segment slips over the lower vertebral segment. Spondylolisthesis is graded by the Meyerding or Wiltse-Newman classification system, which assigns a grade based on the degree of anterior vertebral displacement.[7,9] The degree of slippage of the posteroinferior corner of the upper vertebral body relative to the lower vertebral body determines the grade of slippage: grade 1 represents less than 25% displacement; grade 2, 25%–50% displacement; grade 3, 50%–75% displacement; and grade 4, 75%–100% displacement. Discovery of spondylolysis in asymptomatic patients undergoing imaging for another reason has been reported, with an incidence of 2.5%–3.5%.[7,20,21] There are several etiologies of spondylolysis, but the most common is a stress fracture of the pars interarticularis, thought due to repetitive hyperextension and rotational stress on the spine, especially in sports.[1,13] The lumbar spine is the most commonly affected portion of the spine.[1] The pain produced by spondylolysis can range from mild to severe and is exacerbated by lumbar spine extension.[1] Interestingly, the degree of slippage does not always correlate with the degree of reported pain and most patients do not seem to progress in severity of their slippage.[22]

The management of spondylolysis includes both surgical and nonsurgical options. Nonsurgical management includes use of NSAIDs, bracing, rest, and physical therapy.[1,7,13,23] Surgical management is typically reserved for patients with persistent symptoms despite appropriate nonsurgical management.[1,7,23] Patients with high-grade spondylolisthesis are often treated surgically to prevent further slippage,[1,7,13,23,24] although determining which patients will have worsening of their slippage is a matter of debate.[7,13,23] Consultation with Pediatric Orthopedics is appropriate in cases of spondylolysis with or without spondylolisthesis.

IMAGING PEARLS

1. Not all pediatric patients with nontraumatic back pain require imaging. Consider imaging studies in patients with back pain who have persistent symptoms, worsening symptoms, neurologic findings, or other concerning historical or physical examination findings.
2. Plain radiography is a reasonable first-line imaging modality to employ in patients with back pain in whom imaging is indicated. Two views (PA or AP and lateral) are often sufficient. Oblique views can be added as needed.
3. CT is not a first-line imaging modality for nontraumatic back pain but is excellent at detecting spondylolysis and spondylolisthesis and may be useful if plain radiography is negative or equivocal. Combined nuclear medicine SPECT/CT can detect spondylolysis, including early stress reactions. Obtaining SPECT/CT or CT imaging of the spine may also be indicated if plain radiography is nondiagnostic and there are concerning historical or physical examination findings.
4. MRI is also not a first-line imaging modality for nontraumatic back pain. However, MRI can detect spondylolysis, can depict stress reactions in the pars interarticularis prior to development of an osseous defect, and can identify alternative diagnosis. Obtaining an MRI is reasonable if plain radiography is unremarkable and there are concerning historical or physical examination findings, particularly if there are neurologic symptoms.

References

1. Shah SA, Saller J. Evaluation and diagnosis of back pain in children and adolescents. *J Am Acad Orthop Surg.* 2016;24(1):37-45.
2. Ramirez N, Flynn M, Hill BW, et al. Evaluation of a systematic approach to pediatric back pain: the utility of magnetic resonance imaging. *J Pediatr Orthop.* 2015;35(1):28-32.
3. Bhatia NN, Chow G, Timon SJ, et al. Diagnostic modalities for the evaluation of pediatric back pain: a prospective study. *J Pediatr Orthop.* 2008;28(2):230-233.
4. Feldman DS, Straight JJ, Badra MI, et al. Evaluation of an algorithmic approach to pediatric back pain. *J Pediatr Orthop.* 2006;26(3):353-357.
5. Miller R, Beck NA, Sampson NR, et al. Imaging modalities for low back pain in children: a review of spondylolysis and undiagnosed mechanical back pain. *J Pediatr Orthop.* 2013;33(3):282-288.
6. Selbst SM, Lavelle JM, Soyupak SK, et al. Back pain in children who present to the emergency department. *Clin Pediatr (Phila).* 1999;38(7):401-406.
7. Randall RM, Silverstein M, Goodwin R. Review of pediatric spondylolysis and spondylolisthesis. *Sports Med Arthrosc Rev.* 2016;24(4):184-187.
8. Beck NA, Miller R, Baldwin K, et al. Do oblique views add value in the diagnosis of spondylolysis in adolescents? *J Bone Joint Surg Am.* 2013;95(10):e65(1)-e65.
9. Cavalier R, Herman MJ, Cheung EV, et al. Spondylolysis and spondylolisthesis in children and adolescents: I. diagnosis, natural history, and nonsurgical management. *J Am Acad Orthop Surg.* 2006;14(7):417-424.
10. Trout AT, Sharp SE, Anton CG, et al. Spondylolysis and beyond: value of SPECT/CT in evaluation of low back pain in children and young adults. *Radiographics.* 2015;35(3):819-834.
11. Morimoto M, Sakai T, Goto T, et al. Is the Scotty Dog sign adequate for diagnosis of fractures in pediatric patients with lumbar spondylolysis? *Spine Surg Relat Res.* 2018;3(1):49-53.
12. Spencer HT, Sokol LO, Glotzbecker MP, et al. Detection of pars injury by SPECT in patients younger than age 10 with low back pain. *J Pediatr Orthop.* 2013;33(4):383-388.
13. Tsirikos AI, Garrido EG. Spondylolysis and spondylolisthesis in children and adolescents. *J Bone Joint Surg Br.* 2010;92(6):751-759.
14. Rush JK, Astur N, Scott S, et al. Use of magnetic resonance imaging in the evaluation of spondylolysis. *J Pediatr Orthop.* 2015;35(3):271-275.
15. Sairyo K, Katoh S, Takata Y, et al. MRI signal changes of the pedicle as an indicator for early diagnosis of spondylolysis in children and adolescents: a clinical and biomechanical study. *Spine (Phila Pa 1976).* 2006;31(2):206-211.
16. Jeffries LJ, Milanese SF, Grimmer-Somers KA. Epidemiology of adolescent spinal pain: a systematic overview of the research literature. *Spine (Phila Pa 1976).* 2007;32(23):2630-2637.
17. Skaggs DL, Early SD, D'Ambra P, et al. Back pain and backpacks in school children. *J Pediatr Orthop.* 2006;26(3):358-363.
18. Watson K, Papageorgiou A, Jones G, et al. Low back pain in schoolchildren: occurrence and characteristics. *Pain.* 2002;97(1-2):87-92.
19. Gilbert FJ, Grant AM, Gillan M, et al. Low back pain: influence of early MR imaging or CT on treatment and outcome-multicenter randomized trial. *Radiology.* 2004;231(2):343-351.
20. Ramadorai U, Hire J, DeVine JG, et al. Incidental findings of magnetic resonance imaging of the spine in the asymptomatic pediatric population: a systematic review. *Evid Based Spine Care J.* 2014;5(2):95-100.
21. Urrutia J, Cuellar J, Zamora T. Spondylolysis and spina bifida occulta in pediatric patients: prevalence study using computed tomography as a screening method. *Eur Spine J.* 2016;25(2):590-595.
22. Beutler WJ, Fredrickson BE, Murtland A, et al. The natural history of spondylolysis and spondylolisthesis: 45-year follow-up evaluation. *Spine (Phila Pa 1976).* 2003;28(10):1027-1035.
23. Cheung EV, Herman MJ, Cavalier R, et al. Spondylolysis and spondylolisthesis in children and adolescents: II. Surgical management. *J Am Acad Orthop Surg.* 2006;14(8):488-498.
24. Lundine KM, Lewis SJ, Al-Aubaidi Z, et al. Patient outcomes in the operative and nonoperative management of high-grade spondylolisthesis in children. *J Pediatr Orthop.* 2014;34(5):483-489.

71 Achy Muscles: Pyomyositis/Myositis

ROBERT VEZZETTI, MD, FAAP, FACEP

Case Presentation

A previously healthy 14-year-old male presents with left lower quadrant pain, difficulty bearing weight, and fever. He awoke 6 days ago with sharp left lower quadrant pain. At that time, he was seen at an Emergency Department where abdominal computed tomography (CT) and bloodwork were obtained, which were reported to be normal. He was diagnosed with abdominal wall strain and was discharged home with ibuprofen. He reports that this medication has not helped his pain. He went to his primary care provider the following day, who diagnosed mesenteric adenitis and prescribed hydrocodone. The patient reports that the pain has persisted despite this additional medicine. Several days ago, he developed fever, which has been intermittent since then. He states that he has had progressive difficulty with ambulation secondary to pain. He returned to his primary care provider 2 days ago, who obtained plain radiography of the pelvis, which was normal by report. He has not had preceding trauma, although he states that he is a track and field runner, has an extensive exercise routine, and is unsure if he "pulled something" prior to his current symptoms. He denies vomiting, diarrhea, dysuria, or back pain.

He is febrile to 103 degrees Fahrenheit, has a pulse of 106 beats per minute, a respiratory rate of 24 breaths per minute, and a blood pressure of 109/54 mm Hg. He is not in distress but complains of left-sided hip pain, radiating to the left anterior thigh. His abdominal examination reveals tenderness to the left lower quadrant without rebound or guarding. He has exquisite pain with manipulation of his left leg, pointing to the left hip and left thigh. There is no erythema, swelling, fluctuance, or warmth, but he is tender to palpation over the left anterior thigh.

A review of the outside CT report does not mention any abnormalities. Laboratory work is obtained, revealing a total white blood cell count of 15,000 cc/mm, normal urinalysis, a C-reactive protein (CRP) level of 35 mg/dL, an erythrocyte sedimentation rate (ESR) of 90 mm/hour, and a creatine phosphokinase (CK) level of 299 units/L.

Imaging Considerations

PLAIN RADIOGRAPHY

This imaging modality is the first-line choice for patients presenting with musculoskeletal complaints.[1-4] Plain radiography is useful in detecting fractures, radioopaque foreign bodies, tumors, and changes associated with infection, such as osteomyelitis. It is readily available, exposes the patient to minimal amounts of ionizing radiation, and does not require sedation to complete a meaningful study.

COMPUTED TOMOGRAPHY

This modality can identify fluid collections and the contents of the collection and assist in determining if an abscess exists.[1] Pyomyositis on CT imaging may demonstrate enlargement and decreased attenuation of the affected muscle with effacement of surrounding fat planes.[2] The presence of disproportionate muscular involvement compared to subcutaneous soft tissue can help to distinguish pyomyositis from cellulitis.[2] Using intravenous contrast material, a rim-enhancing abscess may be identified.[2] This modality may be useful to help guide drainage of an identified abscess.[2]

However, CT is inferior to magnetic resonance imaging (MRI) for soft tissue infection evaluation and is not the recommended follow-up study in these patients. If soft tissue or bone infection is suspected, then MRI is the modality of choice.

MAGNETIC RESONANCE IMAGING

MRI has excellent capability in identifying fluid collections such as an abscess and associated anatomy surrounding the abscess.[1,3,4] This modality, preferably with imaging with and without intravenous contrast, is the imaging study of choice for patients with suspected soft tissue infections, including pyomyositis, and bone infections.[2-4] T1-weighted images demonstrate localized areas of hypointensity and T2-weighted images demonstrate hyperintense areas; with abscess, gadolinium-enhanced images will demonstrate an enhancing peripheral rim surrounding a fluid collection, without central enhancement of fluid contents.[4] Limitations for use of MRI include availability and the likely need for sedation in younger patients.

ULTRASOUND (US)

There are several advantages to this imaging modality: availability, lack of ionizing radiation, no requirement for intravenous contrast, and US can identify soft tissue foreign bodies. US has proven useful in assisting with the diagnosis of soft tissue infections; in one study, it outperformed physical examination in the detection of patients with this diagnosis.[5,6] There are reports on the use of US to successfully diagnose pyomyositis in adult patients.[1,5] On US, an abscess may show localized edema, linear plane distortion, and a hypoechoic center area, but this center may be more complex in echotexture. Compression of the abscess during imaging may allow confirmation of fluid contents and may show mobile purulent material.[1,7,8] There are limitations to the use of US in patients with suspected soft tissue infection. This modality is operator dependent. Due to the depth of the abscess in pyomyositis (involving the muscle layer), the clinician employing US should identify the striation of muscle to ensure proper visualization of the muscle layers. US may also underestimate the size of the abscess, and while US can detect fluid collections, identifying the contents of the collection can be difficult.[1]

Imaging Findings

With the history, physical examination findings and laboratory results, and negative plain radiography evaluation, the decision was made to obtain MRI of the pelvis and femur, with and without intravenous contrast. Selected images from this study are provided. Findings of pyomyositis are noted, with muscular edema in pelvic musculature bilaterally, left greater than right, with a loculated fluid collection in the left pectineus muscle, most consistent with abscess (Fig. 71.1). There is also bone marrow edema in the medial left acetabulum suggestive of osteomyelitis (Figs. 71.2 and 71.3).

Case Conclusion

The patient was evaluated by Pediatric Orthopedics and Pediatric Infectious Disease. The patient was taken to the operating suite and had drainage of the fluid collection. Postoperatively, the patient was placed on clindamycin and cefazolin. Cultures obtained from the drainage procedure yielded *Staphylococcus aureus*, which was pan-sensitive to antibiotics. Blood cultures obtained prior to antibiotic administration also yielded this organism.

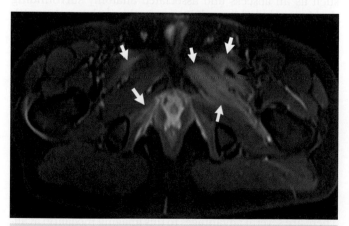

Fig. 71.1 Axial contrast-enhanced T1-weighted magnetic resonance imaging shows abnormal bright signal consistent with abnormal increased contrast enhancement in pelvic musculature bilaterally, left greater than right *(white arrows)*. A low signal fluid collection with surrounding enhancement in the left pectineus muscle is consistent with abscess *(black arrow)*.

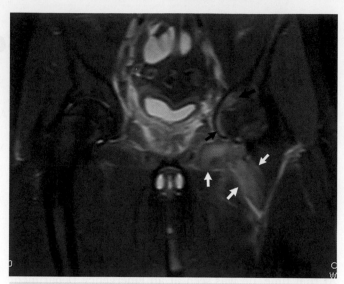

Fig. 71.2 Coronal T2-weighted magnetic resonance imaging shows abnormal increased signal intensity consistent with edema in the musculature of the pelvis, greater on the left *(white arrows)*. In addition, there is abnormal increased signal intensity of bone marrow edema in the left acetabulum *(black arrow)*, most suggestive of osteomyelitis.

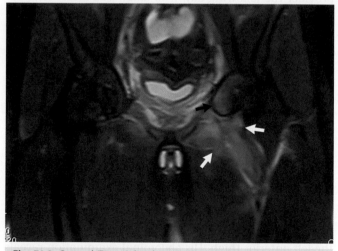

Fig. 71.3 Coronal T2-weighted magnetic resonance imaging shows abnormal increased signal intensity consistent with edema in the musculature of the pelvis, greater on the left *(white arrows)*. In addition, there is abnormal increased signal intensity of bone marrow edema in the left acetabulum *(black arrow)*, most suggestive of osteomyelitis.

Pyomyositis is a bacterial infection of striated muscle that may result from multiple etiologies, including trauma, connective tissue disorders, and immunosuppressive disorders.[3,5,9] *Staphylococcus aureus* is the most common bacterial agent, but case reports exist of other causative organisms, including *Borrelia burgdorferi*.[1,3,5,10] Reported overall mortality in the literature has been reported to be 1.5% to up to 27%; patients with underlying comorbidities have an increased risk.[1,11]

While there may be a paucity of clinical signs, pyomyositis has been identified to progress in three distinct stages:[1,9]

Stage 1—The infection is confined by the muscle aponeurosis and deep fascia without any overlying dermatologic extension.

Stage 2—There may be clinical signs of infection, including signs of inflammation that may appear to be cellulitis.

Stage 3—There is development of extensive infection, which may be life-threatening.

Pyomyositis may be primary (resulting from hematogenous spread from another source) or secondary (due to direct extension from an infectious source, such as Crohn disease, appendicitis).[3,9]

Because clinical symptoms are often nonspecific, pyomyositis may be diagnosed as a viral infection, muscle strain, or other process. However, fever is present in the majority of patients in addition to pain out of proportion to the examination findings.[1,12] In a study of adult patients with pyomyositis, the majority of patients were found to, in addition to fever, have frequent involvement of the quadriceps muscle, be unifocal in location, have elevated leukocytes, and, interestingly, the majority of these patients had a normal creatine kinase level.[1,13]

Acute myositis due to a viral infection is benign, self-limited, and distinct from pyomyositis. Benign childhood myositis is typically seen in school-age children.[14] There are multiple reports in the literature of patients refusing to ambulate secondary to pain usually during a viral infection, particularly influenza.[14–17] The classic complaint is bilateral lower leg pain with systemic symptoms suggestive of a viral infection, such as cough, congestion, sore throat, fever, and malaise.[14] If obtained, a CK level is often elevated (usually in the thousands) and may persist for as long as 2 weeks.[14] This illness is self-limited, with symptomatic and supportive care all that are indicated for management.[14] Notably, if there is focal weakness, neurologic signs, or indications of myoglobinuria, further investigation for other diagnoses is indicated.[14]

Management of pyomyositis depends on clinical stage but consists of antimicrobial therapy with or without surgical drainage. In the early stage, which is inflammatory and prior to organized abscess formation, antimicrobial therapy alone is indicated.[9,18] Abscess formation requires drainage in addition to antibiotic therapy, the duration of which is debatable but can range from 1 to 6 weeks, depending on disease severity and clinical response.[9] One study that examined 15 pediatric patients found that 5 were able to be managed with intravenous antimicrobial therapy alone and improvement was usually seen within the first 3 days of treatment initiation.[3] Treatment course was continued for a total course of 3 to 4 weeks (1 to 2 weeks intravenous therapy followed by 2 weeks of oral antimicrobial therapy).[3] However, the other 10 patients required abscess drainage.[3] Complications from pyomyositis include associated osteomyelitis, muscle scarring, and functional impairments.[9]

IMAGING PEARLS

1. Plain radiography is often the first imaging modality employed in investigating musculoskeletal complaints and is appropriate. Fever, pain out of proportion to the clinical examination, or concerning laboratory values (elevated white blood cell count, ESR, CRP, and/or CK) should prompt the clinician to consider advanced imaging.

2. MRI is an excellent imaging modality to evaluate soft tissues and identify abscesses and is considered the test of choice when pyomyositis is a diagnostic possibility.

3. CT can identify an abscess but does not provide the soft tissue detail of MRI.

4. US is an emerging modality that can readily identify a soft tissue abscess and signs of infection. However, this is operator dependent and skill is required to properly identify and characterize an abscess, which may be difficult in pyomyositis.

References

1. Kumar MP, Seif D, Perera P, et al. Point-of-care ultrasound in diagnosing pyomyositis: a report of three cases. *J Emerg Med.* 2014; 47(4):420-426.
2. Fayad LM, Carrino JA, Fishman EK. Musculoskeletal infection: role of CT in the emergency department. *Radiographics.* 2007;27(6): 1723-1736.
3. Elzohairy MM. Primary pyomyositis in children. *Orthop Traumatol Surg Res.* 2018;104(3):397-403.
4. Soler R, Rodríguez E, Aguilera C, et al. Magnetic resonance imaging of pyomyositis in 43 cases. *Eur J Radiol.* 2000;35(1):59-64.
5. Levitt DL, Byer R, Miller AF. Point-of-care ultrasound to diagnose pyomyositis in a child. *Pediatr Emerg Care.* 2019;35(1):69-71.
6. Iverson K, Haritos D, Thomas R, et al. The effect of bedside ultrasound on diagnosis and management of soft tissue infections in a pediatric ED. *Am J Emerg Med.* 2012;30(8):1347-1351.
7. Robben SG. Ultrasonography of musculoskeletal infections in children. *Eur Radiol.* 2004;14(suppl 4):L65-L77.
8. Tichter A, Riley DC. Emergency department diagnosis of a quadriceps intramuscular loculated abscess/pyomyositis using dynamic compression bedside ultrasonography. *Crit Ultrasound J.* 2013;5(1):3.
9. Taksande A, Vilhekar K, Gupta S. Primary pyomyositis in a child. *Int J Infect Dis.* 2009;13(4):e149-e151.
10. Marin JR, Dean AJ, Bilker WB, et al. Emergency ultrasound-assisted examination of skin and soft tissue infections in the pediatric emergency department. *Acad Emerg Med.* 2013;20(6):545-553.
11. Chiu SK, Lin JC, Wang NC, et al. Impact of underlying diseases on the clinical characteristics and outcome of primary pyomyositis. *J Microbiol Immunol Infect.* 2008;41(4):286-293.
12. Crum NF. Bacterial pyomyositis in the United States. *Am J Med.* 2004;117(6):420-428.
13. Bickels J, Ben-Sira L, Kessler A, et al. Primary pyomyositis. *J Bone Joint Surg Am.* 2002;84(12):2277-2286.
14. Magee H, Goldman RD. Viral myositis in children. *Can Fam Physician.* 2017;63(5):365-368.
15. Agyeman P, Duppenthaler A, Heininger U, et al. Influenza-associated myositis in children. *Infection.* 2004;32(4):199-203.
16. Szenborn L, Toczek-Kubicka K, Zaryczański J, et al. Benign acute childhood myositis during influenza B outbreak. *Adv Exp Med Biol.* 2018;1039:29-34.
17. Paul SP, Fillon G, Heaton PA. Benign acute childhood myositis secondary to parainfluenza A virus. *Br J Hosp Med (Lond).* 2017;78(7):410-411.
18. Peckett WR, Butler-Manuel A, Apthorp LA. Pyomyositis of the iliacus muscle in a child. *J Bone Joint Surg Br.* 2001;83(1):103-105.

72 'Lil Stuffy Noses: Sinusitis

ROBERT VEZZETTI, MD, FAAP, FACEP

Case Presentation

A 15-year-old male presents to the Emergency Department with a complaint of "severe headaches" for the past week. He states he has had cough, which is worse at night, and congestion for the past 2 weeks. He has had minimal rhinorrhea that was initially clear, then green, and is now clear again. He initially had a temperature of 101 degrees Fahrenheit, but this resolved after 2 days. He denies vomiting, sore throat, ear pain, vision changes, weakness, difficulty ambulating, or neck pain. There is no report of trauma. He states that the headache has been waking him up from sleep and has been present in the morning for the past 3 days. There is minimal relief with over-the-counter ibuprofen. His physical examination reveals a well-appearing patient who is afebrile and has unremarkable vital signs. He is normocephalic and atraumatic. There is no photophobia and his extraocular muscles are intact without proptosis or conjunctival erythema. There is no cobblestoning. He has mild nasal congestion with rhinorrhea; the nasal turbinates are mildly edematous. There is no facial edema, tenderness, signs of trauma, or erythema. His neurologic examination is nonfocal.

Imaging Considerations

Routine imaging for suspected routine sinusitis is not recommended, as this is a clinical diagnosis that follows strict criteria.[1–3] The majority of children with uncomplicated upper respiratory tract infection who undergo imaging of the paranasal sinuses, whether plain radiography, noncontrast computed tomography (CT), or magnetic resonance imaging (MRI), will have abnormal findings, including air-fluid levels and mucosal thickening.[1,3] While the findings of clear paranasal sinuses may exclude sinusitis, abnormal findings do not secure a diagnosis of sinusitis.[1] Imaging should be reserved for patients with potential sinusitis who have a suspected complication from sinusitis or if surgical intervention is planned.

PLAIN RADIOGRAPHY

The American Academy of Otolaryngology and Head and Neck Surgery does not recommend the routine use of radiography for the diagnosis of uncomplicated acute bacterial sinusitis.[2,4] Plain radiographs have been reported to have a sensitivity of 76% in acute bacterial sinusitis.[2,4,5]

COMPUTED TOMOGRAPHY

The sinuses can be visualized with non–contrast-enhanced CT, which provides an excellent assessment of bony detail.

However, routine use is not indicated to diagnose clinical sinusitis. Rather, this modality should be reserved for patients with suspected complications from sinusitis, and intravenous contrast–enhanced CT is appropriate in these cases. The most common complication from acute bacterial sinusitis involves the orbit and occurs in children younger than 5 years of age who have ethmoid sinusitis.[1,6,7] Intracranial complications, such as subdural empyema, epidural empyema, venous thrombosis, and brain abscess, have been described in the literature and should be considered in patients who present with severe headache, photophobia, or focal neurologic findings.[1,4,7,8] Non–contrast-enhanced CT may be utilized when planning sinus surgical procedures.[4]

MAGNETIC RESONANCE IMAGING

This imaging modality is not usually utilized in imaging acute sinusitis.[4] However, in patients with suspected intracranial complications, intravenous contrast–enhanced MRI is an appropriate imaging modality to utilize.[1,2]

CT VERSUS MRI

Intravenous contrast–enhanced CT has been the most commonly utilized imaging modality in patients with sinusitis who have suspected complicatons.[1–3] However, in cases of suspected intracranial complications, MRI is preferred.[1,2]

Imaging Findings

Given the patient's concerning history of wakening in the middle of the night and first morning headache, there was concern that the headache was not related to the patient's apparent upper respiratory tract infection. The physical examination was not suggestive of an infectious complication, such as orbital cellulitis or brain abscess. It was decided to obtain a non–contrast-enhanced CT scan of the head. Selected images are provided here. There is extensive mucosal thickening and areas of sinus opacification throughout the paranasal sinuses (Figs. 72.1 and 72.2), but the brain, ventricles, and skull are all unremarkable on imaging.

Case Conclusion

The patient was prescribed amoxicillin and was discharged with close monitoring and follow-up with his primary care provider.

Acute bacterial sinusitis is a complication of a viral upper respiratory infection, and an estimated 7% of pediatric patients seeking care for respiratory symptoms have an illness

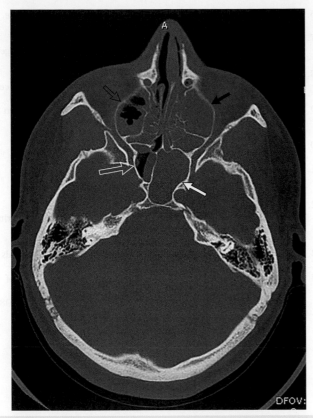

Fig. 72.1 Axial computed tomography image demonstrates opacification of the left maxillary and ethmoid sinuses *(black arrow)* and of the left sphenoid sinus *(white arrow)*. Opacification is seen of the right ethmoid sinus, and mucosal thickening is seen in the right maxillary sinus *(open black arrow)* and the right sphenoid sinus *(open white arrow)*.

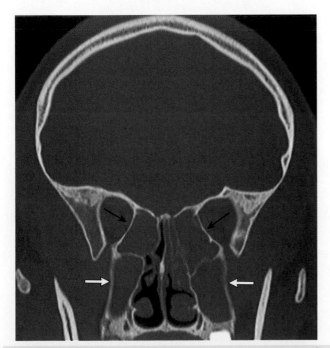

Fig. 72.2 Coronal computed tomography image demonstrates opacification of bilateral posterior ethmoid sinuses *(black arrows)* and maxillary sinuses *(white arrows)*.

that is consistent with sinusitis.[1,9] Symptoms of an acute viral upper respiratory tract infection and those of acute bacterial sinusitis are very similar. Symptoms include nasal discharge (the color, consistency, or quantity may be of any type) and cough (throughout the day but worse at night), and both symptoms may be present.[1] Other symptoms and physical examination findings, including palpation of the sinuses and transillumination of the sinuses, are not specific for sinusitis nor are they helpful in making the diagnosis; nasal cultures are not routinely recommended.[1,10] There are clinical situations that suggest sinusitis in children older than 1 year of age[1]:

1. Persistent illness, i.e., nasal discharge (of any quality) or daytime cough or both lasting more than 10 days without improvement; OR
2. Worsening course, i.e., worsening or new onset of nasal discharge, daytime cough, or fever after initial improvement; OR
3. Severe onset, i.e., concurrent fever (temperature $\geq 39°C/$ 102.2°F) and purulent nasal discharge for at least 3 consecutive days.

Noninfectious rhinitis due to seasonal allergies should also be considered in patients presenting with cough and congestion. Initially, symptoms of an allergic etiology may be mistaken for acute sinusitis; a history of an atopic dermatitis, seasonal variation of symptoms, and stigmata of an allergic condition can assist the clinician in determining if an underlying allergic condition exists.[1]

Management of acute sinusitis is based on several recommendations. In cases of severe onset, worsening clinical course, or persistent illness, antibiotic therapy should be initiated; in cases where symptoms are persistent, the option of continued monitoring of symptoms and withholding antibiotic treatment is appropriate as well.[1] Notably, antibiotic therapy is commonly prescribed for sinusitis in pediatric patients; one study reported that 82% of patients were prescribed antibiotics.[1,11] The American Academy of Pediatrics treatment guidelines note that pediatric patients with sinusitis may defervesce on their own and highlight an opportunity for shared decision making between health care providers and caregivers regarding the initiation of antibiotics versus continued observation.[1] If antimicrobial therapy is initiated, amoxicillin with or without clavulanate is the recommended first-line agent, which will be effective against the most common bacterial organisms causing sinusitis (*Streptococcus pneumonia*, *Moraxella catarrhalis*, and non-typable *Haemophilus influenzae*).[1] Patients allergic to penicillin can be treated with cephalosporins; clindamycin is also an alternative.[1,12] Due to resistance patterns, trimethoprim-sulfamethoxazole and azithromycin should generally not be used.[1,13] Duration of treatment is 7 to 28 days, but a reasonable alternative is to treat for 7 days more after the resolution of symptoms; if there is no improvement within 72 hours of initiation of antibiotic therapy or clinical symptoms are worsening, reassess if the diagnosis of sinusitis is correct, and if so, consider changing antibiotics.[1,14] The use of saline irrigation, oral antihistamines, oral steroids, and nasal steroids has not been extensively studied in the pediatric population, and while no evidence of harm has been noted, their routine use is not supported in the management of sinusitis.[1,3]

1. Routine imaging is not indicated to diagnose clinical sinusitis.
2. CT is appropriate to obtain when there are suspected complications of sinusitis. Non–contrast-enhanced imaging may be employed if surgical management is planned. Contrast-enhanced imaging may be utilized if there are concerns for infectious complications.
3. MRI is appropriate for suspected intracranial complications of sinusitis or as a complement to CT findings.

References

1. Wald ER, Applegate KE, Bordley C, et al. Clinical practice guideline for the diagnosis and management of acute bacterial sinusitis in children aged 1 to 18 years. *Pediatrics*. 2013;132(1):e262-e280.
2. Expert Panel on Neurologic Imaging, Kirsch CFE, Bykowski J, et al. ACR Appropriateness Criteria® sinonasal disease. *J Am Coll Radiol*. 2017;14(11S):S550-S559.
3. Arora HS. Sinusitis in children. *Pediatr Ann*. 2018;47(10):e396-e401.
4. Rosenfeld RM, Piccirillo JF, Chandrasekhar SS, et al. Clinical practice guideline (update): adult sinusitis. *Otolaryngol Head Neck Surg*. 2015 Apr;152:S1–S39.
5. Lau J, Zucker D, Engels EA, et al. *Diagnosis and Treatment of Acute Bacterial Rhinosinusitis. Evidence Report/Technology Assessment No. 9 (Contract 290-97-0019 to the New England Medical Center)*. Rockville, MD: Agency for Health Care Policy and Research; 1999.
6. Wald ER. Periorbital and orbital infections. *Infect Dis Clin North Am*. 2007;21(2):393-408.
7. Brook I. Microbiology and antimicrobial treatment of orbital and intracranial complications of sinusitis in children and their management. *Int J Pediatr Otorhinolaryngol*. 2009;73(9):1183-1186.
8. Kombogiorgas D, Seth R, Modha J, et al. Suppurative intracranial complications of sinusitis in adolescence. Single institute experience and review of the literature. *Br J Neurosurg*. 2007;21(6):603-609.
9. Kakish KS, Mahafza T, Batieha A, et al. Clinical sinusitis in children attending primary care centers. *Pediatr Infect Dis J*. 2000;19(11):1071-1074.
10. Shaikh N, Wald ER. Signs and symptoms of acute sinusitis in children. *Pediatr Infect Dis J*. 2013;32(10):1061-1065.
11. Shapiro DJ, Gonzales R, Cabana MD, et al. National trends in visit rates and antibiotic prescribing for children with acute sinusitis. *Pediatrics*. 2011;127(1):28-34.
12. Pichichero ME. A review of evidence supporting the American Academy of Pediatrics recommendation for prescribing cephalosporin antibiotics for penicillin-allergic patients. *Pediatrics*. 2005;115(4):1048-1057.
13. Jacobs MR. Antimicrobial-resistant *Streptococcus pneumoniae*: trends and management. *Expert Rev Anti Infect Ther*. 2008;6(5):619-635.
14. American Academy of Pediatrics, Subcommittee on Management of Sinusitis and Committee on Quality Improvement. Clinical practice guideline: management of sinusitis. *Pediatrics*. 2001;108(3):798-808.

73 *Who's Brodie? Brodie Abscess*

ROBERT VEZZETTI, MD, FAAP, FACEP

Case Presentation

A 14-month-old previously healthy male presents with limping for the past 5 days. Prior to this symptom, he had cough, congestion, and subjective fever, which his primary care provider had diagnosed as a viral upper respiratory infection. He appeared to be improving when he developed a left-sided limp, which appeared at times to be painful, although over-the-counter ibuprofen seemed to help with pain.

On examination, he is afebrile and has age-appropriate vital signs. Physical examination is unremarkable other than a painful gait when he attempts to ambulate. He had no tenderness in his knee or his hip, and he had a full range of motion on examination.

Imaging Considerations

PLAIN RADIOGRAPHY

Plain radiography is an excellent first-line imaging modality for children with presumed skeletal pain. Ionizing radiation exposure is low and the modality is readily available. Two views of the extremity (anteroposterior and lateral) are sufficient in most cases.

A Brodie abscess will often appear as a distinct, well-demarcated intramedullary lesion. There may be surrounding sclerosis and cortical thickening; cortical destruction may be seen; and periosteal reaction is typically present.[1] Notably, plain radiographs may be unremarkable during the initial stages of abscess development, and radiographic changes may be delayed up to 10 days.[2]

COMPUTED TOMOGRAPHY (CT)

This modality is useful in defining the extent of the lesion but is less useful for defining an inflammatory process. CT is excellent at detecting cortical destruction and periosteal reaction, although is not a first-line imaging modality.[2]

MAGNETIC RESONANCE IMAGING (MRI)

MRI is an excellent modality to visualize and define inflammatory processes, particularly early in the course of illness. This modality has a high sensitivity in detecting the pathology of bone and soft tissue and can define the extent of a pathologic process. Availability and the possible need for sedation may limit immediate use. MRI is typically used as a follow-up study when plain radiography demonstrates a

lesion. Non–contrast-enhanced and contrast-enhanced imaging is employed.

A Brodie abscess visualized with MRI appears as a well-defined lesion with a central area that is hypointense on T1-weighted images but hyperintense on T2-weighted images; the surrounding bone marrow will also enhance; associated surrounding edema is hypointense on T1-weighted images but hyperintense on T2-weighted images.[1–4]

Imaging Findings

Due to the painful gait and history of subjective fevers, the child had bloodwork and plain radiography of the left lower extremity performed. The peripheral white blood cell count was 11,700/mm^3, the erythrocyte sedimentation rate was 26 mm/hour, and the C-reactive protein was 1.4 mg/dL. His gait improved after he was administered ibuprofen. The images were reported to be unremarkable (not provided here). He was discharged with a diagnosis of toxic synovitis and appropriate follow-up instructions were provided.

The child returned 10 days later with worsening and now persistent pain. In the interim period, he had days where the pain waxed and waned and initially was improved with ibuprofen, as before, but now there was no symptomatic improvement. Repeat bloodwork and imaging were obtained. The peripheral white blood cell count was 11,300/mm^3, the erythrocyte sedimentation rate was 35 mm/hour, and the C-reactive protein was 0.8 mg/dL. Plain radiography demonstrates a 9-mm lytic proximal tibial metaphyseal lesion with slightly ill-defined sclerotic borders, and subtle proximal tibial periostitis (Figs. 73.1 and 73.2). MRI was subsequently performed; selected images are provided here. The lesion in the proximal left tibial metaphysis is of low signal intensity on T1-weighted images and high signal intensity on T2-weighted images and shows rim enhancement. On MRI, the lesion extends through the physis and has an irregular extension into the epiphysis. The surrounding bone marrow and soft tissues show edema and mild enhancement, with no soft tissue mass (Figs. 73.3–73.5).

Case Conclusion

The child was admitted to the hospital, and because he was not toxic and in no distress, antibiotic therapy was held, and the child was taken to the operating room after consultation with Pediatric Orthopedics and Pediatric Infectious Disease. During surgical exploration, a well-demarcated

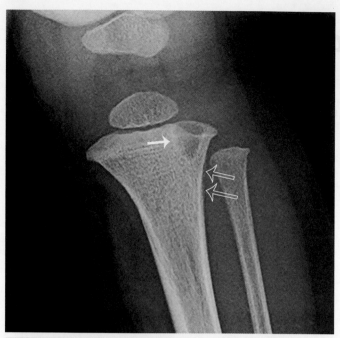

Fig. 73.1 Anterior-posterior view of the proximal tibia and fibula demonstrates a relatively well-defined lytic lesion *(arrow)* of the lateral proximal tibial metaphysis, abutting the physis, with a subtle sclerotic border. Subtle periosteal new bone is seen laterally *(open arrows)*.

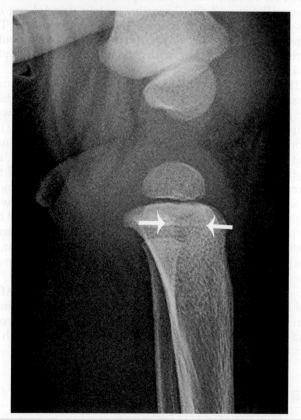

Fig. 73.2 Lateral view of the proximal tibia demonstrates the lytic lesion of the proximal tibial metaphysis *(arrows)*, although the lesion is not as well visualized as on the anterior-posterior view.

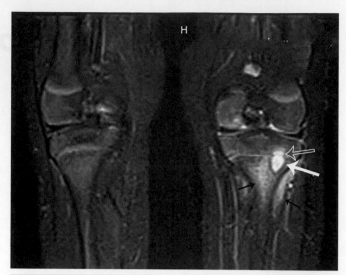

Fig. 73.3 Coronal inversion recovery magnetic resonance image shows a well-defined high signal left tibial metaphyseal lesion *(white arrow)* consistent with a Brodie abscess, crossing the physis into the epiphysis *(open arrow)*. Surrounding high signal bone marrow and soft tissue edema are also seen *(black arrows)*.

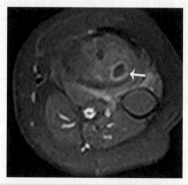

Fig. 73.4 Axial contrast-enhanced T1-weighted image demonstrates high signal rim enhancement *(arrow)* of the Brodie abscess lesion in the proximal left tibial metaphysis. Mild increased signal in the surrounding bone marrow is consistent with increased bone marrow enhancement around the lesion.

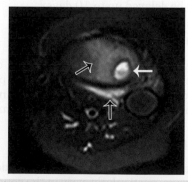

Fig. 73.5 Axial T2-weighted image demonstrates high signal centrally within the Brodie abscess lesion and a low signal rim *(white arrow)*. There is high signal edema in the surrounding bone marrow and soft tissues *(black arrows)*, but no evidence of a soft tissue mass.

area of abscess in the lateral proximal tibia adjacent to and entering the periosteum of the growth plate was discovered and removed without complication. Cultures were sent and antibiotics (clindamycin and ceftriaxone) were initiated. Cultures grew Gram-negative rods (ultimately identified as *Kingella kingae*) and single coverage with ceftriaxone was continued. The child was discharged on postoperative day 2 with continued ceftriaxone for 1 month. He recovered uneventfully.

The first description of a Brodie abscess was by Sir Benjamin Brodie in 1832.[5,6] In this report, Brodie described a young adult who had chronic pain and swelling of the lower leg, just above the right ankle and despite several treatments, there was no success in alleviating the man's condition, leading to a decision to amputate the leg; a post-procedure examination revealed a collection of pus corresponding to the area of the man's symptoms.[5,6] This discovery led Brodie to propose incision and drainage of the area as a future (and limb-sparing) treatment.[5,6]

Development of a Brodie abscess is insidious, and symptoms vary. Patients generally do not appear ill. There is a predilection for more vascularized areas of bone. Both preceding upper respiratory infection (presumed clinically to be viral) and trauma have been implicated in abscess formation.[1,5,7–10] A retrospective review of 21 patients reported pain and limp as common presenting symptoms (80% and 60%, respectively).[11] Other case series have reported localized swelling as a near-universal symptom (10 of 11 patients in this review) with pain and limping present in only half of the cases.[8]

In a recent large systematic review, symptoms consisted of pain (98% of cases) or swelling (54% of cases); 84% of cases were afebrile and less than half of patients in this review had elevated serum inflammatory markers—white blood cell count, C-reactive protein, and erythrocyte sedimentation rate.[5] The mean time from development of symptoms to diagnosis was 12 weeks and the most frequent site of involvement was the femur.[5] Imaging modalities utilized in this review consisted primarily of plain radiography (96% of patients) and MRI (16% of patients); CT was utilized in less than 10% of patients.[5]

The bacterial pathogen associated with Brodie abscess is primarily *Staphylococcus aureus*, although methicillin-resistant *Staphylococcus aureus* and *Salmonella* spp. have been reported.[1,4,5,8,12]

An interesting trend is the role that *K. kingae* appears to be playing in pediatric osteoarticular infections.[7,9,10] *K. kingae* is part of the nasopharyngeal flora of children. This organism has been reported to be commonly involved as a pathogen for osteoarticular infections in children younger than 4 years of age.[13] *K. kingae* has previously been noted to cause invasive upper respiratory tract infection,[14] and the thought is that mucosal damage from this infection allows *K. kingae* to spread hematogenously, resulting in osteoarticular infections.[7,10] *K. kingae* should be considered when deciding on antibiotic therapy for these patients.

Treatment for Brodie abscess is accomplished with surgical drainage and antibiotics.[1,5,11] In van der Naald et al.'s review, treatment consisted primarily of surgical drainage (94% of cases), with the majority of cases in combination with antibiotics (77% of cases); very few cases were treated solely with antibiotics or surgery alone.[5] Recurrence rates are not high (15%) and outcomes are generally good.[5,11,15,16]

IMAGING PEARLS

1. Plain radiography is the first-line imaging modality for pediatric musculoskeletal complaints.
2. A Brodie abscess often appears as a well-demarcated intramedullary lesion with periosteal reaction. Initial radiography may be unremarkable and repeat radiography may be indicated.
3. CT may be utilized as an adjunct study but is not a first-line imaging modality in pediatric musculoskeletal complaints.
4. MRI is usually employed as an adjunct study to further define an abnormal imaging finding, such as a Brodie abscess. This lesion has typical findings on MRI that suggest an infectious process.

References

1. Abdulhadi MA, White AM, Pollock AN. Brodie abscess. *Pediatr Emerg Care*. 2012;28(11):1249-1251.
2. Pöyhiä T, Azouz EM. MR imaging evaluation of subacute and chronic bone abscesses in children. *Pediatr Radiol*. 2000;30(11): 763-768.
3. Bohndorf K. Infection of the appendicular skeleton. *Eur J Radiol*. 2004;14(3):e53-e63.
4. Jaramillo D, Dormans JP, Delgado J, et al. Hematogenous osteomyelitis in infants and children: imaging of a changing disease. *Radiology*. 2017;283(3):629-643.
5. van der Naald N, Smeeing DPJ, Houwert RM, et al. Brodie abscess: a systematic review of reported cases. *J Bone Jt Infect*. 2019;4(1): 33-39.
6. Brodie BC. An account of some cases of chronic abscess of the tibia. *Med Chir Trans*. 1832;17:239-249.
7. Ruttan TK, Higginbotham E, Higginbotham N, et al. Invasive *Kingella kingae* resulting in a brodic abscess. *J Pediatric Infect Dis Soc*. 2015;4(2):e14-e16.
8. Kolowski K. Brodie abscess in the first decade of life. Report of eleven cases. *Pediatr Radiol*. 1980;10(1):33-37.
9. Yagupsky P. *Kingella kingae*: from medical rarity to an emerging paediatric pathogen. *Lancet Infect Dis*. 2004;4(6):358-367.
10. Yagupsky P, Porsch E, St Geme JW. *Kingella kingae*: an emerging pathogen in young children. *Pediatrics*. 2011;127(3):557-565.
11. Foster CE, Taylor M, Schallert EK, et al. Brodie abscess in children: a 10-year single institution retrospective review. *Pediatr Infect Dis J*. 2019;38(2):e32-e34.
12. Tien I. Update on the management of skin, soft tissue, and osteoarticular infections in children. *Curr Opin Pediatr*. 2006;18(3):254-259.
13. Spyropoulou V, Dhouib CA, Merlini L, et al. Primary subacute hematogenous osteomyelitis in children: a clearer bacteriological etiology. *J Child Orthop*. 2016;10(3):241-246.
14. Basmaci R, Ilharreborde B, Doit C, et al. Two atypical cases of *Kingella kingae* invasive infection with concomitant human rhinovirus infection. *J Clin Microbiol*. 2013;51(9):3137-3139.
15. Dartnell J, Ramachandran M, Katchburian M. Haematogenous acute and subacute paediatric osteomyelitis: a systematic review of the literature. *J Bone Joint Surg Br*. 2012;94(5):584-595.
16. Olasinde AA, Oluwadiya KS, Adegbehingbe OO. Treatment of Brodie abscess: excellent results from curettage, bone grafting and antibiotics. *Singapore Med J*. 2011;52(6):436-439.

74 *I Feel It in My Bones: Osteomyelitis*

ROBERT VEZZETTI, MD, FAAP, FACEP

Case Presentation

A 13-year-old male is referred to the Emergency Department by his primary care provider. The patient has had left hip pain for the past week, which has progressively interfered with his daily activities, such as sports, and now has made ambulation difficult. He has had subjective fever but no recent illness and denies any trauma. There has been no back pain, abdominal pain, incontinence, weakness, or numbness. The pain radiates from his left hip to the superior aspect of his left knee.

On examination, the patient is a pleasant teenager in no distress. He has a temperature of 100.2 degrees Fahrenheit, a heart rate of 112 beats per minute, a respiratory rate of 20 breaths per minute, and a blood pressure of 120/76 mm Hg. His physical examination reveals no obvious abnormalities, as he is sitting up on the hospital bed. His leg lengths are equal. He is able to ambulate but when doing so states that this produces left lateral hip pain, pointing to the anterior-lateral aspect of the superior iliac crest. When his left leg is examined, he has good range of motion of the leg at the hip joint; he is able to flex and extend the leg without difficulty, but when the knee is flexed and the leg (at the hip joint) is either abducted or adducted, pain is produced at the superior aspect of the left hip. There is no erythema, swelling, warmth, or signs of trauma. He has no abdominal pain or back pain and has a normal genital examination.

Imaging Considerations

PLAIN RADIOGRAPHY

This imaging modality is most commonly employed in patients with musculoskeletal complaints, given the low ionizing radiation exposure relative to other modalities and general availability. Plain radiography is useful in investigating alternative causes of pain in patients with suspected osteomyelitis, such as fractures. For osteomyelitis, however, radiography is less useful in the acute period. Changes associated with osteomyelitis will not be evident on plain radiography immediately. Associated soft tissue swelling may be seen approximately 3–4 days into the course of the illness and cortical destruction may not be evident for 10–14 days after onset of the infection. Osteopenia may generally be seen after 30%–50% loss of mineralization.[1–4] Osseous radiographic findings of osteomyelitis initially include subperiosteal resorption, followed by bone lucencies, then irregular destruction with new periosteal bone formation.[1]

COMPUTED TOMOGRAPHY (CT)

CT is not a first-line imaging modality for pediatric musculoskeletal infection, as magnetic resonance imaging is a superior modality for this purpose and also due to ALARA principles. CT may be employed as a follow-up examination once the diagnosis of osteomyelitis has been established.[1] This modality may be useful to delineate cortical destruction, periosteal reaction, and the presence of an abscess; intravenous contrast should be used.[2,3,5]

MAGNETIC RESONANCE IMAGING (MRI)

Magnetic resonance (MR) imaging is the imaging modality of choice to detect osteomyelitis.[6] This modality can detect cortical changes associated with edema and destruction and can also be used to differentiate between acute and chronic osteomyelitis.[1–5,7,8] Contrast-enhanced (gadolinium) and noncontrast images may be obtained, but gadolinium use will delineate abscesses.[2,4,6,7] There have been conflicting reports on the routine use of gadolinium for the detection of osteomyelitis. One study found that the sensitivity of osteomyelitis detection using pregadolinium and postgadolinium images was 89% and 91% and the specificity was 96% and 96%, respectively, although gadolinium did increase the ability to detect abscesses.[7,9] However, a study of patients 18 months of age and younger with *Staphylococcus aureus* osteomyelitis found that gadolinium-enhanced imaging significantly improved the detection (100% sensitivity) of osteomyelitis either isolated to the epiphyseal cartilage or combined with metaphyseal and diaphyseal involvement over noncontrast imaging. As the noncontrast imaging showed only a 22% sensitivity for isolated epiphyseal disease and a 44% sensitivity for epiphyseal and metadiaphyseal involvement, the authors recommended contrast-enhanced imaging in children under 18 months of age in communities where community-acquired *Staphylococcus aureus* is endemic.[10] In general, if there is suspicion of an abscess in very young children with osteomyelitis, or if spinal osteomyelitis is suspected, gadolinium should be used.[1,5,6] The decision to use gadolinium can be made jointly by consulting Pediatric Radiology and Pediatric Orthopedics and may be institution dependent. While MRI is an excellent imaging test to detect osteomyelitis, disadvantages include availability and, often, the need for sedation.

ULTRASOUND (US)

This modality is generally available, avoids ionizing radiation, and is less costly than MRI. US has been used to evaluate patients for osteomyelitis and subperiosteal abscess.[2,11–13] Sonographic features suggestive of osteomyelitis include muscle thickening, soft tissue swelling, thickening of the periosteum, and periosteal elevation.[2] US cannot distinguish between pus and sterile fluid.[2,13]

RADIONUCLEOTIDE SCANNING (BONE SCAN)

Utilizing technetium 99 m methylene disphosphonate, bone scanning can demonstrate hyperemia and focal increased uptake of this bone agent suggestive of infection and can be utilized to detect multiple areas of possible infection.[1–3] A three-phase technique (angiographic phase, blood pool phase, and late phase) is used.[2] However, it can be more difficult with this modality to distinguish between other etiologies that will produce abnormal scan findings, such as neoplasm or trauma.[1,2,5]

Imaging Findings

Plain radiography of the pelvis (two views: anterior-posterior and frog lateral) was obtained and no radiographic abnormality was noted (Figs. 74.1 and 74.2). Laboratory studies were obtained, and given these results, MRI of the hips and femurs was performed. Selected images from this study are provided. There is abnormal bone marrow signal intensity and abnormal enhancement in the left femur, greatest proximally but extending into the diaphysis. Within the proximal femoral diaphysis a focal fluid collection with surrounding enhancement suggests a bone abscess. Surrounding edema in the soft tissues is greatest proximally, with edema and enhancement in adjacent musculature, also consistent with myositis (Figs. 74.3–74.8).

Case Conclusion

After initial imaging, laboratory studies were performed, including a complete blood count, C-reactive protein (CRP), erythrocyte sedimentation rate (ESR), and creatine kinase

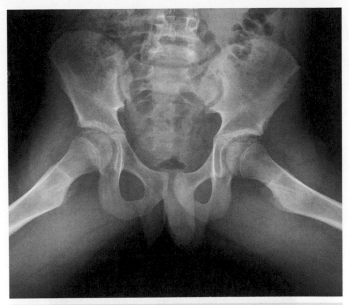

Fig. 74.2 Plain radiographic frog leg view of the pelvis is normal.

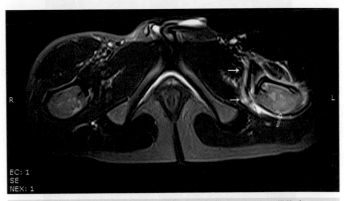

Fig. 74.3 Axial T2-weighted MR image with fat saturation (FS) demonstrating abnormal high signal edema (*arrows*) around the proximal left femur and surrounding adjacent hip musculature. The mild increased signal within the bone marrow of the proximal left femur (*open arrow*) compared to the right femur is consistent with bone marrow edema of osteomyelitis.

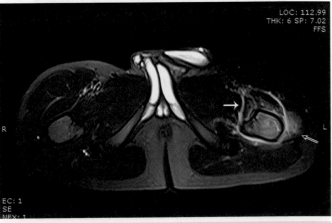

Fig. 74.4 Axial T2-weighted MR image with fat saturation (FS) demonstrating high signal edema fluid (*white arrow*) around the proximal left femur and around adjacent hip musculature, as well as increased signal within the musculature consistent with myositis (*open white arrow*).

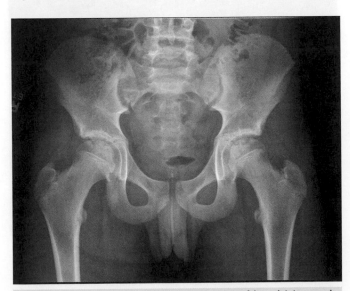

Fig. 74.1 Plain radiographic anterior-posterior view of the pelvis is normal.

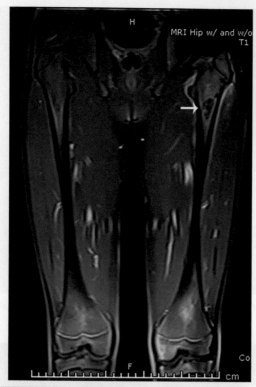

Fig. 74.5 Coronal contrast-enhanced T1-weighted MR image with fat saturation (FS) demonstrating an area of low signal intensity and non-enhancement in the left femoral shaft , with mild surrounding increased enhancement (*arrow*), suggesting abscess.

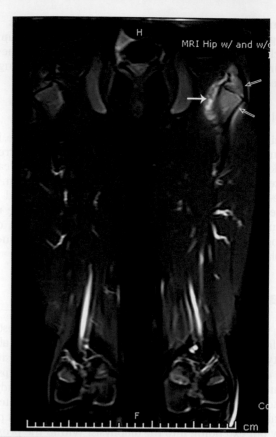

Fig. 74.7 Coronal T1-weighted MR image with fat saturation (FS) demonstrating high signal edema around the proximal left femur (*white arrow*), and asymmetric increased enhancement of the bone marrow of the proximal left femur (*open arrows*) compared to the right femur. These findings are consistent with osteomyelitis.

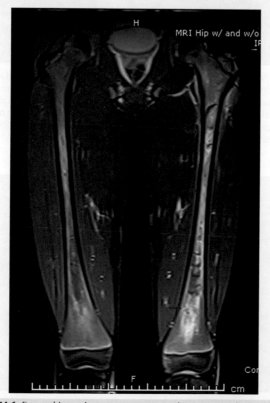

Fig. 74.6 Coronal inversion recovery magnetic resonance image demonstrating a diffusely abnormal increased marrow signal intensity throughout the left femoral shaft, consistent with extension of bone marrow edema.

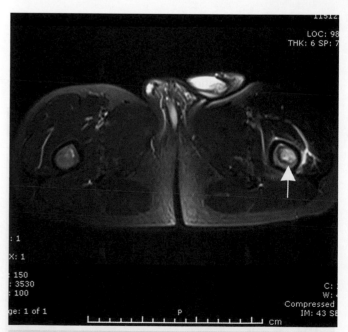

Fig. 74.8 Axial T2-weighted magnetic resonance image with fat saturation (FS) demonstrating a focal well-defined high signal fluid collection in the proximal left femur (*arrow*), consistent with abscess and corresponding to the abnormality seen on contrast-enhanced imaging in Fig. 74.5.

(CK). A blood culture was obtained as well. While the white blood cell count was unremarkable with a slight left shift (6,100 cc/mm with 61% neurophils), the CRP level was markedly elevated at 9.8 mg/dL (normal is less than 1 mg/dL), the ESR was elevated at 65 mm/hour (normal is < 20 mm/hour), and the CK level was normal. These abnormal laboratory findings prompted further imaging with MRI. The patient was admitted to the hospital. Pediatric Orthopedics and Pediatric Infectious Disease were both consulted. The patient was taken to the operating room for debridement of the abscess, which was done uneventfully. Postoperatively, the patient was given cefazolin and clindamycin. Cultures obtained from the abscess showed pan-sensitive *S. aureus*, and antibiotic therapy was tailored to these results. A blood culture obtained during initial evaluation also grew pan-sensitive *S. aureus*. The patient was discharged with an appropriate course of antibiotic therapy and close follow-up.

Pediatric osteomyelitis can develop via several mechanisms, including hematogenous spread (most common), contiguous spread from an infection (such as skin cellulitis), or due to localized trauma.[1,2,14] Osteomyelitis can be classified as:[1,4]

1. Acute—This form of osteomyelitis commonly involves the metaphysis of the bones. In very young children, infection can spread by transphyseal vessels into the growth cartilage of the epiphysis. But this is less common after the age of 2 years as these vessels diminish.[1,2]
2. Chronic—This form of osteomyelitis is characterized by the potential development of bone necrosis embedded in the inflammatory process and periosteal new bone formation.[1] Acute exacerbations followed by remission have been described.[1] Long bone metaphyses of multiple bones are commonly involved.[1]
3. Subacute—This form is insidious in onset, often with symptoms of more than 2 weeks' duration.[1] Brodie abscess is a classic example of subacute osteomyelitis.[1,2]

The majority of cases of osteomyelitis involve the long bones, with the rapidly growing areas of bone more likely to be affected and the infection usually confined to one bone.[1] Roughly one-third of cases occur in the first 2 years of life.[1] Commonly involved organisms are *S. aureus* and Group B *Streptococcus*. In immunocompromised patients, one should consider fungal species; in patients with sickle cell disease, *Salmonella* is common.[1,2,4] An emerging pathogen is *Kingella kingae*, which is primarily seen in children under the age of 4 years. It is difficult to culture but can be identified by polymerase chain reaction techniques.[3,14,15] Recently, there has been the emergence of Panton-Valentine leucocidin (VPL)–producing strains of *S. aureus*. VPL produces tissue necrosis, and infections with this organism tend to produce a more aggressive clinical course and have higher rates of associated complications, such as subperiosteal abscess, pyomyositis, and necrotizing fasciitis, requiring aggressive antimicrobial therapy and, commonly, surgical debridement.[14,16,17]

In addition to imaging studies, blood testing can be helpful in diagnosing osteomyelitis. A complete blood count, CRP, ESR, and blood cultures should be obtained.[3] Patients with osteomyelitis often have an elevated peripheral white blood cell count (approximately one-third), an elevated CRP level (80%), and elevated ESR (90%).[3,18] CRP is an excellent marker of treatment response and can be used for this purpose during a patient's management.[19]

Management of osteomyelitis involves antibiotic treatment and, if clinically applicable, surgical debridement of formed abscess. Antibiotic administration should begin, preferably, once an abscess has undergone surgical intervention and cultures are obtained.[3,14] The decision whether to perform aspiration of easily accessible bones with abscesses in the Emergency Department under sedation or in the operative suite is best left to a consulting pediatric orthopedic surgeon or an orthopedic surgeon comfortable with the management of pediatric osteomyelitis. Empiric antibiotic therapy should be initiated as soon as possible once cultures have been obtained. The choice of antibacterial agent should cover likely pathogens and can be guided by history, the age of the child, underlying comorbidities, and local antimicrobial resistance patterns.[3] Cefazolin is a typical initial choice.[3,4,14] Some studies have recommended clindamycin as initial therapy, but there are rising rates of resistance among *Staphylococcus* species, and *Kingella* is typically resistant to this agent.[3,14,20] The decision to utilize vancomycin is somewhat controversial, but if chosen, coverage for *Kingella* should be included since this organism is also resistant to vancomyin.[3] Additionally, Gram-negative coverage should be included in neonates and infants.[3] The length of antibiotic therapy has traditionally been 4–6 weeks, although there are studies suggesting that a shorter duration of treatment may be acceptable with monitoring for clinical improvement and decreasing CRP values.[3,4,20,21] Consultation with a pediatric infectious disease specialist can help the clinician in antimicrobial agent choice, best route of therapy, and duration of therapy.

Most patients with osteomyelitis have good outcomes. Complications from osteomyelitis including leg-length discrepancies, arthritis, and disturbance in bone growth have been associated with delay in diagnosis, short (<2 weeks) duration of therapy, and younger age.[3,4] Chronic osteomyelitis has been reported in approximately 5% of patients, is more often seen in cases of contiguous osteomyelitis, and often requires prolonged medical and surgical management.[4,22]

IMAGING PEARLS

1. Plain radiography is the initial imaging modality in pediatric patients with musculoskeletal complaints, including patients with suspected osteomyelitis. Other causes of pain, such as fractures, can be identified and this modality is widely available.
2. In the early phase of osteomyelitis, plain radiographs may be normal and evidence of cortical destruction may not be evident until 10–14 days after onset of infection.
3. CT is not considered a first-line imaging modality for osteomyelitis but has shown a role in follow-up examinations once treatment has been initiated.
4. Three-phase bone scanning can be used to detect osteomyelitis in the pediatric population and is useful in detecting multiple areas of infection or in patients with poorly localized symptoms. However, it is more difficult with this modality to distinguish between infection and other causes of increased uptake, such as neoplasm.

Bone scan is not the preferred modality for the evaluation of the pediatric patient presenting in the emergency department with suspected osteomyelitis.
5. US is not currently a standard imaging modality for osteomyelitis but can potentially identify subperiosteal abscess.
6. MRI is the modality of choice for suspected osteomyelitis. The use of gadolinium is somewhat controversial but is recommended in children less than 18 months of age, in cases of suspected abscess, or if spinal osteomyelitis is suspected. If there is uncertainty whether contrast use is indicated, consultation with Pediatric Radiology and/or Pediatric Orthopedics is recommended.

References

1. Blickman JG, van Die CE, de Rooy JW. Current imaging concepts in pediatric osteomyelitis. *Eur Radiol.* 2004;14(suppl 4):L55-L64.
2. Schmit P, Glorion C. Osteomyelitis in infants and children. *Eur Radiol.* 2004;14(suppl 4):L44-L54.
3. Dodwell ER. Osteomyelitis and septic arthritis in children: current concepts. *Curr Opin Pediatr.* 2013;25(1):58-63.
4. Gutierrez K. Bone and joint infections in children. *Pediatr Clin North Am.* 2005;52(3):779-794.
5. Oudjhane K, Azouz EM. Imaging of osteomyelitis in children. *Radiol Clin North Am.* 2001;39(2):251-266.
6. Pugmire BS, Shailam R, Gee MS. Role of MRI in the diagnosis and treatment of osteomyelitis in pediatric patients. *World J Radiol.* 2014;6(8):530-537.
7. Montgomery NI, Rosenfeld S. Pediatric osteoarticular infection update. *J Pediatr Orthop.* 2015;35(1):74-81.
8. Mazur JM, Ross G, Cummings J, et al. Usefulness of magnetic resonance imaging for the diagnosis of acute musculoskeletal infections in children. *J Pediatr Orthop.* 1995;15(2):144-147.
9. Kan JH, Young RS, Yu C, et al. Clinical impact of gadolinium in the MRI diagnosis of musculoskeletal infection in children. *Pediatr Radiol.* 2010;40(7):1197-1205.
10. Browne LP, Guillerman RP, Orth RC, et al. Community-acquired staphylococcal musculoskeletal infection in infants and young children: necessity of contrast-enhanced MRI for the diagnosis of growth cartilage involvement. *AJR Am J Roentgenol.* 2012;198(1):194-199.
11. Abernathy L, Lee Y, Cole W. Ultrasound localisation of subperiosteal abscesses in children with late-acute osteomyelitis. *J Pediatr Orthop.* 1993;13(6):766-768.
12. Kaiser S, Rosenborg M. Early detection of subperiosteal abscesses by ultrasonography. *Pediatr Radiol.* 1994;24(5):336-339.
13. Howard C, Einhorn M, Dagan R, et al. Ultrasonic features of acute osteomyelitis. *J Bone Joint Surg Br.* 1995;77(4):663-664.
14. Castellazzi L, Mantero M, Esposito S. Update on the management of pediatric acute osteomyelitis and septic arthritis. *Int J Mol Sci.* 2016;17(6):e855.
15. Ceroni D, Cherkaoui A, Ferey S, et al. *Kingella kingae* osteoarticular infections in young children: clinical features and contribution of a new specific real-time PCR assay to the diagnosis. *J Pediatr Orthop.* 2010;30(3):301-304.
16. Sdougkos G, Chini V, Papanastasiou DA, et al. Methicillin-resistant *Staphylococcus aureus* producing Panton-Valentine leukocidin as a cause of acute osteomyelitis in children. *Clin Microbiol Infect.* 2007;13(6):651-654.
17. Elledge RO, Dasari KK, Roy S. Panton-Valentine leukocidin-positive Staphylococcus aureus osteomyelitis of the tibia in a 10-year-old child. *J Pediatr Orthop.* 2014;23(4):358-363.
18. Dartnell J, Ramachandran M, Katchburian M. Haematogenous acute and subacute paediatric osteomyelitis: a systematic review of the literature. *J Bone Joint Surg Br.* 2012;94(5):584-595.
19. Paakkonen M, Kallio MJ, Kallio PE, et al. Sensitivity of erythrocyte sedimentation rate and C-reactive protein in childhood bone and joint infections. *Clin Orthop Relat Res.* 2010;468(3):861-866.
20. Peltola H, Paakkonen M, Kallio P, et al, OM-SA Study Group. Clindamycin vs. first-generation cephalosporins for acute osteoarticular infections of childhood: a prospective quasi-randomized controlled trial. *Clin Microbiol Infect.* 2012;18(6):582-589.
21. Jagodzinski NA, Kanwar R, Graham K, Bache CE. Prospective evaluation of a shortened regimen of treatment for acute osteomyelitis and septic arthritis in children. *J Pediatr Orthop.* 2009;29(5):518-525.
22. Ramos OM. Chronic osteomyelitis in children. *Pediatr Infect Dis J.* 2002;21(5):431-432.

75 More Than an Achy Back: Spinal Epidural Abscess

ROBERT VEZZETTI, MD, FAAP, FACEP

Case Presentation

A 4-year-old female presents with 1 week of left-sided abdominal and hip pain. She was evaluated at an outside facility 5 days ago, had plain abdominal radiography, and was diagnosed with constipation. She then returned 2 days later with continued fever but was noted to have difficulty ambulating and reported generalized back pain. She had a urinalysis done that was reportedly concerning for a urinary tract infection. She was prescribed antibiotics but continued to have fever and back pain. She was then evaluated by her primary provider, who noted that the child was not toxic-appearing but did have difficulty ambulating secondary to pain, which she apparently localized to her left hip and lower back. The physician obtained plain radiographs of the lumbar spine and a one-view image of the pelvis. A diagnosis of toxic synovitis was made and scheduled ibuprofen was recommended.

Despite scheduled ibuprofen, the child continued to have intermittent febrile episodes and pain, prompting a visit to the emergency department. On examination, she is well appearing and in no acute distress. Her temperature is 98 degrees Fahrenheit, heart rate is 130 beats per minute, respiratory rate is 22 breaths per minute, and blood pressure is 102/75 mm Hg. She has no abnormal abdominal findings. Her musculoskeletal examination shows no signs of trauma, swelling, or erythema. She has good range of motion of all her extremities, including the lower ones, and there is no tenderness to palpation of the extremity or the joints. She has no spinal tenderness. When you ask the child to walk, she refuses at first but then walks several steps and stops, complaining of lower back and left hip pain.

The mother states that the child has been in good health and denies prior illness or trauma. There is no report of dysuria, incontinence, weakness, numbness, or difficulty with balance.

Imaging Considerations

PLAIN RADIOGRAPHY

Plain radiography is often obtained as a first-line imaging modality for patients with back pain and difficulty ambulating. However, it is not useful in the detection of a spinal epidural abscess. If there is associated osteomyelitis, cortical changes to the bone may be seen 2–3 weeks after the onset of illness.[1,2] The disc space may be narrowed on plain radiography, but this is not sensitive or specific for a spinal epidural abscess.[3,4]

COMPUTED TOMOGRAPHY (CT)

CT is not a first-line imaging modality in patients with a suspected infectious spinal process, such as a spinal epidural abscess. However, if magnetic resonance imaging (MRI) is not available, CT may be an alternative and is often obtained when another process is being considered, such as appendicitis or another intra-abdominal condition, that may make ambulation difficult. CT may be able to visualize a spinal abnormality due to infection, but it lacks sensitivity and specificity.[5,6] CT may be used to guide abscess drainage.[7,8]

MAGNETIC RESONANCE IMAGING

Gadolinium-enhanced MRI is the modality of choice for patients with suspected spinal epidural abscess and has a reported sensitivity and specificity of greater than 90%.[5–10] A spinal epidural abscess appears as an isointense or hypointense collection on T1-weighted images and hyperintense on T2-weighted images.[11]

ULTRASOUND

This modality is not recommended for the evaluation and detection of a spinal epidural abscess.

RADIONUCLEOTIDE SCANNING (BONE SCAN)

This modality is not a first-line imaging test, having been replaced by MRI, and has little role in the diagnosis of an epidural abscess.[6] However, a bone scan may be indicated in cases where there is clinical suspicion of distantly located osteomyelitis. Some authors have advocated obtaining a bone scan if there is abscess-associated osteomyelitis, given the anatomic field limitations of MRI.[8,12]

Imaging Findings

The initial imaging studies obtained by the primary care physician were reviewed. These images are presented here: one view of the pelvis and two views of the lumbar spine (Figs. 75.1–75.3). These images reveal no acute fracture or dislocation and normal bony alignment; however, there is subtle disc space narrowing at L3–4, better appreciated after the MRI examination is reviewed. There is a normal bowel gas pattern.

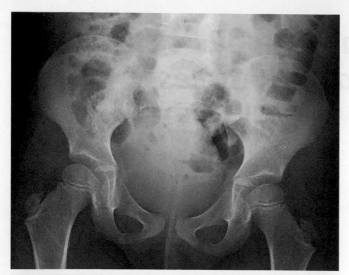

Fig. 75.1 Anterior-posterior view of the pelvis shows normal appearance of osseous structures of the pelvis and hips.

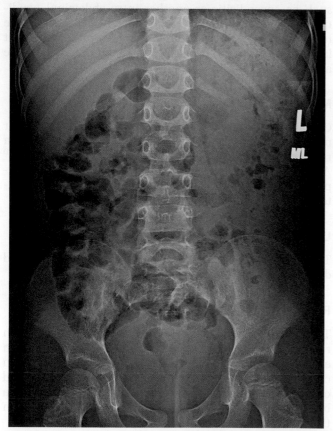

Fig. 75.2 Anterior-posterior view of the lumbosacral spine shows normal appearance of osseous structures.

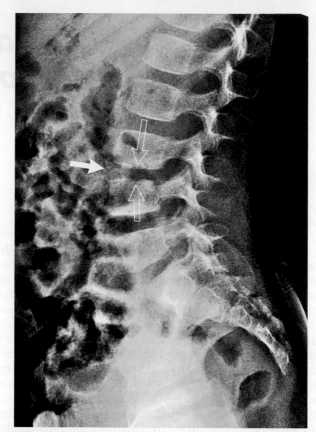

Fig. 75.3 Lateral view of the lumbosacral spine shows normal osseous alignment; however, on the lateral view, there is a very subtle loss of intervertebral disc space height at L3–4 *(white arrow)* with subtle findings of irregularity of the superior end plate of L4 and possibly of the inferior end plate of L3 *(open arrows)*. These latter findings are made more difficult to discern by overlying bowel gas.

Case Conclusion

The history of fever and back pain, along with the child's discomfort during ambulation, was concerning. Laboratory studies were obtained. These revealed an unremarkable complete blood count (including total white blood cell count and differential), normal creatine kinase level, and a normal urinalysis. The erythrocyte sedimentation rate (ESR) was 92 mm/hour (normal for this laboratory is <10) and the C-reactive protein (CRP) was 3.5 mg/dL (normal for this laboratory is <1 mg/dL).

With the history, physical examination, and laboratory values, further imaging was obtained. The child had MRI (with and without intravenous gadolinium contrast) of the lumbar spine. A selected view is presented here. There is L3–4 disc height loss and a fluid collection within the posterior aspect of the L3–4 disc space extending into the epidural space (Fig. 75.4).

Pediatric Orthopedic Surgery and Pediatric Infectious Disease were consulted to assist in the management of this patient. Arrangements were made for CT-guided drainage of the abscess, which was performed without incident. Per infectious disease guidance, appropriate antibiotics were initiated. Over the course of several days, the patient's symptoms improved and she was able to ambulate. Her inflammatory markers (ESR and CRP) trended downward and she was discharged home to complete a 6-week course of antibiotics. Blood cultures and cultures from the abscess did not yield an organism (perhaps due to pretreatment with antibiotics for the previously-diagnosed urinary tract infection). Interestingly, the mother did recall that the child had fallen and struck her lumbar area on a wooden table 2–3 weeks prior to the development of the fever.

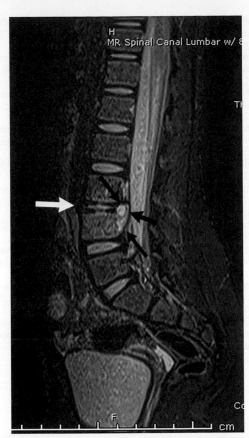

Fig. 75.4 Inversion recovery sagittal image of the spine demonstrates L3–4 disc height loss *(white arrow)*, with a high signal fluid collection extending from the posterior L3–4 disc space into the anterior spinal epidural space *(black arrows)*, consistent with discitis and an epidural abscess (measured 13 × 9 mm).

Spinal epidural abscess is not common. Risk factors for the development of a spinal epidural abscess include spine trauma, previous skin infections, intravenous drug use, and immunodeficiency.[7,11,13] Pediatric patients are less likely to have these risk factors, or underlying conditions[8]; however, spinal epidural abscess has been reported in association with vesicoureteral reflux due to posterior urethral valves, sickle cell disease, and myelogenous leukemia.[8,14] Common presenting symptoms are fever, back pain, refusal to ambulate, refusal to bear weight, and pain with movement, although the diagnosis can be delayed because initial symptoms are often nonspecific.[7,8] A posterior lumbar location is common and this may be due to the anatomic and physiologic characteristics of the developing pediatric spine.[8,15,16] These infections are usually the result of hematogenous spread or direct extension into the epidural space.[8,9,14]

The diagnosis of an epidural abscess is based on clinical, laboratory, and imaging findings.[11] Acute phase reactants, such as the ESR and CRP, can be helpful in the diagnosis of an inflammatory process, such as epidural abscess; ESR has been shown to be a better indicator of disease than white blood cell count.[7,9,13,17,18] CRP is more responsive to therapy than ESR.[8] Elevated inflammatory markers in patients with concerning clinical signs, such as back pain, should prompt the clinician to consider imaging.[7,13]

Staphylococcus aureus (both the methicillin-sensitive and methicillin-resistant species) is the most common organism isolated in patients with a spinal epidural abscess.[7–10,18] Initial antibiotic therapy should be tailored toward this organism, but other pathogens should be considered, based on the current and medical history of the patient. A thorough medical history can provide assistance to the clinician regarding coverage for other organisms, which have been implicated in epidural abscesses formation, such as *Bartonella*, *Aspergillus*, *Salmonella*, and group B *Streptococcus*.[8,9,14,19]

The management of a spinal epidural abscess is traditionally a combination of medical and surgical therapies.[8–10,13] However, current treatment options include antimicrobial therapy alone, in combination with CT-guided drainage, or in combination with operative incision and drainage. The duration of antimicrobial therapy is based on clinical improvement and improvement in laboratory inflammatory markers.[7,18] Some studies have suggested 4 to 6 weeks.[7,8,10,19] One study examined the treatment of a small number of pediatric patients with spinal epidural abscess (nine patients, all under the age of 18 years old), and the majority (seven of the nine patients) did not undergo neurosurgical intervention, although four patients of these seven had CT-guided abscess drainage.[7] All received systemic antibiotics and all recovered without sequelae.[7] Of the two patients who had neurosurgical intervention, laminectomy and incision and drainage of the abscess were the procedures performed.[7] Another small study demonstrated good outcomes and no deaths in pediatric patients who were treated primarily with neurosurgical intervention (six of eight patients), one patient treated with medical therapy after CT-guided drainage, and one patient treated with medical therapy alone. Antibiotic therapy in this series lasted for a mean of 6 weeks.[8] Some authors have suggested consideration of nonsurgical management in patients who have no neurologic deficits or with complete deficit for >3 days, patients with extensive abscesses, or patients who are high surgical risks.[8,10,20] Another study found that management with antimicrobial therapy alone or in combination with CT-guided abscess drainage produced outcomes similar to those of patients managed with antimicrobial therapy and surgical intervention, regardless of patient age, presence of comorbid illness, disease onset, neurologic abnormality at time of presentation, or abscess size.[18] Others have reported success with antimicrobial therapy alone.[9,20] Pediatric Neurosurgery or Orthopedics and Pediatric Infectious Disease should be consulted early when considering management options in patients with spinal epidural abscess, noting that while antimicrobial therapy is universally accepted, surgical or drainage procedures are not necessarily indicated.

Outcomes are based on several factors, with the length of time before initiation of therapy and the severity of neurologic deficit being the two most important outcome predictors.[7,17] Children tend to have better outcomes compared to adult patients.[8]

IMAGING PEARLS

1. Plain radiography is often obtained as a first-line imaging modality in patients with back pain. However, for infectious processes, it is not as useful and is not helpful in diagnosing spinal epidural abscess.
2. CT is often used to guide spinal epidural abscess drainage but is not as useful in detecting a spinal epidural abscess due to lack of sensitivity and specificity.

3. MRI with intravenous gadolinium contrast is the diagnostic imaging modality of choice to investigate a spinal epidural abscess.

References

1. Gutierrez K. Bone and joint infections in children. *Pediatr Clin North Am.* 2005;52(3):779-794.
2. Oudjhane K, Azouz EM. Imaging of osteomyelitis in children. *Radiol Clin North Am.* 2001;39(2):251-266.
3. Khan SH, Hussain MS, Griebel RW, et al. Comparison of primary and secondary spinal epidural abscesses: a retrospective analysis of 29 cases. *Surg Neurol.* 2003;59(1):28-33.
4. Darouiche RO. Spinal epidural abscess. *N Engl J Med.* 2006;355(19):2012-2020.
5. Sugawara R, Kikkawa I, Watanabe H, et al. Pediatric spinal epidural abscess: a case report of a 12-year-old girl without risk factors. *J Am Acad Orthop Surg Glob Res Rev.* 2019;3(3):e066.
6. Bond A, Manian FA. Spinal epidural abscess: a review with specific emphasis on earlier diagnosis. *Biomed Res Int.* 2016;2016:1614328.
7. Hawkins M, Bolton M. Pediatric spinal epidural abscess: a 9-year institutional review and review of the literature. *Pediatrics.* 2013;132(6):e1680-e1685.
8. Auletta JJ, John CC. Spinal epidural abscesses in children: a 15-year experience and review of the literature. *Clin Infect Dis.* 2001;32(1):9-16
9. Bair-Merritt MH, Chung C, Collier A. Spinal epidural abscess in a young child. *Pediatrics.* 2000;106(3):E39.
10. Houston R, Gagliardo C, Vassallo S, et al. Spinal epidural abscess in children: case report and review of the literature. *World Neurosurg.* 2019;126:453-460.
11. Pradilla G, Nagahama Y, Spivak AM, et al. Spinal epidural abscess: current diagnosis and management. *Curr Infect Dis Rep.* 2010;12(6):484-491.
12. Alazraki NP. Radionuclide imaging in the evaluation of infections and inflammatory disease. *Radiol Clin North Am.* 1993;31(4):783-794.
13. Nussbaum ES, Rigamonti D, Standiford H, et al. Spinal epidural abscess: a report of 40 cases and review. *Surg Neurol.* 1992;38(3):225-231.
14. Martino AM, Winfield JA. Salmonella osteomyelitis with epidural abscess: a case report with review of osteomyelitis in children with sickle cell anemia. *Pediatr Neurosurg.* 1990;16(6):321-325.
15. Newell RLM. The spinal epidural space. *Clin Anat.* 1999;12(5):375-379.
16. Hogan QH. Epidural anatomy examined by cryomicrotome section: influence of age, vertebral level, and disease. *Reg Anesth.* 1996;21(5):395-406.
17. Pereira CE, Lynch JC. Spinal epidural abscess: an analysis of 24 cases. *Surg Neurol.* 2005;63(suppl 1):S26-S29.
18. Siddiq F, Chowfin A, Tight R, et al. Medical vs surgical management of spinal epidural abscess. *Arch Intern Med.* 2004;164(22):2409-2412.
19. Tasher D, Armarnik E, Mizrahi A, et al. Cat scratch disease with cervical vertebral osteomyelitis and spinal epidural abscess. *Pediatr Infect Dis J.* 2009;28(9):848-850.
20. Leys D, Lesoin F, Viaud C, et al. Decreased morbidity from acute bacterial spinal epidural abscesses using computed tomography and nonsurgical treatment in selected patients. *Ann Neurol.* 1985;17(4):350-355.

76 It's Tough Being a Kid: Toddler's Fracture

ROBERT VEZZETTI, MD, FAAP, FACEP

Case Presentation

A 2-year-old female is brought for evaluation for right leg pain. The child was jumping in a trampoline house and fell on her right leg. The parents, who accompany the child, did not witness the mechanism by which the child injured her leg, but they state that the child was on the trampoline with several other children, the oldest of whom is 9 years old and is with the patient and her parents. The family reports that all children were bouncing vigorously when the child's right leg became caught in a gap between the pads. After this event, the patient had pain with ambulation, which localized to the right lower leg. There are no other historical concerns, such as emesis, loss of consciousness, neck pain, or back pain.

The child appears comfortable and is interactive. She has vital signs appropriate for her age. Her examination is unremarkable, except for tenderness over the distal portion of her right lower leg. There is no edema or deformity. The patient is grossly neurovascularly intact. There does not appear to be any neck, hip, or back pain.

Imaging Considerations

PLAIN RADIOGRAPHY

Plain radiography is the initial imaging modality of choice in children with musculoskeletal injury. Exposure to ionizing radiation is low and this resource is widely available. Sedation is not required. A two-view (anteroposterior [AP] and lateral) study should be obtained, but consideration should be given to utilization of an oblique view, as some fractures may be better visualized on this projection.[1] Comparison views of the injured and noninjured extremities are typically not necessary and are not routinely obtained; however, in some cases, comparison views may be helpful if there is a finding that is questionable for injury. Note that toddler's fractures can be subtle on plain radiography, and images can be normal even in the setting of a fracture.

Fractures in nonambulatory children or children in which a given history is not compatible with either physical examination or imaging findings should prompt concerns for nonaccidental trauma. In these children, appropriate imaging, including a skeletal survey and, if indicated, neuroimaging, should be obtained, as recommended by the American Academy of Pediatrics and other organizations.[2–4]

OTHER IMAGING MODALITIES

Interest in the utilization of ultrasound as an imaging modality to detect fractures has grown over the past decades. Advantages of this modality are availability and lack of ionizing radiation. However, this modality is operator dependent, requiring expertise in its use and interpretation of findings. As such, ultrasound use may be limited in detecting fractures, particularly subtle injuries.[5] Other imaging modalities, including computed tomography and magnetic resonance imaging, are not indicated in the acute work up of a suspected toddler's fracture.

Imaging Findings

Two views (AP and lateral) of the involved extremity show a nondisplaced right distal tibia fracture (Fig. 76.1). This fracture is not well visualized on the lateral view, but no signs of angulation or displacement are seen (Fig. 76.2). The visualized portions of the knee and ankle do not show any apparent facture or signs of injury.

Case Conclusion

This child was noted to have a toddler's fracture of the tibia and was placed in a posterior short leg splint, with referral to Pediatric Orthopedics. Repeat imaging approximately 1 month after the injury demonstrated healing of the fracture with no apparent complication (Figs. 76.3 and 76.4).

For comparison, a classic-appearing toddler's fracture is noted in Figs. 76.5 through 76.7.

Nondisplaced tibial fractures in young, ambulatory children, known as "toddler's fractures," are very common in this age population. This fracture was initially described by Dunbar et al. in 1964 as an oblique nondisplaced fracture of the distal third of the tibia occurring in children 9 months to 3 years of age.[6,7] Often, there is a history of trivial trauma. Many children will continue to ambulate but with a limp, favoring the affected leg. There may be no known, definitive history of trauma in many children with toddler's fractures. Concerns for nonaccidental trauma are not generally warranted with this type of fracture, especially with classic radiographic appearance and location. If the fracture is not consistent in this regard, if there are clinical signs of more severe injury, or if the child is not ambulatory, then one should consider nonaccidental trauma.

The majority of children with toddler's fracture require nothing more than symptomatic care. Splinting the extremity is appropriate, which helps with pain control, followed by Pediatric Orthopedic follow-up and casting. Children treated with short leg casting, long leg casting, or no immobilization have

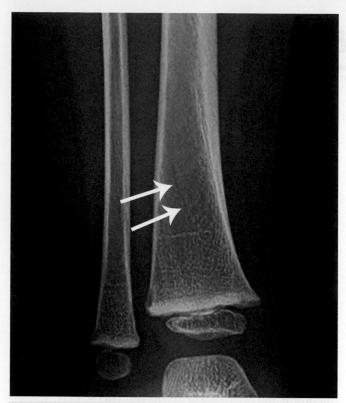

Fig. 76.1 View of the distal tibia from an AP tibia/fibula radiograph demonstrates a subtle nondisplaced oblique distal tibial fracture *(arrows)* consistent with a partially visualized spiral fracture of the tibia.

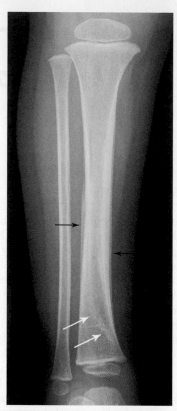

Fig. 76.3 One month post injury, an AP view of the tibia and fibula shows sclerosis about the healing spiral fracture of the distal tibia *(white arrows)* and periosteal new bone along the tibial diaphysis *(black arrows)*.

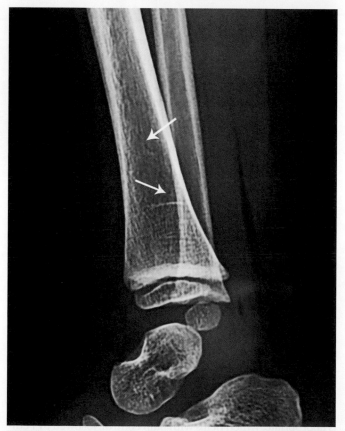

Fig. 76.2 Lateral view of the distal tibia from a tibia/fibula radiograph shows the spiral fracture of the distal tibia *(arrows)* to be very subtle on this view.

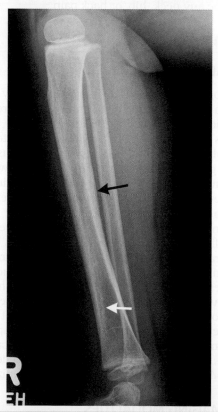

Fig. 76.4 One month post injury, a lateral view of the tibia and fibula shows subtle sclerosis about the healing spiral fracture of the distal tibia *(white arrow)* and periosteal new bone along the tibial diaphysis *(black arrow)*.

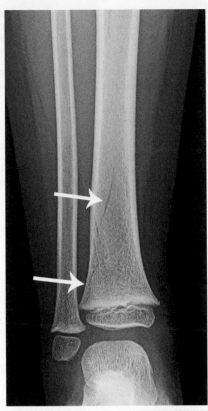

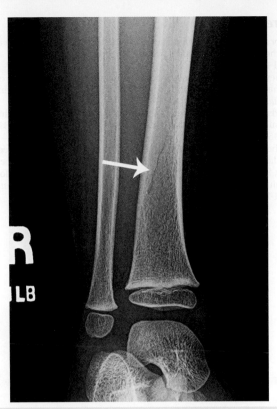

Fig. 76.5 AP view demonstrates a nondisplaced spiral fracture of the distal tibia *(arrows)*, consistent with a classic toddler's fracture.

Fig. 76.7 Oblique view demonstrates a nondisplaced spiral fracture of the distal tibia *(arrow)*, consistent with a classic toddler's fracture.

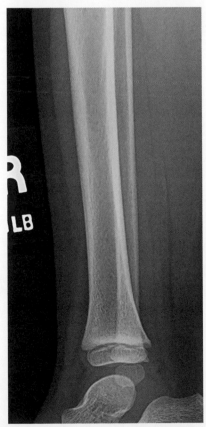

Fig. 76.6 Lateral view shows that the spiral fracture of the tibia is not well seen in lateral projection, despite being well visualized on AP (Fig. 76.5) and oblique (Fig. 76.7) views.

shown to have similar outcomes.[8] Immobilization with casting has been the traditionally advocated treatment, but since fracture displacement is rare, some advocate for either no immobilization or using a boot, rather than splinting or casting, with outcomes reported to be equally satisfactory whether immobilization is used or not.[6] One study of Canadian emergency departments demonstrated that management practices vary widely for both confirmed (39% of respondents utilized immobilization with above-the-knee circumferential casting, 27% with below-knee circumferential casting, and 20% with below-the-knee splinting) and suspected (44% of respondents managed without casting, 22% with below-the-knee splinting, and 14% with above-the-knee circumferential casting) toddler's fractures.[9] It may be appropriate for primary care providers to manage these injuries without orthopedic referral, and clinical pathway management algorithms have been proposed.[10] In the majority of cases, these fractures heal well, and follow-up radiography is not indicated but may be useful if a fracture is suspected and initial imaging is indeterminate.

IMAGING PEARLS

1. Plain radiographs, consisting of two views (AP and lateral) of the affected extremity are generally all that are needed when a toddler's fracture is suspected.
2. An oblique view may be helpful in cases where a fracture is strongly suspected but not evident on other views.
3. Comparison views of the unaffected extremity are not routinely needed but may be indicated in cases where a radiographic finding suggests a fracture.
4. Beware of toddler's type fracture in nonambulatory children. Consideration should be given to nonaccidental trauma with appropriate further workup and imaging.

References

1. Sapru K, Cooper JG. Management of the toddler's fracture with and without initial radiological evidence. *Eur J Emerg Med.* 2014;21(6):451-454.
2. Riney LC, Frey TM, Fain ET, et al. Standardizing the evaluation of nonaccidental trauma in a large pediatric emergency department. *Pediatrics.* 2018;141(1):1-9.
3. Christian CW, Committee on Child Abuse and Neglect. The evaluation of suspected child physical abuse. *Pediatrics.* 2015;135(5):e1337-e1354.
4. Flaherty EG, Perez-Rossello JM, Levine MA, et al. AAP Committee on Child Abuse and Neglect, Section on Radiology, Section on Endocrinology, Section on Orthopedics, and the Society for Pediatric Radiology. Evaluating children with fractures for child physical abuse. *Pediatrics.* 2014;133(2):e477-e489.
5. Lewis D, Logan P. Sonographic diagnosis of toddler's fracture in the emergency department. *J Clin Ultrasound.* 2006;34(4):190-194.
6. Schuh AM, Whitlock KB, Klein EJ. Management of toddler's fractures in the pediatric emergency department. *Pediatr Emerg Care.* 2016;32(7):452-454.
7. Dunbar JS, Owen HF, Nogrady MB, et al. Obscure tibial fracture of infants—the toddler's fracture. *J Can Assoc Radiol.* 1964;15:136-144.
8. Leffler LC, Tanner SL, Beckish ML. Immobilization versus observation in children with toddler's fractures: a retrospective review. *J Surg Orthop Adv.* 2018;27(2):142-147.
9. Seguin J, Brody D, Li P. Nationwide survey on current management strategies of toddler's fractures. *CJEM.* 2018;20(5):739-745.
10. Adamich JS, Camp MW. Do toddler's fractures of the tibia require evaluation and management by an orthopaedic surgeon routinely? *Eur J Emerg Med.* 2018;25(6):423-428.

77 *Hurtn' to Stand: Discitis*

ROBERT VEZZETTI, MD, FAAP, FACEP

Case Presentation

An 18-month-old female presents with 1 to 2 weeks of fussiness and not wanting to ambulate. She has not had any fevers, vomiting, or diarrhea. There is no report of trauma. About 2 weeks prior, she had a cough, congestion, and low-grade fever (100.4 degrees Fahrenheit) that resolved after a few days. She has been healthy since then.

Her primary care physician evaluated the child 1 day after her symptoms began. At that time, the child was complaining of what was thought to be left leg pain (the mother stated that the child cried when attempting to ambulate and did not seem to want to bear weight on the left leg). Plain radiographs of the pelvis (including anterior-posterior [AP] and frog leg views), the left femur, and left tibia-fibula were obtained and were unremarkable. Since that time, the child has refused to ambulate and does not want to bear weight on either leg. Her primary care provider obtained a bilateral hip ultrasound (US), which was unremarkable.

Her physical examination shows a child in no distress. Her temperature is 98 degrees Fahrenheit, heart rate is 101 beats per minute, respiratory rate is 22 breaths per minute, and blood pressure is 90/60 mm Hg. She has an unremarkable examination, including her neurologic examination, which demonstrates no weakness or obvious lack of sensation. When attempting to ambulate, she refuses to do so and in fact cries when standing upright. She does not have any obvious findings on her extremities and range of motion maneuvers at her hip, knees, and ankles are normal. You note that the child prefers to lie down and, when she sits up, appears to be in discomfort.

Imaging Considerations

Gait disturbances in the pediatric patient have a lengthy differential diagnosis to consider. History and physical examination should guide further laboratory and radiographic evaluation.

PLAIN RADIOGRAPHY

Plain radiography is often employed as an initial imaging modality in pediatric patients who have either painful ambulation or who are refusing to ambulate. Obtaining radiographs in children with these symptoms is a reasonable first step, utilizing AP and lateral views.[1,2] Early on in the course of the illness, radiographs usually appear normal. Children who have discitis may demonstrate narrowing of the disc space with varying degrees of vertebral

end plate destruction, resulting in loss of disc space height, usually 2 to 3 weeks after the onset of illness.[1,3–8] Radiography also has the advantage of detecting other possible causes of pain, such as fractures.

ULTRASOUND

The use of US in the evaluation of a patient with suspected discitis has not been established.

COMPUTED TOMOGRAPHY (CT)

CT has a limited role in the initial evaluation of patients with suspected discitis or other infections of the spine, although it can be used to guide biopsy procedures.[9] This modality does have the ability to provide detailed information about anatomy (especially bone detail) but may not detect abnormalities early in the course of illness.[2]

BONE SCAN (TECHNETIUM-99M)

Bone scan is sensitive for the detection of inflammatory processes, such as infection, but is not specific.[2,8,10] This modality has largely been replaced by magnetic resonance imaging (MRI).

MAGNETIC RESONANCE IMAGING

MRI with and without intravenous contrast has become the imaging study of choice to evaluate for discitis or suspected infection of the spine.[2,7,8,10–14] One study showed that MRI has a sensitivity of 97% for the detection of infection[15] and greater than 90% for discitis.[2] This modality has largely superseded nuclear bone scanning and is both sensitive and specific for discitis.[3,5] MRI findings vary depending on when the imaging study is obtained. Early in the process, vertebral end plates, the disc, and subchondral regions show only minor changes, but as the process progresses, the end plates may become irregular and blurred, ultimately becoming dark on T1-weighted images and bright on T2-weighted images; the disc may appear collapsed; and the adjacent vertebrae may show abnormality if the infection spreads.[3,7,9]

Imaging Findings

The patient underwent MRI of the lumbar spine. Selected images from that study are provided here. There is abnormal marrow edema in the L2 and to a lesser extent L3 vertebral bodies. The L2/3 disc demonstrates loss of height, altered signal intensity, and enhancement (Figs. 77.1–77.3).

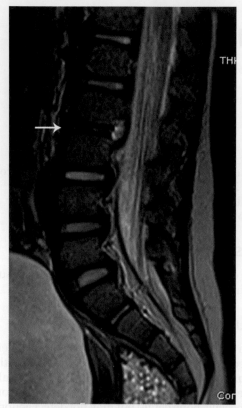

Fig. 77.1 T2-weighted sagittal image demonstrating L2 disc height loss and decreased signal intensity *(arrow)*.

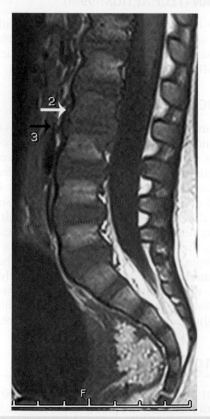

Fig. 77.2 T1-weighted sagittal image demonstrating decreased marrow signal consistent with abnormal marrow edema in the L2 vertebral body *(white arrow)* and decreased disc space height at L2/3 *(black arrow)*.

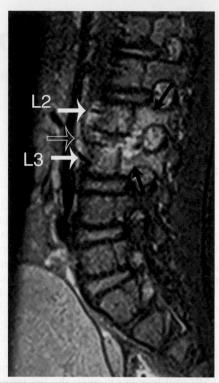

Fig. 77.3 Sagittal STIR sequence demonstrating increased signal of abnormal marrow edema in the L2 and L3 vertebral bodies *(white arrows)*. The L2 disc demonstrates disc height loss and heterogeneous decreased and increased signal *(open arrow)*. Bone marrow edema also extends into the pedicles and posterior elements of L2 and L3 *(black arrows)*.

Case Conclusion

The diagnosis of discitis was made. In addition to imaging, laboratory studies were done, including a complete blood count (CBC), C-reactive protein (CRP), and erythrocyte sedimentation rate (ESR). The white blood cell count was 16×10^9, the ESR was 97 mm/hour, and the CRP level was 2 mg/dL. Pediatric Infectious Disease and Pediatric Orthopedics were both consulted; ceftriaxone and clindamycin were started. The patient improved and by the fifth hospital day had improved ambulation and decreased pain. A peripherally inserted catheter line was placed and she was discharged with a course of antibiotics. Blood cultures that were obtained at admission and prior to antibiotic administration were negative. Surgical intervention was not needed.

Discitis refers to infection of a disc space and adjacent vertebral end plates[9] and is not a common disease in the pediatric population. Discitis has a predilection for children less than 5 years of age and primarily affects the lumbar region.[3–5,7,13,16,17] There may be little to no fever and primary symptoms include a progressive limp or refusal to ambulate. Notably, presenting symptoms of discitis can vary with the developmental age of the child.[3,4,5,7,13,16,17] This is in contrast to vertebral osteomyelitis, which tends to affect older children who are usually febrile, more ill-appearing, and may complain of pain anywhere along the spine, although initially it can be difficult to distinguish between the two entities.[3] Additional symptoms of discitis include irritability and abdominal pain, but symptoms can be vague.[7,9,13] The pathophysiology leading to the development of discitis is not well understood. Discitis is thought to occur due to the presence of a rich blood supply to the disc in younger children, who have cartilaginous vascular channels (that disappear as a patient ages) and robust intraosseous arterial connections (which are not as prevalent in older children).[1,3,8,9,16] Infection with prodromal illness, often diagnosed as viral, has been reported prior to the development of discitis, as well as prior trauma.[8]

Laboratory studies (CBC, ESR, CRP) can be elevated but are nonspecific, and the majority of patients with discitis have negative blood cultures.[3,6,8,18] One study had a negative blood culture rate of 88%.[3] However, obtaining these studies is suggested in children with suspected discitis, since initially distinguishing between discitis and vertebral osteomyelitis can be difficult. Since the rate of positive blood cultures in vertebral osteomyelitis is higher than in discitis[3,6] and laboratory studies are often obtained prior to imaging, it is reasonable to proceed with laboratory studies, including blood culture.

There is no universal management strategy, and even the use of antimicrobial therapy in discitis is somewhat controversial. The course of pediatric discitis is often self-limited.[8,19] Many experts have proposed an infectious cause, however, since the majority of pediatric patients with discitis have negative cultures and patients have been noted to recover without antimicrobial therapy; *routine* use of antimicrobials has come into question but is recommended by some authors.[3,5,6,7] Ideally, cultures should be obtained from the bone, but even then will return an organism in up to 50% of patients.[1,3,18] When an organism is identified, *Staphylococcus aureus* is most commonly isolated.[1,8,13,20] Some authors have recommended biopsy in patients who are not improving despite antibiotic therapy.[1,13] The duration of therapy for discitis has not been universally established, but many centers recommend clinical examination as a guideline for the duration of therapy.[3,6–8,19] Nevertheless, antimicrobial therapy is often initiated when discitis is diagnosed, particularly if there is a focus of infection.[3,6,7,8,13] Previous studies have documented faster improvement in patients who are managed with antibiotics.[8,19]

Bracing, in addition to antibiotic therapy, has also been utilized for discitis treatment. Some authors have utilized bracing without antibiotic therapy in children who are well appearing, have reassuring laboratory values (normal CBC, normal inflammatory markers, a negative blood culture), and have evidence of inflammation without focus of infection.[8] As with antibiotic therapy decisions, consultation with Pediatric Orthopedics and Pediatric Infectious Disease is appropriate if bracing (with or without antibiotic therapy) is considered.

IMAGING PEARLS

1. Plain radiography of the spine, employing AP and lateral views, is the initial imaging modality of choice in patients with suspected discitis.

2. Plain radiography may be unremarkable early in discitis. However, spine radiographs may demonstrate narrowing of the disc space with varying degrees of destruction of vertebral end plate destruction, resulting in loss of disc height, usually 2 to 3 weeks after the onset of illness.

3. MRI is the imaging modality of choice in patients with suspected discitis. MRI findings vary depending on how long the discitis process has been present, but there are characteristic findings that are present on T1- and T2-weighted images.

4. The decision to initiate antibiotics or manage with symptomatic care in patients with discitis may be assisted by a combination of laboratory results and imaging findings in conjunction with the appropriate consultants.

References

1. Kocher MS, Lee B, Dolan M, et al. Pediatric orthopedic infections: early detection and treatment. *Pediatr Ann.* 2006;35(2):112-122.
2. Simpfendorfer CS. Radiologic approach to musculoskeletal infections. *Infect Dis Clin North Am.* 2017;31(2):299-324.
3. Fernandez M, Carrol CL, Baker CJ. Discitis and vertebral osteomyelitis in children: an 18-year review. *Pediatrics.* 2000;105(6):1299-1304.
4. Spencer SJ, Wilson NI. Childhood discitis in a regional children's hospital. *J Pediatr Orthop B.* 2012;21(3):264-268.
5. Date AR, Rooke R, Sivashankar S. Lumbar discitis. *Arch Dis Child.* 2006;91(2):11.
6. Germain ML, Krenzer KA, Hasley BP, et al. 11-month-old child refuses to sit up. *Pediatr Ann.* 2008;37(5):290-293.
7. Tyagi R. Spinal infections in children: a review. *J Orthop.* 2016;13(4):254-258.
8. Chandrasenan J, Klezl Z, Bommireddy R, et al. Spondylodiscitis in children: a retrospective series. *J Bone Joint Surg Br.* 2011;93(8):1122-1125.
9. Offiah AC. Acute osteomyelitis, septic arthritis and discitis: differences between neonates and older children. *Eur J Radiol.* 2006;60(2):221-232.
10. Naranje S, Kelly DM, Sawyer JR. A systematic approach to the evaluation of a limping child. *Am Fam Physician.* 2015;92(10):908-916.
11. Dunbar JA, Sandoe JA, Rao AS, et al. The MRI appearances of early vertebral osteomyelitis and discitis. *Clin Radiol.* 2010;65(12):974-981.
12. Rankine JJ. MRI of spinal infection. *Curr Orthop.* 2004;18(6):426-433.
13. Early SD, Kay RM, Tolo VT. Childhood diskitis. *J Am Acad Orthop Surg.* 2003;11(6):413-420.
14. Brown R, Hussain M, McHugh K, et al. Discitis in young children. *J Bone Joint Surg Br.* 2001;83(1):106-111.
15. Ledermann HP, Schweitzer ME, Morrison WB, et al. MR imaging findings in spinal infections: rules or myths? *Radiology.* 2003;228(2):506-514.
16. Sanapala S, Neelmanee R, Prashant K, et al. Diagnostic use of MRI in the non-mobile infant. *BMJ Case Rep.* 2012;2012:bcr2012007378.
17. Agarwal R, Yousif O, Basu H. An unusual cause of non–weight bearing. *Arch Dis Child.* 2013;98(4):286.
18. Crawford AH, Kucharzyk DW, Ruda R, et al. Diskitis in children. *Clin Orthop.* 1991;266:70-79.
19. Ring D, Johnston CE II, Wenger DR. Pyogenic infectious spondylitis in children: the convergence of discitis and vertebral osteomyelitis. *J Pediatr Orthop.* 1995;15(5):652-660.
20. Dayer R, Alzahrani MM, Saran N, et al. Spinal infections in children: a multicentre retrospective study. *Bone Joint J.* 2018;100-B(4):542-548.

78   *My Knee Won't Stop Swelling! Osteosarcoma*

ROBERT VEZZETTI, MD, FAAP, FACEP

Case Presentation

A 6-year-old female presents with persistent, worsening right knee swelling for the past 2 months. The area has become painful over the past few weeks, especially at night. There has been no fever, erythema, or swelling of the other extremities or joints. There is no report of trauma, but prior to the development of symptoms, the child was quite physically active and it is possible that she may have injured the knee while playing. The child's physical examination is remarkable for generalized swelling of the right knee. She has minimal pain to palpation of the superior aspect of the knee; full extension of the knee produces pain. There is no warmth, erythema, or fluctuance.

Imaging Considerations

PLAIN RADIOGRAPHY

A two-view radiographic examination of the involved extremity is reasonable first-line imaging in pediatric patients with extremity complaints and is often utilized in trauma settings. Clinical prediction rules have been developed to assist the clinician in identifying which trauma patients may benefit from imaging.[1] In selected patients, such as those who have sustained trauma, additional views may be needed. For example, a sunrise view can be used to assess the patella for fracture or subluxation, which may not be visualized on a two-view study.

Children with knee pain, especially chronic pain, who have no signs of abnormality on their clinical examination typically will have imaging of the involved knee. However, the possibility of referred pain should be considered. A common scenario illustrating this is referred pain from the hip with a slipped capital femoral epiphysis or Legg-Calve-Perthes disease. In these cases, imaging of the hip (anterior-posterior [AP] and frog leg views) is appropriate while also imaging the involved knee.

COMPUTED TOMOGRAPHY (CT)

Non–contrast-enhanced CT is generally not a first-line imaging study in pediatric knee complaints. It may be employed to better visualize fractures such as patellar or tibial plateau fractures and to evaluate joint involvement if a fracture is present. In children with identifiable bone masses, CT is used to look for metastatic lesions, especially in the thorax.[2]

MAGNETIC RESONANCE IMAGING (MRI)

While generally not a first-line imaging modality, MRI is a more definitive study to visualize joint spaces, ligaments, and tendons and evaluate tumoral, inflammatory, or infectious processes. MRI is used to further evaluate masses that are initially detected through other modalities.

Imaging Findings

The child had three views performed of the right knee. These images reveal abnormal sclerosis of the distal femoral diaphysis and metaphysis, discontinuous periosteal new bone, and cloudlike calcification around the distal femur, with extension into the surrounding soft tissues (Figs. 78.1A–78.3). Because of the possibility of trauma, a sunrise view was also obtained; there is no fracture (Fig. 78.4). The findings noted on plain radiography suggest an aggressive process, with the ossification extending into the soft tissues most suggestive of osteosarcoma.

Case Conclusion

Osteosarcoma is the most common primary pediatric bone tumor and is highly aggressive, but survival rates (currently approximately 60%–70%) have improved since the introduction of effective treatment, which includes chemotherapy and, in some cases, surgical amputation.[3-5] Overall survival depends on the initial staging of the tumor and the response to treatment. Patients with a nonresectable primary, metastatic, or recurrent disease have a poor prognosis.[3] Most children with osteosarcoma have a history of pain, which may initially be intermittent but over time becomes steady. It is not uncommon for the patient to present with a clinical history of trauma. Osteosarcoma usually involves the metaphysis of long bones. The distal femur, humerus, and proximal tibia are common locations of involvement. Lung is the most common site for metastasis of osteosarcoma and patients with metastatic disease at the time of diagnosis have a lower survival rate (20%–30%) compared to those without metastatic disease; however, those with isolated lung metastases have a better prognosis than those with metastases to the bone or other sites.[4,6,7]

Plain radiography in osteosarcoma often will demonstrate sclerosis of the involved bone and tumoral ossification within the mass, including calcification in the soft tissue

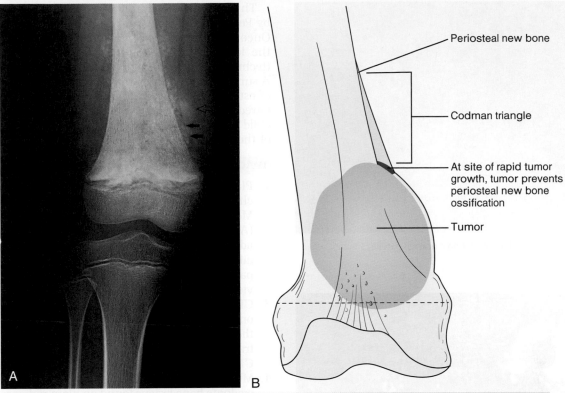

Fig. 78.1 A. Anterior-posterior view of the right knee shows a sclerotic lesion of the distal femoral diaphysis and metaphysis. The periosteal reaction is discontinuous, creating a Codman triangle appearance *(arrows)*. Tumor extending beyond the bone shows cloudlike ossification *(open arrow)*. B. Illustration of a Codman triangle of periosteal new bone related to a bone tumor.

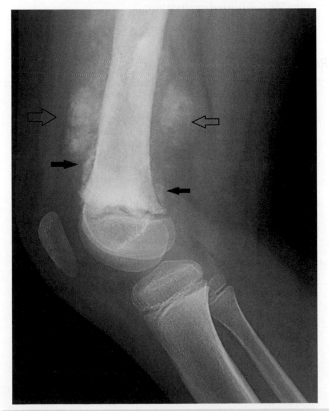

Fig. 78.2 Lateral view of the knee again demonstrates discontinuous periosteal reaction *(arrows)* and tumoral ossification in the soft tissues *(open arrows)*.

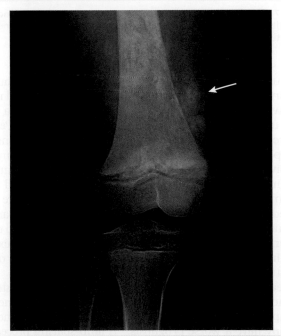

Fig. 78.3 Oblique view shows sclerosis of the distal femur, periosteal reaction, and tumoral ossification characteristic of osteosarcoma *(arrow)*.

mass extending beyond the bone. However, some osteosarcoma lesions, such as telangiectatic osteosarcoma, may present with a lytic appearance and may be subtle on radiography. Periosteal reaction with osteosarcoma reflects the aggressive nature of the lesion and is often discontinuous, as

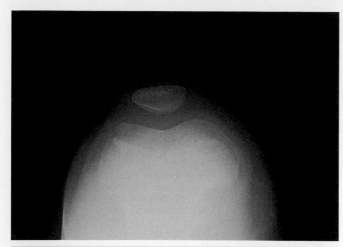

Fig. 78.4 Sunrise view demonstrating a normal patella.

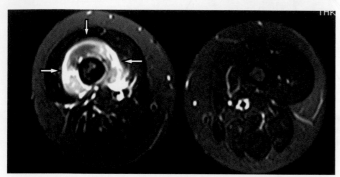

Fig. 78.5 Axial magnetic resonance image shows high signal tumor of the distal right femur extending circumferentially into the surrounding soft tissues *(arrows)*.

This patient was admitted for subspecialty consultation by Pediatric Oncology and Pediatric Orthopedic Surgical Oncology. An MRI was obtained, delineating the extent of the lesion (Fig. 78.5). A nuclear medicine bone scan (technetium 99) showed no indication of bone metastasis. A surgical biopsy was performed, confirming the diagnosis of osteosarcoma. Systemic chemotherapy was initiated, followed by surgical excision of the mass. Unfortunately, the child ultimately required hip disarticulation (amputation) of the extremity.

IMAGING PEARLS

1. Plain radiography is the first-line imaging modality for children with musculoskeletal complaints.
2. Most children with knee symptoms can have two views (AP and lateral) of the knee. If there is a trauma history, additional views may be indicated, as some fractures are difficult to visualize on two-view imaging. For example, patellar pain may necessitate the utilization of a "sunrise view" to better visualize the patella.
3. CT can be utilized to further evaluate findings detected on plain radiographic imaging. This modality is useful for the evaluation of some fractures, employing a noncontrast technique. In cases of suspected osteosarcoma, CT of the thorax is used to detect lung metastasis.
4. MRI is the preferred imaging modality to further evaluate bone lesions found on plain radiography. This study is not typically obtained in an emergency setting, unless imaging findings or clinical presentation suggest infection; children with lesions concerning for an oncologic process are typically admitted to an inpatient service for continued evaluation.

the tumor growth is often too rapid to allow for smooth, continuous periosteal reaction. Instead, the periosteal reaction will be seen to abruptly terminate, often forming a Codman triangle as seen in this patient (see Fig. 78.1B). Periosteal reaction patterns associated with aggressive lesions are not specific for osteosarcoma and may be seen with any aggressive osseous lesion. Once the tumor is detected, further imaging is performed to determine tumor extent and plan treatment. CT and magnetic resonance imaging are employed for this purpose. CT is the current gold standard to evaluate for lung metastases.[4] MRI provides a detailed evaluation of the tumor, including depiction of osseous extent and involvement of surrounding soft tissues and other structures.[4]

Treatment for osteosarcoma is guided by staging. Systemic chemotherapy and surgical resection are cornerstones of therapy. Patients with an initially poor response to chemotherapy have a worse prognosis.[6] A limb-sparing procedure is preferred, but there are cases where this is not possible, particularly if there is a poor response to initial treatment.[6,8]

References

1. Moore BR, Hampers LC, Clark KD. Performance of a decision rule for radiographs of pediatric knee injuries. *J Emerg Med.* 2005;28(3): 257-261.
2. Vijayakumar V, Collier AB, Ruan C, et al. Multimodality imaging in pediatric osteosarcoma in the era of image gently and image wisely campaign with a close look at the CT scan radiation dose. *J Pediatr Hematol Oncol.* 2016;38(3):227-231.
3. Kager L, Tamamyan G, Bielack S. Novel insights and therapeutic interventions for pediatric osteosarcoma. *Future Oncol.* 2017;13(4):357-368.
4. Bielack SS, Hecker-Nolting S, Blattmann C, et al. Advances in the management of osteosarcoma. *F1000Res.* 2016;5:2767.
5. Reed DR, Hayashi M, Wagner L, et al. Treatment pathway of bone sarcoma in children, adolescents, and young adults. *Cancer.* 2017;123(12):2206-2218.
6. Anderson ME. Update on survival in osteosarcoma. *Orthop Clin North Am.* 2016;47(1):283-292.
7. Slade AD, Werneke CL, Hughes DP, et al. Effect of concurrent metastatic disease on survival in children and adolescents undergoing lung resection for metastatic osteosarcoma. *J Pediatr Surg.* 2015;50(1):157-160.
8. Allison DC, Carney SC, Ahlmann ER, et al. A meta-analysis of osteosarcoma outcomes in the modern medical era. *Sarcoma.* 2012;2012:704872.

79 Not THOSE Ewings: Ewing Sarcoma

ROBERT VEZZETTI, MD, FAAP, FACEP

Case Presentation

A 9-year-old male presents with a 4-month history of right upper arm pain. Over the past 2 months, he and his parents have noted the development of swelling to the arm as well. The patient is active in sports, particularly baseball, and the pain started after he pitched a game. He was given ibuprofen with some relief of the pain, but over the past several weeks, this has not been helping. He has not had fever, numbness, weakness, rash, or other symptoms.

Physical examination reveals a well-appearing pleasant patient in no acute distress. His vital signs are unremarkable. He has a normal physical examination with the exception of his right upper arm, where there is swelling, and tenderness of the midshaft of the right humerus. While he has normal gross range of motion, he does complain of pain with movement of the arm. There is no erythema, warmth, or fluctuance. He is neurologically intact.

Imaging Considerations

PLAIN RADIOGRAPHY

Plain radiography is the initial imaging modality of choice in patients with musculoskeletal complaints. Since Ewing sarcoma commonly presents with pain,[1] this modality is the first-line modality utilized in these patients.[2] A two-view imaging study (anteroposterior and lateral) is usually obtained. This study may reveal osteolysis and periosteal reaction. The periosteal reaction of Ewing sarcoma usually reflects the aggressive nature of the lesion and can produce characteristic imaging findings such as the classically described "onion skin" periosteal new bone and the presence of the "Codman triangle." With an aggressive lesion, the periosteal reaction is often discontinuous, as the tumor growth is often too rapid to allow for smooth, continuous periosteal reaction. Instead, the periosteal reaction will be seen to abruptly terminate, forming a Codman triangle, as seen subsequently in this patient and in Chapter 78 (Fig. 78.1). The Codman triangle is an area of new subperiosteal bone created when the tumor raises the periosteum away from the bone and is often accompanied by spicule formation in the soft tissues.[1,3]

COMPUTED TOMOGRAPHY (CT)

This imaging modality may be appropriate as a secondary study when initial plain radiography is abnormal; however, magnetic resonance imaging (MRI) is the most appropriate secondary imaging study for a suspected malignant primary bone tumor.[2] CT may be used in the staging process, including evaluation of metastasis to the lungs, once the diagnosis of Ewing sarcoma is suspected.[1,2] The rapidity and wide availability of this imaging test, as well as the lack of sedation need, are advantages for CT.

MAGNETIC RESONANCE IMAGING

MRI with and without intravenous contrast is the advanced imaging modality of choice when initial plain radiography is abnormal or unremarkable, and a primary bone tumor is otherwise suspected.[2] MRI is excellent at defining intramedullary involvement and depicting the soft tissue extent of a lesion.[1,2] Since this modality is also very good at delineating the anatomic relationships between the tumor and surrounding structures, it is useful at planning operative intervention and biopsies.[1,2,4]

POSITRON EMISSION TOMOGRAPHY (PET)

This modality is used as a follow-up imaging test in the staging and treatment process; it is not a first-line imaging modality.

Imaging Findings

The patient's history and physical examination findings warrant further investigation. Plain radiography of the right humerus was obtained. These images were somewhat difficult to obtain, since the patient had pain with movement of the arm despite pain medication. These images revealed a destructive lesion in the midshaft of the right humerus, with a permeative lytic pattern in the cortex. The periosteal reaction surrounding the lesion was indicative of an aggressive lesion, with a Codman triangle and spiculated periosteal new bone (see Chapter 78 [Osteosarcoma], for further discussion of the Codman triangle). These patterns occur as an aggressive tumor lesion that expands beyond the bone, elevates the periosteum, and lesion growth outpaces the growth of newly-formed subperiosteal bone (Fig. 79.1).

Case Conclusion

The patient was referred to Pediatric Oncology for further evaluation of the bone lesion. He had a metastatic workup

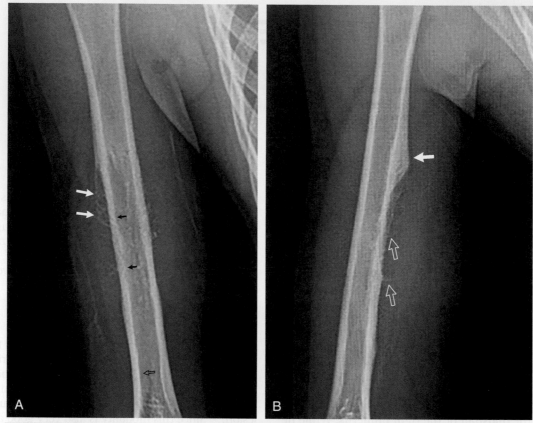

Fig. 79.1 Anteroposterior (A) and lateral (B) radiographic images of the right humerus demonstrate an aggressive-appearing lesion in the mid-diaphysis. There is permeative destruction of the cortical bone, seen as a subtle, moth-eaten appearance of increased lucency in the region of the tumor *(black arrows)* compared to normal cortex *(open black arrow)*. The periosteal reaction is also of an aggressive pattern: with a Codman triangle *(white arrows)* and spicules of periosteal new bone *(open white arrows)*, which are perpendicular to the cortical surface. These patterns of periosteal reaction reflect an aggressive, rapidly growing tumor mass that elevates the periosteum.

with additional imaging, which demonstrated no other areas of disease. A biopsy was obtained, confirming the diagnosis of Ewing sarcoma. An appropriate chemotherapy regimen was initiated and the patient had an excellent response. Surgical excision will subsequently be performed.

Ewing sarcoma is an aggressive form of bone cancer, with a reported incidence of 1–3 per 1 million people per year.[1] It is a tumor of childhood and adolescence, with a median age at diagnosis of 14 to 15 years old in this population,[1] and is most commonly diagnosed in the second decade of life.[2] It represents the second most common primary malignant bone tumor in children.[1,3,5–7]

The most common presenting symptom in patients with Ewing sarcoma is pain, with palpable swelling or mass in many patients.[1,3] The median duration of symptoms prior to diagnosis is between 4 and 6 months; a pathologic fracture may be the initial presenting symptom leading to diagnosis.[1,8,9] Fever and weight loss are not common symptoms but when present correlate with metastatic disease.[1,3] Ewing sarcoma can affect skeletal and extraskeletal soft tissues. In pediatric patients, Ewing sarcoma often affects the axial skeleton (50%), including the flat bones of pelvis and chest wall.[1,3] Long bones are also commonly affected (46% with roughly 20% femoral in location).[1,3] These tumors usually originate in the diaphysis, whereas osteosarcoma tends to be metaphyseal in location.[1,3] Approximately one-fourth of

patients will have metastasis at diagnosis; pulmonary metastasis is the most common site (up to one-third of patients).[1,3,7] Laboratory tests such as erythrocyte sedimentation rate or C-reactive protein may be elevated in Ewing sarcoma.[3]

The diagnosis of Ewing sarcoma consists of clinical and radiologic findings, but biopsy is the gold standard. Because this lesion can demonstrate extensive necrosis, several core biopsies are usually needed to make the diagnosis, and in up to one-third of cases, results may be indeterminate, resulting in a delay in diagnosis.[1] An open biopsy is the preferred method for confirming the diagnosis.[1,3]

Prognostic factors for Ewing sarcoma depend on the age of the patient, tumor site/volume, response to chemotherapy, and the extent and site of metastases.[1,5,6,10] Stage of the disease is the most significant prognostic factor; it has been shown that patients with isolated pulmonary metastases have a better course than those with osseous metastases or bone marrow involvement.[1,5] Chemotherapy response is also an important prognostic factor as chemotherapy-induced tumor necrosis is associated with increased survival.[1,6] In general, patients with disseminated disease or recurrent disease have unfavorable prognoses and there is no standardized treatment protocols for these patients or for those with refractory disease.[1,3,11] The role of imaging to assess patient response to treatment is less clear. Some studies have suggested the use of PET scanning to gauge treatment response.[1,12]

Once the diagnosis of Ewing sarcoma is made, staging is performed. Procedures used in the staging process include chest CT, whole-body bone scintigraphy, and bone marrow biopsy. More recently, PET scan, often used in combination as a PET-CT scan, has been replacing bone scintigraphy.[1,3]

Treatment of Ewing sarcoma is multimodal, consisting of localized and systemic treatment. This has led to increased survival of patients with this tumor, with a cure rate of 50%[1,3] and an overall survival rate of 75%.[7] The usual sequence of therapy includes primary induction chemotherapy, followed by local therapy (surgical excision), then adjuvant chemotherapy.[3] Localized surgery, with or without radiotherapy, has produced good outcomes in patients with small, localized disease, whereas patients with tumors that are less amenable to resection, due to location or size, have less favorable outcomes.[1,3,13,14] However, even in patients with disseminated disease, surgery is still utilized in disease management.[14,15] Limb salvage is generally attempted, although amputation is indicated in some cases where limb salvage would not be satisfactory.[3] Debulking of tumor has not been shown to improve localized control of disease.[3] Radiotherapy is indicated as an initial localized treatment choice when surgical resection is limited, but patients in this category generally do not have a favorable outcome.[3] Systemic chemotherapy is an important aspect of Ewing sarcoma management. There are several treatment protocols available; in North America, a five-drug alternating regimen is typically utilized.[3]

IMAGING PEARLS

1. Plain radiography is the initial imaging modality of choice in patients with musculoskeletal pain.
2. Ewing sarcoma involves the flat bones of the central skeleton or bones of the limbs. In the limbs, this sarcoma usually involves the bone diaphysis.
3. MRI is the advanced imaging modality of choice for patients with Ewing sarcoma. It is excellent for visualizing intramedullary involvement and soft tissue extent of a lesion. This modality may be used in planning local control (i.e., surgical) and for disease surveillance.
4. CT is performed as part of a metastatic workup for patients with Ewing sarcoma.
5. PET may be used for staging and treatment planning. In combination with chest CT, this imaging modality can be used for metastatic evaluation. PET scanning has also been proposed as a means to evaluate treatment response.

References

1. Potratz J, Dirksen U, Jürgens H, et al. Ewing sarcoma: clinical state-of-the-art. *Pediatr Hematol Oncol*. 2012;29(1):1-11.
2. Expert Panel on Musculoskeletal Imaging, Bestic JM, Wessell DE, et al. ACR Appropriateness Criteria primary bone tumors. *J Am Coll Radiol*. 2020;17(5S):S226-S238.
3. Bernstein M, Kovar H, Paulussen M, et al. Ewing's sarcoma family of tumors: current management. *Oncologist*. 2006;11(5):503-519.
4. Paulussen M, Bielack S, Jurgens H, et al. Ewing's sarcoma of the bone: ESMO clinical recommendations for diagnosis, treatment, and follow-up. *Ann Oncol*. 2009;20(suppl 4):140-142.
5. Cotterill SJ, Ahrens S, Paulussen M, et al. Prognostic factors in Ewings tumor of bone: analysis of 975 patients from the European Intergroup Cooperative Ewing's Sarcoma Study Group. *J Clin Oncol*. 2000;18(17):3108-3114.
6. Paulussen M, Ahrens S, Dunst J, et al. Localized Ewing tumor of bone: final results of the Cooperative Ewing's Sarcoma Study CESS 86. *J Clin Oncol*. 2000;19(6):1818-1829.
7. Balamuth NJ, Womer RB. Ewing's sarcoma. *Lancet Oncol*. 2010;11(2):184-192.
8. Widhe B, Widhe, T. Initial symptoms and clinical features in osteosarcoma and Ewing sarcoma. *J Bone Joint Surg Am*. 2000;82(5):667-674.
9. Bramer JAM, Abudu AA, Grimer RJ, et al. Do pathological fractures influence survival and local recurrence rate in bony sarcomas? *Eur J Cancer*. 2007;43(13):1944-1951.
10. Bacci G, Ferrari S, Bertoni F, et al. Prognostic factors in nonmetastatic Ewing's sarcoma of bone treated with adjuvant chemotherapy: analysis of 359 patients at the Instituto Ortopedico Rizzoli. *J Clin Oncol*. 2000;18(1):4-11.
11. Barker L, Pendergrass T, Sanders J, et al. Survival after recurrence of Ewing's sarcoma family of tumors. *J Clin Oncol*. 2005;23(19):4354-4362.
12. Hawkins DS, Schuetze SM, Butrynski JE, et al. [18F]Fluorodeoxyglucose positron emission tomography predicts outcome for Ewing sarcoma family of tumors. *J Clin Oncol*. 2005;23(34):8828-8834.
13. Ginsberg JP, Goodman P, Leisenring W, et al. Long-term survivors of childhood Ewing sarcoma: report from the Childhood Cancer Survivor Study. *J Natl Cancer Inst*. 2010;102(16):1272-1283.
14. Bacci G, Ferrari S, Longhi A, et al. Therapy and survival after recurrence of Ewing's tumors: the Rozzoli experience in 195 patients treated with adjuvant and neoadjuvant chemotherapy from 1979 to 1997. *Ann Oncol*. 2003;14(11):1654-1659.
15. Haeusler J, Ranft A, Boelling T, et al. The value of local treatment in patients with primary, disseminated, multifocal Ewing sarcoma (PDMES). *Cancer*. 2010;116(2):443-450.

80 *What Is This? Bone Cyst*

ROBERT VEZZETTI, MD, FAAP, FACEP

Case Presentation

A 5-year-old male presents with left arm pain after a fall. He was playing soccer when he fell and landed on his left shoulder. He immediately complained of upper arm pain. His examination is significant for focal tenderness to the proximal left humerus with decreased range of motion when he attempts to raise the arm. There is mild edema. He is grossly neurovascularly intact. Imaging is obtained and a proximal humeral fracture is noted. However, the fracture is through a mildly expansile radiolucent lesion.

Prior to this trauma, the child had no symptoms, including fever, pain, or edema of the extremity. He also has no chronic medical conditions.

Imaging Considerations

PLAIN RADIOGRAPHY

As with most pediatric acute musculoskeletal trauma, plain radiography is the initial imaging modality of choice. When imaging the upper extremity in pediatric patients, two views (anteroposterior and lateral) of the involved extremity are appropriate. Consideration of imaging the joint above and below the suspected fracture area should be given, especially if there are historical or clinical indications of a second injury or where pain localization is difficult.

COMPUTED TOMOGRAPHY (CT)

CT, while excellent for evaluating fractures, is not indicated in the initial evaluation of suspected humeral fractures in children.

MAGNETIC RESONANCE IMAGING (MRI)

MRI is not indicated in the initial imaging of musculoskeletal injuries in pediatric patients. This modality may be utilized if there are concerns for neurologic injury or compromise, although it is typically obtained after initial treatment and evaluation. MRI is often not readily available compared to plain radiography and CT. Younger children may require sedation.

Imaging Findings

Two views (anteroposterior and lateral) of the injured arm are obtained. There is a nondisplaced fracture through a lucent lesion involving the proximal humeral metaphysis and diaphysis that is suggestive of a bone cyst (Figs. 80.1

and 80.2). The radiographic appearance of the lesion is consistent with a simple bone cyst.

Case Conclusion

This patient's arm was placed in a sling, and the patient was provided appropriate pain control instructions, and referred to Pediatric Orthopedics for evaluation and follow-up. The child did have advanced imaging as an outpatient (MRI) confirming a simple bone cyst. He was treated with continued sling use and close observation.

Simple bone cysts (also known as unicameral bone cysts, or UBCs) are benign lesions commonly encountered in pediatric patients and are most often found in long bones, most commonly the humerus and the femur, although they can appear anywhere. UBCs are lucent, metadiaphyseal lesions and may be mildly expansile. The etiology of UBC is unknown.[1,2] UBCs are often incidental discoveries when imaging is performed for another reason, such as trauma.[1] They can, as in this patient, serve as a nidus for a pathologic fracture due to cortical thinning but rarely produce pain or swelling without fracture. With UBC, there is no periosteal reaction unless there has been a fracture. A painful lucent lesion without fracture is more likely to be malignant, and not a UBC.[1] Most UBCs are treated conservatively and resolve spontaneously, especially after fracture. Treatment may be indicated for patients with recurrent fractures, continued pain, or for prevention of deformity and includes corticosteroid injection, autologous bone marrow injection, and curettage with bone grafting, although recurrence rates are high.[1,3,4]

In contrast to UBC, aneurysmal bone cyst (ABC) is a locally aggressive, expansile lucent lesion that forms blood-filled cavities in bone. ABC also occurs most often in long bones but can appear in any bone, with approximately 20% involving the spine.[1] While the majority of ABCs are benign, they can be associated with malignant processes; their etiology is unknown but are thought to represent neoplastic processes.[1,5] ABC can be associated with periosteal reaction, pain, and swelling without fracture and can predispose to pathologic fracture. Primary lesions are more common than secondary lesions; secondary lesions can be associated with chondroblastoma, fibrous dysplasia, or nonossifying fibroma.[1,5] MRI and biopsy are used to assist in making the diagnosis of ABC. Aneurysmal bone cysts may be treated conservatively, operatively (curettage and bone grafting or cement), or with radiotherapy; spontaneous resolution has been reported but is not common.[1,5]

In the acute setting, further imaging to investigate simple bone cysts is typically not indicated beyond plain radiography, which demonstrates a radiolucent, well-defined lesion.[1,6] Some cysts will have fracture fragments that migrate within intracystic fluid, the "fallen fragment sign," that is pathognomic for a simple bone cyst.[6] CT can define lesion borders and assess cortical thickness or fracture risk.[1,5,6] Some simple cysts, though, have heterogeneous features and peripheral thickening that may make distinguishing these lesions from ABC lesions difficult.[2]

Aneurysmal bone cysts can be identified on plain radiography. Their appearance is radiolucent and expansile, circumscribed by thin cortical bone, with trabeculations within the lesion.[1,2,5] CT is less accurate in lesion characterization than MRI is but can be used to assess fracture risk.[6] MRI is more useful in distinguishing simple bone cysts from aneurysmal bone cysts and is the imaging modality of choice following plain radiography if further imaging is deemed necessary.[1,5,6] The combination of plain radiography and MRI has been shown to improve specificity and sensitivity in diagnosing aneurysmal bone cysts but is not often indicated in the acute setting.[5–7]

Bone cysts, whether simple or aneurysmal, should be referred to a Pediatric Orthopedist for definitive diagnosis and management.

IMAGING PEARLS

1. Plain radiography is the imaging modality of choice in pediatric musculoskeletal trauma, utilizing two views (anteroposterior and lateral).
2. Bone cysts, whether simple or aneurysmal, may both serve as points for pathologic fractures in children. Distinguishing between the two on initial plain radiography may be difficult and additional testing may be done as an outpatient.
3. MRI may be indicated if an aneurysmal bone cyst is suspected, but this is not an initial test and can be obtained on an outpatient basis.
4. Aneurysmal bone cysts, while generally benign, can be associated with a malignant process.
5. Patients with a bone cyst should be referred to Pediatric Orthopedics.

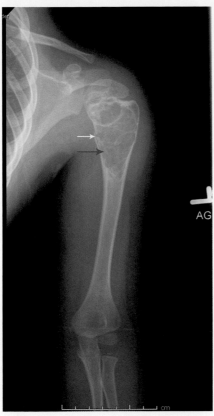

Fig. 80.1 Anteroposterior view demonstrating a nondisplaced fracture *(white arrow)* through a "bubbly" non–aggressive-appearing lesion *(red arrow)*.

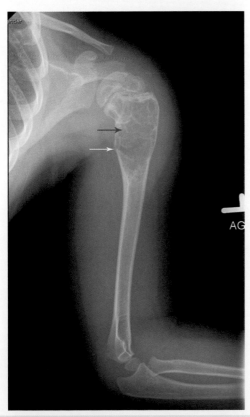

Fig. 80.2 Lateral view of the lesion, which is consistent with a bone cyst *(red arrow)*. The fracture can again be seen *(white arrow)*.

References

1. Rosenblatt J, Koder A. Understanding unicameral and aneurysmal bone cysts. *Pediatr Rev.* 2019;40(2):51-59.
2. Margau R, Babyn P, Cole W, et al. MR imaging of simple bone cysts in children: not so simple. *Pediatr Radiol.* 2000;30(8):551-557.
3. Zhao JG, Wang J, Huang WJ, et al. Interventions for treating simple bone cysts in the long bones of children. *Cochrane Database Syst Rev.* 2017;2:CD010847.
4. Donaldson S, Wirgt JG. Recent developments in treatment for simple bone cysts. *Curr Opin Pediatr.* 2011;23(1):73-77.
5. Park HY, Yang SK, Sheppard WL, et al. Current management of aneurysmal bone cysts. *Curr Rev Musculoskelet Med.* 2016;9(4):435-444.
6. Mascard E, Gomez-Brouchet A, Lambot K. Bone cysts: unicameral and aneurysmal bone cyst. *Orthop Traumatol Surg Res.* 2015;101(suppl 1):S119-S127.
7. Mahnken AH, Nolte-Ernsting CC, Wildberger JE, et al. Aneurysmal bone cyst: value of MRI and conventional radiography. *Eur Radiol.* 2003;13(5):1118-1124.

ENT

81 *Who Let the Dogs Out? Croup*

MICHAEL GORN, MD

ENT

Case Presentation

A 14-month-old, previously healthy child presents to the Emergency Department in the middle of the night with respiratory distress, hoarseness, and a barky cough. He has had mild congestion and a low-grade fever for a day. On physical examination, the child is in moderate respiratory distress and is anxious appearing while struggling to inhale each breath. His respiratory rate is 58 breaths per minute, his pulse oxygenation saturation is 98% on room air, and he has prominent subcostal and suprasternal retractions. He is not febrile. On auscultation, he has stridor, but no wheezing or rales in all lung fields, and breath sounds are equal throughout. The child is looking around anxiously without neck movement restrictions or drooling. The parents are concerned that the child "choked on something" since the child's respiratory distress was so acute in onset. They were seen at an urgent care facility just prior to arrival and had plain chest radiographs performed, which they have provided for review.

Imaging Considerations

PLAIN RADIOGRAPHY

Croup is a clinical diagnosis, and radiographs are not commonly indicated. However, the "steeple sign" is the typical finding on an anterior-posterior (AP) view of the chest or a soft tissue neck radiograph.[1–3] Also called the "wine bottle sign," it is a description of the appearance of the tracheal narrowing in the subglottic area.[1–3] The lateral radiograph may demonstrate narrowing and haziness of the subglottic trachea with overdistention of the hypopharynx.[1–3] If plain radiography is utilized to diagnose suspected croup, a lateral view should be obtained, since epiglottitis has a similar appearance to croup on the AP view. Dedicated soft tissue neck radiographs are useful for this purpose and can provide greater detail.

Advantages of plain radiography include relatively low exposure to ionizing radiation, rapidity, and availability, but imaging should be performed only if the diagnosis of croup is in question or a patient is not responsive to appropriate management for croup. Radiographic findings suggestive of other conditions include swelling of the epiglottis, a foreign body, an asymmetric compromise of the airway, an irregular or edematous trachea, and tracheal compression or deviation.[1–3] If there is concern for a nonradiopaque foreign body, a more serious infectious process (such as tracheitis, or an oropharyngeal or retropharyngeal abscess), or an anatomic issue (such as a vascular ring or sling), then advanced imaging modalities may be indicated.

COMPUTED TOMOGRAPHY (CT)

This imaging modality may be utilized if alternative diagnoses that may present in a manner similar to croup are being considered. These include foreign body ingestion/aspiration, tracheitis, anatomic variants (such as a vascular ring/sling), an airway hemangioma, or conditions causing tracheal compression, such as masses. CT is not otherwise routinely indicated or used.

MAGNETIC RESONANCE IMAGING (MRI)

Similar to CT, MRI is utilized as a secondary or tertiary imaging modality in patients who are suspected to have an alternative diagnosis that requires advanced imaging. This may be the case with anatomic variants or masses.

ULTRASOUND (US)

This imaging test may also be useful to detect etiologies that may mimic the clinical symptoms of croup, in particular, swallowed foreign bodies. The lack of ionizing radiation, availability, and portability of this modality make it particularly attractive in the urgent or emergent setting. However, US is operator dependent and has limited application for infectious cases or patients with complex vascular anatomy that may be causing croup-like symptoms.

Imaging Findings

Two-view radiography of the chest is provided. The lungs demonstrate normal volume without evidence of infiltrate, atelectasis, or air trapping. The heart appears normal. There is mild subglottic narrowing (Figs. 81.1 and 81.2). An illustration comparing the normal radiographic appearance of the subglottic airway to the appearance of the subglottic airway in croup is shown in Fig. 81.3. A different patient, a 4-year-old with findings of croup shown on dedicated soft tissue views of the neck, is presented in Fig 81.4.

Case Conclusion

The patient was administered racemic epinephrine via a nebulizer and monitored carefully. He improved dramatically shortly after treatment completion and was also given an oral dose of dexamethasone. The child was discharged home after a 2-hour period of observation to ensure no recurrence of stridor. He was able to tolerate oral fluids well.

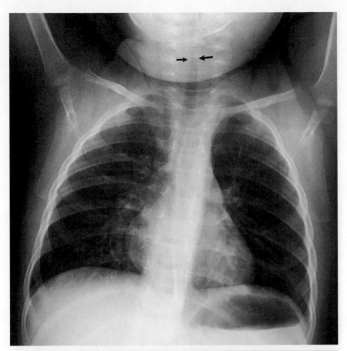

Fig. 81.1 Anterior-posterior (AP) view of the chest demonstrates normal lung volumes without evidence of infiltrate, atelectasis, or air trapping. On this view, there is subglottic narrowing, with a "steeple sign" seen of the subglottic trachea *(arrows)*.

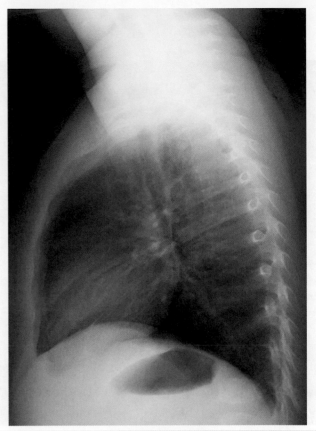

Fig. 81.2 Lateral view of the chest demonstrating normal lung volumes without evidence of infiltrate, atelectasis, or air trapping.

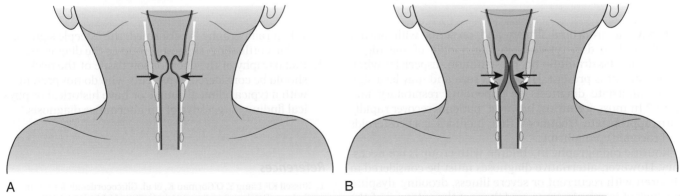

A   B

Fig. 81.3 Comparison of the normal appearance of the subglottic airway to the appearance of the subglottic airway in croup, on an anterior-posterior *(AP)* view of the neck. (A) Note the shoulder-like appearance of the normal subglottic airway *(arrows)*. (B) With croup, this normal appearance is lost and the subglottic airway instead resembles a church steeple *(arrows)*.

The parents were advised to monitor him closely for recurrence of respiratory distress and signs of dehydration.

Laryngotracheitis or croup is a common respiratory illness characterized by inspiratory stridor, barking (seal-like) cough, and hoarseness. The primary pathogens causing this illness are parainfluenza, adenovirus, and respiratory syncytial viruses, although virtually any upper respiratory virus can lead to croup symptoms.[4–6] Croup has a seasonal pattern, is more common in the fall and winter, and is more common in boys, and although it is seen from 3 months to

6 years of age, peak incidence is from age 6 months to 3 years.[4–6] The underlying viral infection causes inflammation of the larynx and subglottic airway and results in extrathoracic tracheal narrowing that causes the classic symptoms of inspiratory stridor and cough. Croup may begin as an upper respiratory infection and a low-grade fever. The barky cough and stridor can begin at any time point during the illness, but severity typically peaks between days 3 and 5.[4,5] A spasmotic variant of croup may be familial or related to atopic conditions.[4–6] This variant does

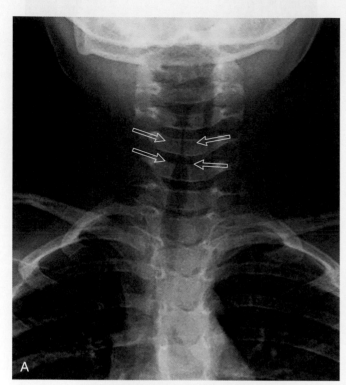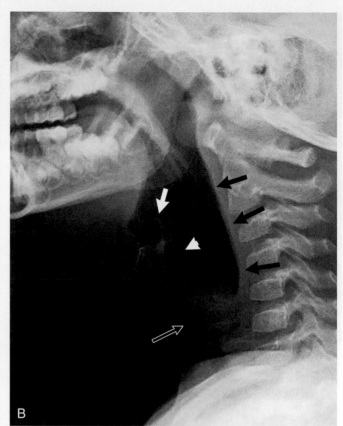

Fig. 81.4 Croup in a 4-year-old. Anterior-posterior and lateral soft tissue neck series shows symmetric subglottic airway narrowing consistent with croup seen on the frontal view as a steeple sign (*open arrows*, A) and seen as near obscuration of the subglottic airway on the lateral view (*open arrow*, B). On the lateral view (B), the epiglottis (*white arrow*) and aryepiglottic folds (*white arrowhead*) have a normal appearance and the hypopharynx is overdistended (*black arrows*).

not have a prodrome illness and presents with abrupt cough and stridor, typically in the middle of the night. Croup may be dramatic on presentation, especially when severe stridor is present. Hypoxia is rare and may be a sign of an alternate diagnosis or impending respiratory failure.[4–6] In most scenarios, however, patients recover rapidly with appropriate treatment that includes corticosteroids and racemic epinephrine.

Routine radiography in children with croup is not necessary. However, alternative diagnoses must be considered in children with recurrent or severe illness, drooling, dysphagia, lack of immunizations, and those at the extremes of the typical age range for croup. The differential diagnosis includes bacterial tracheitis, epiglottitis, foreign body, vocal cord dysfunction, gastroesophageal reflux disease, subglottic hemangiomas, and congenital anomalies of the airway or upper gastrointestinal tract. In rare instances, laryngoscopy or additional radiologic evaluation with CT, MRI, or an upper gastrointestinal series may be needed to evaluate for other etiologies.[1,6,7]

IMAGING PEARLS

1. Radiography is rarely indicated for either classic or spasmotic croup.

2. When radiography is performed, the "steeple sign" or "wine bottle sign" suggests croup as the diagnosis.

3. Radiography of the chest or soft tissue of the neck should be considered in patients who do not present with a typical clinical course or have historical or physical findings suggestive of an alternative diagnosis.

References

1. Russell KF, Liang Y, O'Gorman K, et al. Glucocorticoids for croup. *Cochrane Database Syst Rev.* 2011;(1):CD001955. doi:10.1002/14651858.CD001955.pub3.
2. Hiebert JC, Zhao YD, Willis EB. Bronchoscopy findings in recurrent croup: a systematic review and meta-analysis. *Int J Pediatr Otorhinolaryngol.* 2016;90:86-90.
3. Darras KE, Roston AT, Yewchuk LK. Imaging acute airway obstruction in infants and children. *Radiographics.* 2015;35(7):2064-2079.
4. Choi J, Lee GL. Common pediatric respiratory emergencies. *Emerg Med Clin North Am.* 2012;30(2):529-563.
5. Bjornson CL, Johnson DW. Croup in children. *CMAJ.* 2013;185(15):1317-1323.
6. Petrocheilou A, Tanou K, Kalampouka E, et al. Viral croup: diagnosis and a treatment algorithm. *Pediatr Pulmonol.* 2014;49(5):421-429.
7. Bjornson C, Russell KF, Vandermeer B, et al. Nebulized epinephrine for croup in children. *Cochrane Database Syst Rev.* 2011;(2):CD006619. doi:0.1002/14651858.CD006619.pub2.

82 All That Drools: Retropharyngeal and Peritonsillar Abscess

MICHAEL GORN, MD, and BHAIRAV PATEL, MD

Case Presentation

A 4-year-old child is referred from her primary care provider's office over concerns for meningitis. The patient has had fever and decreased oral intake and has not wanted to move her neck or head for the past 3 days. She has had rhinorrhea and mild cough for the past 3 days. She was seen by her primary care physician initially, who diagnosed an upper respiratory infection. The patient returned to her primary care provider when it was noted she did not want to move her neck or head.

Her physical examination reveals an anxious child in no immediate distress. She has a temperature of 103 degrees Fahrenheit, a heart rate of 120 beats per minute, respiratory rate of 30 breaths per minute, and a blood pressure of 85/40 mm Hg. Her examination reveals a mildly erythematous oropharynx without palatal petechiae or asymmetry. She is tilting her head toward the left and has very limited range of motion of the neck. In fact, she is refusing to move her neck or head. There is scattered anterior cervical lymphadenopathy that is nontender and without fluctuance. Her tympanic membranes are clear and there is no mastoid tenderness, erythema, or fluctuance.

Imaging Considerations

The retropharyngeal space is not usually well visualized on imaging without the presence of a pathologic process.[1,2] Imaging often plays a role in both the diagnosis and the management of patients with suspected deep soft tissue neck infections.

PLAIN RADIOGRAPHY

This imaging modality can be useful in assessing for the presence of an infection in the deep spaces of the neck. Plain radiography is available and rapid and has minimal exposure to ionizing radiation with adherence to pediatric imaging protocols. The presence of an increase in the width of the soft tissue space anterior to the cervical spine with narrowing of the oropharyngeal airway should prompt the clinician to consider such infections.[3–5] In children younger than 5 years of age, the retropharyngeal space normally measures one-half of the full width of the adjacent vertebral body; in older children, a second cervical (C2) prevertebral width of greater than 7 mm and sixth cervical (C6) width of

up to 14 mm are acceptable.[3,6–8] Some authors propose that prevertebral space measurements greater than these measurements, with clinical findings to support a deep neck space infection, are sufficient to make the diagnosis of a retropharyngeal abscess (RPA).[3,9,10] However, obtaining lateral neck radiographs can be challenging in pediatric patients, who may not cooperate behaviorally to produce a meaningful study. Flexion of the neck, crying, swallowing, and rotational artifacts can lead to difficulty interpreting these radiographs.[3,6–8,11] Additional indications of a deep neck infection may include gas within the soft tissues of the neck, prevertebral or retropharyngeal soft tissue thickening, cervical spine straightening (loss of lordosis) on the lateral view, and torticollis on anterior-posterior projections.[1,6–8]

COMPUTED TOMOGRAPHY (CT)

Intravenous contrast-enhanced CT is the study of choice for imaging patients with suspected neck deep tissue infection.[1,3,6–8,12] Patients with an RPA will demonstrate characteristic fluid in the retropharyngeal space and peripheral rim-like enhancement, defining the abscess, which appears as a homogenous area of hypodensity.[1,3] CT can have difficulty in distinguishing between RPA and cellulitis but remains the imaging modality of choice for these patients.[13] If a peritonsillar abscess is suspected, CT is an excellent modality to visualize this disease process. A peritonsillar abscess will be seen as diffuse enlargement and enhancement of the affected tonsil with an associated fluid collection surrounded by rim-like enhancement, although sometimes, the differentiation between a peritonsillar abscess and a necrotic retropharyngeal lymph node may be difficult.[1–3]

CT can be utilized to make management decisions in patients with deep soft tissue neck infections (i.e., antibiotics versus surgical intervention). This modality is also useful when evaluating the relationship between the infection and surrounding anatomic structures, including proximity to the great blood vessels and other vascular structures.[1,3,6–8,12] CT also has the advantage of narrowing the differential diagnosis by detecting trauma, foreign bodies, and congenital anatomic abnormalities (such as branchial cleft cysts and thyroglossal duct cysts, both of which can become infected). This modality does expose the patient to ionizing radiation, which can be minimized by adherence to As Low As Reasonably Achievable (ALARA) principles. The test is rapid and sedation is not generally needed.

ULTRASOUND

Ultrasound has the advantages of rapidity and availability while not requiring sedation or exposing the child to ionizing radiation. This imaging modality has been utilized for superficial neck infections in pediatric patients, decreasing the need for CT use, but is not helpful in evaluating suspected deep space infections.[1,14,15] However, ultrasound can miss a significant subset of patients who have lateral neck infections associated with deep coexisting retropharyngeal infection ultimately detected by CT (10%), and these patients require repeat imaging, the majority of the time (80%) employing CT.[15]

MAGNETIC RESONANCE IMAGING (MRI)

MRI is not used as a first-line imaging modality in patients with suspected deep soft tissue infections of the neck. However, MRI may be indicated in patients with suspected complications of such neck infections, particularly if there is concern for vascular complications such as jugular venous thrombosis.[3]

Imaging Findings

The history and physical examination findings were suspicious for a deep soft tissue neck infection, rather than meningitis. Therefore, CT imaging with intravenous contrast was obtained. Selected images from that study are included here. These images demonstrate a large right retropharyngeal hypodensity extending from the nasopharynx to the level of the hyoid bone, compatible with retropharyngeal phlegmon, extending along the right aspect of the skull base, C1, and C2 vertebral bodies (Fig. 82.1).

Case Conclusion

The patient was given intravenous clindamycin and admitted for intravenous fluids. Pediatric Otolaryngology was consulted, and recommended continuation of the clindamycin. Over 48 hours, the patient improved and was able to take oral fluids. She was discharged with oral antibiotics to complete a 10-day course and recovered uneventfully.

RPA is uncommon, mostly seen in children between the ages of 2 and 4 years, but can occur in all age groups from neonates to adults.[4,6,12,16,17] The retropharyngeal space extends from the base of the skull to the posterior mediastinum and laterally into the pharyngeal space. In children, lymphatic chains that drain the upper airway respiratory structures are located within this space and are the typical source of infection, which can extend into the potential spaces within the layers of the deep cervical facia and down into the mediastinum.[4,6,12,16,17] Infection is thought to begin as an upper respiratory infection (usually viral) leading to a suppurative process of these regional lymph nodes, culminating in abscess formation.[4] Abscess formation can also be associated with trauma to the area or a foreign body.[4]

The clinical presentation of an RPA can vary and the differential diagnosis is broad, which can include infectious

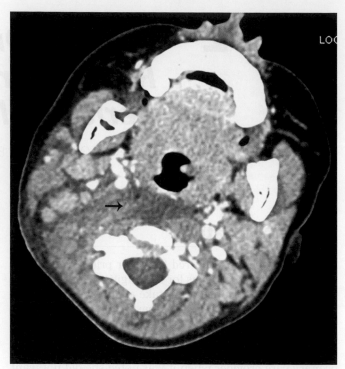

Fig. 82.1 Axial contrast-enhanced computed tomography scan of the neck at the level of the oropharynx demonstrates prominent retropharyngeal edema without peripherally enhancing fluid collection *(black arrow)*.

processes (meningitis, for example), trauma, tumors/masses, and congenital anomalies. A thorough history and physical examination will help narrow the differential diagnosis. There are no specific diagnostic symptoms. Fever, neck pain, and dysphagia are common symptoms; in infants, decreased oral intake, drooling, fussiness, and limited neck motion may also be seen. Some patients may present with signs of upper airway obstruction, such as stridor or respiratory distress. In these patients, great care must be taken during the physical examination not to exacerbate potential airway compromise, which can lead to patient decompensation; in some cases, examination in the operating suite under sedation with a controlled airway may be indicated in toxic-appearing patients who may have tenuous airways or signs of impending airway compromise.[4,6,12,16,17]

Management of an RPA is dependent on the size of the abscess as well as associated complications. Management involves both medical and surgical options.

Medical Management

Small abscesses (less than 2 cm) and associated retropharyngeal cellulitis without associated complications are usually treated with intravenous antibiotics.[1,2,18,19] In one series, failure of medical management was based on the size of the abscess alone, with medical management likely to fail in patients with abscess size greater than 2 cm; these patients subsequently required surgical intervention.[18] Antibiotic choice should cover Gram-positive and anaerobic organisms, although infections are typically polymicrobial, with *Streptococcus* species, *Fusobacterium*, and *Peptostreptococcus* species as common culprits.[13] Antibiotic regimen should be guided by local antibiograms and preferences.

Surgical Management

Large abscesses (≥2 cm), the presence of airway compromise, and failing intravenous antibiotic therapy are indications for surgical management in patients with RPA.[3,4,6–8,12] Patients in whom it is difficult to reach the abscess may benefit from CT-guided abscess drainage.[4] It may be appropriate to utilize 24 to 48 hours of intravenous broad-spectrum antibiotic therapy prior to surgical intervention.[4,6,12,16,17]

Complications from an RPA, aside from airway obstruction, include aspiration pneumonia, carotid artery pseudoaneurysm, septic thrombophlebitis of the internal jugular vein (Lemierre syndrome), atlantoaxial dislocation, and mediastinitis.[4,6,12,16,17]

COROLLARY CASE: PERITONSILLAR ABSCESS

These are common deep space neck infections in the pediatric population. These infections have a reported incidence of 9 out of 100,000 patients younger than 20 years of age and peak in the adolescent time period.[4,20] As with RPA, these infections are often polymicrobial. Clinical presentation is also similar to RPA and common symptoms are sore throat with fever. Dysphagia, voice changes, and trismus may be present. A classic physical examination finding is unilateral uvular deviation and unilateral posterior pharyngeal fullness,[4,21] corresponding to abscess location. Interestingly, younger children are more likely to have a neck mass.[22]

Imaging may play a role in the diagnosis of a peritonsillar abscess. However, patients with a clinical history and examination consistent with a peritonsillar abscess do not generally require imaging. If the diagnosis is in question, imaging is appropriate. Oral ultrasonography may be utilized and has been demonstrated effective for evaluating and detecting peritonsillar abscesses.[4,23] However, young patients may not tolerate this procedure well. CT with intravenous contrast can be utilized in cases where the diagnosis is in question, since this modality is excellent for detecting a deep neck abscess or identifying an alternative diagnosis.[4,21] MRI is superior to CT for delineating soft tissues and identifying complications from a peritonsillar abscess.[21,24] Management consists of drainage (either aspiration or incision),[4] which in adolescents and cooperative older children may be done at the bedside, but younger children may require performance of this procedure in the operating suite. Antibiotic choice is the same as with RPA. As with a small (less than 2 cm) RPA, intravenous antibiotics may be initially used without surgical treatment for 24 to 48 hours with close monitoring; if there is a lack of response or worsening clinical condition, then surgical management is indicated.[21,22] Older patients in whom bedside drainage is tolerated, have adequate pain control, and adequate oral intake can often be discharged with appropriate antibiotics.[21,25] Complications associated with a peritonsillar abscess are similar to those of an RPA.

A 15-year-old patient presented with 4 days of sore throat and voice change. The physical examination was remarkable for pharyngeal erythema but minimal asymmetry of the oropharynx. An intravenous contrast-enhanced CT examination was obtained and a selected image is presented here (Fig. 82.2). There is a 1.9 × 3.1 × 3.4-cm peripherally enhancing fluid collection with mild mass effect in the right retropharyngeal space with deviation of the oropharyngeal

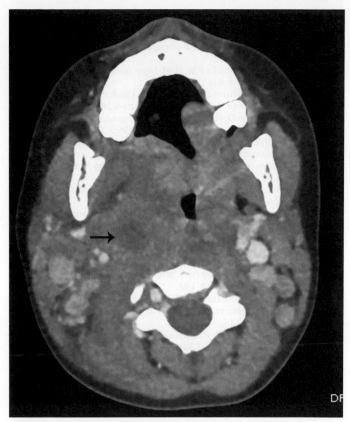

Fig. 82.2 Axial contrast-enhanced computed tomography scan of the neck demonstrates a small peripherally enhancing mass in the right lateral retropharyngeal space consistent with a suppurative node of Rouviere (*black arrow*).

airway to the left. This is consistent with an abscess secondary to a suppurative lymph node. Pediatric Otolaryngology was consulted and the decision was made to perform drainage in the operating suite. This was done without incident.

IMAGING PEARLS

1. Plain radiography of the soft tissues of the neck may be a good imaging modality in patients with low suspicion for a deep space soft tissue neck infection, evaluating the width of the prevertebral spaces of the cervical vertebrae. However, this modality can be difficult to obtain in young children, complicating interpretation of the study.
2. CT with intravenous contrast is the imaging modality of choice when RPA, peritonsillar abscess, or deep tissue neck infection is suspected.
3. Imaging may not be indicated in patients with a history and examination consistent with a peritonsillar abscess and can be obtained if there is concern for an associated complication.
4. Ultrasound has proven effective for superficial lateral neck infections and, in some older pediatric patients, peritonsillar abscess. However, ultrasound is not useful for deep soft tissue infections.
5. MRI is not a first-line imaging modality but is useful if there are concerns for complications, such as vascular involvement.

References

1. Ludwig BJ, Foster BR, Saito N, et al. Diagnostic imaging in nontraumatic pediatric head and neck emergencies. *Radiographics*. 2010;30(3):781-799.
2. Vieira F, Allen SM, Stocks RM, et al. Deep neck infection. *Otolaryngol Clin North Am*. 2008;41(3):459-483.
3. Philpott CM, Selvadurai D, Banerjee AR. Paediatric retropharyngeal abscess. *J Laryngol Otol*. 2004;118(12):919-926.
4. Boucher C, Dorion D, Fisch C. Retropharyngeal abscesses: a clinical and radiologic correlation. *J Otolaryngol*. 1999;28(3):134-137.
5. Hartmann RW. Recognition of retropharyngeal abscess in children. *Am Fam Physician*. 1992;46(1):193-196.
6. Li RM, Kiemeney M. Infections of the neck. *Emerg Med Clin North Am*. 2019;37(1):95-107.
7. Virk JS, Pang J, Okhovat S, et al. Analysing lateral soft tissue neck radiographs. *Emerg Radiol*. 2012;19(3):255-260.
8. Vural C, Gungor A, Comerci S. Accuracy of computerized tomography in deep neck infections in the pediatric population. *Am J Otolaryngol*. 2003;24(2):143-148.
9. Goldenberg D, Golz A, Joachims HZ. Retropharyngeal abscess: a clinical review. *J Laryngol Otol*. 1997;111(6):546-550.
10. Sethi DS, Stanley RE. Deep neck abscesses-changing trends. *J Laryngol Otol*. 1994;108(2):138-143.
11. Ravindranath T, Janakiraman N, Harris V. Computed tomography in diagnosing retropharyngeal abscess in children. *Clin Pediatr (Phila)*. 1993;32(4):242-244.
12. Stoner MJ, Dulaurier M. Pediatric ENT emergencies. *Emerg Med Clin North Am*. 2013;31(3):795-808.
13. Dudas R, Serwint JR. In brief: retropharyngeal abscess. *Pediatr Rev*. 2006;27(6):e45-e46.
14. Sethia R, Mahida JB, Subbarayan RA, et al. Evaluation of an imaging protocol using ultrasound as the primary diagnostic modality in pediatric patients with superficial soft tissue infections of the face and neck. *Int J Pediatr Otorhinolaryngol*. 2017;96:89-93.
15. Quinn NA, Olson JA, Meier JD, et al. Pediatric lateral neck infections—computed tomography vs ultrasound on initial evaluation. *Int J Pediatr Otorhinolaryngol*. 2018;109:149-153.
16. Brook I. Fusobacterial head and neck infections in children. *Int J Pediatr Otorhinolaryngol*. 2015;79(7):953-958.
17. Ali NE, Alyono JC, Koltai PJ. Neonatal retropharyngeal abscess with complications: apnea and cervical osteomyelitis. *Int J Pediatr Otorhinolaryngol*. 2019;126:109613.
18. Kosko J, Casey J. Retropharyngeal and parapharyngeal abscesses: factors in medical management failure. *Ear Nose Throat J*. 2017;96(1):E12-E15.
19. Wong DKC, Brown C, Mills N, et al. To drain or not to drain—management of pediatric deep neck abscesses: a case-control study. *Int J Pediatr Otorhinolaryngol*. 2012;76(12):1810-1813.
20. Novis SJ, Prichett CV, Thorne MC, et al. Pediatric deep space neck infections in US children, 2000-2009. *Int J Pediatr Otorhinolaryngol*. 2014;78(5):832-836.
21. Galioto N. Peritonsillar abscess. *Am Fam Physician*. 2017;95(8):501-506.
22. Hsaio HJ, Huang YC, Hsia SH, et al. Clinical features of peritonsillar abscess in children. *Pediatr Neonatol*. 2012;53(6):366-370.
23. Huang Z, Vintzileos W, Gordish-Dressman H, et al. Pediatric peritonsillar abscess: outcomes and cost savings from using transcervical ultrasound. *Laryngoscope*. 2017;127(8):1924-1929.
24. Powell J, Wilson JA. An evidence-based review of peritonsillar abscess. *Clin Otolaryngol*. 2012;37(2):136-145.
25. Yaghchi A, Cruise A, Kapoor K, et al. Out-patient management of patients with a peritonsillar abscess. *Clin Otolaryngol*. 2008;33(1):52-55.

83 Frog in Your Throat: Supraglottic Infections and Bacterial Tracheitis

ROBERT VEZZETTI, MD, FAAP, FACEP, and BHAIRAV PATEL, MD

Case Presentation

A 10-year-old female presents with 2–3 weeks of progressively worsening throat pain and dysphagia. She was diagnosed 2 weeks ago with *Streptococcal* pharyngitis by her primary care provider. She was treated with a 10-day course of amoxicillin and had mild improvement, but her symptoms returned. She was evaluated by her physician again and told she had a viral infection, since her rapid strep test was negative. Over the past 3–4 days, she has had fever to 103 degrees Fahrenheit; the throat pain and dysphagia have worsened considerably. Her parents note she has had "voice changes"—the child's voice has taken on a "muffled" quality. She has had no other symptoms, has had no travel, and has been otherwise in her usual state of health.

Physical examination reveals an uncomfortable appearing child; she appears ill. She prefers to sit up, stating that lying down makes it "more difficult for me to breathe." Her temperature is 101 degrees Fahrenheit, her heart rate is 120 beats per minute, respiratory rate is 25 breaths per minute, blood pressure is 120/80 mm Hg, and oxygen saturation is 95% on room air. She has an erythematous posterior oropharynx without obvious asymmetry, but her examination is limited secondary to difficulty opening her mouth, which she states hurts her throat. Her chest examination is clear, but there is transmitted upper airway noise. There is no obvious stridor.

Imaging Considerations

Acutely ill, toxic-appearing children should have immediate treatment, including airway stabilization if clinically indicated. While having an imaging study to assist in diagnosis is advantageous, delaying care to obtain such a study is not advisable, since these children can decompensate quickly. Once a clinician deems it safe, then appropriate imaging studies may be performed.

PLAIN RADIOGRAPHY

Plain radiography has the advantage of being readily accessible and providing relatively low ionizing radiation exposure. Anteroposterior and lateral views are usually performed. Depending on the etiology, plain radiography may demonstrate findings in certain clinical scenarios. For

example, narrowing of the proximal trachea may be seen in croup (the classic "steeple sign"), radio-opaque foreign bodies may be visualized, and exudative tracheitis may show linear airway filling defects, irregularity, or asymmetric subglottic narrowing.[1,2] Interpretation of plain radiography should be performed in the context of the child's history, clinical examination, and clinician suspicion for a particular disease process.

COMPUTED TOMOGRAPHY (CT)

CT can detect various pathologies, including tracheitis, epiglottitis, abscess, and foreign bodies.[3] However, CT involves ionizing radiation exposure, and is not portable, requiring the patient to go to the CT scanner. In patients with potential airway compromise, this can complicate completing a CT study.

MAGNETIC RESONANCE IMAGING (MRI)

MRI is not a first-line modality in the acutely ill patient. However, it is excellent at imaging anatomic and infectious causes of upper airway problems.[3] Availability and the need for sedation are limiting factors to more immediate use.

Imaging Findings

While the child did appear uncomfortable, she was deemed stable to undergo imaging. In this case, the decision was made to obtain an intravenous (IV) contrast–enhanced CT study of the soft tissues of the neck. Selected images are provided. There is no evidence of abscess, but there is diffuse edema in the hypopharyngeal and laryngeal region extending along the visualized upper trachea, producing severe airway narrowing, greatest in the hypopharyngeal and laryngeal regions. These findings are consistent with severe supraglottic swelling (Figs. 83.1A, 83.2A and 83.3A). For comparison, CT images demonstrating normal views of these structures are provided (Figs. 83.1B, 83.2B, and 83.3B).

Case Conclusion

The child was admitted to the Pediatric Intensive Care Unit (PICU) for close respiratory monitoring. Laboratory

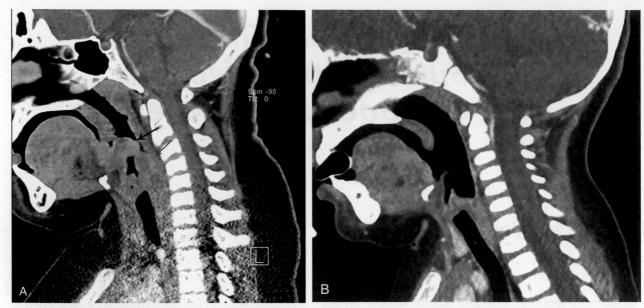

Fig. 83.1 Selected computed tomography sagittal view (A) of a swollen epiglottis *(black arrow)*, supraglottis, and hypopharynx *(red arrow)*. (B) Normal structures.

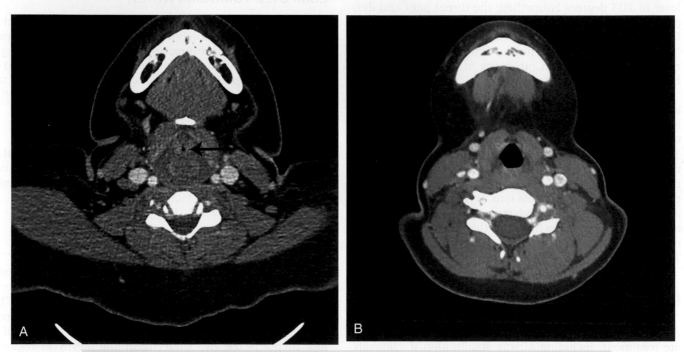

Fig. 83.2 Selected computed tomography axial image (A) of a swollen supraglottis with edematous (low attenuation) soft tissues and near complete airway narrowing *(arrow)*. (B) Normal structures.

testing was performed. Her complete blood count and comprehensive metabolic profile were both unremarkable (total white blood cell count was 9500 cc mm with a neutrophilic predominance), and rapid strep testing was negative. Vancomycin, pipercillin/tazobactam, and dexamethasone were initiated. Pediatric Otolaryngology and Pediatric Infectious Disease were consulted. The child had laryngoscopy performed, which demonstrated exudate visible in the nasopharynx, oropharynx, and supraglottic regions with diffuse edema involving the epiglottis, arytenoids, and trachea. Over the next several days, the child improved and did not require intubation. She was transitioned to oral antibiotics (amoxicillin-clavulanate) and was followed closely by Pediatric Otolaryngology. Cultures obtained during laryngoscopy grew *Staphylococcus pseudointermedius* only.

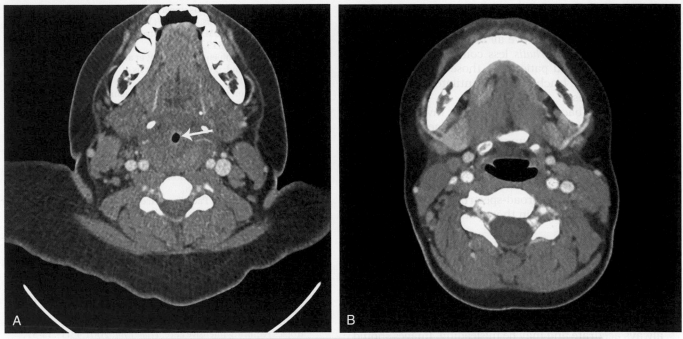

Fig. 83.3 Selected computed tomography axial view (A) demonstrating a swollen supraglottis with edematous (low attenuation) soft tissues and near complete airway narrowing *(arrow)*. (B) Normal structures.

SUPRAGLOTTITIS/EPIGLOTTITIS

Supraglottitis refers to inflammation of the supraglottic region and includes the epiglottis, vallecula, arytenoids, and aryepiglottic folds. This process places affected patients at high risk for airway obstruction and death.[4] The diagnosis is established by direct or indirect visualization of the inflamed supraglottic structures during laryngoscopic examination.[4] Prior to the introduction of the *Haemophilus influenza* type B vaccine in the late 1980s, this clinical entity was commonly encountered in the pediatric population as epiglottitis, although now it is not as often seen in immunized pediatric populations and is more commonly encountered in adult populations.[4,5] The annual incidence of epiglottitis has been reported to be 0.6–0.8/100,000 immunized patients, making the vaccine against *Haemophilus influenza* type B extremely effective.[5] Etiologies leading to infection include bacterial organisms, such as *Haemophilus influenzae* type B (still seen), *Streptococcus pneumoniae*, and viral organisms such as Epstein-Barr virus, varicella-zoster virus, parainfluenza, and herpes simplex virus.[5,6]

Classically, acute onset of drooling, dysphagia, and distress are consistent with supraglottic infection, with rapid progression to a toxic-appearing child.[6] A viral prodrome is not uncommon prior to the development of supraglottic infection. Symptoms suggestive of this disease process in adult populations include sore throat, dysphagia, fever, muffled voice, and dyspnea.[4,7,8] This differs slightly in pediatric patients, who are more likely to present with fever (83%), tachycardia (83%), and stridor (83%); sore throat and dysphagia are not as common.[8]

Management of patients with supraglottitis or epiglottitis consists of keeping the patient calm (so not to worsen what may be a tenuous airway and lead to clinical decompensation), IV antibiotics (to cover *Streptococcus* and *Staphylococ*-

cus species—ceftriaxone [or other third-generation cephalosporin] or ampicillin/tazobactam is typically utilized, with the addition of clindamycin if anaerobic bacteria are a concern, and vancomycin for toxic-appearing patients), and hospital admission.[4,5,8] Stridor, hypoxia, and drooling have been noted to be risk factors for necessity of airway intervention.[4] Corticosteroid use is somewhat controversial, but in one study, the majority of both adult and pediatric patients did receive corticosteroids.[4] Many studies have not shown corticosteroid administration to positively impact length of hospital stay, period of intubation, or duration of stay in the intensive care unit, but there may be selection bias due to the severity of illness in study patients.[4,5] Consultation with Pediatric Otolaryngology is recommended. If the patient is toxic-appearing or there is concern for airway decompensation, admission to a PICU is appropriate.

BACTERIAL TRACHEITIS

Bacterial tracheitis is not commonly seen but is potentially life-threatening. One study reported that bacterial tracheitis was three times more likely to cause respiratory failure in pediatric patients than croup and epiglottitis combined.[9,10] It accounts for up to 14% of upper airway obstruction in pediatric patients.[11,12] The disease usually presents as an ill-appearing child, in whom fever and respiratory distress (including dyspnea and stridor) are seen; voice changes may be reported; children usually do not present with drooling.[2,10,13,14] Bacterial tracheitis is thought to be secondary to bacterial overgrowth in the context of a prodromal viral upper respiratory infection.[2,10,11,13–16] A definitive diagnosis can be made by direct laryngoscopy, which, if utilized, should be performed by a Pediatric Otolaryngologist in an operative setting, during which a Gram stain and cultures can be obtained.[2,3,11,16]

The etiology of bacterial tracheitis varies. *Staphylococcus aureus, Haemophilus influenzae, Moraxella catarrhalis*, and *Streptococcus pneumoniae* have all been implicated, with *H. influenzae* and *M. catarrhalis* less commonly seen.[2,10,11,13] Immunocompromised patients or those who are technology dependent (i.e., tracheostomy, ventilator use) may have atypical pathogens.

Treatment for bacterial tracheitis first involves securing the patient's airway. Patients may not immediately require intubation, but this can change. Consultation with a Pediatric Intensivist is a good approach. Many patients with this illness are admitted to the PICU; one study reported a PICU admission rate of 94% and intubation rates range from 50% to 83%.[9,11,12,15,17] Broad-spectrum antibiotics are a mainstay of management in these patients.[2,6]

IMAGING PEARLS

1. Initial stabilization, including addressing airway compromise, is the first step in treatment of a patient with suspected supraglottic infection or bacterial tracheitis.
2. Plain radiography can suggest abnormalities of the trachea and other structures of the upper airway but is not always accurate and may be misleading. Images should be interpreted in the context of the clinical history and physical examination. In a patient who is deemed too unstable for CT, plain radiography has the advantages of availability and speed of study completion.
3. CT is excellent at visualizing upper airway pathology. An IV contrast–enhanced study should be obtained. However, this study necessitates the patient leaving the acute care area and great care should be taken to ensure that a patient is stable enough to undergo this study.

References

1. Walner DL. Utility of radiographs in the evaluation of pediatric upper airway obstruction. *Ann Otol Rhinol Laryngol.* 1999;108(4):378-383.
2. Loftis, L. Acute infectious upper airway obstructions in children. *Semin Pediatr Infect Dis.* 2006;17(1):5-10.
3. Ida JB, Thompson DM. Pediatric stridor. *Otolaryngol Clin North Am.* 2014;47(5):795-819.
4. Bizaki AJ, Numminen J, Vasama JP, et al. Acute supraglottitis in adults in Finland: review and analysis of 308 cases. *Laryngoscope.* 2011;121(10):2107-2113.
5. Glynn F, Fenton J. Diagnosis and management of supraglottitis (epiglottitis). *Curr Infect Dis Rep.* 2008;10(3):200-204.
6. Kasem AJ. Case report of a 5-year-old with epiglottitis: an atypical presentation of an uncommon disease. *Pediatr Emerg Care.* 2018;34(1):e11-e13.
7. Guardiani E, Bliss M, Harley E. Supraglottitis in the era following widespread immunization against *Haemophilus influenzae* type B: evolving principles in diagnosis and management. *Laryngoscope.* 2010;120(1): 2183-2188.
8. Baird SM, Marsh PA, Padiglione A, et al. Review of epiglottitis in the post *Haemophilus influenzae* type-b vaccine era. *ANZ J Surg.* 2018;88(11):1135-1140.
9. Hopkins A, Lahiri T, Salerno R, et al. Changing epidemiology of life-threatening upper airway infections: the reemergence of bacterial tracheitis. *Pediatrics.* 2006;118(4):1418-1421.
10. Miranda AD, Valdez TA, Pereira KD. Bacterial tracheitis: a varied entity. *Pediatr Emerg Care.* 2011;27(10):950-953.
11. Graf J, Stein F. Tracheitis in pediatric patients. *Semin Pediatr Infect Dis.* 2006;17(1):11-13.
12. Chan PW, Goh M, Lum L. Severe upper airway obstruction in the tropics requiring intensive care. *Pediatr Int.* 2001;43(1):53-57.
13. Casazza G, Graham ME, Nelson D, et al. Pediatric bacterial tracheitis-a variable entity: case series with literature review. *Otolaryngol Head Neck Surg.* 2019;160(3):546-549.
14. Gallagher PG, Myer CM. An approach to the diagnosis and treatment of membranous laryngotracheobronchitis in infants and children. *Pediatr Emerg Care.* 1991;7(6):337-342.
15. Salamone FN, Bobbitt DB, Myer CM, et al. Bacterial tracheitis reexamined: is there a less severe manifestation? *Otolaryngol Head Neck Surg.* 2004;131(6):871-876.
16. Stroud RH, Friedman NR. An update on inflammatory disorders of the pediatric airway: Epiglottitis, croup and tracheitis. *Am J Otolaryngol.* 2001;22(4):268-275.
17. Marcos Alonso S, Molini Menchon N, Rodriguez Nunez A, et al. Bacterial tracheitis; an infectious cause of upper airway obstruction to be considered in children. *An Pediatr (Barc).* 2005;63(2):164-168.

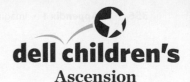

dell children's
Ascension

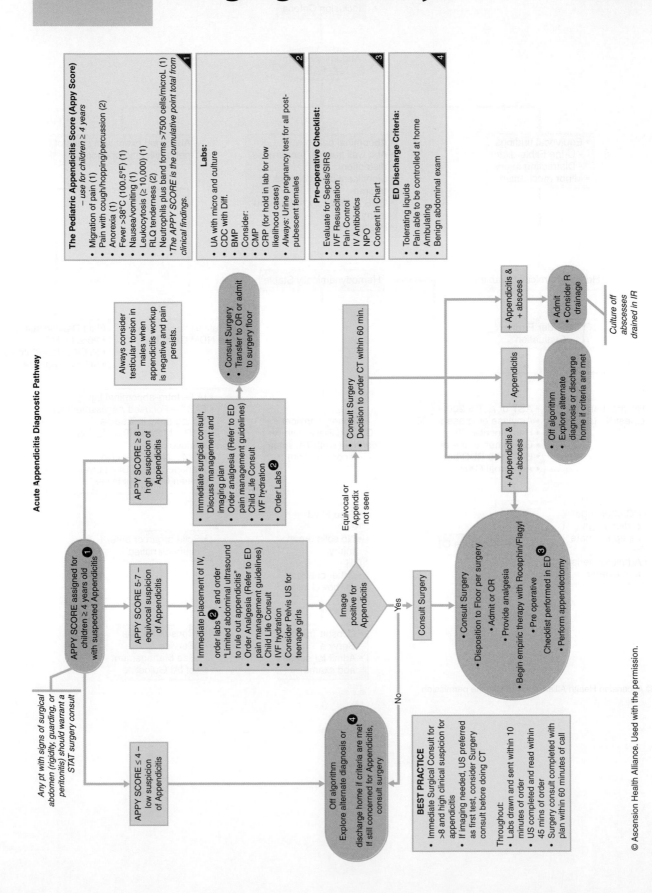

The Pediatric Appendicitis Score (Appy Score)
-- use for children ≥ 4 years
- Migration of pain (1)
- Pain with cough/hopping/percussion (2)
- Anorexia (1)
- Fever >38°C (100.5°F) (1)
- Nausea/vomiting (1)
- Leukocytosis (≥ 10,000) (1)
- RLQ tenderness (2)
- Neutrophils plus band forms >7500 cells/microL (1)
The APPY SCORE is the cumulative point total from clinical findings.

Labs:
- UA with micro and culture
- CDC with Diff.
- BMP
- Consider:
  - CMP
  - CRP (for hold in lab for low likelihood cases)
- Always: Urine pregnancy test for all post-pubescent females

Pre-operative Checklist:
- Evaluate for Sepsis/SIRS
- IVF Resuscitation
- Pain Control
- IV Antibiotics
- NPO
- Consent in Chart

ED Discharge Criteria:
- Tolerating liquids
- Pain able to be controlled at home
- Ambulating
- Benign abdominal exam

Acute Appendicitis Diagnostic Pathway

Any pt with signs of surgical abdomen (rigidity, guarding, or peritonitis) should warrant a STAT surgery consult

APPY SCORE assigned for children ≥ 4 years old with suspected Appendicitis ❶

Always consider testicular torsion in males when appendicitis workup is negative and pain persists.

APPY SCORE ≥ 8 – high suspicion of Appendicitis

- Immediate surgical consult, Discuss management and imaging plan
- Order analgesia (Refer to ED pain management guidelines)
- Child Life Consult
- IVF hydration
- Order Labs ❷

- Consult Surgery
- Transfer to OR or admit to surgery floor

APPY SCORE 5-7 – equivocal suspicion of Appendicitis

- Immediate placement of IV, order labs ❷, and order "Limited abdominal ultrasound to rule out appendicitis"
- Order Analgesia (Refer to ED pain management guidelines)
- Child Life Consult
- IVF hydration
- Consider Pelvis US for teenage girls

Image positive for Appendicitis

Equivocal or Appendix not seen

- Consult Surgery
- Decision to order CT within 60 min.

Yes

Consult Surgery

No

APPY SCORE ≤ 4 – low suspicion of Appendicitis

Off algorithm
Explore alternate diagnosis or discharge home if criteria are met If still concerned for Appendicitis, consult surgery ❹

BEST PRACTICE
- Immediate Surgical Consult for >8 and high clinical suspicion for appendicitis
- If imaging needed, US preferred as first test, consider Surgery consult before doing CT

Throughout:
- Labs drawn and sent within 10 minutes of order
- US completed and read within 45 mins of order
- Surgery consult completed with plan within 60 minutes of call

- Consult Surgery
- Disposition to Floor per surgery
- Admit or OR
- Provide analgesia
- Begin empiric therapy with Rocephin/Flagyl
- Pre operative Checklist performed in ED ❸
- Perform appendectomy

+ Appendicitis & - abscess

- Appendicitis

+ Appendicitis & + abscess

Off algorithm
- Explore alternate diagnosis or discharge home if criteria are met

Admit
- Consider R drainage

Culture off abscesses drained in IR

© Ascension Health Alliance. Used with the permission.

355

Evaluation of Blunt Abdominal Trauma

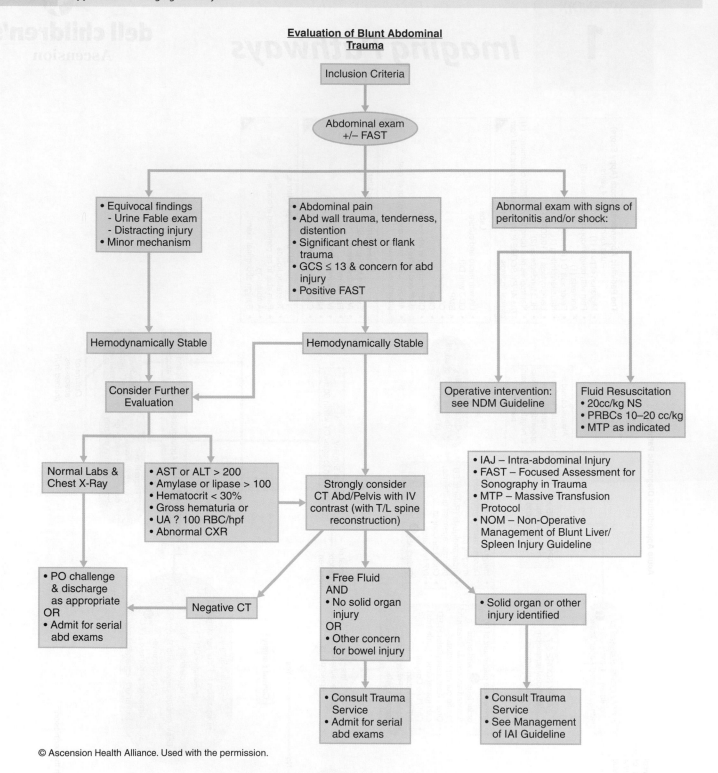

Inclusion Criteria

Abdominal exam +/– FAST

Equivocal findings
- Equivocal findings
  - Urine Fable exam
  - Distracting injury
- Minor mechanism

Abdominal pain
- Abdominal pain
- Abd wall trauma, tenderness, distention
- Significant chest or flank trauma
- GCS ≤ 13 & concern for abd injury
- Positive FAST

Abnormal exam with signs of peritonitis and/or shock:

Hemodynamically Stable

Hemodynamically Stable

Consider Further Evaluation

Operative intervention: see NDM Guideline

Fluid Resuscitation
- 20cc/kg NS
- PRBCs 10–20 cc/kg
- MTP as indicated

Normal Labs & Chest X-Ray

- AST or ALT > 200
- Amylase or lipase > 100
- Hematocrit < 30%
- Gross hematuria or
- UA ? 100 RBC/hpf
- Abnormal CXR

Strongly consider CT Abd/Pelvis with IV contrast (with T/L spine reconstruction)

- IAJ – Intra-abdominal Injury
- FAST – Focused Assessment for Sonography in Trauma
- MTP – Massive Transfusion Protocol
- NOM – Non-Operative Management of Blunt Liver/Spleen Injury Guideline

- PO challenge & discharge as appropriate
OR
- Admit for serial abd exams

Negative CT

- Free Fluid AND
- No solid organ injury
OR
- Other concern for bowel injury

- Solid organ or other injury identified

- Consult Trauma Service
- Admit for serial abd exams

- Consult Trauma Service
- See Management of IAI Guideline

VERY LOW RISK FOR INTRA-ABDOMINAL INJURY (IAI)
Clinical Risk Stratification

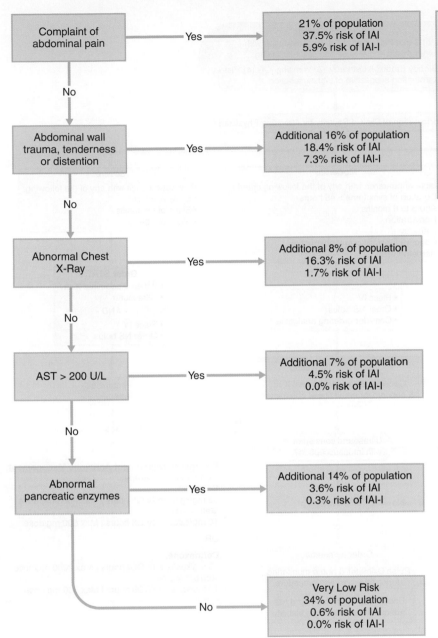

| Complaint of abdominal pain | —Yes→ | 21% of population
37.5% risk of IAI
5.9% risk of IAI-I |

No ↓

| Abdominal wall trauma, tenderness or distention | —Yes→ | Additional 16% of population
18.4% risk of IAI
7.3% risk of IAI-I |

No ↓

| Abnormal Chest X-Ray | —Yes→ | Additional 8% of population
16.3% risk of IAI
1.7% risk of IAI-I |

No ↓

| AST > 200 U/L | —Yes→ | Additional 7% of population
4.5% risk of IAI
0.0% risk of IAI-I |

No ↓

| Abnormal pancreatic enzymes | —Yes→ | Additional 14% of population
3.6% risk of IAI
0.3% risk of IAI-I |

—No→

| Very Low Risk
34% of population
0.6% risk of IAI
0.0% risk of IAI-I |

- Patients with only 1 positive variable had IAI 4.5% of the time.
- Patients with 2 positive variables had IAI 16.8% of the time.
- Patients with >2 positive variables had IAI 37.8% of the time.

- IAI – Intra-abdominal Injury
- IAI-I – Intra-abdominal Injury patients receiving acute intervention (transfusion, embolization, or surgery)
- Abnormal pancreatic enzymes = amylase or lipase higher than lab reported norms

Acute Intussusception <u>Emergency Department</u> Pathway

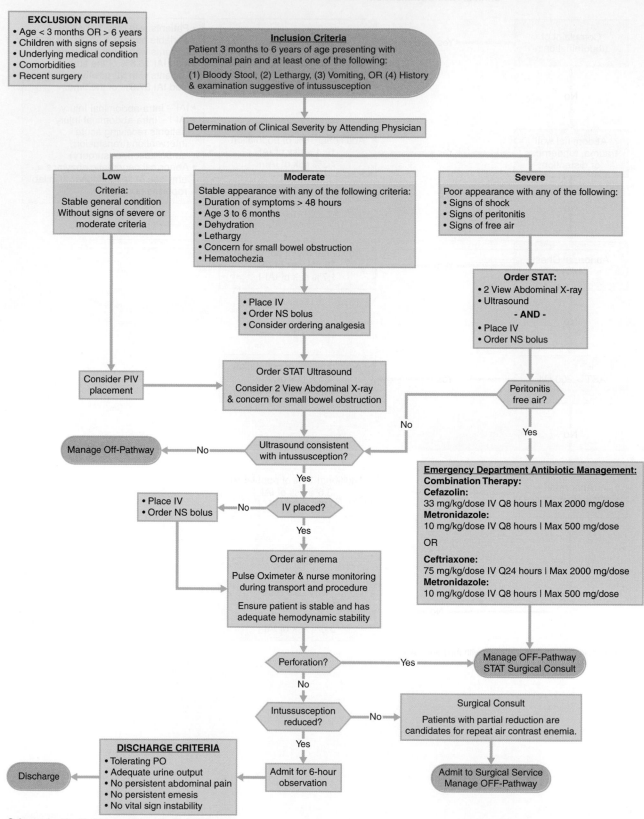

EXCLUSION CRITERIA
- Age < 3 months OR > 6 years
- Children with signs of sepsis
- Underlying medical condition
- Comorbidities
- Recent surgery

Inclusion Criteria
Patient 3 months to 6 years of age presenting with abdominal pain and at least one of the following:
(1) Bloody Stool, (2) Lethargy, (3) Vomiting, OR (4) History & examination suggestive of intussusception

Determination of Clinical Severity by Attending Physician

Low
Criteria:
Stable general condition
Without signs of severe or moderate criteria

Moderate
Stable appearance with any of the following criteria:
- Duration of symptoms > 48 hours
- Age 3 to 6 months
- Dehydration
- Lethargy
- Concern for small bowel obstruction
- Hematochezia

Severe
Poor appearance with any of the following:
- Signs of shock
- Signs of peritonitis
- Signs of free air

Order STAT:
- 2 View Abdominal X-ray
- Ultrasound
- AND -
- Place IV
- Order NS bolus

- Place IV
- Order NS bolus
- Consider ordering analgesia

Consider PIV placement

Order STAT Ultrasound
Consider 2 View Abdominal X-ray & concern for small bowel obstruction

Peritonitis free air?

Manage Off-Pathway ← No — Ultrasound consistent with intussusception?

No

Yes

Emergency Department Antibiotic Management:
Combination Therapy:
Cefazolin:
33 mg/kg/dose IV Q8 hours | Max 2000 mg/dose
Metronidazole:
10 mg/kg/dose IV Q8 hours | Max 500 mg/dose

OR

Ceftriaxone:
75 mg/kg/dose IV Q24 hours | Max 2000 mg/dose
Metronidazole:
10 mg/kg/dose IV Q8 hours | Max 500 mg/dose

- Place IV
- Order NS bolus

← No — IV placed?

Yes

Order air enema
Pulse Oximeter & nurse monitoring during transport and procedure
Ensure patient is stable and has adequate hemodynamic stability

Perforation? — Yes → Manage OFF-Pathway STAT Surgical Consult

No

Intussusception reduced? — No → Surgical Consult
Patients with partial reduction are candidates for repeat air contrast enemia.

Yes

DISCHARGE CRITERIA
- Tolerating PO
- Adequate urine output
- No persistent abdominal pain
- No persistent emesis
- No vital sign instability

Discharge ← Admit for 6-hour observation

Admit to Surgical Service Manage OFF-Pathway

PEDIATRIC CERVICAL SPINE CLEARANCE ALGORITHM
LOW-RISK MECHANISM OF INJURY

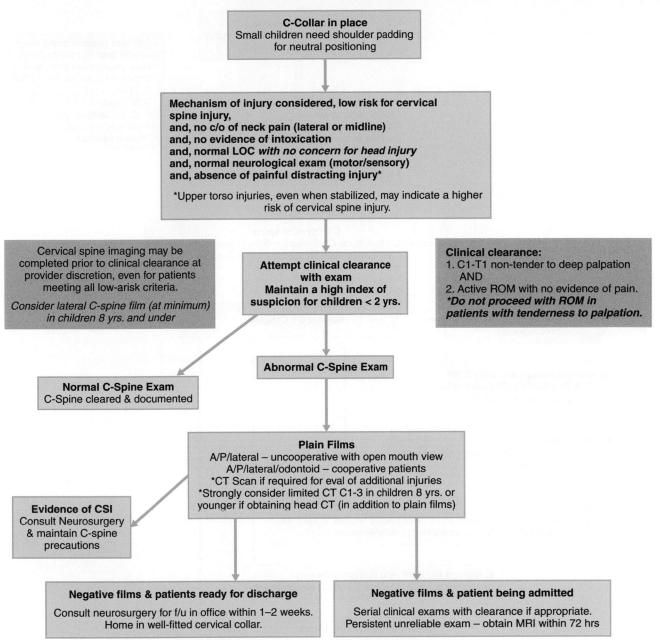

C-Collar in place
Small children need shoulder padding
for neutral positioning

Mechanism of injury considered, low risk for cervical spine injury,
and, no c/o of neck pain (lateral or midline)
and, no evidence of intoxication
and, normal LOC *with no concern for head injury*
and, normal neurological exam (motor/sensory)
and, absence of painful distracting injury*

*Upper torso injuries, even when stabilized, may indicate a higher risk of cervical spine injury.

Cervical spine imaging may be completed prior to clinical clearance at provider discretion, even for patients meeting all low-arisk criteria.

Consider lateral C-spine film (at minimum) in children 8 yrs. and under

Attempt clinical clearance with exam
Maintain a high index of suspicion for children < 2 yrs.

Clinical clearance:
1. C1-T1 non-tender to deep palpation AND
2. Active ROM with no evidence of pain.
Do not proceed with ROM in patients with tenderness to palpation.

Abnormal C-Spine Exam

Normal C-Spine Exam
C-Spine cleared & documented

Plain Films
A/P/lateral – uncooperative with open mouth view
A/P/lateral/odontoid – cooperative patients
*CT Scan if required for eval of additional injuries
*Strongly consider limited CT C1-3 in children 8 yrs. or younger if obtaining head CT (in addition to plain films)

Evidence of CSI
Consult Neurosurgery & maintain C-spine precautions

Negative films & patients ready for discharge
Consult neurosurgery for f/u in office within 1–2 weeks.
Home in well-fitted cervical collar.

Negative films & patient being admitted
Serial clinical exams with clearance if appropriate.
Persistent unreliable exam – obtain MRI within 72 hrs

PEDIATRIC CERVICAL SPINE CLEARANCE ALGORITHM
HIGH-RISK MECHANISM OF INJURY

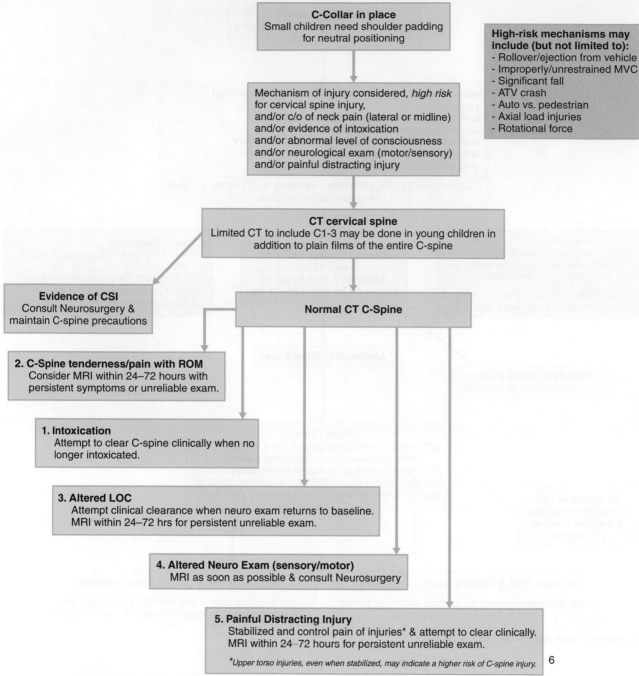

C-Collar in place
Small children need shoulder padding for neutral positioning

High-risk mechanisms may include (but not limited to):
- Rollover/ejection from vehicle
- Improperly/unrestrained MVC
- Significant fall
- ATV crash
- Auto vs. pedestrian
- Axial load injuries
- Rotational force

Mechanism of injury considered, *high risk* for cervical spine injury,
and/or c/o of neck pain (lateral or midline)
and/or evidence of intoxication
and/or abnormal level of consciousness
and/or neurological exam (motor/sensory)
and/or painful distracting injury

CT cervical spine
Limited CT to include C1-3 may be done in young children in addition to plain films of the entire C-spine

Evidence of CSI
Consult Neurosurgery & maintain C-spine precautions

Normal CT C-Spine

2. C-Spine tenderness/pain with ROM
Consider MRI within 24–72 hours with persistent symptoms or unreliable exam.

1. Intoxication
Attempt to clear C-spine clinically when no longer intoxicated.

3. Altered LOC
Attempt clinical clearance when neuro exam returns to baseline.
MRI within 24–72 hrs for persistent unreliable exam.

4. Altered Neuro Exam (sensory/motor)
MRI as soon as possible & consult Neurosurgery

5. Painful Distracting Injury
Stabilized and control pain of injuries* & attempt to clear clinically.
MRI within 24–72 hours for persistent unreliable exam.

*Upper torso injuries, even when stabilized, may indicate a higher risk of C-spine injury.

6

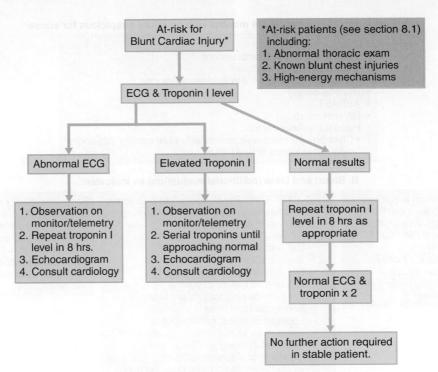

A. Evaluation of children 12–24 months with an injury suspicious for abuse:

- Thorough history
- Head to toe physical assessment
- Social services consultation
- Photodocumentation of any cutaneous injuries
- Skeletal survey
- ALT/AST
- UA with micro
- Head CT without contrast
  - Children with neurologic abnormality (*see section 7.2*) and/or external evidence of head injury

B. Blood and urine (additional evaluation) as indicated:

Urine & serum toxicology
- Concern for ingestion
- Evidence of neurologic abnormality (if head CT is obtained)
- Report or suspicion of substance abuse in caregiver by history or presentation.

CBC, PT/PTT, vW Panel, Factor VIII & IX levels
- Intracranial hemorrhage (ICH) *concerning for abusive head trauma*
  - Diffuse ICH
  - ICH with mixed density blood
  - Bilateral ICH
  - ICH with altered mental status
  - ICH with no history of trauma
- Bruising concerning for inflicted injury
  - Non-ambulatory child
  - Location: buttocks, genitals, ears, hands, feet, torso
  - Patterned bruising
  - Extensive or clustered bruising
- Other injury associated with bleeding such as solid organ injury
- *For clinically significant bleeding, see "Screening for bleeding disorders guideline."*
- *Consider for patients with diffuse cerebral edema and no intracranial hemorrhage*

Bone abnormality evaluation - 25-hydroxy-Vit D, intact PTH, Alkaline Phosphatase, Calcium, Phosphorus levels
- Children with > 1 fracture
- Radiographic concern for osteopenia or metabolic bone disease

C. Consultation as indicated:

Neurosurgical Consultation
All patients with skull fractures (including convexity and base) must have a neurosurgical consultation prior to discharge from the hospital.

Orthopedic Consultation
Non-ambulatory children with a long bone fracture must have orthopedic consultation prior to disposition from the ED.

Ophthalmology Consultation
Patients with ICH; also consider for injuries to the face/neck or eyes and eye findings concerning for genetic disorders. Ophthalmology may be consulted after admission.

D. Diagnostic imaging (additional) as indicated:

CT Abdomen/Pelvis with IV contrast
- Abnormal chest or abdominal exam
- Consider with >10 RBCs per HPF on urinalysis
- ALT OR AST >80 mg/dl
  - Or admit to Trauma Service for observation and serial abdominal exams
- May be indicated by the CARE Team

MRI brain/spine with and without contrast
- May be indicated with ICH to further delineate injury, per neurosurgery or CARE team.

Non-Accidental Trauma (NAT)
< 12 months

A. Evaluation of children who meet <u>at least one</u> of the following criteria sets:
    1. < 12 months with either a skeletal fracture or other injury suspicious for abuse
    2. Non-ambulatory with either a skeletal fracture or other injury suspicious for abuse

- Thorough history
- Head to toe physical assessment
- Social services consultation
- Photo documentation of any cutaneous injuries
- Skeletal survey
- ALT/AST
- UA with micro
- Head CT without contrast
  - All children less than 6 mos
  - Children with neurologic abnormality (*see section 7.2*) and/or external evidence of head injury

B. Blood and urine (additional evaluation) as indicated:

Urine & serum toxicology
- Concern for ingestion
- Evidence of neurologic abnormality (if head CT is obtained)
- Report or suspicion of substance abuse in caregiver by history or presentation.

CBC, PT/PTT, vW Panel, Factor VIII & IX levels
- Intracranial hemorrhage (ICH) *concerning for abusive head trauma*
  - Diffuse ICH
  - ICH with mixed density blood
  - Bilateral ICH
  - ICH with altered mental status
  - ICH with no history of trauma
- Bruising concerning for inflicted injury
  - < 9 mos of age
  - Non-ambulatory child
  - Location: buttocks, genitals, ears, hands, feet, torso
  - Patterned bruising
  - Extensive or clustered bruising
- Other injury associated with bleeding such as solid organ injury
- *For clinically significant bleeding, see Screening for Bleeding Disorders guideline.*
- *Consider for patients with diffuse cerebral edema and no introcranial hemorrhage*

Bone abnormality evaluation - 25-hydroxy-Vit D, intact PTH, Alkaline Phosphatase, Calcium, Phosphorus levels
- Children with > 1 fracture
- Radiographic concern for osteopenia or metabolic bone disease

C. Consultation as indicated:

Neurosurgical Consultation
All patients with <u>skull fractures</u> (including convexity and base) must have a neurosurgical consultation prior to discharge from the hospital.

Orthopedic Consultation
Children < 12 mos. or non-ambulatory children with a long bone fracture must have orthopedic consultation prior to disposition from the ED.

Ophthalmology Consultation
Patients with ICH; also consider for injuries to the face/neck or eyes and eye findings concerning for genetic disorders. Ophthalmology may be consulted after admission.

D. Diagnostic imaging (additional) as indicated:

CT Abdomen/Pelvis with IV contrast
- Abnormal chest or abdominal exam
- Consider with >10 RBCs per HPF on urinalysis
- ALT OR AST >80 mg/dl
  - Or admit to Trauma Service for observation and serial abdominal exams
- May be indicated by the CARE Team

MRI brain/spine with and without contrast
- May be indicated with ICH to further delineate injury, per neurosurgery or CARE team.

A. Evaluation of children >24 months with an injury suspicious for abuse:

- Thorough history
- Head to toe physical assessment
- Social services consultation
- Photo documentation of any cutaneous injuries
- Skeletal survey – indicated up to 5 yrs., only on a case by case basis:
  - Unconscious patient, non-verbal patient or inadequate exam
- ALT/AST & UA with micro
  - Multiple or severe injuries or with concern for abdomen/pelvic trauma
- Head CT without contrast
  - Children with neurologic abnormality (*see section 7.2*) and/or external

B. Blood and urine (additional evaluation) as indicated:

Urine & serum toxicology
- Concern for ingestion
- Evidence of neurologic abnormality (if head CT is obtained)
- Report or suspicion of substance abuse in caregiver by history or presentation.

CBC, PT/PTT, vW Panel, Factor VIII & IX levels
- Intracranial hemorrhage (ICH) *concerning for abusive head trauma*
  - Diffuse ICH
  - ICH with mixed density blood
  - Bilateral ICH
  - ICH with altered mental status
  - ICH with no history of trauma
- Bruising concerning for inflicted injury
  - Non-ambulatory child
  - Location: buttocks, genitals, ears, hands, feet, torso
  - Patterned bruising
  - Extensive or clustered bruising
- Other injury associated with bleeding such as solid organ injury
- *For clinically significant bleeding, see "Screening for bleeding disorders guideline."*
- *Consider for patients with diffuse cerebral edema and no introcranial hemorrhage*

Bone abnormality evaluation - 25-hydroxy-Vit D, intact PTH, Alkaline Phosphatase, Calcium, Phosphorus levels
- Children with > 1 fracture
- Radiographic concern for osteopenia or metabolic bone disease

C. Consultation as indicated:

Neurosurgical Consultation
All patients with skull fractures (including convexity and base) must have a neurosurgical consultation prior to discharge from the hospital.

Orthopedic Consultation
Non-ambulatory children with a long bone fracture must have orthopedic consultation prior to disposition from the ED.

Ophthalmology Consultation
Patients with ICH; also consider for injuries to the face/neck or eyes and eye findings concerning for genetic disorders. Ophthalmology may be consulted after admission.

D. Diagnostic imaging (additional) as indicated:

CT Abdomen/Pelvis with IV contrast
- Abnormal chest or abdominal exam
- Consider with >10 RBCs per HPF on urinalysis
- ALT OR AST >80 mg/dl
  - Or admit to Trauma Service for observation and serial abdominal exams
- May be indicated by the CARE Team

MRI brain/spine with and without contrast
- May be indicated with ICH to further delineate injury, per neurosurgery or CARE team.

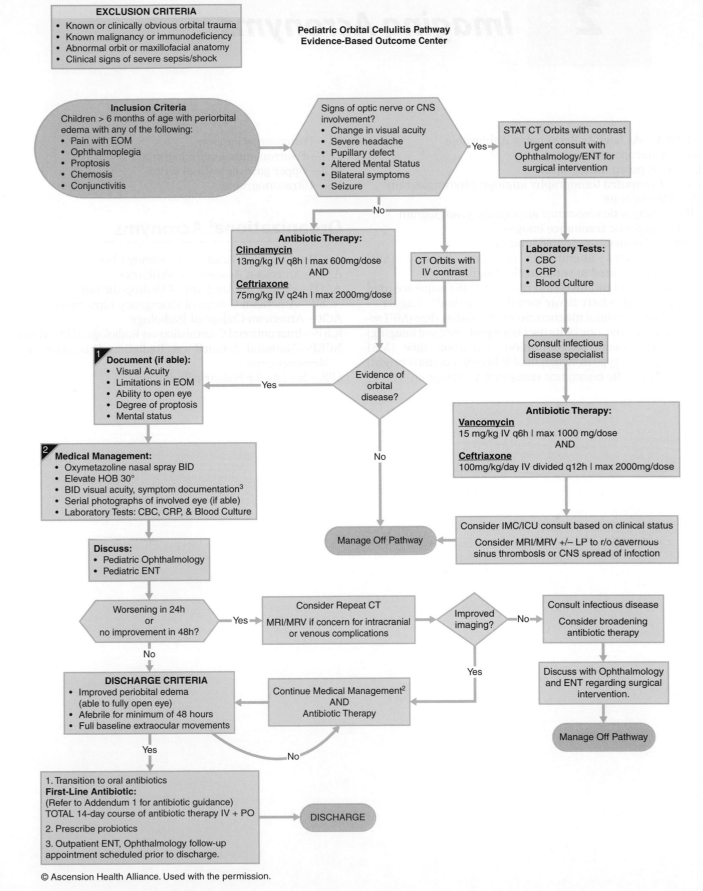

EXCLUSION CRITERIA
- Known or clinically obvious orbital trauma
- Known malignancy or immunodeficiency
- Abnormal orbit or maxillofacial anatomy
- Clinical signs of severe sepsis/shock

Pediatric Orbital Cellulitis Pathway
Evidence-Based Outcome Center

Inclusion Criteria
Children > 6 months of age with periorbital edema with any of the following:
- Pain with EOM
- Ophthalmoplegia
- Proptosis
- Chemosis
- Conjunctivitis

Signs of optic nerve or CNS involvement?
- Change in visual acuity
- Severe headache
- Pupillary defect
- Altered Mental Status
- Bilateral symptoms
- Seizure

Yes →

STAT CT Orbits with contrast
Urgent consult with Ophthalmology/ENT for surgical intervention

No ↓

Antibiotic Therapy:
Clindamycin
13mg/kg IV q8h | max 600mg/dose
AND
Ceftriaxone
75mg/kg IV q24h | max 2000mg/dose

CT Orbits with IV contrast

Laboratory Tests:
- CBC
- CRP
- Blood Culture

Consult infectious disease specialist

1 **Document (if able):**
- Visual Acuity
- Limitations in EOM
- Ability to open eye
- Degree of proptosis
- Mental status

← Yes

Evidence of orbital disease?

No ↓

Antibiotic Therapy:
Vancomycin
15 mg/kg IV q6h | max 1000 mg/dose
AND
Ceftriaxone
100mg/kg/day IV divided q12h | max 2000mg/dose

2 **Medical Management:**
- Oxymetazoline nasal spray BID
- Elevate HOB 30°
- BID visual acuity, symptom documentation[3]
- Serial photographs of involved eye (if able)
- Laboratory Tests: CBC, CRP, & Blood Culture

Discuss:
- Pediatric Ophthalmology
- Pediatric ENT

Manage Off Pathway ←

Consider IMC/ICU consult based on clinical status
Consider MRI/MRV +/− LP to r/o cavernous sinus thrombosis or CNS spread of infection

Worsening in 24h or no improvement in 48h?

Yes →

Consider Repeat CT
MRI/MRV if concern for intracranial or venous complications

→ **Improved imaging?**

No →

Consult infectious disease
Consider broadening antibiotic therapy

↓

Discuss with Ophthalmology and ENT regarding surgical intervention.

↓

Manage Off Pathway

Yes ↓ (from Improved imaging?)

No ↓ (Worsening)

DISCHARGE CRITERIA
- Improved periobital edema (able to fully open eye)
- Afebrile for minimum of 48 hours
- Full baseline extraocular movements

← Continue Medical Management[2] AND Antibiotic Therapy

No

Yes ↓

1. Transition to oral antibiotics
First-Line Antibiotic:
(Refer to Addendum 1 for antibiotic guidance)
TOTAL 14-day course of antibiotic therapy IV + PO
2. Prescribe probiotics
3. Outpatient ENT, Ophthalmology follow-up appointment scheduled prior to discharge.

→ DISCHARGE

2 *Imaging Acronyms*

ALARA—As Low As Reasonably Achievable
AP—Anteroposterior view
CT—Computed tomography
CTA—Computed tomography angiography/angiogram
IV—Intravenous
MRA—Magnetic resonance angiography/angiogram
MRI—Magnetic resonance imaging
　DWI—Diffusion-weighted imaging
　FLAIR—Fluid attenuated inversion recovery (MRI sequence used to suppress fluid signal)
　STIR—Short tau inversion recovery (MRI sequence used to suppress fatty tissue signal, hence fluid is bright)
　T1—Longitudinal magnetization relaxation time (MRI sequence type, one of its uses is for post-contrast imaging)
　T2—Transverse magnetization relaxation time (MRI sequence type in which fluid is bright, edema is bright)
MRV—Magnetic resonance venography/venogram

PA—Posteroanterior view
PET—Positron emission tomography
UGI—Upper gastrointestinal series
US—Ultrasonography

Organizational Acronyms

AAFP—American Academy of Family Physicians
AAP—American Academy of Pediatrics
AAOS—American Academy of Orthopedic Surgery
ACEP—American College of Emergency Physicians
ACR—American College of Radiology
ICRP—International Commission on Radiological Protection
NCRP—National Council on Radiation Protection and Measurements
SPR—Society for Pediatric Radiology

Index

Page numbers followed by "b", "f" and "t" indicate boxes, figures and tables, respectively.